Headache

Series Editor

Paolo Martelletti, Roma, Italy

The purpose of this Series, endorsed by the European Headache Federation (EHF), is to describe in detail all aspects of headache disorders that are of importance in primary care and the hospital setting, including pathophysiology, diagnosis, management, comorbidities, and issues in particular patient groups. A key feature of the Series is its multidisciplinary approach, and it will have wide appeal to internists, rheumatologists, neurologists, pain doctors, general practitioners, primary care givers, and pediatricians. Readers will find that the Series assists not only in understanding, recognizing, and treating the primary headache disorders, but also in identifying the potentially dangerous underlying causes of secondary headache disorders and avoiding mismanagement and overuse of medications for acute headache, which are major risk factors for disease aggravation. Each volume is designed to meet the needs of both more experienced professionals and medical students, residents, and trainees.

Derya Uludüz • Marcelo Valença
Aynur Özge • Mario Fernando Prieto Peres
Editors

Rare Causes of Headache Disorders

Case Based Diagnostic Approach

Springer

Editors
Derya Uludüz
School of Medicine, Neurology Department
Istanbul University Cerrahpasa
Samatya, Türkiye

Aynur Özge
Mersin State Hospital
Mersin, Turkey

Marcelo Valença
Neurology and Neuroscience
Federal University of Pernambuco
Recife, Brazil

Mario Fernando Prieto Peres
Universidade de São Paulo
São Paulo, SP, Brazil

ISSN 2197-652X ISSN 2197-6538 (electronic)
Headache
ISBN 978-3-032-10241-6 ISBN 978-3-032-10242-3 (eBook)
https://doi.org/10.1007/978-3-032-10242-3

This Springer imprint is published by the registered company Springer Nature Switzerland AG
The registered company address is: Gewerbestrasse 11, 6330 Cham, Switzerland

Foreword

When we think about headaches, our minds naturally go to the common culprits: the dull ache of a tension headache, the throbbing misery of a migraine, the searing pain of a cluster headache, or the stuffy pressure of a sinus issue. These are the daily realities for more than a billion people. But beyond this familiar landscape exists a rarer and more complex territory—the realm of uncommon headache disorders. These are not merely *bad headaches* but often distinct medical conditions or symptoms of a serious underlying problem. Understanding them is crucial because they challenge both patients and doctors to look deeper. They remind us that the sensation of head pain can be a messenger for a wide array of intricate physiological malfunctions.

Consider, for instance, headaches that are intimately tied to the very pressure that surrounds our brain. There are conditions where the body produces too much cerebrospinal fluid or fails to absorb it properly, leading to a build-up of pressure inside the skull. This can cause a persistent, daily headache often worse in the morning, and crucially, it can threaten vision by swelling the optic nerves. Conversely, the opposite problem can occur—a leak of this same fluid, perhaps from a tiny tear in the spine's lining. This results in a profound low-pressure headache, one with a telltale signature: it is excruciating when you sit or stand but vanishes almost completely when you lie flat. Then there are the vascular crises, where the blood vessels in the brain itself suddenly constrict in a wave of spasms, leading to a sudden, explosive *thunderclap* headache that can peak in seconds, often triggered by something as simple as an orgasm or a moment of exertion.

Beyond pressure and blood vessels, the structure of the nervous system itself can be a source. A congenital malformation where brain tissue extends into the spinal canal can cause headaches triggered by coughing or straining. While the fear of a brain tumor is common, it is a rare cause of headache; when it does occur, the pain is usually part of a larger picture, including personality changes, seizures, or weakness. We must also include the searing, electric shock-like pains of cranial neuralgias, which are less a constant ache and more a series of lightning strikes to the face, triggered by the slightest touch or gust of wind.

The overarching theme with these rare headache disorders is that they are frequently *red flags*. They demand medical attention not because the pain itself is always worse but because what they represent is a system in distress. A headache that is new and progressive in an older person, one that comes with fever and confusion, or one that changes dramatically with posture, is the brain's way of signaling that something specific and potentially dangerous is wrong. In essence, exploring these rare causes expands our understanding of headache from a simple condition to a complex language of symptoms, urging us to listen carefully to what the pain is trying to say.

This book superbly addresses and catalogs this wealth of clinical information and represents a veritable goldmine for the clinician. Tackling diagnostic uncertainties in this area of headache medicine is the real challenge. The more well-known primary headaches belong to patients who navigate life with established diagnoses, whereas the rare forms, being sometimes life-threatening, require impeccable clinical knowledge. It is a reference volume that is essential for the physical or virtual library of every clinician who, from whatever discipline, approaches rare headaches and for whom a missed diagnosis is not an option.

Unitelma Sapienza Università di Roma Paolo Martelletti
Roma, Italy

Contents

Part I
Migraine

Chapter 1
Hemiplegic Migraine

Elcio Juliato Piovesan and Marco Antonio Takashi Utiumi

1.1 Introduction

Hemiplegic migraine (HM) is a rare migraine subtype marked by transient motor auras with or without headache, typically starting in childhood or adolescence [1, 2]. It is linked to ion channel gene mutations that disrupt neuronal excitability and lower thresholds for cortical spreading depolarization (CSD). The classic triad includes non-motor aura, motor aura, and headache, though presentations vary widely even within families carrying the same mutation. HM may also involve ataxia, epilepsy, and cognitive symptoms, with a tendency to diminish in severity over time [2]. Diagnosis is clinical in familial cases (FHM), but sporadic forms (SHM) often require imaging and genetic testing. Treatment options remain limited, and preventive strategies lack robust evidence.

1.2 Pathophysiology

HM is an autosomal dominant disorder with 80–90% penetrance [3], caused by mutations in known genes such as the CACNA1A (FHM Type 1 [FHM1]), ATP1A2 (FHM2), SNC1A (FHM3), and, more recently, PRRT2 [4, 5]. However, in up to 80% of the cases, no genetic mutation is identified (classified as Familial hemiplegic migraine, other loci) [6], suggesting that the genetic heterogeneity of HM extends beyond a Mendelian inheritance [7].

E. J. Piovesan (✉)
Universidade Federal do Paraná, Curitiba, Brazil

M. A. T. Utiumi
Clínica de Neurologia São José, São José, Brazil

D. Uludüz et al. (eds.), *Rare Causes of Headache Disorders*, Headache,
https://doi.org/10.1007/978-3-032-10242-3_1

From a neurophysiological perspective, the auras accompanying HM attacks, including the motor ones, are triggered by CSD [8]. This phenomenon might activate the trigeminal nerve at a peripheral level and provoke headaches [9]. CSD may be succeeded by vascular changes and the production of proinflammatory molecules, leading to a state of parenchymal inflammation with the opening of pannexin-1 channels and inflammasome activation [8]. The motor weakness that can develop into hemiplegia in HM attacks is possibly the result of a prolonged aura since the same patient can have typical FHM attacks interspersed with attacks of non-hemiplegic migraine with aura (MA) [8, 9].

FHM1 is caused by mutations in the CACNA1A gene (19p13.1) that encodes the voltage-gated calcium channels alpha 1A subunit ($Ca_v2.1$). A gain-of-function leads to their frequent opening and activation at lower voltages than those required by channels in individuals without HM [8, 9]. An increase in glutamate secretion [10] might, finally, favor the occurrence of CSD (Fig. 1.1). FHM2 is associated with the ATP1A2 gene (1q23.2), which encodes the alpha-2 subunit of the Na^+/K^+ ATPase pump. The loss-of-function effect may sustain a state of cortical hyperexcitability [10], which would explain epilepsy in cases of FHM [10]. On the other hand, in FHM3 (SCN1A gene [2q24.3], alpha-1 subunit of the voltage-gated Na^+ channel [$Na_v1.1$]), the resulting gain-of-function may converge in a hyperexcitability state [10].

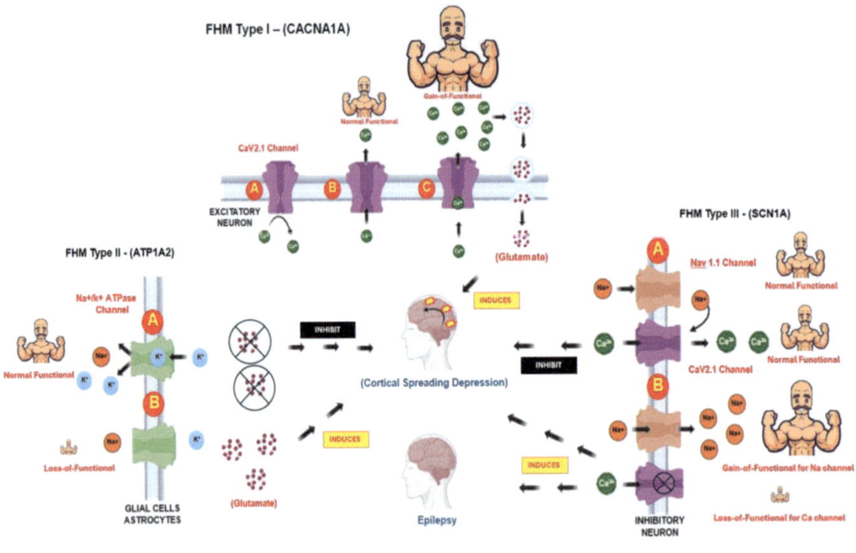

Fig. 1.1 Flow chart illustrating three types of Familial Hemiplegic Migraine (FHM) mechanisms. 1. **FHM Type I (CACNA1A):** Shows a gain-of-function in the CaV2.1 channel of excitatory neurons, leading to increased glutamate release. 2. **FHM Type II (ATP1A2):** Depicts a Na+/K+ ATPase channel in glial cells with normal and loss-of-function states, affecting glutamate regulation and inducing cortical spreading depression. 3. **FHM Type III (SCN1A):** Illustrates Nav 1.1 and CaV2.1 channels in inhibitory neurons, with gain-of-function in Ca channels and loss-of-function in Na channels, leading to epilepsy. Arrows indicate the flow of ions and neurotransmitters, with labels for normal and dysfunctional states

The propagation of CSD reaching the corticostriatal regions could explain the severe motor deficits in FHM1 [10]. During CSD, an increase in $Ca2^+$ concentration in cortical neurons is observed, which is expected with a gain-of-function mutation of $Ca_v2.1$ in pyramidal cells [10]. There is an increase in oxygen consumption and a consequent reduction in tissue O_2 during vigorous CSD [10]. In these experimental models, multiple CSDs may occur more frequently in homozygous models than in heterozygous ones [10]. In FHM1, it is possible to observe glutamatergic changes while the GABAergic release is unaltered [10]. In addition, specialized core microcircuits of inhibitory interneurons may be involved and responsible for maintaining the excitatory–inhibitory balance pathways necessary to transfer information while preventing runaway excitation [10]. These microcircuits are essential for the correct processing of sensory information (control of sensory gain, suppression, synchronization and generation of cortical rhythms, formation of cell assemblies, and transfer of information to higher areas) [1]. They are likely dysfunctional in FHM, leading to alterations in cortical function and contributing to the development of FHM [1].

1.3 Case Presentation

A 15-year-old female student with a history of paroxysmal headaches for 8 years presented at the headache clinic. She reported a sensation of water drops dripping down her right arm, which quickly evolved into a loss of muscle strength in the lower and upper right limbs, followed by difficulty walking and moving her arm. A few minutes later, visual changes appeared, consisting of images of lights and lines. She also reported difficulty speaking. The reduction in strength, the visualization of lights, and the difficulty in speaking lasted about an hour and a half. However, the line images persisted for 24 h in her field of vision. A moderate headache with nausea, photophobia, and phonophobia followed all these symptoms. The pain worsened with body movements. She reported significant cognitive impairment lasting up to 36 h. Previous attempts to control the disease had already been made with propranolol and lamotrigine.

The patient's mother has suffered from migraine with visual aura and sensation of loss of muscle strength since she was 12 years old. The patient had no history of seizures. In the first attack, she was hospitalized and underwent magnetic resonance imaging (MRI) and arterial and venous phase magnetic resonance angiography (MRA) with no abnormal findings. Lumbar puncture and transcranial Doppler showed no abnormalities. Autonomic system disorders were investigated using a tilt table test, but no abnormalities were found. Hematological and metabolic/endocrinological tests were all normal. The patient underwent a genetic study that revealed alterations in the CACNA1A gene and was subsequently diagnosed with FHM1. She started calcium channel blockers (flunarizine) as a prophylactic treatment. In 6 months, she had three moderate-intensity attacks and one of greater magnitude with hemiparesis.

1.4 Case Discussion

This case demonstrates the complexity of HM. The motor aura aggregated with visual, sensory, or speech symptoms in a patient with a migraine-type headache is highly suggestive of HM. The diagnosis is based on the family history and, whenever possible, genetic testing. The results of prophylactic treatment are usually suboptimal. The acute treatment depends on the presentation of symptoms, primarily whether cognitive dysfunction is present or not.

1.5 Clinical Characteristics

Like other migraine types, HM can present with four stages: (1) a premonitory phase with non-headache symptoms; (2) an aura that includes motor symptoms; (3) the headache phase; and (4) a recovery or postdromic stage (Fig. 1.2). Generally, the first attack consists of a headache with aura but no hemiplegia. The number of attacks throughout life varies, reaching up to 0.4/year [11]. Triggering factors include physical and emotional stress and even pregnancy.

Premonitory Phase The semiological information on the premonitory phase is lacking. This stage typically presents with symptoms such as insomnia, yawning, fatigue, and irritability [12], indicating hypothalamic involvement.

Aura Phase The characteristics of the aura phase are fundamental for a correct clinical diagnosis, as elegantly demonstrated by Bonemazzi [13]. The HM "core" is the presence of two or more aura symptoms—TOGETHER, CONCOMITANT, AGGREGATED—which differentiates it from other types of MA in which, when more than one aura symptom occurs, they usually follow one another (each symptom in isolation) [1, 14] (Fig. 1.2). In HM, four or more types of aura can occur in the same attack in up to 72% of cases, three types in 30%, and, rarely, only one type of aura in up to 5% of cases [1, 14, 15].

The total duration of all aura symptoms can vary from 10 min to 7 days, although the most typical duration is 60–120 min [14, 15]. Each symptom typically lasts between 5 and 30 min [1, 14, 15]. The classic sequence of aura presentation begins with visual, sensory, motor, aphasic, and basilar manifestations. There may be other types of aura with different combinations [1, 14].

Visual aura is reported in 74–97% of cases [1, 12, 14–16]. The symptoms include impaired central vision, hemianopsia, blurred vision, scintillating scotoma, phosphenes, flickering lines, and zig-zag lines [14]. The symptom duration ranges from 5 min to 12 h (average of 2 h) [1, 14, 15, 17].

Sensorial symptoms occur in up to 97% of patients and are characterized by hypoesthesia, numbness, and paresthesia. The symptoms spread gradually and may be ipsilateral or contralateral to the motor symptoms, and less frequently, bilateral [1, 14–16]. The symptoms occur more frequently in the arms, hands, face, tongue, legs, and body [14, 15]. It usually lasts 1–12 h (average of 4 h) [1, 14, 15, 17].

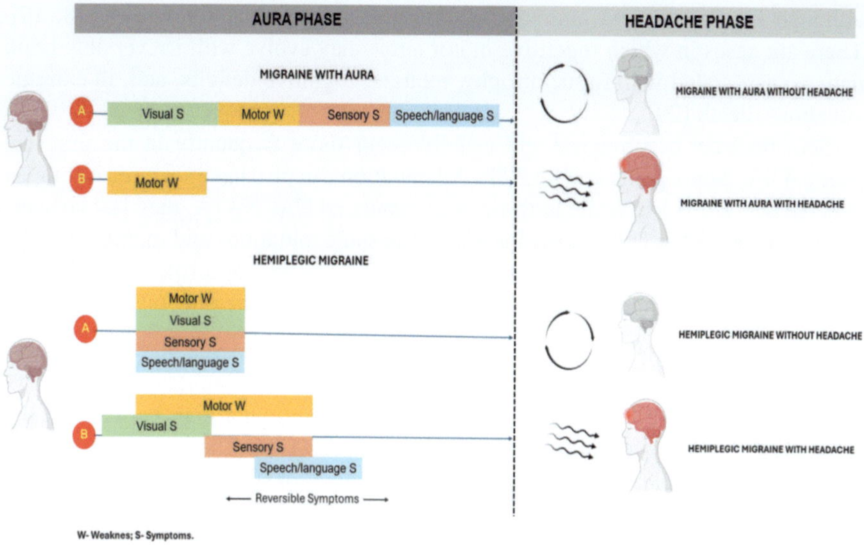

Fig. 1.2 Diagram illustrating the phases of migraines. The left side shows the "Aura Phase" with two types: "Migraine with Aura" and "Hemiplegic Migraine." Each type is divided into sections labeled with symptoms: Visual, Motor, Sensory, and Speech/Language, marked as either weakness (W) or symptoms (S). The right side depicts the "Headache Phase," showing outcomes: "Migraine with Aura without Headache," "Migraine with Aura with Headache," "Hemiplegic Migraine without Headache," and "Hemiplegic Migraine with Headache." Arrows indicate reversible symptoms.

Motor symptoms are characterized by weakness or paralysis in the hands, arms, feet, legs, tongue, face, and body [1, 14–16]. The weakness, which is typically unilateral in most cases, has a gradual onset and usually lasts for ≥5 min [1, 14, 15]. The motor deficit can spread to the other side [16]. Unlike the different forms of aura described above, motor aura can last from 30 min to 24 h (an average of 5 h). It may last longer than 24 h in 8% and 2% of those with sporadic and familial forms, respectively [1]. Language symptoms occur in 60–81% of cases [1, 14–16] and are characterized by alterations such as dysphasia, aphasia, dysarthria, and dysnomia. Aphasia can be sensory or motor [1, 14–16]. Its duration varies from 1 to 12 h [1, 14, 15, 17].

Brainstem aura symptoms are reported in 60–73% of cases, with manifestations as diverse as decreased hearing, dizziness, tinnitus, a sensation of pressure and pain in the ear, loss of balance, vertigo, clumsiness in the hands, dropping of objects, dysarthria, diplopia, tongue stiffness, pharyngeal and tongue numbness, swallowing difficulties, drop attacks, and decreased level of consciousness [1, 13–16].

Some semiological aspects may be more suggestive of an HM aura than other types of MA. Sensory symptoms are more extensive in HM, spreading through the face, arms, feet, and legs [1]. Visual symptoms begin peripherally as a scotoma, whereas with MA, the onset of symptoms is more central, characterized by zig-zag lines [1, 14]. In aphasic aura, the MA patient complains of language changes; in HM, impaired comprehension is more common. In HM, the motor aura can last much longer. The typical clinical pattern is complete recovery of symptoms, although hemiplegia and altered consciousness may persist for weeks [18, 19]. There are cases in which repetitive motor auras may evolve with irreversible brain damage associated with tissue atrophy, infarcts, cognitive deficits, and, in extreme situations, death [20].

Seizures may be observed and usually occur more frequently in the first few years of life. Some patients with ATP1A2 mutation can also have seizures lasting an average of 3.8 ± 6.1 h, while in those with a mutated CACNA1A, they last an average of 24.3 ± 23.5 h [11]. Individuals with the same mutations and members of the same family may also exhibit clinical variability, suggesting a role for additional factors (e.g., environmental elements) in the expression of the phenotype [3].

Headache Phase Headaches facilitate the diagnosis; however, the patient may present with aura but no pain complaints [15]. The headache is unilateral in 50–80% and bilateral in 40–50% of cases [1, 14, 15]. Unilateral pain may be fixed on the same side or shift to the other side between attacks [16]. The headache may be described as pulsatile, pressure, squeezing, throbbing, or stabbing.

The pain is of moderate to severe intensity and worsens with physical activity. It starts during or after the visual aura or, very rarely, before [14, 15]. Its duration varies from 4 to 72 h, with some cases lasting from 5 min to 5 days [1, 14, 15]. Non-headache symptoms might occur during headache attacks and include nausea (84–94%), vomiting (58–80%), phonophobia (70–92%), photophobia (70–99%), fever (8–58%), and mental confusion and disorientation (36–81%). Other manifestations have been reported, including autonomic symptoms (e.g., nasal congestion, lacrimation), motion sickness, Raynaud's syndrome, loss of consciousness, and seizures [17]. In the pediatric population, irritability, agitation, and drowsiness may occur [17]. More severe symptoms include visual hallucinations, meningismus, limb alienation, apraxia, hyperacusis, and torticollis [21].

Postdromic Phase The postdromic stage is the least understood. The non-painful symptoms include motor, cognitive, and cerebellar clinical manifestations. They can last from a few hours to several days.

Interictal Phase Patients may present abnormal functioning between attacks, a common finding in familial forms, emphasizing the role of the underlying genetic alteration in other physiological processes and increasing the burden on patients. Cerebellar signs are frequently found in FHM1, characterized by downbeat positioning nystagmus associated with ataxia in up to 60% of cases. In FHM2, these findings are rare [1, 22].

Some CACNA1A and ATP1A2 mutations are associated with mental retardation and cognitive impairment after recurrent severe seizures [23, 24]. Those with symptom onset in the first few years of life may present severe manifestations such as coma and seizures, predictive symptoms of an unfavorable clinical evolution [1]. Patients with a mutated CACNA1A between 3 and 18 years old with HM, torticollis, vertigo, and tonic upward gaze showed progression to cognitive dysfunction and cerebellar atrophy (vermis) [25]. Seizures in HM patients can be of the partial or generalized type, associated or not with fever [26]. Epilepsy begins in childhood and usually precedes the onset of HM attacks [2]. It generally has a benign course, with more frequent events occurring in FHM2. Epileptic seizures are generally independent of migraine attacks [20].

1.6 Diagnostic Algorithm

Step 1: Clinical suspicion

- *Identify key symptoms:*
  - Migraine with motor aura plus visual, sensory, and/or speech or language aura; together, concomitant, or aggregated (Fig. 1.2).
  - Family history of HM.
  - Semiological cyclical behaviors start in life's first and second decades. It is possible to observe a reduction in intensity and severity over time.

Step 2: Initial diagnostic workup

- *Perform brain MRI:*
  - Assess for white matter hyperintensities (WMHs).
    Cerebellar atrophy (with or without ataxia).
  - Unilateral cytotoxic edema has been observed during attacks in the sporadic type.
  - Middle cerebral artery vasospasm has been described in a third of patients, with 12.5% evolving into vasogenic edema.

Step 3: Consider genetic testing

- *Conduct genetic testing:*
  - Test for CACNA1A (FHM1), ATP1A2 (FHM2), SCN1A (FHM3), or PRRT2 gene mutations. Offspring of patients with FHM have a 50% chance of inheriting the disorder.

Step 4: Additional diagnostic evaluations

- *Perform EEG:*
  - Abnormalities during or immediately after the end of seizures might be observed in up to 85% of cases (asymmetry of the tracing, diffuse slow waves on the symptomatic side, and slowing occipital activity).
- *Cerebrospinal fluid analysis:*
  - Exclude other differential diagnoses such as meningoencephalitis and subarachnoid hemorrhage. Consider Headache and Neurological Deficits with Cerebrospinal Fluid Lymphocytosis (HaNDL), but note that the symptoms are typically limited to 3 months in this syndrome.

Table 1.1 Diagnostic criteria for the diagnosis of hemiplegic migraine [27]

1.2.3 Hemiplegic migraine
A. Attacks fulfilling criteria for 1.2 *Migraine with aura* and criterion B below
B. Aura consisting of both of the following:
C. Fully reversible motor weakness[a,b]
D. Fully reversible visual, sensory, and/or speech/language symptoms
1.2.3.1 Familial hemiplegic migraine
A. Attacks fulfilling criteria for 1.2.3 *Hemiplegic migraine*
B. At least one first- or second-degree relative has had attacks fulfilling criteria for 1.2.3 *Hemiplegic migraine*
1.2.3.2 Sporadic hemiplegic migraine
A. Attacks fulfilling criteria for 1.2.3 *Hemiplegic migraine*
B. No first- or second-degree relative fulfils criteria for 1.2.3 *Hemiplegic migraine*

[a]The term *plegic* means paralysis in most languages, but most attacks are characterized by motor weakness

[b]Motor symptoms generally last less than 72 h but, in some patients, motor weakness may persist for weeks

Step 5: Apply the International Classification of Headache Disorders, third edition (ICHD-3) Diagnostic Criteria (Table 1.1)

Step 6: Confirm diagnosis

- *Confirm hemiplegic migraine:*
  - CACNA1A (FHM1), ATP1A2 (FHM2), SCN1A (FHM3), or PRRT2 (other types) gene mutations or sporadic types.

Step 7: Classification re-evaluation

- *Reassess headache classification for other secondary types of headache.*
  - See below (Sect. "Differential Diagnosis").

1.7 Differential Diagnosis

Differential diagnosis is essential in patients with no affected relatives (sporadic forms) or when a reliable family history is lacking. The type and magnitude of HM symptoms make ruling out other significant disorders necessary, including diseases such as cerebrovascular events, infectious conditions, inflammatory diseases, epilepsy with hemiparesis, and tumors [28].

In cases of transient ischemic attacks (TIA) and strokes, the condition is sudden, while in HM, the neurological symptoms evolve gradually [1]. Motor aura may start in the hand, spread to the arm, and finally reach the face. The manifestation is sudden in all regions in neurovascular conditions. Headaches precede weakness in cases of vascular syndromes, while they occur closer in time in cases of HM [29].

Headache is rare in cases of TIA but common in patients with hemorrhagic stroke and young patients with HM [29].

Other vascular disorders discussed elsewhere include hereditary cerebral angiopathy [30] and cerebral autosomal dominant arteriopathy with subcortical infarcts (CADASIL).

Seizures followed by Todd's syndrome (motor weakness secondary to a seizure) can be confused with motor auras [1, 30]. Approximately 7% of those with FHM may also have epilepsy, which often makes the differential diagnosis challenging [26]. HM motor symptoms can last from 30 min to days, while seizures usually last only a few minutes. The typical motor patterns of seizures include limb spasms, head-turning, and loss of consciousness at their onset [2]. Todd's syndrome can be as long-lasting as HM, and this differential diagnosis is often complex.

In infectious cases, the patient typically presents with fever and some degree of altered mental status. Differential diagnosis with hypo- or hyperactive delirium of infectious origin may be necessary. The diagnostic workup includes neuroimaging to rule out structural lesions and the analysis of the cerebrospinal fluid [31] when the condition is unclear.

Stroke-like migraine attacks after radiation therapy (SMART) syndrome is a rare condition that may occur in patients with a history of brain radiotherapy 20–30 years before the onset of symptoms. Imaging tests may show thick cortical gyral enhancement [32].

Alternating hemiplegia of childhood is a rare genetic disorder of childhood caused by mutations in the ATP1A3 gene that produces periodic episodes of hemi- or quadriplegia, associated with dystonia, epilepsy, and cognitive alterations [33].

HaNDL is a rare sporadic condition characterized by hemiparesis and aphasia, associated with changes in cerebral blood flow and an increase in the lymphocyte count in the cerebrospinal fluid [34]. This condition can be related to FHM1 [23]. However, HaNDL is monophasic and lasts up to 3 months, while FHM recurs for years and is associated with frequent visual symptoms [17].

Mitochondrial disorders [35] can present with recurrent migraine-like headaches, neurological deficits, neuroimaging, and genetic findings. Sturge-Weber disorder may manifest with symptoms like HM, although typical dermatological changes help differentiate the disease [36]. Hypercapnia, hyponatremia, hypocalcemia, hepatic and renal failure, carotid dissection, antiphospholipid syndrome, systemic lupus erythematosus, and ornithine transcarbamylase deficiency can all present with symptoms that suggest HM [13].

1.8 Management

Non-pharmacological treatment begins by avoiding exposure to potentially seizure-generating factors, including pharmacological substances. The triggering factors can be emotional and intense physical stress, viral infections, and head trauma [37].

In isolated reports, the use of vasoconstrictive drugs (ergotamine and dihydroergotamine) in the acute phase of the disease can exacerbate the aura [30]. During the interictal periods, the use of topiramate [38] and glucagon-like peptide-1 (GLP-1) agonist (liraglutide) [39] can also worsen the HM evolution. An isolated case of regadenoson use, a selective A2A adenosine receptor agonist, triggering HM was reported [40].

In the acute phase with altered consciousness (brain edema), we favor a more aggressive intervention. Magnesium sulfate 2 g intravenous (IV) every 8 h (3 doses) and dexamethasone were administered, followed by 0.1 mg/kg IV every 6 h for 5 days, resulting in complete improvement [41]. In cases of cerebral edema, we may use dexamethasone 0.5 mg/kg/day IV in 3 pulses/day for 3 days, followed by gradual oral tapering and hypertonic solution at 3% 1.5 mL/kg/h, maintaining Na^+ between 145 and 155 mEq/L [42].

In acute cases without altered consciousness, triptans can produce good or excellent symptom control in up to 62% of cases [43]. Nasal administration of ketamine reduced the duration of aura in those with FHM by 42% [44]. Verapamil 5 mg IV over 5 min, followed by an oral maintenance dose of 120 mg/day, reduced headache symptoms but had little impact on hemiplegia [45].

Some oral drugs can be used for prophylactic management. Verapamil 120 mg, administered two to three times a day [24, 46, 47], reduced the intensity and impact of HM. Acetazolamide, 250–500 mg, reduces the burden of attacks and nystagmus and is primarily used in cases related to the CACNA1A gene [22, 38]. Flunarizine 10 mg daily [48], lamotrigine [42], and propranolol 10 mg three to four times a day [46] have been tried. Memantine 10 mg twice daily and dextromethorphan have been primarily used in individuals with the ATP1A2 variant [49]. Telcagepant [50] showed some therapeutic effects.

Botulinum neurotoxin type A utilizing the PREEMPT protocol, has shown improvement in patients with HM [51]. The use of CGRP (calcitonin gene-related peptide) monoclonal antibodies such as galcanezumab in a family with PRRT2 mutation caused a >50% reduction of auras and pain frequency, analgesics consumption, and functional improvement. In another study, administering galcanezumab for 3 months in six patients reduced the severity of the attacks to moderate in half of them, motor weakness in four, and the MIDAS (Migraine Disability Assessment Test) score improved in five. There was no change in the number of days with headache and the characteristics of aura [52].

Gepants, small molecules with CGRP receptor antagonism activity, should be avoided during HM attacks due to the risk of worsening cerebral vasospasm [53]. Promising treatments, such as foramen ovale closure, have been described in five different cases, potentially providing control over HM [54]. No studies have evaluated the presence of patent foramen ovale in groups of patients with HM to date.

1.9 Conclusion

Hemiplegic migraine is a rare disorder whose main clinical feature is the presence of motor symptoms frequently associated with other types of aura. The differential diagnosis, including stroke, epilepsy, and other conditions, is an important step. Because it is a disorder associated with ion channel disturbances, cortical spreading depression is the primary pathophysiological mechanism. Symptoms can be as severe as mental confusion, coma, and seizures. Acute treatment includes calcium channel blockers, but prophylaxis is limited. Natural history consists of a typical dramatic phase during the first few years of life, with a favorable course afterward.

References

1. Russell MB, Ducros A. Sporadic and familial hemiplegic migraine: pathophysiological mechanisms, clinical characteristics, diagnosis, and management. Lancet Neurol. 2011;10:457–70. https://doi.org/10.1016/S1474-4422(11)70048-5.
2. Di Stefano V, Rispoli MG, Pellegrino N, Graziosi A, Rotondo E, Napoli C, Pietrobon D, Brighina F, Parisi P. Diagnostic and therapeutic aspects of hemiplegic migraine. J Neurol Neurosurg Psychiatry. 2020;91(7):764–71. https://doi.org/10.1136/jnnp-2020-322850.
3. Sutherland HG, Albury CL, Griffiths LR. Advances in genetics of migraine. J Headache Pain. 2019;20:72. https://doi.org/10.1186/s10194-019-1017-9.
4. van den Maagdenberg AMJM, Haan J, Terwindt GM, Ferrari MD. Migraine: gene mutations and functional consequences. Curr Opin Neurol. 2007;20:299–305. https://doi.org/10.1097/WCO.0b013e3281338d1f.
5. Riant F, Roos C, Roubertie A, Barbance C, Hadjadj J, Auvin S, Baille G, Beltramone M, Boulanger C, Cahn A, Cata F, Cheuret E, Cuvellier JC, Defo A, Demarquay G, Donnet A, Gaillard N, Massardier E, Guy N, Lamoureux S, Le Moigno L, Lucas C, Ratiu D, Redon S, Rey C, Thauvin C, Viallet F, Tournier-Lasserve E, Ducros A. Hemiplegic migraine associated with *PRRT2* variations: a clinical and genetic study. Neurology. 2022;98(1):e51–61. https://doi.org/10.1212/WNL.0000000000012947.
6. Sutherland HG, Maksemous N, Albury CL, Ibrahim O, Smith RA, Lea RA, Haupt LM, Jenkins B, Tsang B, Griffiths LR. Comprehensive exonic sequencing of hemiplegic migraine related genes in a cohort of suspected probands identifies known and potential pathogenic variants. Cells. 2020;9(11):2368. https://doi.org/10.3390/cells9112368.
7. Alfayyadh MM, Maksemous N, Sutherland HG, Lea RA, Griffiths LR. PathVar: a customisable NGS variant calling algorithm implicates novel candidate genes and pathways in hemiplegic migraine. Clin Genet. 2025;107(2):157–68. https://doi.org/10.1111/cge.14625.
8. Pietrobon D, Moskowitz MA. Chaos and commotion in the wake of cortical spreading depression and spreading depolarizations. Nat Rev Neurosci. 2014;15:379–93. https://doi.org/10.1038/nrn3770.
9. Kaag Rasmussen M, Møllgård K, Bork PAR, Weikop P, Esmail T, Drici L, Wewer Albrechtsen NJ, Carlsen JF, Huynh NPT, Ghitani N, Mann M, Goldman SA, Mori Y, Chesler AT, Nedergaard M. Trigeminal ganglion neurons are directly activated by influx of CSF solutes in a migraine model. Science. 2024;385(6704):80–6. https://doi.org/10.1126/science.adl0544.
10. Pietrobon D, Brennan KC. Genetic mouse models of migraine. J Headache Pain. 2019;20:79. https://doi.org/10.1186/s10194-019-1029-5.

11. Mangano GD, Capizzi MR, Mantuano E, Veneziano L, Santangelo G, Quatrosi G, Nardello R, Raieli V. Familial hemiplegic migraine in pediatric patients: a genetic, clinical, and follow-up study. Headache. 2023;63(7):889–98. https://doi.org/10.1111/head.14582.
12. Marconi R, De Fusco M, Aridon P, Plewnia K, Rossi M, Carapelli S, Ballabio A, Morgante L, Musolino R, Epifanio A, Micieli G, De Michele G, Casari G. Familial hemiplegic migraine type 2 is linked to 0.9Mb region on chromosome 1q23. Ann Neurol. 2003;53(3):376–81. https://doi.org/10.1002/ana.10464.
13. Bonemazzi I, Brunello F, Pin JN, Pecoraro M, Sartori S, Nosadini M, Toldo I. Hemiplegic migraine in children and adolescents. J Clin Med. 2023;12(11):3783. https://doi.org/10.3390/jcm12113783.
14. Thomsen LL, Ostergaard E, Olesen J, Russell MB. Evidence for a separate type of migraine with aura: sporadic hemiplegic migraine. Neurology. 2003;60:595–601. https://doi.org/10.1212/01.wnl.0000046524.25369.7d.
15. Lykke Thomsen L, Kirchmann Eriksen M, Faerch Romer S, Andersen I, Ostergaard E, Keiding N, Olesen J, Russell MB. An epidemiological survey of hemiplegic migraine. Cephalalgia. 2002;22(5):361–75. https://doi.org/10.1046/j.1468-2982.2002.00371.x.
16. Barros J, Ruano L, Domingos J, Tuna A, Damásio J, Alonso I, Silveira I, Sequeiros J, Coutinho P. The prevalence of familial hemiplegic migraine with cerebellar ataxia and spinocerebellar ataxia type 6 in Portugal. Headache. 2014;54(5):911–5. https://doi.org/10.1111/head.12260.
17. Toldo I, Brunello F, Morao V, Perissinotto E, Valeriani M, Pruna D, Tozzi E, Moscano F, Farello G, Frusciante R, Carotenuto M, Lisotto C, Ruffatti S, Maggioni F, Termine C, Di Rosa G, Nosadini M, Sartori S, Battistella PA. First attack and clinical presentation of hemiplegic migraine in pediatric age: a multicenter retrospective study and literature review. Front Neurol. 2019;10:1079. https://doi.org/10.3389/fneur.2019.01079.
18. Kumar G, Topper L, Maytal J. Familial hemiplegic migraine with prolonged aura and multimodality imaging: a case report. Headache. 2009;49:139–42. https://doi.org/10.1111/j.1526-4610.2008.01180.x.
19. Saleh C, Pierquin G, Beyenburg S. Hemiplegic migraine presenting with prolonged somnolence: a case report. Case Rep Neurol. 2016;8:204–10. https://doi.org/10.1159/000448473.
20. Kumar A, Samanta D, Emmady PD, Arora R. Hemiplegic migraine. In: StatPearls. Treasure Island (FL): StatPearls Publishing; 2025.
21. Cuenca-León E, Corominas R, Fernàndez-Castillo N, Volpini V, Del Toro M, Roig M, Macaya A, Cormand B. Genetic analysis of 27 Spanish patients with hemiplegic migraine, basilar-type migraine and childhood periodic syndromes. Cephalalgia. 2008;28(10):1039–47. https://doi.org/10.1111/j.1468-2982.2008.01645.x.
22. Suzuki M, Fujiwara K, Tsubuku T, Yabe I, Sasaki H, Fukuda S. Time course of downbeat positioning nystagmus in familial hemiplegic migraine type 1 treated with acetazolamide. J Neurol Sci. 2016;368:206–8. https://doi.org/10.1016/j.jns.2016.07.020.
23. Vahedi K, Denier C, Ducros A, Bousson V, Levy C, Chabriat H, Haguenau M, Tournier-Lasserve E, Bousser MG. CACNA1A gene de novo mutation causing hemiplegic migraine, coma, and cerebellar atrophy. Neurology. 2000;55(7):1040–2. https://doi.org/10.1212/wnl.55.7.1040.
24. Rispoli MG, Di Stefano V, Mantuano E, De Angelis MV. Novel missense mutation in the ATP1A2 gene associated with atypical sporapedic hemiplegic migraine. BMJ Case Rep. 2019;12(10):e231129. https://doi.org/10.1136/bcr-2019-231129.
25. Humbertclaude V, Riant F, Krams B, Zimmermann V, Nagot N, Annequin D, Echenne B, Tournier-Lasserve E, Roubertie A, Episodic Syndrome Consortium. Cognitive impairment in children with CACNA1A mutations. Dev Med Child Neurol. 2020;62(3):330–7. https://doi.org/10.1111/dmcn.14261.
26. Prontera P, Sarchielli P, Caproni S, Bedetti C, Cupini LM, Calabresi P, Costa C. Epilepsy in hemiplegic migraine: genetic mutations and clinical implications. Cephalalgia. 2018;38(2):361–73. https://doi.org/10.1177/0333102416686347.

27. International Headache Society. Headache classification committee of the International Headache Society (IHS) the international classification of headache disorders, 3rd edition. Cephalalgia. 2018;38:1–211. https://doi.org/10.1177/0333102417738202.
28. Pelzer N, Stam AH, Haan J, Ferrari MD, Terwindt GM. Familial and sporadic hemiplegic migraine: diagnosis and treatment. Curr Treat Options Neurol. 2013;15(1):13–27. https://doi.org/10.1007/s11940-012-0208-3.
29. Terrin A, Toldo G, Ermani M, Mainardi F, Maggioni F. When migraine mimics stroke: a systematic review. Cephalalgia. 2018;38(14):2068–78. https://doi.org/10.1177/0333102418767999.
30. Black DF. Sporadic hemiplegic migraine. Curr Pain Headache Rep. 2004;8:223–8. https://doi.org/10.1007/s11916-004-0056-2.
31. Ohmura K, Suzuki Y, Saito Y, Wada T, Goto M, Seto S. Sporadic hemiplegic migraine presenting as acute encephalopathy. Brain Dev. 2012;34(8):691–5. https://doi.org/10.1016/j.braindev.2011.11.002.
32. Zheng Q, Yang L, Tan LM, Qin LX, Wang CY, Zhang HN. Stroke-like migraine attacks after radiation therapy syndrome. Chin Med J. 2015;128(15):2097–101. https://doi.org/10.4103/0366-6999.161393.
33. Kansagra S, Mikati MA, Vigevano F. Alternating hemiplegia of childhood. Handb Clin Neurol. 2013;112:821–6. https://doi.org/10.1016/B978-0-444-52910-7.00001-5.
34. Yilmaz A, Kaleagasi H, Dogu O, Kara E, Ozge A. Abnormal MRI in a patient with 'headache with neurological deficits and CSF lymphocytosis (HaNDL)'. Cephalalgia. 2010;30(5):615–9. https://doi.org/10.1111/j.1468-2982.2009.01950.x.
35. Montagna P, Gallassi R, Medori R, Govoni E, Zeviani M, Di Mauro S, Lugaresi E, Andermann F. MELAS syndrome: characteristic migrainous and epileptic features and maternal transmission. Neurology. 1988;38(5):751–4. https://doi.org/10.1212/wnl.38.5.751.
36. Planche V, Chassin O, Leduc L, Regnier W, Kelly A, Colamarino R. Sturge-Weber syndrome with late onset hemiplegic migraine-like attacks and progressive unilateral cerebral atrophy. Cephalalgia. 2014;34(1):73–7. https://doi.org/10.1177/0333102413505237.
37. Hansen JM, Hauge AW, Ashina M, Olesen J. Trigger factors for familial hemiplegic migraine. Cephalalgia. 2011;31:1274–81. https://doi.org/10.1177/0333102411415878.
38. Striano P, Zara F, Santorelli FM, Striano S. Topiramate-associated worsening symptoms in a patient with familial hemiplegic migraine. J Neurol Sci. 2008;272:194–5. https://doi.org/10.1016/j.jns.2008.05.015.
39. Modestino EJ, Bowirrat A, Lewandrowski KU, Sharafshah A, Badgaiyan RD, Thanos PK, Baron D, Dennen CA, Elman I, Sunder K, Murphy KT, Blum K. Hemiplegic migraines exacerbated using an injectable GLP-1 agonist for weight loss. Acta Sci Neurol. 2024;7(5):12–8. https://doi.org/10.31080/asne.2024.07.0731.
40. Elsadany M, McMahon SR, Mehla S, Duvall WL. Hemiplegic migraine episode triggered by regadenoson. J Nucl Cardiol. 2022;29:3469–73. https://doi.org/10.1007/s12350-021-02736-1.
41. Turner C, Campbell L, Fung R, Desai S, Oyenubi A, Cayabyab F, Huntsman RJ. Treatment of CACNA1A encephalopathy and cerebral edema with magnesium and dexamethasone. Can J Neurol Sci. 2024;52(2):314–7. https://doi.org/10.1017/cjn.2024.52.
42. Camia F, Pisciotta L, Morana G, Schiaffino MC, Renna S, Carrera P, Ferrari M, Baglietto MG, Veneselli E, Siri L, Mancardi MM. Combined early treatment in hemiplegic attacks related to CACNA1A encephalopathy with brain oedema: blocking the cascade? Cephalalgia. 2017;37(12):1202–6. https://doi.org/10.1177/0333102416668655.
43. Artto V, Nissilä M, Wessman M, Palotie A, Färkkilä M, Kallela M. Treatment of hemiplegic migraine with triptans. Eur J Neurol. 2007;14(9):1053–6. https://doi.org/10.1111/j.1468-1331.2007.01900.x.
44. Kaube H, Herzog J, Käufer T, Dichgans M, Diener HC. Aura in some patients with familial hemiplegic migraine can be stopped by intranasal ketamine. Neurology. 2000;55(1):139–41. https://doi.org/10.1212/wnl.55.1.139.

45. Yu W, Horowitz SH. Familial hemiplegic migraine and its abortive therapy with intravenous verapamil. Neurology. 2001;57:1732–3. https://doi.org/10.1212/wnl.57.9.1732.
46. Lai CW, Ziegler DK, Lansky LL, Torres F. Hemiplegic migraine in childhood: diagnostic and therapeutic aspects. J Pediatr. 1982;101:696–9. https://doi.org/10.1016/s0022-3476(82)80293-x.
47. Hsu DA, Stafstrom CE, Rowley HA, Kiff JE, Dulli DA. Hemiplegic migraine: hyperperfusion and abortive therapy with intravenous verapamil. Brain Dev. 2008;30(1):86–90. https://doi.org/10.1016/j.braindev.2007.05.013.
48. Tobita M, Hino M, Ichikawa N, Takase S, Ogawa A. A case of hemiplegic migraine treated with flunarizine. Headache. 1987;27(9):487–8. https://doi.org/10.1111/j.1526-4610.1987.hed2709487.x.
49. Ueda K, Serajee F, Huq AM. Clinical benefit of NMDA receptor antagonists in a patient with ATP1A2 gene mutation. Pediatrics. 2018;141:S390–4. https://doi.org/10.1542/peds.2017-0852.
50. Ho TW, Connor KM, Zhang Y, Pearlman E, Koppenhaver J, Fan X, Lines C, Edvinsson L, Goadsby PJ, Michelson D. Randomized controlled trial of the CGRP receptor antagonist telcagepant for migraine prevention. Neurology. 2014;83(11):958–66. https://doi.org/10.1212/WNL.0000000000000771.
51. Chen TY, Garza I, Dodick DW, Robertson CE. The effect of OnabotulinumtoxinA on aura frequency and severity in patients with hemiplegic migraine: case series of 11 patients. Headache. 2018;58:973–85. https://doi.org/10.1111/head.13317.
52. Danno D, Ishizaki K, Kikui S, Takeshima T. Treatment of hemiplegic migraine with anti-calcitonin gene-related peptide monoclonal antibodies: a case series in a tertiary-care headache center. Headache. 2008;63:984–9. https://doi.org/10.1111/head.14591.
53. Mulder IA, Li M, de Vries T, Qin T, Yanagisawa T, Sugimoto K, van den Bogaerdt A, Danser AHJ, Wermer MJH, van den Maagdenberg AMJM, MaassenVanDenBrink A, Ferrari MD, Ayata C. Anti-migraine calcitonin gene-related peptide receptor antagonists worsen cerebral ischemic outcome in mice. Ann Neurol. 2020;88(4):771–84. https://doi.org/10.1002/ana.25831.
54. Wang P, Yao F, Zhang H, Yu Q, Wang Y. Disappearance of aura symptoms in patients with hemiplegic migraine after patent foramen ovale closure: a case report and literature review. Front Neurol. 2023;14:1267100. https://doi.org/10.3389/fneur.2023.1267100.

Chapter 2
Migrainous Status

Mauro Eduardo Jurno and Ligia Barros de Oliveira

2.1 Introduction

Migrainous status is one of the most debilitating complications of migraine, characterized by a migraine attack lasting more than 72 h, with persistent and uncontrollable symptoms resulting in significant functional incapacitation. Although recognized by the International Classification of Headache Disorders (ICHD-3; code 1.4.1. Migrainous Status) [1], its pathophysiology and epidemiology remain poorly understood, with significant gaps in its investigation and effective treatment [2, 3].

This chapter aims to discuss status migrainosus, using a clinical case observed by the authors as the foundation for the discussion.

2.2 Pathophysiology

The exact pathophysiology of migrainous status is not fully understood, but it shares several characteristics with common migraine, such as activation of the trigeminovascular system and central and peripheral sensitization [4].

Evidence suggests that migrainous status may have a biological basis distinct from common migraine, representing a more refractory and prolonged state that does not respond well to conventional therapies. Genetic studies indicate that specific genetic variants may be associated with a higher susceptibility to more severe and prolonged migraine attacks [4].

M. E. Jurno (✉) · L. B. de Oliveira
Barbacena School of Medicine – FUNJOB and Minas Gerais State Hospital Foundation – FHEMIG, Barbacena, Brazil

D. Uludüz et al. (eds.), *Rare Causes of Headache Disorders*, Headache,
https://doi.org/10.1007/978-3-032-10242-3_2

Furthermore, some research indicates that migrainous status may cause reversible structural changes in the brain, such as vasogenic edema and hypoperfusion, suggesting deeper involvement than typical migraine. However, such findings are still rare and require validation through larger, controlled studies [4].

2.3 Case Presentation

The patient, a female, 35 years old, reports having experienced a severe unilateral headache on the right side 4 days before admission. The headache was characterized as pulsatile, accompanied by intense nausea, photophobia, and phonophobia. She denies having osmophobia. The episode began similarly to her usual migraine attacks. Still, this time the pain persisted for over 72 h, continuously, despite using her routine medications, which include sumatriptan and non-steroidal anti-inflammatory drugs (NSAIDs). She also took dipyrone and rested in a dark place, but found no relief from her painful symptoms and general malaise.

The patient notes that before the current episode, she had been experiencing episodic headaches two to three times a month, always triggered by stress and sleep deprivation. Typically, her episodes lasted between 12 and 24 h, but they had never exceeded 48 h. In the last 24 h, she reported increasing difficulty sleeping due to persistent pain and nausea, having vomited twice.

The patient has been diagnosed with migraine without aura since the age of 25. She reports that her most common triggers are stress, irregular sleep, and the menstrual period. She has no other significant clinical comorbidities and denies chronic medication use except for migraine control. Patient's mother has a history of migraine, controlled with preventive medications.

On physical examination, the patient was afebrile, with a blood pressure of 120/80 mmHg and a heart rate of 76 bpm. She appeared lucid and oriented but was visibly distressed, holding her head and adopting a posture suggestive of significant discomfort. Neurological examination revealed no focal deficits, and fundoscopy showed no abnormalities. There were no signs of neck stiffness or other meningeal irritation.

Based on the report of severe headache persisting for over 72 h with inadequate response to usual treatment, the probable diagnosis is Migrainous Status. This condition is exacerbated by associated vomiting and other debilitating symptoms, characterizing a medical emergency.

2.4 Case Discussion

This is a typical case of status migrainosus in a patient with a history of migraine, triggered by stress and sleep deprivation. The progression to a prolonged crisis unresponsive to standard medications justifies the need for a more aggressive approach, including intravenous (IV) therapies and hospital observation. Proper management can prevent complications such as the progression to chronic migraine and reduce the severe functional impact associated with the condition [3–7]. Given the refractoriness of the headache to standard treatments and its prolonged duration, a more intensive management strategy in a hospital setting was warranted. The proposed plan included intravenous hydration with a saline solution to address potential electrolyte imbalances and dehydration resulting from vomiting. Dexamethasone (8 mg IV) was administered to reduce neuroinflammation and lower the risk of recurrence. Metoclopramide (10 mg IV) was used to manage associated nausea and vomiting. Intravenous magnesium sulfate was added for its known prophylactic and crisis-modulating effects in refractory migraine. Additionally, an anticonvulsant such as intravenous valproic acid was considered due to its reported efficacy in treatment-resistant attacks. The patient was admitted for observation over the first 24 h to monitor clinical response and allow for timely adjustment of therapy as needed. With appropriate treatment, it is expected that the patient will show improvement within 24–48 h, with a gradual resolution of symptoms. However, a subsequent evaluation should be considered to review long-term preventive medication and discuss the management of comorbid conditions.

2.5 Clinical Characteristics

Epidemiological studies indicate that migrainous status is relatively uncommon, although it is often underreported. A survey conducted in Olmsted County, Minnesota, identified an age- and sex-adjusted incidence rate of 26.6 per 100,000 individuals per year, with a peak between the ages of 40 and 49, and a predominance among women.

Other studies suggest that between 3% and 20% of individuals with migraine may experience migrainous status at some point [5].

Risk factors for developing this condition include excessive use of pain medications during attacks, sleep disturbances, stress, and lack of effective treatment for migraine attacks. One of the primary triggers includes irregular sleep patterns, both excess and deprivation, which are strongly associated with the risk of migrainous status recurrence. Patients with episodic migraine are also more likely to progress to chronic migraine if they experience recurrent migrainous status.

Additionally, migraine attacks resistant to acute pharmacological therapy increase the likelihood of complications, such as progression to chronic migraine and the development of medication dependency [6].

2.6 Diagnostic Algorithm

The diagnostic approach to status migrainosus begins with a careful evaluation of the clinical history, with particular attention to the duration and course of the headache. According to the International Classification of Headache Disorders (ICHD-3), status migrainosus is defined as a migraine attack lasting longer than 72 h, with either continuous pain or only brief periods of remission. In most cases, patients have a pre-existing diagnosis of migraine, and the episode typically evolves from a standard migraine attack that fails to resolve with usual treatment.

The symptom profile is essential in guiding the diagnosis. Common features include severe, often unilateral, pulsatile headache, accompanied by nausea, vomiting, photophobia, and phonophobia. Patients often report worsening of symptoms with routine physical activity and significant impairment in daily functioning. Disruption of sleep and emotional distress are also frequently observed. The presence of these typical features, in the absence of alarming neurological signs, supports the diagnosis of a primary migraine complication rather than a secondary headache disorder.

An important step in the diagnostic process is assessing the response to standard acute migraine treatments, such as triptans, NSAIDs, or rest in a dark room. In status migrainosus, these measures typically fail to provide relief. This lack of therapeutic response is a hallmark of the condition and indicates the need for more aggressive management.

A neurological examination should always be performed to exclude secondary causes of prolonged headache. In status migrainosus, the examination is usually normal, without focal deficits, meningeal signs, or altered mental status. However, if any of these findings are present, clinicians must consider other serious etiologies such as subarachnoid hemorrhage, central nervous system infections, or space-occupying lesions, and order appropriate investigations.

Neuroimaging, particularly magnetic resonance imaging (MRI), may be indicated in patients with atypical features, a first-time prolonged headache episode, or poor response to treatment. This helps to rule out secondary causes and may occasionally reveal reversible changes associated with prolonged migraine attacks, such as cortical spreading depression or mild vasogenic edema. In cases of persistent vomiting, laboratory investigations including electrolytes, renal function, and inflammatory markers may also be useful to assess for dehydration and systemic effects.

Finally, the application of ICHD-3 diagnostic criteria (code 1.4.1) helps confirm the diagnosis. These include: a prior diagnosis of migraine, an attack lasting more than 72 h, continuous or nearly continuous headache, and significant functional impairment that is unresponsive to acute treatment. Recognizing this condition early is critical, as delayed diagnosis can lead to hospitalization, medication overuse, and progression to chronic migraine.

2.7 Management

The management of migrainous status is not yet standardized, and different approaches are used in outpatient and hospital settings. In the early stages of this condition, many specialists recommend treating the crisis within 72 h, using medications such as corticosteroids, NSAIDs, neuroleptics, and triptans [4].

In refractory cases, where patients no longer respond to traditional therapies, treatment in a hospital setting with intravenous medication administration is recommended. Commonly used options include intravenous fluids, magnesium sulfate, anticonvulsants, and serotonergic agents such as sumatriptan [6].

In emergencies, the primary focus is to alleviate pain and associated symptoms such as nausea and vomiting. Some studies suggest that a combination of different classes of medications, including antiemetics, NSAIDs, and corticosteroids, may be effective in reducing symptoms [6]. Nonetheless, there is a notable lack of high-quality clinical trials exploring the efficacy of the various available therapies.

For patients with chronic status migrainosus, prolonged use of migraine medications without an effective prophylactic approach may exacerbate the condition, leading to medication overuse headache. In these cases, a gradual discontinuation of medications, combined with an appropriate preventive therapy, may prove to be an effective strategy [6, 7].

Although status migrainosus is a temporary condition, its recurrence is associated with a poorer prognosis for patients with migraine. One study indicated that approximately 15% of patients experiencing an episode of status migrainosus have a recurrence within 1 year [3]. Furthermore, these patients are at increased risk of developing chronic migraine, particularly if triggering factors, such as sleep disorders and inappropriate medication use, are not managed [5].

Status migrainosus is also linked to high hospitalization and treatment costs, reflecting its severity and the complexity of its management. Studies estimate that the average price of hospitalization for the treatment of status migrainosus can range from US$3800 to US$7000 per episode, depending on the severity and treatments utilized [5].

2.8 Conclusion

Status migrainosus is a debilitating condition, the pathophysiology of which is not yet fully understood. While several therapeutic options are available, there remains a need for high-quality randomized clinical trials to determine the best management strategies. Early treatment and personalized use of prophylactics appear to be key in preventing the evolution to this complication, thereby reducing both morbidity and the economic impact of the condition.

References

1. Olesen J. Headache classification committee of the international headache society (IHS) the international classification of headache disorders. Cephalalgia. 2018;38(1):1–211.
2. Karlsson WK, Ostinelli EG, Zhuang ZA, Kokoti L, Christensen RH, Al-Khazali HM, Deligianni CI, Tomlinson A, Ashina H, Ruiz de la Torre E, Diener HC, Cipriani A, Ashina M. Comparative effects of drug interventions for the acute management of migraine episodes in adults: systematic review and network meta-analysis. BMJ. 2024;386:e080107. https://doi.org/10.1136/bmj-2024-080107.
3. Vander Pluym JH, Mangipudi K, Mbonde AA, Gritsch D, Caronna E, Halker Singh RB, Butterfield RJ, Smith JH. Incidence of status migrainosus in Olmsted County, Minnesota, United States: characterization and predictors of recurrence. Neurology. 2023;100(3):e255–63. https://doi.org/10.1212/WNL.0000000000201382.
4. Kamourieh S, Rozen T, Anderson JM. Status migrainosus. Handb Clin Neurol. 2024;199:413–39.
5. Orr SL. Status migrainosus: one of the most poorly understood but important complications of migraine. Neurology. 2023;100(3):107–8. https://doi.org/10.1212/WNL.0000000000201477.
6. Vécsei L, Szok D, Nyári A, Tajti J. Treating status migrainosus in the emergency setting: what is the best strategy? Expert Opin Pharmacother. 2018;19(14):1523–31. https://doi.org/10.1080/14656566.2018.1516205.
7. Robblee J, Orlova YY, Ahn AH, Ali AS, Birlea M, Charleston L 4th, Singh NN, Souza MNP. Real-world approaches to outpatient treatment of status migrainosus: a survey study. Headache. 2024;64(8):1040–8. https://doi.org/10.1111/head.14769.

Chapter 3
Migrainous Infarction

Alessandro Borrelli, Fabiana Ursitti, and Massimiliano Valeriani

3.1 Introduction

Migrainous infarction is an ischemic stroke that originates during a typical migraine with aura attack. It initially presents with the usual features of previous episodes but lasts longer (more than 60 min), is often accompanied by new symptoms, and may be associated with greater headache severity. It must be distinguished from ischemic strokes of other causes that mimic migraine symptoms, as well as from ischemic strokes occurring in patients with a concurrent diagnosis of migraine with aura [1]. Thus, migrainous infarction represents a distinct clinical entity among the possible ischemic stroke manifestations in patients with migraine with aura. Based on the few available studies, the prevalence of ischemic strokes is estimated to be between 0.05% and 0.8%.

A. Borrelli · F. Ursitti
Developmental Neurology Unit, Bambino Gesù Children's Hospital IRCCS, Rome, Italy

M. Valeriani (✉)
Developmental Neurology Unit, Bambino Gesù Children's Hospital IRCCS, Rome, Italy

Systems Medicine Department, Tor Vergata University of Rome, Rome, Italy

Translational Pain Neuroscience and Precision Medicine, CNAP, Department of Health Science and Technology, School of Medicine, Aalborg University, Aalborg, Denmark
e-mail: valeriani@opbg.net; massimiliano.valeriani@opbg.net

D. Uludüz et al. (eds.), *Rare Causes of Headache Disorders*, Headache,
https://doi.org/10.1007/978-3-032-10242-3_3

3.2 Pathophysiology

The relationship between migraine and stroke is complex. Migraine with aura is recognized as an independent risk factor for ischemic stroke, while data regarding migraine without aura are less indicative [2, 3]. Cortical spreading depolarization (CSD) is an essential electrophysiological phenomenon underlying aura. Its relationship with ischemia is ambivalent: CSD increases metabolic demands while reducing cerebral blood flow, potentially damaging metabolically compromised brain tissue and leading to ischemia [4], but it can also be induced by ischemia itself [5], thus worsening brain tissue damage and neurologic outcomes [4]. The complex mechanisms underlying the association between migraine and ischemic stroke are largely unidentified; however, endothelial dysfunction, hormones (especially estrogens), and genetic factors may play essential roles in this relationship, which is beyond the scope of this chapter [3, 4].

Most reported cases in the literature do not indicate a precise underlying pathophysiological mechanism. While cases of migraine-related strokes with associated vasospasm were described [6–9], adherence to the diagnostic criteria for a migrainous infarction could be found only in one patient [9]. Lebedeva et al. described signs of multiple microemboli in the middle cerebral artery of a patient experiencing migrainous infarction, though no clear embolic source was identified [10].

3.3 Case Presentation

Our exemplary patient is a 32-year-old non-smoking woman in good health. She does not take any medications, except for an oral contraceptive pill containing drospirenone and ethinyl estradiol. The patient has been suffering from occasional headache attacks since her adolescence. Her attacks are sometimes preceded by visual symptoms such as fortification spectra or scintillating scotomas. Her headaches are typically unilateral, pulsatile, and associated with photophobia, occurring approximately once per week. She usually takes naproxen, with good effectiveness.

One evening, she experienced a right-sided scintillating scotoma, accompanied by the occurrence, after 40 min, of a bilateral parietal headache, associated with nausea and photophobia. She was not particularly concerned by these symptoms, as they resembled her usual migraine with aura episodes. Still, she noticed that the visual symptoms progressively evolved into a negative scotoma, which persisted throughout the headache. She went to bed expecting that these symptoms would disappear during sleep. Upon waking the following morning, her right visual field defect had worsened, along with increased headache intensity, prompting her to present to the emergency department. Clinical examination revealed a right homonymous hemianopia. Her blood pressure was normal. As her headache persisted, she was administered intravenous ketorolac. After neurological consultation, the patient underwent a contrast-enhanced brain CT (computed tomography) scan, which revealed a hypodensity in the left occipital lobe. A migraine-related ischemic stroke was suspected and secondary prevention with aspirin 100 mg was started. Later that day, brain MRI (magnetic resonance imaging) with angiography confirmed an infarction in the left occipital cortex and excluded major vascular disease. Laboratory testing showed normal glucose, cholesterol, and triglyceride levels. A complete hypercoagulation panel of laboratory tests was negative, including Protein C, Protein S, prothrombin time (PT), activated partial thromboplastin time (aPTT), antithrombin III, Factors II and VII, D-dimer, antiphospholipid, anticardiolipin, and anti-β2-glycoprotein antibodies, lupus anticoagulant, MTHFR gene mutations, and Factor V Leiden. Transesophageal echocardiography and Holter electrocardiography yielded unremarkable findings. Oral contraception was discontinued. On follow-up, the patient gradually regained normal vision.

3.4 Case Discussion

This case illustrates the typical features of migrainous infarction. The patient had a history of migraine with aura and use of oral contraception, with no additional stroke risk factors identified. Her symptoms initially presented with the typical characteristics of her migrainous attacks, but persisted throughout the headache phase. She sought medical attention after several hours, reporting the development of an atypical symptom (homonymous hemianopia) and aura persistence beyond 1 h. Neuroimaging confirmed an infarction in the occipital cortex, a location consistent with the clinical presentation. Secondary prevention with aspirin was initiated.

3.5 Clinical Characteristics

Episodes begin with the typical symptoms of previous aura attacks, with additional symptoms potentially arising due to the extension of brain involvement to other areas. Although the definition of migrainous infarction requires one or more aura symptoms to persist for more than 1 h, many patients may seek medical attention after hours or days. Additionally, patients may report increased headache severity or experience unusually intense nausea, phonophobia, or photophobia [11] or resistance to the usual medications [6].

The infarction most commonly occurs in the territory supplied by the posterior cerebral artery. Scotomas, positive visual symptoms, and sensory deficits are common early manifestations, often progressing to homonymous hemianopia in many patients. The majority of cases involve the posterior cerebral vascular territory, as this was the case in 84% of patients in the most extensive case series [12], particularly the vertebrobasilar system. Localization in the anterior and middle cerebrovascular systems is less common, causing different clinical manifestations [6, 10–15].

Interestingly, a reduction in both the frequency and severity of headaches has been reported in the months following migrainous infarction [16, 17]. This phenomenon may not be specific to migrainous infarction, as a reduction in headache frequency has also been observed in migraine patients with ischemic stroke, regardless of etiology [18].

We reviewed the frequency of various traditional risk factors in cases of migrainous infarction (as outlined in the inclusion criteria). Most patients were female (60%), and 31% of them used oral contraceptives. The age of patients reported in the literature ranges from 18 to 93 years, with a weighted median of 39 years and an interquartile range (IQR) of 22.5 (inclusive of extremes). Hyperlipidemia was present in 23%, a smoking habit in 24%, and hypertension in 12%. A patent foramen ovale (PFO) was not consistently investigated across all articles; however, when considering only patients who underwent an echocardiogram, it was present in 24%. Notably, two case series reported a high prevalence of PFO. Wolf et al. reported that 64.7% of patients with migraine-related stroke had a PFO [19]. In comparison, Laurell et al. reported a prevalence of 40% among the 30 patients with migrainous infarction who underwent echocardiography [12]. PFO persistence into adulthood is more common among patients with migraine with aura than in the general population (Table 3.1).

Traditional cardiovascular risk factors, such as diabetes, hypertension, and dyslipidemia, appear to play a less significant role when compared with other types of ischemic strokes. Case-series reports a low prevalence of these factors, while oral contraceptives and smoking are both common. A retrospective study of 33 Scandinavian patients with migrainous infarction found a statistically significant lower frequency of current smoking, hypertension, hyperlipidemia, and diabetes compared to a cohort of 1008 young Finnish patients with stroke of any cause [12]. Similarly, in a vast cohort of 17,633 young patients aged 18–50 years with ischemic stroke due to any cause, there were higher frequencies of hypertension (36.6%), diabetes (13.8%), dyslipidemia (31.7%), and smoking (49.2%) [33].

Female sex and young age (<45 years) are established risk factors for ischemic stroke in migraine patients [34, 35], with the risk further increasing in combination with oral contraceptive use and smoking [34].

The use of vasoactive medications, such as triptans and ergotamines, has been proposed as a potential risk factor for migrainous infarction, and caution has been advised regarding their use in patients with migraine with aura [4]. Despite their widespread use, limited data exist concerning cardiovascular risk in the use of both classes of drugs. A meta-analysis by Roberto et al., which synthesized data from four studies, was unable to draw definitive conclusions due to variations in study design and potential biases [36]. More recently, an extensive retrospective case-crossover study identified an increased risk of myocardial and cerebral infarction following triptan initiation [37]. However, this risk was exceptionally low in patients without other cardiovascular risk factors (1) new case per 30,000 patients). Still, other sources reported that a higher rate of major cardiovascular events was observed with the use of triptans in patients with previous cardiovascular risk factors [38].

Table 3.1 Risk factors reported in cases of migrainous infarction in the literature

	Total	Male	Female	Age	HT	Smoking	Diabetes	OC	Dyslipidemia	PFO
Kandemir Yılmaz and Kirikli [20]	1	1		71						
Lebedeva et al. [10]	1		1	18						
Lebedeva et al. (2015) as reported in Lebedeva et al. [10]	2	1	1	54 and 53	2			1	1	EC NR
Bylund et al. [21]	1	1		49					1	1
Terrin et al. [22]	1		1	56						
Vinciguerra et al. [9]	1		1	44						
Mancini et al. [15]	1	1		32			1			
Serrano et al. [17]	15	7	8	34.8 median; range 18–55	2	4		4	5	
Morais et al. [23]	1		1	37				1		
Khardenavis et al. [14]	1		1	27						
Campagna et al. [24]	1		1	47	1		1	1	1	
Renard et al. [25]	1	1		47						EC NR
Lai and Hong [26]	1	1		60	1	1				
Wolf et al. [19]	11	NR	NR	NR	5	4		5	3	8
Laurell et al. [12]	33	13	20	39 median; range 19–76	4	7	1	6	10	12 (EC only in 30 patients)
Decima et al. [7]	1	1		41		1			1	
Arai et al. [27]	1	1		64	1					
Liang and Scott [28]	1		1	57						
Tzoulis et al. [11]	1		1	93						
Frigerio et al. [13]	6	1	5	Female: 29 median; range 23–40 Male: 36		3		2		Unclear number of patients who underwent EC

(continued)

Table 3.1 (continued)

	Total	Male	Female	Age	HT	Smoking	Diabetes	OC	Dyslipidemia	PFO
Tang et al. [29]	1		1	29						
Arboix et al. [30]	9	3	6	32 median; range 24–60		1		2	1	
Linetsky et al. [16]	6	1	5	56 median; range 39–65						
Sacquegna et al. [31]	1		1	31		1				
Moen et al. [32]	1	1		37		1				
Total	**100**	**34**	**55**	**39 weighted median; IQR 22.5**	**16**	**24**	**3**	**22**	**23**	**21**
Prevalence	/	**37%**	**60%**	/	**16%**	**24%**	**3%**	**31%[a]**	**23%**	**24%[b]**

Note: This list includes all articles stating adherence to ICHD-3 criteria and available in English language. We excluded works that clearly reported in the text features not meeting ICHD-3 criteria (e.g., patients who did not experience migraine with aura attacks previously)

EC echocardiogram, *HT* hypertension, *ICHD-3* International Classification of Headache Disorders-III, *IQR* interquartile range (including extremes), *NR* not reported, *OC* oral contraception, *PFO* patent foramen ovale

[a]Percentage of total female patients, with the exclusion of cases by Wolf et al. [19] who do not report the share of female patients

[b]Percentage of patients who underwent an echocardiogram

Other conditions are associated with both migraine and stroke and could explain some cases of migrainous infarction: atrial fibrillation, hereditary small vessel diseases, dissection of cervical artery, antiphospholipid syndrome [4].

Further research is needed to elucidate the role and prevalence of risk factors in migrainous infarction, as well as the underlying pathophysiological mechanisms.

International Classification of Headache Disorders III (ICHD-3) Criteria for Migrainous Infarction [1]

A. A migraine attack fulfilling criteria B and C
B. Occurring in a patient with 1.2 Migraine with aura and typical of previous attacks except that one or more aura symptoms persist for >60 min[1]
C. Neuroimaging demonstrates ischemic infarction in a relevant area
D. Not better accounted for by another ICHD-3 diagnosis

Note: 1. There may be additional symptoms attributable to the infarction

3.6 Diagnostic Algorithm

A diagnosis of migrainous infarction primarily demands the clinical distinction from transient ischemic attacks (TIAs) and uncomplicated attacks of migraine with aura. After this distinction has been made, neuroimaging can confirm the presence of ischemia and rule out vascular diseases. It is also recommended to rule out hypercoagulation disorders, cardioembolism, and rare genetic causes of stroke, like CADASIL (Cerebral Autosomal Dominant Arteriopathy with Subcortical Infarcts and Leukoencephalopathy) and MELAS (Mitochondrial Encephalopathy, Lactic Acidosis, Stroke).

A distinction from a typical attack of migraine with aura is difficult. Migraine is implicated in both false positives ("stroke mimics") and false negatives ("stroke chameleons"), with misdiagnoses being relatively common [3]. Clinical suspicion of migrainous infarction should be guided by the long duration of aura symptoms, especially if they persist after headache relief, and presence of unusual accompanying manifestations. Sometimes the attack is more severe than usual, leading patients to seek medical attention. Hemiplegic migraine and migraine with unilateral motor symptoms are two conditions that can be mistaken for migrainous infarction and must be thoughtfully excluded.

TIA symptoms typically manifest suddenly and tend to appear simultaneously from the onset, whereas aura symptoms usually develop more gradually and evolve [39]. Patients with migrainous infarction initially present with their typical aura symptoms, followed by the progressive emergence of additional symptoms depending on the extent of brain involvement. TIA symptoms are typically negative in nature, whereas aura must include at least one positive manifestation [1].

Additionally, TIA, by definition, lasts less than 24 h; therefore, prolonged symptoms necessitate the exclusion of an infarction.

Neuroimaging is essential for confirming the diagnosis of infarction. As in other forms of ischemic stroke, the choice of the most appropriate brain imaging technique depends on a multifactorial evaluation. MRI or CT with angiography is indicated to exclude atherosclerosis, arterial dissection, or vasospasm. The use of MRI with DWI (diffusion weighted imaging) sequences may be beneficial in the acute phase, as it is the most sensitive within the first 24 h. Patients arriving at the emergency department in the first few hours may benefit from a CT or MRI with DWI and fluid-attenuated inversion recovery (FLAIR) sequences to be evaluated for thrombolysis. However, to date, there is no literature on the use of thrombolysis for this indication, as most patients present to the emergency department hours or even days after symptom onset [19].

The diagnostic workup must include laboratory tests to rule out underlying thrombophilia, such as PT, aPTT, Factor V Leiden, protein C and S activity levels, MTHFR mutations, antithrombin III, antiphospholipid, anticardiolipin, and anti-β2 glycoprotein antibodies, lupus anticoagulant, and homocysteine levels. To exclude cardiac embolism, echocardiography (preferably transesophageal) along with prolonged electrocardiographic monitoring or Holter electrocardiogram (ECG) is mandatory: these can exclude a right-to-left shunt (patent foramen ovale) or arrythmias such as cardiac fibrillation [4].

Step 1: Clinical suspicion

- *Identify key clinical characteristics*
  - History of migraine with aura, particularly in young females, but not exclusively
  - Episode resembling previous ones, but longer in duration (by definition, more than 60 min), with the possible addition of the following characteristics:
    - Additional symptoms (from the onset or starting progressively)
    - Greater intensity of the attack

Step 2: Diagnostic workup

- *Perform brain imaging*: CTA or MRA; MRI with DWI and FLAIR is functional in the first 24 h
- *Confirm infarction*: Primarily in the posterior cerebrovascular territory, but not exclusively
- *Rule out vascular disease* (atherosclerosis, arterial dissection, vasospasm)
- *Assess hypercoagulability*
  - Laboratory tests: PT, aPTT, Factor V Leiden, protein C and S activity levels, MTHFR mutations, antithrombin III, antiphospholipid, anticardiolipin, anti-β_2 glycoprotein antibodies, lupus anticoagulant, and homocysteine levels.

- *Rule out cardiac embolism (cardiac fibrillation, right-to-left shunt)*
  - Transesophageal (preferred) or transthoracic echocardiography
  - Prolonged ECG or Holter ECG

  Consider genetic testing for rare causes of migraine and stroke when appropriate, such as CADASIL and MELAS
- *Assess risk factors for stroke:*
  - Blood pression monitoring
  - Laboratory testing for dyslipidemia and diabetes
  - Oral contraception
  - Smoking

3.7 Management

Antiplatelet therapy with aspirin or clopidogrel is advisable for the prevention of recurrences [4]. Dual antiplatelet therapy has never been studied explicitly in migrainous infarction. However, aspirin and clopidogrel are recommended by the American Heart Association American Stroke Association (AHA/ASA) ASA guidelines for minor non-cardioembolic ischemic stroke or high-risk TIA for a maximum of 90 days [40]. They may also be a plausible choice for non-cardioembolic migrainous infarction.

Assessment of modifiable cardiovascular risk factors is also essential. As already pointed out, traditional risk factors such as diabetes, hypertension, and dyslipidemia are less frequent (and possibly less significant) compared to other young stroke patients. At the same time, oral contraception and smoking are more important. Oral contraception is currently contraindicated by the U.S. Medical Eligibility Criteria for Contraceptive Use in patients with migraine with aura, and its discontinuation is recommended [41].

Preventive therapy for migraine is generally advised after ischemic brain events. Although an association between migraine frequency and stroke risk has been observed [42], there is no consistent evidence that migraine prevention reduces the risk of stroke [43]. A 19-year cohort study, however, showed that migraine patients who are treated with a combination of two or more preventive medications have a reduced risk of stroke when compared to patients using only one medication [44]. Further studies are needed to clarify the role of migraine prevention in the risk of ischemic stroke. Calcium channel blockers may be a suitable preventive option for patients with migraine and a history of stroke, due to their vasodilatory effects and anti-ischemic properties, which are mediated by interactions with GABA-A (gamma-aminobutyric acid) receptors in the brain. Melatonin, valproic acid, and onabotulinumtoxinA can be considered safe alternatives.

Regarding acute treatments, extreme caution is advised when using triptans and ergotamines in patients with prolonged aura, due to a potential increased risk of stroke [4]. Furthermore, triptans are currently contraindicated in patients with a history of cardiovascular ischemic events, including cerebral infarction.

Most patients have a favorable outcome, with either complete remission or minor residual symptoms. However, some cases of permanent significant disability have been reported. To the best of our knowledge, only one fatal case has been reported in the literature: a 57-year-old woman who was admitted for a headache of greater intensity than usual, and whose evaluation revealed signs of vasospasm and multifocal infarcts in the occipital and insular cortices as well as in the deep white matter [6]. However, this case does not appear to meet all the criteria for migrainous infarction [10], and may be more appropriately classified as a migraine-related stroke with different characteristics.

Rates of complete recovery after migrainous infarction vary widely in the literature. Arboix et al. reported that 67% of their patients were symptom-free at discharge, after 9.75 ± 6.2 days [30]. In a Scandinavian cohort of 33 patients evaluated after 3 months, only 3 (9%) had complete remission, while 28 (85%) had residual symptoms (including visual field defects), and 2 (6%) had significant disability—these two cases involved brainstem infarcts, resulting in tetraparesis and cranial nerve involvement [12]. Serrano et al. reported that 67% of patients with migraine-related stroke had mild symptoms at discharge (modified Rankin Scale 0–2), increasing to 71% at 90 days and 80% at the end of follow-up (mean: 7.5 years; range: 12–240 months) [17]. Further data and analyses are needed to better understand the prognostic factors and natural history of migrainous infarction.

3.8 Conclusion

Migrainous infarction is a rare ischemic complication of migraine with aura, defined by strict diagnostic criteria. It represents a specific entity within the complex and still largely unexplored relationship between migraine and stroke. Here, we presented an exemplary case along with a discussion of the main clinical and pathophysiological characteristics, including recommendations for diagnostic workup and management. However, these considerations are limited by the current literature, which consists predominantly of case reports and a few case series, with inconsistent or unverifiable adherence to ICHD-3 criteria. Moreover, based on current knowledge, the distinction between migrainous infarction and migraine-related stroke does not appear to influence the diagnostic approach or management strategy.

References

1. Headache Classification Committee of the International Headache Society (IHS). The international classification of headache disorders, 3rd edition. Cephalalgia. 2018;38(1):1–211.
2. Hu X, Zhou Y, Zhao H, Peng C. Migraine and the risk of stroke: an updated meta-analysis of prospective cohort studies. Neurol Sci. 2017;38(1):33–40.

3. Ravi V, Osouli Meinagh S, Bavarsad SR. Reviewing migraine-associated pathophysiology and its impact on elevated stroke risk. Front Neurol. 2024;15:1435208.
4. Chiang CC, Chen SP. Migrainous infarction. In: Handbook of clinical neurology [Internet]. Elsevier; 2024 [cited 2024 Oct 1]. p. 465–74. Available from: https://linkinghub.elsevier.com/retrieve/pii/B9780128233573000215.
5. Tietjen GE, Khubchandani J. Vascular biomarkers in migraine. Cephalalgia. 2015;35(2):95–117.
6. Marshall N, Maclaurin WA, Koulouris G. MRA captures vasospasm in fatal migrainous infarction. Headache. 2007;47(2):280–3.
7. Decima D, Cavallo M, Leotta MR, Gaballo A. Migrainous infarction: association with vascular risk factors in a male subject. Neurol Sci. 2009;30(S1):145–6.
8. Tsai CF, Chen CC, Wang SC, Yip PK. Reversible vasospasm in migrainous infarction. J Ultrasound Med. 2010;29(3):481–4.
9. Vinciguerra L, Cantone M, Lanza G, Bramanti A, Santalucia P, Puglisi V, et al. Migrainous infarction and cerebral vasospasm: case report and literature review. J Pain Res. 2019;12:2941–50.
10. Lebedeva ER, Gurary NM, Olesen J. Diagnosis of migrainous infarction: a case report and analysis of previously published cases. Diagnostics. 2023;13(15):2502.
11. Tzoulis C, Naess H, Thomassen L. Migrainous cerebral infarction in a previously healthy 93-year-old female patient with no risk factors for stroke. Cephalalgia. 2006;26(7):894–5.
12. Laurell K, Artto V, Bendtsen L, Hagen K, Kallela M, Meyer EL, et al. Migrainous infarction: a Nordic multicenter study. Eur J Neurol. 2011;18(10):1220–6.
13. Frigerio R, Santoro P, Ferrarese C, Agostoni E. Migrainous cerebral infarction: case reports. Neurol Sci. 2004;25(S3):s300–1.
14. Khardenavis V, Karthik DK, Kulkarni S, Deshpande A. Cortical laminar necrosis in a case of migrainous cerebral infarction. Case Rep. 2018;2018:bcr.
15. Mancini V, Mastria G, Frantellizzi V, Troiani P, Zampatti S, Carboni S, et al. Migrainous infarction in a patient with sporadic hemiplegic migraine and cystic fibrosis: a 99mTc-HMPAO brain SPECT study. Headache. 2019;59(2):253–8.
16. Linetsky E, Leker RR, Ben-Hur T. Headache characteristics in patients after migrainous stroke. Neurology. 2001;57(1):130–2.
17. Serrano F, Arauz A, Uribe R, Becerra LC, Mantilla K, Zermeño F. Long-term follow-up of patients with migrainous infarction. Clin Neurol Neurosurg. 2018;165:7–9.
18. Censori B, Partziguian T, Poloni M. Migraine improves after ischemic stroke. J Stroke Cerebrovasc Dis. 2013;22(8):e338–42.
19. Wolf ME, Szabo K, Griebe M, Förster A, Gass A, Hennerici MG, et al. Clinical and MRI characteristics of acute migrainous infarction. Neurology. 2011;76(22):1911–7.
20. Kandemir Yılmaz M, Kirikli P. Bilateral occipital infarcts due to persistent migraine with aura in an elderly. Agri. 2024;36(4):281–4.
21. Bylund W, Patrick R, Macdonald A. Detection of migrainous infarction with formal visual field testing: a case report. Clin Pract Cases Emerg Med. 2020;4(3):366–70.
22. Terrin A, Mainardi F, Maggioni F. The pathological spectrum behind migraine aura status: a case series. Neurol Sci. 2019;40(4):861–4.
23. Morais R, Sobral F, Cunha G, Brito O, Santana I. Advanced MRI study of migrainous infarction presenting as cortical laminar necrosis—case report and literature review. Clin Neurol Neurosurg. 2018;167:82–5.
24. Campagna G, Vickers A, Ponce CMP, Lee AG. Homonymous hemianopsia as the presenting sign of migrainous infarction. Can J Ophthalmol. 2018;53(6):e229–32.
25. Renard D, Nerrant E, Freitag C. Early recurrence of migrainous infarction. Acta Neurol Belg. 2015;115(4):675–6.
26. Lai TH, Hong CT. Prolonged symptoms in sporadic hemiplegic migraine: aura or migrainous infarction? Acta Neurol Taiwan. 2012;21(3):129–32.
27. Arai S, Utsunomiya H, Arihiro S, Arakawa S. Migrainous infarction in an adult: evaluation with serial diffusion-weighted images and cerebral blood flow studies. Radiat Med. 2008;26(5):313–7.
28. Liang Y, Scott TF. Migrainous infarction with appearance of laminar necrosis on MRI. Clin Neurol Neurosurg. 2007;109(7):592–6.

29. Tang SC, Jeng JS, Liu HM, Yip PK. Migrainous infarction involving two different arterial territories: report of two cases. Acta Neurol Taiwan. 2004;13(1):20–3.
30. Arboix A, Massons J, García-Eroles L, Oliveres M, Balcells M, Targa C. Migrainous cerebral infarction in the Sagrat Cor Hospital of Barcelona stroke registry. Cephalalgia. 2003;23(5):389–94.
31. Sacquegna T, Andreoli A, Baldrati A, Lamieri C, de Carolis P, Pasquale GD, et al. Ischemic stroke in young adults: the relevance of migrainous infarction. Cephalalgia. 1989;9:255–8.
32. Moen M, Levine SR, Newman DS, Dull-Baird A, Brown GG, Welch KM. Bilateral posterior cerebral artery strokes in a young migraine sufferer. Stroke. 1988;19(4):525–8.
33. Jacob MA, Ekker MS, Allach Y, Cai M, Aarnio K, Arauz A, et al. Global differences in risk factors, etiology, and outcome of ischemic stroke in young adults—a worldwide meta-analysis. Neurology. 2022;98(6):e573–88.
34. Schürks M, Rist PM, Bigal ME, Buring JE, Lipton RB, Kurth T. Migraine and cardiovascular disease: systematic review and meta-analysis. BMJ. 2009;339:b3914.
35. Zhao W, Wang D, Tan Y, Yang J, Zhang S. Migraine and the correlation between stroke: a systematic review and meta-analysis. Medicine (Baltimore). 2024;103(45):e40315.
36. Roberto G, Raschi E, Piccinni C, Conti V, Vignatelli L, D'Alessandro R, et al. Adverse cardiovascular events associated with triptans and ergotamines for treatment of migraine: systematic review of observational studies. Cephalalgia. 2015;35(2):118–31.
37. Petersen CL, Hougaard A, Gaist D, Hallas J. Risk of stroke and myocardial infarction among initiators of triptans. JAMA Neurol. 2024;81(3):248.
38. Wang Z, VanderPluym JH, Halker Singh RB, Alsibai RA, Roellinger DL, Firwana M, et al. Safety of triptans in patients who have or are at high risk for cardiovascular disease. Mayo Clin Proc. 2024;99(11):1722–31.
39. Nadarajan V, Perry RJ, Johnson J, Werring DJ. Transient ischaemic attacks: mimics and chameleons. Pract Neurol. 2014;14(1):23.
40. Kleindorfer DO, Towfighi A, Chaturvedi S, Cockroft KM, Gutierrez J, Lombardi-Hill D, et al. 2021 guideline for the prevention of stroke in patients with stroke and transient ischemic attack: a guideline from the American Heart Association/American Stroke Association. Stroke [Internet]. 2021 [cited 2024 Nov 15];52(7). Available from: https://www.ahajournals.org/doi/10.1161/STR.0000000000000375.
41. Nguyen AT, Curtis KM, Tepper NK, Kortsmit K, Brittain AW, Snyder EM, et al. U.S. medical eligibility criteria for contraceptive use, 2024. MMWR Recomm Rep. 2024;73(4):1–126.
42. Kurth T, Schürks M, Logroscino G, Buring JE. Migraine frequency and risk of cardiovascular disease in women. Neurology. 2009;73(8):581–8.
43. Gryglas A, Smigiel R. Migraine and stroke: what's the link? What to do? Curr Neurol Neurosci Rep. 2017;17(3):22.
44. Liao CC, Chien CH, Shih YH, Tsai FJ, Li JM. Acupuncture is effective at reducing the risk of stroke in patients with migraines: a real-world, large-scale cohort study with 19-years of follow-up. Int J Environ Res Public Health. 2023;20(3):1690.

Chapter 4
Migraine Aura-Triggered Seizure

Ilaria Notaristefano, Valentina Baglioni, and Vincenzo Guidetti

4.1 Introduction

A migraine aura-triggered seizure, formerly known as migralepsy, is a rare condition characterized by a seizure occurring during or within 1 h after a migraine attack with aura [1]. Lennox and Lennox first described this condition in their textbook *Epilepsy and Related Disorders*, reporting a case of "ophthalmic migraine with perhaps nausea and vomiting followed by symptoms characteristic of epilepsy" [2].

The term *migralepsy* is a historical portmanteau of *migraine* and *epilepsy*, coined by Dr. Douglas Davidson to describe this phenomenon better. Notably, such cases are more common in children than in adults [3]. However, due to significant diagnostic confusion caused by the term *migralepsy*, it has been replaced by *migraine aura-triggered seizure* in more recent classifications. The original term led to misdiagnosis in numerous cases where patients had both migraine with aura and epilepsy, resulting in an inaccurate classification of their condition. Additionally, visual migraine aura and occipital seizures can be mistaken for one another, particularly in cases of prolonged seizures [4]. Although headaches and seizures are, respectively, the first and third most common reasons for a referral from a general practitioner to a neurologist [5], *migraine aura-triggered seizure* remains a rare condition [6].

This chapter aims to clarify the nature of this condition, including its characteristics, diagnostic challenges, and key differences from other similar disorders.

I. Notaristefano · V. Baglioni · V. Guidetti (✉)
Child and Adolescent Neuropsychiatry, Sapienza University of Rome, Rome, Italy

D. Uludüz et al. (eds.), *Rare Causes of Headache Disorders*, Headache,
https://doi.org/10.1007/978-3-032-10242-3_4

4.2 Pathophysiology

The pathophysiological causes underlying *migraine aura-triggered seizures* are still unclear. For this condition to arise, both a migraine aura that induces rapid shifts in cortical excitability and a brain predisposed to synchronized discharges, as seen in epilepsy, must be present. Recent research suggests that both migraine and epilepsy may share a common underlying mechanism of neocortical hyperexcitability, which—when combined with specific genetic and molecular predispositions—can lead to distinct downstream phenomena. In epilepsy, this hyperexcitability is thought to produce a paroxysmal depolarizing shift that directly triggers a seizure, whereas, in migraine, it evolves into cortical spreading depression (CSD), which is subsequently followed by cortical suppression [7].

Moreover, the hypothesis that migraine aura may represent a preictal state further unifies these observations. According to this view, the neurovascular coupling mechanisms that underlie the migraine aura—beginning with an initial wave of hyperexcitability and followed by massive ionic shifts across neuronal membranes—can facilitate seizure onset in a cortex already predisposed to epilepsy. Essentially, when the rapid changes induced by a migraine aura occur in a brain susceptible to synchronized discharges, they may pave the way for a seizure [8, 9]. Thus, both hypotheses converge on the idea that a hyperexcitable cortex is central to the pathogenesis of these conditions. Depending on individual susceptibility and the dynamics of the underlying neurovascular processes, this hyperexcitability may manifest as either a migraine with aura, an epileptic seizure, or even a scenario where the migraine aura itself triggers the seizure.

An alternative hypothesis proposes that aura-triggered seizures represent a form of reflex epilepsy, in which activation of a task-specific neural network induces excessive neuronal synchronization, ultimately leading to a seizure. However, this explanation appears less effective in accounting for the observed phenomena [8].

4.3 Case Presentation

An 11-year-old girl has experienced recurrent headaches since she was 4 years old. In her early years, the headaches were relatively mild in severity and accompanied by nausea and showed improvement with acute treatment with paracetamol. In her family history, a high frequency of migraine and epileptic conditions was reported: her mother suffers from migraine with aura and vasculitis, her maternal grandmother has migraine without aura, and an aunt has been diagnosed with epilepsy. By the age of eight, the patient's headaches had become more frequent and severe, prompting a thorough clinical evaluation. She was diagnosed with migraine with aura following the International Classification of Headache Disorders-III (ICHD-3) criteria. Her migraine episodes are described as intense, throbbing pain localized to the right frontal and temporal regions, often accompanied by photophobia, phonophobia, facial flushing, and nausea. These attacks occurred approximately two to four times per month and were disruptive enough to interfere with her daily activities significantly. In response to her worsening symptoms, prophylactic treatment with flunarizine was started, leading to a notable improvement in her condition. Given the strong family history of migraines, a genetic diagnostic evaluation was performed by a Next Generation System (NGS) panel to explore potential inherited causes. However, the genetic investigation revealed no pathogenic variants among the genes examined. Despite the improvement with flunarizine, at the age of 10, the patient experienced 2 distinct episodes where her typical aura was followed in less than 20 min by a sudden loss of consciousness, with a tonic–clonic seizure, which resolved spontaneously. A similar episode occurred during a subsequent febrile illness the following year. In light of these seizure episodes, further neurological evaluation was pursued. An interictal electroencephalography (EEG) revealed the presence of sharp waves, in particular in the centrotemporal regions, while a brain MRI returned normal findings.

These investigations led to the initiation of topiramate therapy at a dose of 2 mg/kg/day. More recent EEG assessments have not demonstrated any epileptiform abnormalities, and, currently, the patient remains free from clinical seizures.

4.4 Case Discussion

This clinical case illustrates a migraine aura-triggered seizure, which led to the young girl's diagnosis. Several key features can be identified:

1. The presence of migraine with aura symptoms (including throbbing pain, photophobia, phonophobia, facial flushing, and nausea).
2. The occurrence of an epileptic seizure within 1 h of the headache onset.
3. A favorable response to antiseizure medication.

4.5 Diagnostic Criteria and Differential Diagnosis

Per ICHD-3 [1], the diagnosis of *migraine aura-triggered seizure* is possible in case of:

A. A seizure fulfilling diagnostic criteria for one type of epileptic attack, and criterion B below.
B. Occurring in a patient with 1.2 Migraine with aura, and during or within 1 h after an attack of migraine with aura.
C. Not better accounted for by another ICHD-3 diagnosis.

As observed, migraine aura-triggered seizure is a diagnosis of exclusion, meaning that other potential conditions must be ruled out first. Therefore, it is essential to

Table 4.1 Differential features of migraine visual aura and occipital lobe seizures

Migraine visual aura [11]	Occipital lobe seizure [12]
Fluttering, uncolored, zigzag Develops gradually over 5–30 min Acute onset is rare Total duration <60 min Emerges in the center of the visual field and gradually shifts to the outer edges of a visual hemi-field, often leaving a blind spot Followed by migraine without aura Spots, circles, and beads with or without colors may be experienced, but not dominant	Mainly colored circular patterns Develop rapidly within seconds Brief duration (2–3 min) Frequently appear in the outer regions of a temporal visual hemi-field, increasing in size and multiplying during the seizure, often shifting horizontally toward the opposite side Postictal headache frequently occurs 3–15 min after the seizures end Progress to other occipital and extra-occipital manifestations and convulsions

exclude confounding factors such as visual phenomena of epileptic origin (e.g., occipital lobe epilepsy), syncope, and psychogenic non-epileptic seizures (PNES) [10]. Additionally, for this diagnosis, the association between epileptic seizures and migraine without aura remains unclear.

In particular, to differentiate visual aura from visual epileptic phenomena, it is necessary to know their features, as described in Table 4.1.

Also, the Visual Aura Rating Scale (VARS) is a validated instrument in which scores of ±5 are considered indicative of migraine aura [13].

To simplify the approach, a diagnostic algorithm has been proposed for cases suspected of migraine aura-triggered seizures.

4.6 Diagnostic Algorithm

Step 1: Clinical suspicion.

- Identify key symptoms:
  - Migraine with aura (evaluate frequency and intensity).
  - Epileptic seizure during or within 1 h after an attack of migraine with aura.

Step 2: Initial diagnostic workup.

- Perform EEG, if possible, during migraine.
- Brain imaging.

Step 3: Additional diagnostic evaluations for the differential diagnosis.

- Performed VARS scale.
  - Score ≥5 points: probably migraine visual aura.
  - Score ≤5 points: improbable migraine visual aura.
- Differential diagnosis from syncope and PNES.

Step 3: Confirm diagnosis.

- Confirm diagnosis of exclusion, considering that it is rarer than the other conditions.

4.7 Management

Nowadays, there is no specific treatment for migraine aura-triggered seizures. Some researchers emphasize the importance of preventing migraine onset; however, most patients respond poorly to traditional migraine treatments such as flunarizine and propranolol [14]. Some evidence suggests that opioids, when used as monotherapy, may effectively prevent both migraines and subsequent seizures [15]. Other clinicians highlight the strong clinical and EEG response to antiseizure treatment [14], with the choice of medication depending on the type of seizures presented. Among available treatments, topiramate has demonstrated efficacy in both migraine and epilepsy through randomized controlled trials and is approved for both conditions [16]. For these reasons, it is often the preferred therapeutic option in this context.

4.8 Conclusion

Migraine aura-triggered seizure remains a rare and complex phenomenon at the intersection of migraine and epilepsy. Despite historical diagnostic confusion surrounding the term "migralepsy," this condition is now recognized as a diagnosis of exclusion, requiring careful differentiation from other pathologies. While the underlying mechanisms remain incompletely understood, research suggests that cortical hyperexcitability plays a central role, with migraine aura potentially acting as a seizure trigger in predisposed individuals. Management remains challenging, with conventional migraine prophylaxis often proving insufficient. However, antiseizure drugs—particularly topiramate—have shown efficacy in reducing both migraine attacks and seizure occurrence, making them a preferred therapeutic option.

References

1. Headache Classification Committee of the International Headache Society (IHS). The international classification of headache disorders, 3rd edition. Cephalalgia. 2018;38(1):1–211. https://doi.org/10.1177/0333102417738202. PMID: 29368949.
2. Lennox WG. Epilepsy and related disorders. Boston: Little; 1960.
3. Davies PTG, Panayiotopoulos CP. Migraine triggered seizures and epilepsy triggered headache and migraine attacks: a need for re-assessment. J Headache Pain. 2011;12(3):287–8. https://doi.org/10.1007/s10194-011-0344-2. PMID: 21516466.

4. Demarquay G, Rheims S. Relationships between migraine and epilepsy: pathophysiological mechanisms and clinical implications. Rev Neurol (Paris). 2021;177(7):791–800. https://doi.org/10.1016/j.neurol.2021.06.004. PMID: 34340811.
5. Stone J, Carson A, Duncan R, Roberts R, Warlow C, Hibberd C, Coleman R, Cull R, Murray G, Pelosi A, Cavanagh J, Matthews K, Goldbeck R, Smyth R, Walker J, Sharpe M. Who is referred to neurology clinics?—the diagnoses made in 3781 new patients. Clin Neurol Neurosurg. 2010;112(9):747–51. https://doi.org/10.1016/j.clineuro.2010.05.011. PMID: 20646830.
6. Vercueil L. Migralepsy, what it is and what it is not. Rev Neurol (Paris). 2022;178(7):654–8. https://doi.org/10.1016/j.neurol.2022.01.006. PMID: 35148906.
7. Garg D, Tripathi M. Borderlands of migraine and epilepsy. Neurol India. 2021;69(Suppl 1):S91–7. https://doi.org/10.4103/0028-3886.315994. PMID: 34003153.
8. Lucas C. Migraine with aura. Rev Neurol (Paris). 2021;177(7):779–84. https://doi.org/10.1016/j.neurol.2021.07.010. PMID: 34384631.
9. Berger M, Speckmann EJ, Pape H, Gorji A. spreading depression enhances human neocortical excitability *in vitro*. Cephalalgia. 2008;28(5):558–62. https://doi.org/10.1111/j.1468-2982.2008.01556.x. PMID: 18399818.
10. Sances G, Guaschino E, Perucca P, Allena M, Ghiotto N, Manni R. Migralepsy: a call for a revision of the definition. Epilepsia. 2009;50(11):2487–96. https://doi.org/10.1111/j.1528-1167.2009.02265.x. PMID: 19694799.
11. Russell MB, Olesen J. A nosographic analysis of the migraine aura in a general population. Brain. 1996;119(2):355–61. https://doi.org/10.1093/brain/119.2.355.
12. Panayiotopoulos CP. Visual phenomena and headache in occipital epilepsy: a review, a systematic study and differentiation from migraine. Epileptic Disord. 1999;1(4):205–16. PMID: 10937155.
13. Eriksen M, Thomsen L, Olesen J. The Visual Aura Rating Scale (VARS) for migraine aura diagnosis. Cephalalgia. 2005;25(10):801–10. https://doi.org/10.1111/j.1468-2982.2005.00955.x. PMID: 16162257.
14. Hanci F, Turay S, Dilek M, Bektas M, Kabakus N. Migralepsy; clinical and electroencephalography findings in children. Exp Biomed Res. 2019;2(1):20–4. https://doi.org/10.30714/j-ebr.2019147579.
15. Derakhshan I. Successful opioid monotherapy in migralepsy: a case series. J Neurol Disord [Internet] 2016 [cited 3 March 2025];4(4). Avaible on: http://www.esciencecentral.org/journals/successful-opioid-monotherapy-in-migralepsy-a-case-series-2329-6895-1000275.php?aid=77120. https://doi.org/10.4172/2329-6895.1000275.
16. Colombo B, Dalla Libera D, Volontè MA, Spagnolo F, Dalla Costa G, Martinelli V, Comi G. Migralepsy: a new case confirming the existence of this migraine complication and proposing therapy. Neurol Sci. 2013;34(8):1465–6. https://doi.org/10.1007/s10072-012-1212-9. PMID: 23124486.

Chapter 5
Episodic Syndromes That May Be Associated with Migraine: Recurrent Gastrointestinal Disturbance

Toshiyuki Hikita

5.1 Introduction

The third edition of the International Classification of Headache Disorders (ICHD-3) lists recurrent gastrointestinal disturbance as a subsection of 1.6 Episodic syndromes that may be associated with migraine [1]. It states that such syndromes often precede or coincide with the onset of migraine [2]. Subsection 1.6.1 Recurrent gastrointestinal disturbance comprises 1.6.1.1 Cyclical vomiting syndrome and 1.6.1.2 Abdominal migraine. These conditions are discussed in Chaps. 6 and 7 of this publication, "Migraine: Episodic Syndromes That May Be Associated with Migraine: Cyclical Vomiting Syndrome," and "Migraine: Episodic Syndromes That May Be Associated with Migraine: Abdominal Migraine."

In the second edition of the International Classification of Headache Disorders (ICHD-2), cyclical vomiting, abdominal migraine, and benign paroxysmal vertigo of childhood were listed as subcategories of childhood periodic syndrome that are commonly precursors of migraine [3]. Recurrent gastrointestinal disturbance was added as a subcategory in the ICHD-3, which also provided the diagnostic criteria. These are shown in Table 5.1. Previously used terms for this condition have included chronic abdominal pain, functional abdominal pain, functional dyspepsia, irritable bowel syndrome, and functional abdominal pain syndrome. The ICHD-3 description of recurrent gastrointestinal disturbance is: "Recurrent episodic attacks of abdominal pain and/or discomfort, nausea and/or vomiting, occurring infrequently, chronically or at predictable intervals, that may be associated with migraine."

T. Hikita (✉)
Department of Pediatrics, Teikyo University School of Medicine, Itabashi-Ku, Tokyo, Japan

Hikita Pediatric Clinic, Kiryu City, Gunma, Japan
e-mail: t-hikita@ra2.so-net.ne.jp

D. Uludüz et al. (eds.), *Rare Causes of Headache Disorders*, Headache,
https://doi.org/10.1007/978-3-032-10242-3_5

Table 5.1 International Classification of Headache Disorders-3 diagnostic criteria for recurrent gastrointestinal disturbance

A. At least five attacks with distinct episodes of abdominal pain and/or discomfort and/or nausea and/or vomiting
B. Normal gastrointestinal examination and evaluation
C. Not attributed to another disorder

5.2 Pathophysiology

Although the pathophysiology of recurrent gastrointestinal disturbance is unclear, it is thought to be related to migraine. Symptoms may be intensified by stress, and it is believed to have a neurological etiology. Cases have been reported in which triptan preparations, which are used to treat migraine, are effective. These studies suggest that serotonin metabolism may be involved [2, 4–8]. Primary headache disorders, including migraine, are among the most common neurological diseases. Episodic syndromes that may be related to migraine, including recurrent gastrointestinal disturbances such as abdominal migraine and cyclical vomiting, often precede the onset of migraine or co-occur. They also may resemble the pathology of migraine [9].

5.3 Case Presentation

A 3-year and 5-month-old girl presented with recurrent upper abdominal pain occurring one to three times per week, with each episode lasting between 10 min and 1 h. These episodes were sometimes accompanied by diarrhea or vomiting. Before the onset of pain, she often stopped eating and would lie down. She occasionally reported headaches and showed signs of photophobia and reduced appetite. During episodes, she preferred quiet environments and sometimes had difficulty sleeping due to the discomfort. Her medical history included atopic dermatitis and car sickness. There was a positive family history of typical migraine with aura in her mother. The patient was diagnosed with recurrent abdominal pain by the pediatrician and was monitored clinically, though no specific diagnostic investigations were performed. Until she was 6 years and 10 months old, the patient experienced episodes of abdominal pain around her navel. This was accompanied by nausea, but no vomiting or diarrhea. She would sometimes complain of headaches when she had abdominal pain. There were no warning signs preceding the episodes. During the periods of pain, the patient was sensitive to sound and light, and her face was pale. From around the age of 8 years and 10 months, the patient complained of severe pulsating pain in the left temporal region that occurred approximately twice a month for 2–4 h. The pain worsened with routine physical activity and was accompanied by photophobia, phonophobia, and nausea. The patient was diagnosed with migraine without aura. Acetaminophen was effective against the headaches.

The patient did not experience abdominal pain after the age of 9 years and 6 months. However, since the age of 9 years and 6 months, the patient has continued to experience migraines, with headaches occurring approximately twice a month at 15 years and 2 months. Acetaminophen remains effective, and the patient is under ongoing outpatient observation.

5.4 Case Discussion

Based on the intensity and duration of abdominal pain and the frequency of vomiting, this case did not meet the diagnostic criteria for abdominal migraine or cyclical vomiting syndrome. Although the patient in this case also complained of headaches, in some cases of recurrent gastrointestinal disturbance, headaches do not accompany the abdominal pain. This case met the diagnostic criteria for recurrent gastrointestinal disturbance (Table 5.1) [1]. Provided organic disease is ruled out, patients with recurrent abdominal pain are observed, but no further examinations are required. If the diagnostic criteria for abdominal migraine are met during the course of the disease, the patient is treated for abdominal migraine. In the ICHD-2, the diagnostic criterion for abdominal migraine was abdominal pain for 1 h or more, but this was changed to 2 h or more in the ICHD-3 [1, 3]. A previous study of recurrent abdominal pain and abdominal migraines found that recurrent abdominal pain, which is relatively mild, is more common than abdominal migraines [10]. When the duration of abdominal migraine was extended from 1 to 2 h in the diagnostic criteria, the number of cases decreased. Relatively mild cases that do not meet the diagnostic criteria for abdominal migraine or cyclical vomiting syndrome should be diagnosed as recurrent gastrointestinal disturbance and observed for any progression. A previous study of cyclical vomiting syndrome conducted by the authors followed 25 cases for >5 years. Among these, 4 (16%) patients developed abdominal migraine and 11 (44%) developed migraine (Fig. 5.1) [11]. This suggests a strong relationship among cyclical vomiting syndrome, a subtype of recurrent gastrointestinal disturbance, abdominal migraine, and migraine. In addition, cases have been reported in which sumatriptan, a migraine medication, was effective against cyclical vomiting syndrome and abdominal migraine [4–8]. Other drugs that are effective in the prevention of migraine headaches have also been found effective in the treatment of cyclical vomiting syndrome. This suggests that these conditions share a common pathophysiology.

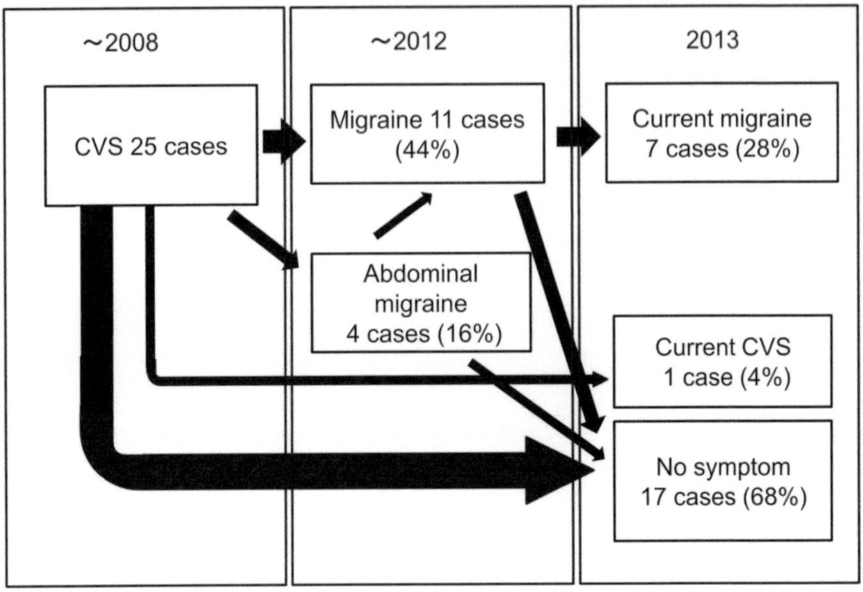

Fig. 5.1 Outcomes of 25 patients with cyclical vomiting syndrome. In 2008, all 25 patients had cyclical vomiting syndrome and did not have migraines at that time. Over the next 5 years, 11 patients (44%) developed migraines, and 4 patients (16%) developed abdominal migraines. By 2013, more than 5 years after 2008, 1 patient (4%) still had cyclical vomiting syndrome, 7 patients (28%) had migraines, and 17 patients (68%) had no symptoms

5.5 Diagnostic Algorithm

Step 1: Clinical suspicion.

- *Identify key symptoms:*
  - Recurrent distinct episodes of abdominal pain and/or discomfort and/or nausea and/or vomiting.
  - Family history of migraine.

Step 2: Initial diagnostic workup.

- *Inspection, auscultation, palpation:*
  - No organic cause of the symptom.
  - No trauma.

Step 3: Apply ICHD-3 diagnostic criteria (Table 5.1) [1]
Step 4: Classification re-evaluation.

- *Reassess headache classification for episodic syndrome that may be associated with migraine.*
  - See Chaps. 6 and 7.

Table 5.2 Differential diagnosis and useful examinations for recurrent gastrointestinal disturbance

Digestive disease: Chronic appendicitis, abnormality (intestinal malrotation), mucosal disorder (ulcer, esophagitis, Crohn's disease), pancreatitis, hepatobiliary disease (cholelithiasis, choledochal cyst)
Blood examination: Blood count, ALT, γ-GTP, amylase, lipase.
Urinalysis: VMA, HVA,.
Fecal examination: Fecal culture.
Diagnostic imaging: Abdominal ultrasonography, abdominal ultrasonography, esophagogastroduodenoscopy, upper GI series.
Neurological disorder: Brain tumor, intracranial hypertension, abdominal migraine, abdominal epilepsy
Diagnostic imaging: Brain MRI and/or CT, electroencephalogram.
Otolaryngologic disorder: Chronic sinusitis, vestibular disorder
Diagnostic imaging: Paranasal sinus CT.
Urological diseases: Kidney stones, hydronephrosis, etc.
Diagnostic imaging: Abdominal ultrasonography.
Urinalysis: Uric acid, ca/Cr ratio.
Metabolic or endocrine disease: Mitochondrial disease, urea cycle disorder, fatty acid metabolism disease, acute intermittent porphyria, diabetes mellitus, Addison disease, pheochromocytoma, hereditary angioedema
Blood examination: Electrolyte, blood glucose, catecholamine, blood gas, lactic acid, amino acid, ammonia, ACTH, ADH.
Urinalysis: Ketone body, organic acid, carnitine, porphobilinogen.
Other: Munchausen syndrome, anxiety, depression, pregnancy
Blood examination: hCG
Urinalysis: Drug test.
Other: Psychological consult.

ACTH adrenocorticotropic hormone, *ADH* antidiuretic hormone, *ALT* alanine aminotransferase, *CT* computed tomography, *GI* gastrointestinal, *γ-GTP* gamma-glutamyl transpeptidase, *HVA* homovanillic acid, *MRI* magnetic resonance imaging, *VMA* vanillylmandelic acid

Diagnostic criteria for recurrent gastrointestinal disturbance have been described in the ICHD-3. An essential step in diagnosing recurrent gastrointestinal disturbance is to rule out organic diseases. For example, the criteria presented in ICHD-3 are in Table 5.1 [1]. It is always necessary to perform appropriate examinations before making a diagnosis of recurrent gastrointestinal disturbance. Differential diagnosis and practical examinations are described in Table 5.2. There is no specific examination for recurrent gastrointestinal disturbance; a combination of examinations, as in Table 5.2, must be conducted.

5.6 Management

In cases of recurrent gastrointestinal disturbance where the abdominal pain is severe or lasts for extended durations, blood tests and imaging are required. In such cases, the same examinations as those for abdominal migraine and cyclical vomiting syndrome are performed to rule out other conditions (Chaps. 6 and 7). One of the diagnostic criteria for recurrent gastrointestinal disturbance is normal gastrointestinal examination and evaluation results. In this case, the mother had migraines, and the child suffered from car sickness. Although the child's condition in this case persisted for a long time, it did not worsen. No medication was prescribed for the abdominal pain, and the patient was monitored without blood or imaging examination. Eventually, the pain improved. In mild cases of recurrent gastrointestinal disturbance, routine examination is not necessary.

5.7 Conclusion

Recurrent gastrointestinal disturbances include cyclical vomiting syndrome and abdominal migraine. However, it also includes cases of recurrent abdominal pain and vomiting that do not meet the diagnostic criteria for these conditions. Patients may have a family history of migraine. Some cases progress to migraine during follow-up. If no neurological findings are found on examination, symptoms often improve with careful follow-up without unnecessary examination. However, it is advisable to explain to the family that, if the condition persists, the patient may develop migraine in the future.

References

1. Headache Classification Committee of the International Headache Society (IHS). Headache Classification Committee of the International Headache Society (IHS): the international classification of headache disorders, 3rd edition. Cephalalgia. 2018;38(1):1–211. https://doi.org/10.1177/0333102417738202.
2. Irwin S, Barmherzig R, Gelfand A. Recurrent gastrointestinal disturbance: abdominal migraine and cyclic vomiting syndrome. Curr Neurol Neurosci Rep. 2017;17:21. https://doi.org/10.1007/s11910-017-0731-4.
3. Headache Classification Subcommittee of the International Headache Society. The international classification of headache disorders: 2nd edition. Cephalalgia. 2004;24(Suppl):1–160.
4. Benson JM, Zorn SL, Book LS. Sumatriptan in the treatment of cyclic vomiting. Ann Pharmacother. 1995;29:997–9. https://doi.org/10.1177/106002809502901008.
5. Kowalczyk M, Parkman H, Ward L. Adult cyclic vomiting syndrome successfully treated with intranasal sumatriptan. J Gen Intern Med. 2010;25:88–91. https://doi.org/10.1007/s11606-009-1162-y.
6. Kakisaka Y, Wakusawa K, Haginoya K, Saito A, Uematsu M, Yokoyama H, Sato T, Tsuchiya S. Efficacy of sumatriptan in two pediatric cases with abdominal pain-related functional gastrointestinal disorders: does the mechanism overlap that of migraine? J Child Neurol. 2010;25:234–7. https://doi.org/10.1177/0883073809336875.
7. Hikita T, Kodama H, Kaneko S, Amakata K, Ogita K, Mochizuki D, Kaga F, Nakamoto N, Fujii Y, Kikuchi A. Sumatriptan as a treatment for cyclic vomiting syndrome: a clinical trial. Cephalalgia. 2011;31:504–7. https://doi.org/10.1177/0333102410390398.

8. Calhoun AH, Pruitt AP. Injectable sumatriptan for cyclic vomiting syndrome in adults: a case series. Headache. 2014;54:1526–30. https://doi.org/10.1111/head.12444.
9. Abu-Arafeh I, Gelfand AA. The childhood migraine syndrome. Nat Rev Neurol. 2021;17:449–58. https://doi.org/10.1038/s41582-021-00497-6.
10. Hikita T. Prevalence of abdominal migraine and recurrent abdominal pain in a Japanese clinic. Pediatr Int. 2016;58:669–71. https://doi.org/10.1111/ped.13005.
11. Hikita T, Kodama H, Ogita K, Kaneko S, Nakamoto N, Mimaki M. Cyclic vomiting syndrome in infants and children: a clinical follow-up study. Pediatr Neurol. 2016;57:29–33. https://doi.org/10.1016/j.pediatrneurol.2016.01.001.

Chapter 6
Episodic Syndromes That May Be Associated with Migraine: Cyclical Vomiting Syndrome

Ishaq Abu-Arafeh

6.1 Introduction

Cyclical vomiting syndrome (CVS) is a childhood syndrome related to migraine. CVS presents with specific clinical features and follows a defined clinical pattern in its prognosis and response to treatment, similar to those of childhood migraine. CVS is characterised by recurrent stereotypical episodes of intense nausea and vomiting lasting between 2 and 72 h, interspaced by periods of full return to normal health. Children continue to have normal general health, growth and development. Although interest in CVS and research into its clinical characteristics have increased over the past 20–30 years, the initial description of the condition dates back to the late nineteenth century [1]. CVS has attracted the attention of general paediatricians, paediatric gastroenterologists, neurologists and headache specialists. The definition and criteria for the diagnosis, therefore, were developed as a migraine disorder within the International Classification of Headache Disorders (ICHD) and as a Functional Gastrointestinal Disorder by Gastroenterologists [2, 3]. CVS has also been reported in adult patients of all ages and is increasingly recognised as an common cause for patients referred for gastroenterology clinics [4].

This review will cover the epidemiology, pathogenesis, clinical features, prognosis, treatment and the impact of CVS on patients' quality of life.

The onset of CVS can occur at any age, but is most common during early childhood. Several studies reported the peak age of onset of CVS to be around 5–6 years [5]. Both male and female children are affected almost equally. CVS have been reported from all over the world with a comparable prevalence regardless of ethnic or socio-economic background. The prevalence of CVS is estimated at around 2% in children between the ages of 5–15 years in Scotland, Australia and Turkey [5–7],

I. Abu-Arafeh (✉)
Paediatric Neurosciences Unit, Royal Hospital for Children, Glasgow, UK
e-mail: ishaq.abu-arafeh2@nhs.scot

D. Uludüz et al. (eds.), *Rare Causes of Headache Disorders*, Headache,
https://doi.org/10.1007/978-3-032-10242-3_6

with an estimated incidence of 3.15/100,000 children per year [8]. The prevalence of CVS in adult patients is not known, but at least one in ten new patients referred to a gastroenterology clinic may have CVS [9]. There is a very close and consistent relationship between CVS and migraine. Children with a personal or family history of migraine have an increased risk of presenting with CVS, and children with CVS have an increased risk of developing migraine late in childhood or in early adult life.

6.2 Pathogenesis

Despite the close relationship between migraine and CVS, the pathogenesis of CVS continues to be a subject of speculation and controversy. Underlying genetic predisposition for CVS has been shown in clinical and epidemiological studies to be closely associated with migraine. The molecular genetics of both migraine and CVS are very likely to be complex and polygenic, and continue to be a target for research. However, single-gene mutations have been reported in patients with familial hemiplegic migraine involving the voltage-gated calcium channel (CACNA1A), sodium-potassium ATPase channels (ATP1A2), and the voltage-gated sodium channels (SCN1A) and PRRT2 [10]. In some patients with CVS, a single-gene mutation on the Ryanodine Receptor 2 (RYR2) has been detected. It may have a significant association with the disease [11].

Mitochondrial gene mutations and polymorphism have also been investigated to delineate the suspected maternal role in the disease inheritance [12–14].

Mechanisms that initiate and maintain an episode of CVS may involve one or more pathways including autonomic and neuroendocrine dysfunction, hypothalamic-pituitary-adrenal axis activation and the dysregulation of the central nervous system emetic centre and chemoreceptor trigger zone (CTZ) [12, 13, 15]. Dysregulation of the cannabinoid type 1 receptor (CB1) in the brain may also play a role in the pathogenesis of CVS, as has been shown in chronic use of cannabis and a possible disorder of endogenous cannabinoid metabolism presenting with a syndrome of recurrent vomiting [16]. Functional MRI (magnetic resonance imaging) studies have shown altered intrinsic connectivity of the sensorimotor network, specifically salience to the mid-posterior insula, in patients with migraine and CVS compared to healthy control individuals [17].

6.3 Case Presentation

Adam presented at the age of 6 years with a chief complaint of recurrent episodes of intense nausea and vomiting with no apparent reason. His parents reported that he had been seen and assessed by physicians many times since he was 3 years old. Adam is well and healthy between episodes, and he has achieved excellent growth and development.

His first episode of vomiting was around the age of 3 years, and it was thought to be due to a viral illness. During the following 2 years, he experienced a total of 5 similar episodes, each lasting up to 24 h, before returning to normal.

Over the past 2 years, vomiting episodes became more frequent, occurring once every 8–10 weeks. Each episode lasts between 12 and 48 h and is often triggered by stressful events, such as school difficulties, excitement for a birthday party, or a family holiday. Parents can predict the onset of the episodes with a change in the child's behaviour. They describe Adam as emotional, moody, tired and not interested in food on the day before the onset of vomiting. The next day, Adam becomes distressed, cries, looks pale, refuses food, feels nauseated and within 1–2 h starts vomiting repeatedly. He vomits four to six times per hour, starting with undigested food, followed by yellow-green fluids, until he gets exhausted and becomes visibly unwell and lethargic. Occasionally, Adam may complain of central abdominal pain and frontal headache.

Adam was born normally at term and had no neonatal problems. He has no family history of similar illnesses. His mother has menstrual migraine. His father and his 8-year-old brother are well and healthy.

Over the past 2 years, Adam was taken to the local hospital on several occasions because of suspected or confirmed dehydration, and he was given intravenous fluids. The physical examination revealed no additional abnormal findings, no fever, and no focus of infection was identified.

During his current assessment, investigations revealed a normal blood count, normal inflammatory markers, normal blood tests for electrolytes, urea, creatinine, liver function tests, and glucose, as well as a negative screen for coeliac disease. No evidence of infection on throat swabs and urine culture. He also had a normal metabolic screen and upper gastrointestinal endoscopy. MRI scan of the brain was also normal.

A diagnosis of CVS was made, and Adam was commenced on prophylactic treatment with pizotifen 0.5 mg per night. Parents were given a written management plan to implement during future episodes, including the administration of ondansetron melt tablets 4 mg as early as possible after the onset of CVS.

6.4 Case Discussion

Adam's clinical case demonstrates the difficulties in making the diagnosis of CVS in early childhood and, especially, in infancy. Although the diagnosis can be suspected early in the course of the disease, it cannot be confirmed until several episodes (at least five) have been assessed and documented, exhibiting typical clinical features, a normal physical examination and normal appropriate investigations. Therefore, it is not surprising that in some cases the diagnosis can be delayed and appropriate treatment is not given until several years later. Several factors may also contribute to late diagnosis, including an atypical clinical presentation, episodes triggered by intercurrent illnesses, long intervals between episodes and possibly a lack of awareness of the condition among clinical personnel.

Taking a thorough clinical history is crucial in assessing a child with CVS. Enquiry about all symptoms throughout the whole duration of the episodes will identify, as seen in the case of Adam above, the several phases of the CVS episode, the trigger factors, premonitory symptoms, associated symptoms, relieving factors, response to treatment and resolution of the episode and return to normal health (Fig. 6.1).

Episodes of CVS can be triggered by stress, anxiety, missing sleep, missing meals and intercurrent illnesses [18]. Premonitory symptoms may be noted 1–2 days before the onset of vomiting and may include excessive tiredness, yawning, a change in mood and behaviour and loss of appetite. After the onset of vomiting, children may complain of intense nausea, pallor, sleepiness, central abdominal pain and frontal headache [19]. Excessive vomiting can cause dehydration, and parents should be vigilant for the warning signs of dehydration, such as dry mouth, a raised heart rate, a fast and weak pulse, a drop in level of consciousness and passing little or no urine. Parents will be advised to seek medical advice if any of these symptoms become apparent.

The start of resolution of the episode is manifested by the child becoming more alert, talkative, and responsive to the family and the environment, followed by a gradual reduction in nausea and vomiting, a return of a good appetite, and asking for fluids, drinks and food to eat. The child may want to sleep for a few hours or overnight. Upon awakening from sleep, the child feels well and gradually returns to normal health.

Following several episodes, patients and parents can recognise the stereotypical and almost identical nature of the episodes in their clinical presentation, duration and frequency. Patients and parents can often predict the date of the next episode with remarkable accuracy. They can also predict the evolution of symptoms and pending dehydration and can appropriately seek medical advice or attend emergency department. Typical episodes are consistent with the International

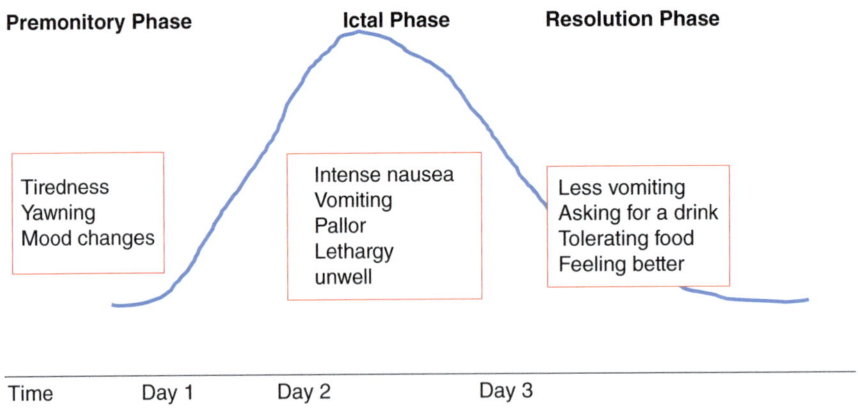

Fig. 6.1 Phases of the CVS episode

Table 6.1 Criteria for the diagnosis of cyclical vomiting syndrome

ICHD-3 (2018) [2]	Rome-IV (2016) [3]
A. At least five attacks of intense nausea and vomiting, fulfilling criteria B and C B. Stereotypical in an individual patient and recurring with predictable periodicity C. All of the following: 1. Nausea and vomiting occur at least four times per hour 2. Attacks last 1 h and up to 10 days 3. Attacks occur at least 1 week apart D. Complete freedom from symptoms between attacks E. Not attributed to another disorder	Must include all of the following: 1. The occurrence of two or more periods of intense, unremitting nausea and paroxysmal vomiting, lasting hours to days, within a 6-month period 2. Episodes are stereotypical in each patient 3. Episodes are separated by weeks to months, with return to baseline health between episodes 4. After appropriate medical evaluation, the symptoms cannot be attributed to another condition

Classification of Headache Disorders' (2018) criteria or Rome-IV (2016) for the diagnosis of CVS, as in Table 6.1.

The clinical presentation of Adam was largely typical of CVS. The episodes are discrete, time limited and resolve completely with return to normal health in between episodes. Additionally, Adam has experienced normal growth, with a normal gain in weight and typical development. He did not have added features to suggest an alternate diagnosis, particularly in renal tract, the gastrointestinal system, the central nervous system or symptoms related to a metabolic disorder. Therefore, it was appropriate to carry out investigations early in the course of the disease when the diagnosis could not be confirmed with certainty. His symptoms were in keeping with the clinical criteria for the diagnosis of CVS (Table 6.1). As in the case above, a positive family history of migraine is common among children with CVS, but it is not necessary to confirm the diagnosis.

6.5 Diagnostic Algorithm

The diagnosis of CVS is usually made by excluding other possible underlying causes, which is an important criterion in both the ICHD-3 and Rome-IV [2, 3]. Some conditions can be excluded on clinical history and physical examination alone. Other conditions that mimic CVS, especially if the presentation is atypical, may require further investigations and should be carried out whenever there is uncertainty about the diagnosis of CVS.

The choice of investigations depends on the predominant symptoms during episodes (Fig. 6.2).

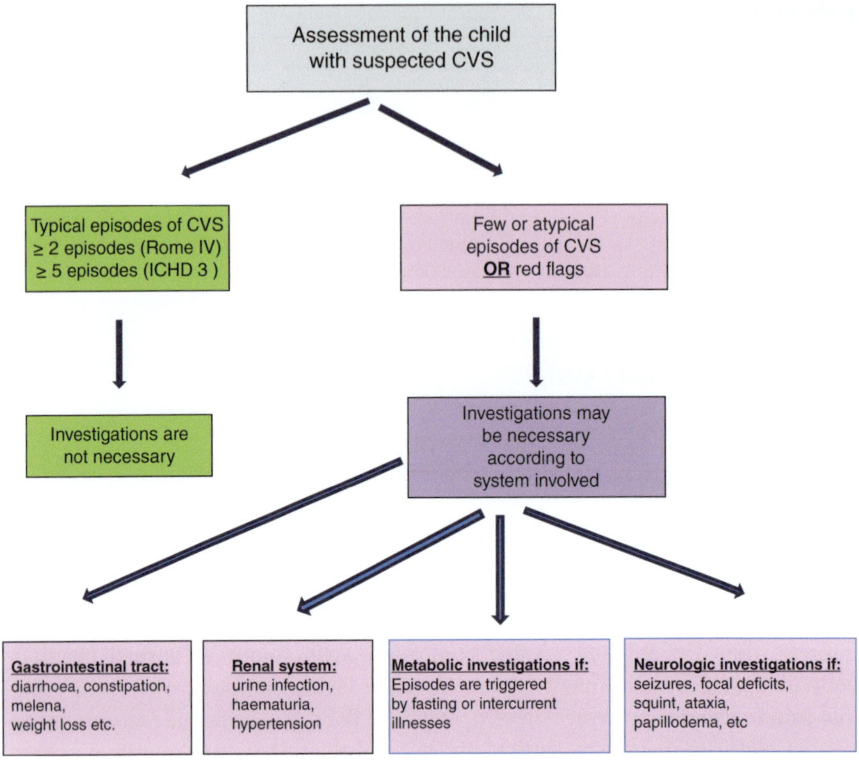

Fig. 6.2 Flow chart on the assessment of the child with possible CVS

- In children with fever, it is prudent to exclude respiratory infections, urinary tract infection and other serious infections such as meningitis and septicaemia.
- In children with episodes that are consistently triggered by missing meals or intercurrent infections, it is important to exclude metabolic causes such as fatty acid oxidation disorders by measuring blood lactate, pyruvate, ammonia, liver function tests and plasma amino acids as well as urinary organic acids.
- Children presenting with abdominal pain, diarrhoea, constipation, food intolerance and weight loss should be investigated with abdominal ultrasound, coeliac screen, inflammatory markers and upper gastrointestinal endoscopy.
- Investigations of the urinary tract should be carried out in children with unilateral loin pain, dysuria, haematuria and recurrent urinary tract infections.
- Neurological investigations with brain imaging are important if the child presents with seizures, new focal neurological deficits, motor incoordination, personality change or papilloedema.

6.6 Management

Once the diagnosis is established, the child and the parents are given verbal and written information about the disease in order for them to prepare and take part in formalising the management plan at home and to liaise with teachers in the management of acute episodes at school. The management plan should take into account the recurrent nature of the syndrome, the severity of illness and potential complications, dehydration and on some occasions the need for hospital admission and administration of intravenous fluids [20, 21]. The chronic nature of the disease may have an adverse impact on the quality of life of the affected children and their families and also on the child's school attendance and education [22].

The earlier the treatment starts after the onset of symptoms the more successful the outcome will be. Children will be taught to recognise the early features of the pending or actual attack and also to inform parents or the adult carers of early symptoms. The child should be allowed to rest in a quiet room and monitored by an adult carer. The child will be given free access to fluids to take small sips, paracetamol, if needed, and anti-emetic. Early administration of anti-emetic medications will help in relieving or reducing nausea and vomiting and also improve gastric emptying in order to allow reliable oral rehydration. The choice of which anti-emetic drug to give depends on local availability, experience and licensing (Table 6.2) [23, 24]. Ondansetron is a 5-Hydroxytriptamin ($5HT_3$) antagonist and has a good safety profile in young children. Other medications can also be used with caution in regard to possible adverse reactions such as cardiac arrhythmia and prolonged QT interval on electrocardiograph recording with chronic use of domperidone and extrapyramidal side effect with metoclopramide.

Children with short and mild episodes may be managed successfully at home as above and with rest, sleep and sips of fluids. In some patients, the episode of vomiting starts suddenly and reaches a peak of intensity over a very short period of time making oral treatment unachievable. In these children there is a high risk of dehydration and medical treatment with intravenous infusion is necessary [21, 25].

Table 6.2 Anti-emetic medications

Drug	Action	Single dose	Maximum daily dose	Minimum interval	Form for dose
Ondansetron	$5HT_3$ antagonist	4 mg	8 mg	12 h	Oral melt tablet; Oral solution; injectable
Metoclopramide	D_2 and $5HT_4$ antagonist	0.5 mg/kg	20 mg	12 h	Oral tablet; Oral suspension; injectable
Domperidone	Dopamine antagonist	10 mg	30 mg	8 h	Oral tablet; Oral suspension
Cyclizine	Anti-histamine	25 mg (6–11 years); 50 mg (12–17 years)	75 mg; 150 mg	8 h	Oral dispersible tablet; injectable

Sumatriptan nasal spray may be administered to children aged 12 years and above, and may help terminate the episode [26].

Children are advised to adopt a healthy lifestyle that reduces the risk and frequency of CVS. The advice includes a regular routine of getting enough sleep, eating regular meals, exercising regularly and getting good rest in between. Children will be advised to monitor for specific triggers and try to avoid them as well as to reduce intake of caffeinated drinks and avoid smoking.

Preventative medications for CVS may also be recommended for children with frequent episodes, prolonged duration, severe risk of dehydration and inadequate response to acute treatment. The decision to start preventive medication should be taken jointly with the child and his parents in order to ensure compliance with the recommendations.

Open observational studies have shown several medications to be effective including the tricyclic antidepressant amitriptyline, the prokinetic erythromycin, the anti-migraine drugs pizotifen, cyproheptadine and propranolol and other drugs such as L-carnitine and coenzyme Q10 [27].

Amitriptyline, pizotifen and cyproheptadine are first-line treatments for many children due to their relatively good response and safety profile, but may need to be avoided in overweight children as they may improve appetite and may lead to weight gain.

Amitriptyline is recommended as the first-line treatment due to its relative ease of administration in a single daily dose at night and very little risk of adverse reactions. The recommended dose is about 0.25 mg/day and can be increased in steps if needed up to 1.0 mg/day. Amitriptyline is available as liquid solution and in tablet forms.

Pizotifen is a safe and effective preventive treatment for migraine in children and can be effective in the prevention of CVS. It is given as a single oral dose of 0.5–1.5 mg at night. It is well tolerated, especially by young children.

Cyproheptadine has a dual action as an anti-histamine and calcium channel antagonist (143, 144). It is administered orally in a daily dose of 0.25–0.5 mg/kg, split into two to three doses per day.

Propranolol, a beta-blocker, is an effective preventive treatment for migraine and was also shown to be useful for the prevention of CVS in children. Propranolol is administered orally in a dose of 1–2 mg/kg, divided into two doses.

Erythromycin is a macrolide antibiotic with a prokinetic property that makes it potentially useful in preventing vomiting, particularly in CVS. Erythromycin has a good safety profile and is given in a dose of 10 mg/kg twice a day.

Other potential preventive treatments include flunarizine, L-carnitine and coenzyme Q10. The use of anti-epileptic drugs sodium valproate and topiramate is not recommended in girls and young women with child-bearing potential.

CVS can have an adverse impact on children's quality of life and education. Children 5–18 years of age with CVS and parents of children (2–18 years old) with CVS scored lower on Health-Related Quality of Life (HRQoL) questionnaire compared to children with irritable bowel syndrome and other organic gastrointestinal disorders [28]. Duration of episodes and missing school days were significantly associated with lower scores by children. Delayed diagnosis and missing school days negatively impacted on parents' scores [28].

It is estimated that in 24% of children with CVS, the condition resolves completely by late adolescence and early adult life. In about 30% the disease continues and in 40–50% CVS will be replaced by migraine with or without aura [29].

6.7 Conclusion

Cyclical vomiting syndrome (CVS) is a relatively common paediatric condition, affecting approximately 2% of children. It occurs equally in boys and girls, with a typical onset between the ages of 5 and 6 years. Diagnosis is based on the fulfilment of either the ICHD-3 or Rome-IV criteria. Early and effective management of acute episodes is essential to prevent complications such as dehydration. Preventive therapies not only reduce the frequency and severity of attacks but also contribute to improved quality of life and better school attendance and educational outcomes. Notably, one-third of affected children achieve complete remission by late adolescence, while nearly 50% go on to develop migraine with or without aura in early adulthood.

References

1. Gee S. On fitful or recurrent vomiting. St Bartholomew's Hosp Rep. 1882;18:1–6.
2. Headache Classification Committee of the International Headache Society. The international classification of headache disorders, 3rd edition. Cephalalgia. 2013;33(9):653.
3. Hyams JS, Di LoRenzo C, Saps M, Shulman RJ, Staiano A, van Tilburg M. Childhood functional gastrointestinal disorders: child/adolescent. Gastroenterology. 2016;150:1456–68.
4. Abell TL, Adams KA, Boles RG, Bousvaros A, Chong SK, Fleisher DR, Hasler WL, Hyman PE, Issenman RM, Li BU, Linder SL, Mayer EA, McCallum RW, Olden K, Parkman HP, Rudolph CD, Taché Y, Tarbell S, Vakil N. Cyclic vomiting syndrome in adults. Neurogastroenterol Motil. 2008;20(4):269–84. https://doi.org/10.1111/j.1365-2982.2008.01113.x.
5. Abu-Arafeh I, Russell G. Cyclical vomiting syndrome in children: a population-based study. J Pediatr Gastroenterol Nutr. 1995;21:454–8.
6. Ertekin V, Selimoglu MA, Altnkaynak S. Prevalence of cyclic vomiting syndrome in a sample of Turkish school children in an urban area. J Clin Gastroenterol. 2006;40:896–8.
7. Cullen K, Macdonald WB. The periodic syndrome. Its nature and prevalence. Med J Aust. 1963;50(2):167–72.
8. Fitzpatrick E, Bourke B, Drumm B, Rowland M. The incidence of cyclic vomiting syndrome in children: population-based study. Am J Gastroenterol. 2008;103(4):991–5; quiz 996. https://doi.org/10.1111/j.1572-0241.2007.01668.x. Epub 2007 Dec 5. PMID: 18070235.

9. Sagar RC, Sood R, Gracie DJ, Gold MJ, To N, Law GR, Ford AC. Cyclic vomiting syndrome is a prevalent and under-recognized condition in the gastroenterology outpatient clinic. Neurogastroenterol Motil. 2018;30(1):e13174. https://doi.org/10.1111/nmo.13174. Epub 2017 Jul 26.
10. Alfayyadh MM, Maksemous N, Sutherland HG, Lea RA, Griffiths LR. Unravelling the genetic landscape of hemiplegic migraine: exploring innovative strategies and emerging approaches. Genes. 2024;15:443.
11. Lee J, Wong SA, Li BU, Boles RG. NextGen nuclear DNA sequencing in cyclic vomiting syndrome reveals a significant association with the stressinduced calcium channel (RYR2). Neurogastroenterol Motil. 2015;27:990–6.
12. Ye Z, Xue A, Huang Y, Wu Q. Children with cyclic vomiting syndrome: phenotypes, disease burden and mitochondrial DNA analysis. BMC Gastroenterol. 2018;18:104.
13. Boles RG, Chun N, Senadheera D, Wong LJ. Cyclic vomiting syndrome and mitochondrial DNA mutations. Lancet. 1997;350:1299–300.
14. Salpietro CD, Briuglia S, Merlino MV, Di Bella C, Rigoli LA. Mitochondrial DNA mutation (A3243GmtDNA) in a family with cyclic vomiting. Eur J Pediatr. 2003;162:727–8.
15. Chelimsky TC, Chelimsky GG. Autonomic abnormalities in cyclic vomiting syndrome. J Pediatr Gastroenterol Nutr. 2007;44:326–30.
16. Fitzpatrick E, Bourke B, Drumm B, Rowland M. Outcome of children with cyclical vomiting syndrome. Arch Dis Child. 2007;92:1001–4.
17. Ellingsen DM, Garcia RG, Lee J, Lin RL, Kim J, Thurler AH, Castel S, Dimisko L, Rosen BR, Hadjikhani N, Kuo B, Napadow V. Cyclic vomiting syndrome is characterized by altered functional brain connectivity of the insular cortex: a cross-comparison with migraine and healthy adults. Neurogastroenterol Motil. 2017;29(6):e13004. https://doi.org/10.1111/nmo.13004. Epub 2016 Dec 1. PMID: 27910222; PMCID: PMC5423835.
18. Abu-Arafeh I, Gelfand AA. The childhood migraine syndrome. Nat Rev Neurol. 2021;17(7):449–58.
19. Raucci U, Borrelli O, Di Nardo G, Tambucci R, Pavone P, Salvatore S, Baldassarre ME, Cordelli DM, Falsaperla R, Felici E, Ferilli MAN, Grosso S, Mallardo S, Martinelli D, Quitadamo P, Pensabene L, Romano C, Savasta S, Spalice A, Strisciuglio C, Suppiej A, Valeriani M, Zenzeri L, Verrotti A, Staiano A, Villa MP, Ruggieri M, Striano P, Parisi P. Cyclic vomiting syndrome in children. Front Neurol. 2020;11:583425. https://doi.org/10.3389/fneur.2020.583425. PMID: 33224097; PMCID: PMC7667239.
20. Beals L, Sarjinsky S, Faltyn M, Issenman RM, Kam AJ. Cyclic vomiting syndrome in the emergency department: a 10-year review of clinical presentation and management. Pediatr Emerg Care. 2022;38(10):e1578–83. https://doi.org/10.1097/PEC.0000000000002694. Epub 2022 May 12.
21. Abdulkader ZM, Bali N, Vaz K, Yacob D, Di Lorenzo C, Lu PL. Predictors of hospital admission for pediatric cyclic vomiting syndrome. J Pediatr. 2021;232:154–8. https://doi.org/10.1016/j.jpeds.2020.11.055. Epub 2020 Nov 28.
22. Wang-Hall J, Li BUK, Tarbell SE. Family health-related quality of life in pediatric cyclic vomiting syndrome. J Pediatr Gastroenterol Nutr. 2018;66(5):738–43. https://doi.org/10.1097/MPG.0000000000001797.
23. Lee LYW, Abbott L, Mahlangu B, Moodie SJ, Anderson S. The management of cyclic vomiting syndrome: a systematic review. Eur J Gastroenterol Hepatol. 2012;24:1001–6.
24. Isoldi S, Di Nardo G, Mallardo S, et al. Cyclic vomiting syndrome in children: a nationwide survey of current practice on behalf of the Italian Society of Pediatric Gastroenterology, Hepatology and Nutrition (SIGENP) and Italian Society of Pediatric Neurology (SINP). Ital J Pediatr. 2022;48(1):156. https://doi.org/10.1186/s13052-022-01346-y. PMID: 36042474; PMCID: PMC9429644.

25. Li BUK. Treating cyclic vomiting syndrome in the emergency department: sooner appears better. J Pediatr. 2021;232:12–4. https://doi.org/10.1016/j.jpeds.2020.12.066. Epub 2020 Dec 26.
26. Hikita T, Kodama H, Kaneko S, Amakata K, Ogita K, Mochizuki D, Kaga F, Nakamoto N, Fujii Y, Kikuchi A. Sumatriptan as a treatment for cyclic vomiting syndrome: a clinical trial. Cephalalgia. 2011;31(4):504–7. https://doi.org/10.1177/0333102410390398. Epub 2010 Dec 8.
27. Tillman EM, Harvath EM. Cyclic Vomiting Syndrome in Pediatric Patients: A Review of Therapeutics. J Pediatr Pharmacol Ther. 2022;27(1):12–8. https://doi.org/10.5863/1551-6776-27.1.12. Epub 2021 Dec 22. PMID: 35002554; PMCID: PMC8717616.
28. Tarbell SE. LI BUK, health -related quality of life in children and adolescents with cyclic vomiting syndrome: a comparison with published data on youth with irritable bowel syndrome and organic gastrointestinal disorders. J Pediatr. 2013;163:493–7.
29. Dignan F, Symon DNK, Abu-Arafeh I, Russell G. The prognosis of cyclical vomiting syndrome. Arch Dis Child. 2001;84:55–7.

Chapter 7
Episodic Syndromes That May Be Associated with Migraine: Abdominal Migraine

Arife Cimen Atalar, Ebru Nur Vanli-Yavuz, and Pinar Topaloğlu

7.1 Introduction

Abdominal migraine (AM) is a member of a group of syndromes known as "the episodic syndromes associated with migraine" including recurrent gastrointestinal (GI) disturbance (1.6.1) (cyclic vomiting syndrome [1.6.1.1] and AM [1.6.1.2]), benign paroxysmal vertigo (1.6.2), and benign paroxysmal torticollis (1.6.3) [1].

AM is considered the most common childhood periodic syndrome seen in a pediatric headache clinic, accounting for 48.9% of cases in one study [2]. Studies suggest a higher prevalence in girls, though some indicate equal distribution between genders [3].

Although it is recognized as a disorder of childhood, it can also be encountered in adults where it is frequently underrecognized and can be quite challenging for clinicians dealing with these patients [4]. According to the latest version of the International Classification of Headache Disorders (ICHD-3), it is defined as an idiopathic condition of recurrent attacks of midline abdominal pain with moderate-to-severe intensity concomitant with vasomotor symptoms such as anorexia, pallor, nausea, and vomiting [1]. The presence of renal or gastrointestinal disease should be ruled out for accurate diagnosis; hence a detailed differential diagnosis should be

A. C. Atalar
Department of Neurology, Istanbul Physical Therapy and Rehabilitation Training and Research Hospital, Istanbul, Turkey

E. N. Vanli-Yavuz
Mediclinic City Hospital Dubai, Dubai, UAE

P. Topaloğlu (✉)
Division of Child Neurology, Department of Neurology, Istanbul Faculty of Medicine, Istanbul University, Istanbul, Turkey

D. Uludüz et al. (eds.), *Rare Causes of Headache Disorders*, Headache,
https://doi.org/10.1007/978-3-032-10242-3_7

performed. The attacks can be so severe that they might interfere with everyday activities and impair school performance of affected children, decreasing their quality of life [5].

Although the presence of this condition has been acknowledged since the early 1900s, the initial definition as a separate condition appeared in the ICHD second edition in 2004 under the "Childhood Periodic Syndromes" section, as a precursor of migraine headache [6, 7], followed by the Rome Classification of Functional Gastrointestinal Disorders in 2006 [8]. The prevalence in school-aged children (3–15 years old) is estimated between 1% and 4.5%, with a predominance of females (3/2 female/male) [9], while the exact prevalence in adulthood remains scarce [4].

There is a handful of extensive research about abdominal migraine and a significant gap of knowledge regarding the pathophysiology, epidemiology, pathogenesis, and management, which limits awareness and recognition of this condition [7]. In this chapter, AM will be reviewed comprehensively in separate subsections in the light of the latest scientific literature to emphasize this important but underdiagnosed condition.

7.2 Pathophysiology

Multiple hypotheses have been proposed to explain the pathophysiology of AM, but none have been conclusively proven.

Most comprehensive explanation for functional gastrointestinal disorders (FGIDs), emphasizes the strong connection between the enteric and central nervous systems (CNS), which share a common embryonic origin. Individuals with FGIDs have an increased sensitivity to nociceptive stimuli, influenced by genetic, environmental, and psychosocial factors like early-life stressors, leading to visceral hyperalgesia.

Proposed mechanisms for visceral hyperalgesia include increased sensitivity of primary sensory and central spinal neurons, impaired inhibitory pain control, and a dysfunctional stress response. These disruptions affect the gut–brain axis, resulting in abnormal secretion of excitatory neurotransmitters such as serotonin, a key regulator of gastrointestinal (GI) motility, secretion, and sensation. The continuous communication between the brain and gut through neural and hormonal pathways may contribute to changes in the CNS, causing symptoms like headaches. Additionally, autonomic nervous system stimulation and heightened sympathetic activity may explain associated symptoms like pallor.

Advanced imaging techniques, including functional MRI (magnetic resonance imaging), have revealed abnormalities in visceral pain processing pathways in FGID patients. Although the visceral hyperalgesia theory has not been specifically validated in abdominal migraine (AM) patients, it remains the most well-supported explanation for FGIDs [10].

Abnormal gut motility is another potential factor in the pathophysiology of AM. It is thought that gastrointestinal distension and irregular contractions could lead to functional abdominal pain, increasing the sensitivity to pain (hyperalgesia).

A study conducted in Sri Lanka between 2007 and 2012 assessed gastric motility in 17 children with AM (ages 4–12) and compared them to healthy controls. The findings revealed significantly slower gastric emptying rates and reduced antral motility in the children with AM. Furthermore, a slower gastric emptying rate was linked to longer pain episodes, while weaker antral contractions correlated with more severe symptoms. These results suggest that disruptions in gastric motility might contribute to the onset and progression of AM [10].

Patients with AM may experience altered gut permeability, as mucosal permeability serves as an indirect indicator of overall gut health. A 1995 study by Bentley et al. examined gut mucosal permeability in 11 children diagnosed with AM, comparing them to healthy controls. The results showed a significant increase in gut permeability among AM patients.

Longitudinal follow-ups of three patients over 3 years, with assessments conducted three times annually, revealed a correlation between permeability changes and symptom severity. As symptoms improved, gut permeability decreased, and vice versa. This observation may help explain why non-steroidal anti-inflammatory drugs (NSAIDs) are ineffective in AM management, as these drugs are known to increase mucosal permeability.

Despite these findings, no further research has been conducted to confirm this hypothesis or explore its clinical relevance in treating AM. Additionally, this study was conducted before formal diagnostic criteria for AM were established [11].

Dietary influences may play a role in the development and severity of AM symptoms. Studies on cephalic migraines have shown a notably higher prevalence among individuals with atopy and other allergic conditions, suggesting a possible link between dietary allergens and migraine episodes. Similarly, in AM, specific food allergens may trigger an immune response in the gut, leading to inflammation and symptom manifestation in predisposed individuals.

This theory is reinforced by the observation that some AM patients experience symptom relief when following an oligoantigenic diet, which removes common dietary triggers. The diet's effectiveness suggests that food sensitivities or immune-mediated reactions might contribute to AM.

While this connection is promising, further research is necessary to better understand the role of diet in AM and to develop targeted dietary interventions for affected individuals [11–13].

In 1995, Bentley et al. studied IgE levels and positive radioallergosorbent (RAST) test results in 14 patients with AM and a group of healthy individuals. Their findings showed no significant differences in IgE levels or RAST test results between the two groups. Additionally, skin prick tests did not identify any dietary allergens in patients with AM. This suggests that AM may mainly cause a localized immune response in the gut rather than affecting the whole immune system.

Laboratory studies have shown that enterocytes (intestinal cells) can express Major Histocompatibility Complex (MHC) class II antigens and release certain chemical signals, which stimulate immune cells in the gut lining when exposed to dietary antigens. More recent research highlights the mucosal immune system as a key regulator of the gut–brain axis. Both the adaptive immune system (especially T-cells) and the innate immune system (such as mucosal lymphoid cells, mast cells, and mononuclear phagocytic cells) help maintain gut–brain balance. When this balance is disrupted, it has been linked to functional gastrointestinal disorders (FGIDs). A similar immune system dysfunction is also involved in cephalic migraines.

Further studies on immune system changes in AM patients could help improve understanding of the condition and lead to better treatment options [14–16].

Disruptions in neurotransmitter metabolism, resulting in an imbalance between excitatory and inhibitory amino acids, have been widely investigated in cephalic migraine. A comparable process may contribute to the development of AM [17, 18].

In the central nervous system (CNS), glutamic acid and aspartic acid act as key excitatory neurotransmitters, while gamma-aminobutyric acid (GABA) plays a major role as an inhibitory neurotransmitter.

Phenol sulfotransferase (PST) enzymes (S and P) are essential for metabolizing catecholamines and other amine neurotransmitters. Studies indicate that individuals with diet-induced migraines have significantly reduced PST enzyme activity. This decline results in the accumulation of inflammatory neuropeptides and neurotransmitters, disrupting the balance between excitatory and inhibitory signals and affecting brain circuits associated with dopamine, serotonin, and norepinephrine. CNS hyperexcitability is considered a crucial factor in cephalic migraine.

A range of factors—including genetic predisposition, environmental influences, dietary triggers, and psychosocial stress—can activate the trigeminovascular system, leading to the release of inflammatory neuropeptides and neurotransmitters like calcitonin gene-related peptide (CGRP), substance P, serotonin, and nitric oxide, all of which contribute to migraine development. A similar mechanism involving heightened excitatory amino acid activity may also play a role in AM. This could potentially explain the effectiveness of certain treatments, such as valproate, which enhances GABA levels in AM patients [19–21].

In 1995, Bentley et al. reviewed the platelet expression of the two PST isoenzymes (S and P) in 21 patients with AM, comparing them to normal subjects. No significant change in enzyme activity was noted between the two groups. However, the level of enzyme activity in platelets might not accurately reflect the levels in the enteric nervous system. Further studies are needed to confirm this hypothesis [14].

7.2.1 Genetic and Psychosocial Factors in AM Pathogenesis

Genetic mutations and polymorphisms, though not yet fully understood, play a role in regulating ion channels, neurotransmitter metabolism, and mitochondrial function in the central nervous system (CNS), contributing to the development of migraine headaches. There is also strong evidence suggesting a genetic predisposition to functional abdominal pain. A 2017 study indicated that Y2 receptor antagonism and YY gene deletion might be associated with visceral hypersensitivity. The link between genetics and AM is further supported by the fact that many patients have a family history of migraines or chronic abdominal pain. However, more research is needed to identify the specific genetic factors involved.

Psychosocial factors such as hormonal changes (menstrual cycle and pregnancy), lifestyle, diet, anxiety, and chronic stress are known to influence cephalic migraines. Similarly, stress and anxiety have been associated with functional gastrointestinal disorders (FGIDs). While the role of these factors in AM is not yet fully understood, future research may provide more insights into their impact [22].

Other theories about the causes of FGIDs and cephalic migraine suggest that factors such as autonomic instability, problems with the hypothalamus–pituitary axis, changes in the gut microbiome, small intestinal bacterial overgrowth, previous infections with long-term effects, lactose intolerance, and abnormal mitochondrial function may play a role. More research is needed to fully understand how these factors contribute to cephalic migraine [22].

7.3 Case Presentation

A 9-year-old girl was referred to our pediatric clinic with a 6-month history of recurrent severe abdominal pain. The pain was midline and periumbilical in location, described as dull and moderate-to-severe in intensity, lasting 8–12 h per episode. Attacks occurred approximately twice monthly, often disrupting school attendance.

Associated symptoms included nausea, reduced appetite, and noticeable pallor during episodes. No headaches occurred during these attacks. Between episodes, she was completely asymptomatic and had normal growth and development.

Her medical history was unremarkable. Family history revealed that her mother had migraine without aura. Physical examination was normal.

Extensive investigations were performed by her primary physician before referral, including complete blood count, inflammatory markers, celiac serology, liver and renal function tests, abdominal ultrasound, and urinalysis—all of which were normal.

Given the clinical history and symptom pattern, abdominal migraine was considered. The diagnosis was confirmed based on ICHD-3 criteria: ≥5 attacks of midline abdominal pain lasting 2–72 h with associated vasomotor symptoms and complete return to baseline between attacks.

Management included education about the diagnosis, lifestyle modifications (regular meals and sleep hygiene), and identification of potential triggers (caffeine-containing soft drinks and skipped meals). Due to attack frequency and severity, prophylactic therapy with cyproheptadine was initiated at 0.25 mg/kg/day. At follow-up after 3 months, the patient reported a marked reduction in attack frequency (one mild episode) and severity, with no significant side effects from treatment.

7.4 Clinical Characteristics and Diagnosis

Diagnosing abdominal migraine is challenging, as recurrent abdominal pain is common in childhood and can be caused by various systemic diseases, including gastrointestinal system disorders [23]. A correct clinical diagnosis is essential for preventing patients from excess and unnecessary diagnostic interventions and treatments hence a detailed differential diagnosis is needed [4].

Currently, two separate sets of diagnostic criteria are proposed for AM: the International Classification of Headache Disorders third edition (ICHD-3) criteria [1] and the Rome Foundation, Rome-IV Functional GI Disorders criteria [24, 25]. Although both set of diagnostic criteria share some common points in terms of abdominal pain and associated symptoms, there are certain variations regarding the details.

Both criteria accept AM as a childhood disorder, and it is widely accepted that AM resolves over time as the patient reaches adulthood and evolves into migraine thus might be accepted as "a migraine precursor of childhood" [4, 26]. Contrary to this belief, cases regarding patients with AM of adulthood are increasingly being reported although the exact prevalence is still not known due to the lack of extensive research and the under-recognition of this condition in adulthood [4].

According to the ICHD-3 criteria, AM is classified under the heading of "1.6 Episodic syndromes that may be associated with migraine" as a subheading with the code 1.6.1.2 [1]. The main properties of AM are listed as, an idiopathic disorder with recurrent attacks of moderate-to-severe abdominal pain coexisting with vasomotor symptoms, nausea, and vomiting that lasts for 2–72 h. The patient should be asymptomatic and completely normal between the episodes [1]. As a rule, headache should not exist during these episodes.

The Rome-IV criteria have been published in 2016 [25] and has similar points to that of ICHD-3 criteria [4]. The criteria can be summarized as follows: paroxysmal episodes of intense periumbilical, midline, or diffuse abdominal pain lasting equal to or more than 1 h. Abdominal pain is very severe and interferes with normal everyday activities and these symptoms are not related with another medical condition. There are some associated symptoms such as anorexia, nausea, vomiting, headache, photophobia, or pallor. At least two of these symptoms should accompany to abdominal pain and a minimum of two episodes in 6 months are mandatory for exact diagnosis [24].

The major differences between these two sets of criteria are in terms of pain duration and the number of episodes to confirm the diagnosis. In addition, the obligatory "lack of headaches during the episodes" in ICHD-3 [4] is another important point.

These main differences can be summarized as follows:

1. Pain duration should be between 2 and 72 h in ICHD-3 criteria whereas it was stated as 1 h or more in Rome-IV criteria.
2. Five attacks are mandatory for diagnosis in ICHD-3 whereas 2 episodes are enough in Rome-IV criteria.

3. Headache was defined as an associated symptom in Rome-IV whereas lack of headache is obligatory for diagnosis in ICHD-3.
4. At least 6 months of period is needed for diagnosis in Rome-IV but in ICHD-3 no time period was reported.
5. Gastrointestinal and renal diseases should be ruled out for diagnosis in ICHD-3 criteria but in Rome-IV it was reported as "other medical conditions" that should be ruled out.

The final diagnosis is made clinically and there are no certain biomarkers or symptoms that point out to an exact diagnosis of AM in a child/adolescent. A detailed anamnesis and a thorough systemic and neurological examination are the hallmarks of diagnosis along with necessary diagnostic interventions. The questioning of dietary habits, the history of medical and neurological conditions, and triggers of the abdominal pain is essential. The most common triggers of AM are light (bright or flickering), lack of sleep/poor sleep, fasting, traveling, stressful life events, and certain dietary habits (citrus food, caffeine, cheese, chocolate, carbonated drinks, colorings, and flavorings) [5]. Once identified, avoiding these triggers can be beneficial in order to minimize the attacks [3].

The questioning of pain characterization and associated symptoms is important. The localization of pain can be either periumbilical (65–80%) or diffuse (16%) and the pain quality can be dull (60%) or colicky (22%) [9]. Some children can express behavioral irritability before the attacks as a premonitory symptom [9, 27, 28]. The average duration of episodes is between 1 and 17 h and the patient can experience 2–20 attacks per month [5]. The child should be neurologically normal between the attacks.

7.5 Differential Diagnosis

It is imperative that a detailed differential diagnosis including evaluation for secondary and treatable causes of recurrent abdominal pain is performed [9]. The following medical conditions should be investigated thoroughly before making AM diagnosis in a child with recurrent abdominal pain [5].

- Gastrointestinal disorders (pancreatitis, small bowel obstruction, pseudo-obstruction), acid peptic disease (esophagitis, gastritis, peptic ulcer disease), eosinophilic diseases (esophagitis, gastritis, enteropathy), celiac disease, gall bladder disease (choledochal cyst, cholelithiasis, cholecystitis), inflammatory bowel disease, pancreatitis, other functional abdominal pain disorders (functional dyspepsia, irritable bowel syndrome, cyclic vomiting syndrome [CVS], functional abdominal pain), lactose intolerance, chronic hepatitis
- Surgical causes (hernia, appendicitis, intussusception)
- Renal disorders (obstructive uropathy, urinary tract infections, nephrolithiasis, etc.)

- Central nervous system disorders (intracranial hypertension, posterior fossa disorders, hematoma or familial dysautonomia, cerebral venous sinüs thrombosis, epilepsy)
- Endocrine disorders (diabetes, adrenal insufficiency)
- Metabolic diseases (methylmalonic acidemia, acute intermittent porphyria, ornithine transcarbamylase deficiency, lead poisoning, etc.)

The following investigations/interventions can be helpful to rule out the possible alternative diagnoses when evaluating a patient with recurrent abdominal pain:

- Routine blood examinations (full blood count, erythrocyte sedimentation rate [ESR], C-reactive protein [CRP], electrolytes, urea and creatinine, glucose levels), liver and renal function tests, celiac antibodies
- Pregnancy test
- Urine and stool studies (microscopy, culture, and sensitivity, stool occult blood and microscopy, etc.)
- Radiological studies (abdominal X-ray, pelvis and abdominal ultrasound investigations)
- Brain magnetic resonance imaging
- Contrast study of upper gastrointestinal tract and small bowel
- Endoscopic interventions (esophagogastroduodenoscopy, colonoscopy, etc.) [5]

Cyclic vomiting syndrome (CVS) is another important migraine equivalent in children, which can easily be confused with AM and should be differentiated. It is characterized by episodic attacks of intense nausea and vomiting (at least five attacks), with predictably cyclical timing of episodes (periodic), and the child is completely normal between attacks [1]. The major difference between these two syndromes is that vomiting is the hallmark symptom in CVS but is less prominent in AM. Vomiting is most intense at the start of the episode especially within the first hour, and gradually decreases at the following 4–8 h [9]. CVS is a benign disorder and can sometimes overlap with AM.

AM is often seen as an early indicator of cephalic migraine, even though most patients eventually outgrow the condition. Main outcomes of a study by Dignan et al. focused on whether abdominal migraine persisted or resolved and whether participants had a past or present history of migraine headaches, based on International Headache Society (IHS) criteria. Results showed that 31 cases (61%) experienced a complete resolution of abdominal migraine. However, 70% of those previously diagnosed with abdominal migraine had either current (52%) or past (18%) migraines that met IHS criteria, compared to only 20% of the control group [29].

However, 70% of these individuals later developed migraines, with or without aura, compared to just 20% in the control group [30]. While AM can occasionally persist into adulthood, further longitudinal research is necessary to better understand its long-term prognosis and progression from childhood into adulthood.

7.6 Management of Abdominal Migraine

Different strategies may be used to treat abdominal migraine but double-blind, placebo-controlled trials are still inadequate. Treatment of abdominal migraine is very similar to all pediatric migraine patient profile although there are some details to give attention to [31].

Management of abdominal migraine focuses on acute symptom relief, prophylaxis, lifestyle modifications, and patient education. Before trying pharmacological agents, it is very important to take developmental growth status, lifestyle characteristics, school work scheme, and accompanying activities into consideration [32].

7.7 The Following Strategies Are Essential

7.7.1 Acute Symptom Relief

Before pharmacological methods, ensuring adequate hydration and allowing the patient to rest in a quiet, dark environment may help reduce symptom severity.

7.7.1.1 Pharmacological Treatment

First-line medications used in acute attacks include paracetamol/acetaminophen (10–15 mg/kg/dosage) and non-steroidal anti-inflammatory drugs (NSAIDs), such as ibuprofen (7.5–10 mg/kg/dosage) for pain relief. In cases with nausea and vomiting, antiemetics (e.g., ondansetron) can be beneficial but it is better to use them as additives to other acute medications [33].

Triptans are being more widely used in all migraine patients as published data increase our experience. Though primarily used for classic migraines, triptans (such as sumatriptan) may help alleviate abdominal migraine episodes, especially in older children and adults. Four important agents—Almotriptan (ages 12–17), Rizatriptan (ages 6–17), Zolmitriptan nasal spray (ages 12–17), and Sumatriptan/Naproxen combination (ages 12–17)—are available for pediatric age groups [34].

A 5HT-1F agonist Lasmiditan is a relatively new molecule with triptan-like effect by decreasing Calcitonin Gene Releasing Peptide (CGRP) release from presynaptic vesicles [35].

Although there is limited knowledge about CGRP antagonists such as rimegepant, ubrogepant, and zavegepant among pediatric population, they may take part in future treatment strategies of abdominal migraine.

7.7.2 *Prophylaxis of Abdominal Migraine*

For patients experiencing frequent or severe abdominal migraine episodes, prophylactic treatment is necessary to reduce occurrence and intensity. During deciding pharmacological prophylaxis, it is also important to make lifestyle modifications such as:

Dietary Adjustments: Identifying and avoiding trigger foods (e.g., chocolate, caffeine, processed meats) can help prevent recurrent episodes [32]. There are also some oral nutraceuticals such as Riboflavin (50–400 mg/day), Vitamin D, Magnesium (up to 9 mg/kg/day as magnesium oxide), which are well tolerated and shorten attacks and reduce symptom severity [36].

Regular Sleep Patterns: Establishing a consistent sleep schedule and ensuring sufficient rest play a crucial role in preventing migraine attacks. Melatonin (0.3 mg/kg) may be used to regulate sleep patterns.

Mind–body therapies such as cognitive-behavioral therapy (CBT), mindfulness (MDT), and biofeedback (BFB) help patients cope with stressors that may trigger migraine episodes. Published data suggest that they have minimal side effects in adult patients but pediatric group data are still missing [31]. These methods can be beneficial in children and adolescents to help control physiological responses associated with migraines. Stress management techniques such as cognitive-behavioral therapy (CBT), meditation, and relaxation exercises can be beneficial in reducing attack frequency [32].

Non-invasive neuromodulation techniques are non-invasive vagal nerve stimulator (nVNS), transcranial magnetic stimulator (TMS), remote electrical neuromodulation (REN), transcutaneous supraorbital electrostimulation, and external trigeminal nerve stimulator (eTNS). Transcranial direct current stimulation (tDCS) is also another inexpensive and portable method that shows some beneficial effect among adults. REN has FDA approval above 12 years of age and eTNS has approval above 8 years of age, but there are no published data of these non-invasive methods in abdominal migraine cohort.

7.7.2.1 Pharmacologic Prophylaxis

Classical and approved drugs for pediatric migraine can also be used for abdominal migraine prophylaxis. Beta-blockers (propranolol, 2–4 mg/kg/day) have been commonly used since many years but sometimes they are ineffective among severe recurrent attacks [31].

Antiepileptic drugs, especially topiramate (1–10 mg/kg/day) and valproic acid (20–40 mg/kg/day), have been found effective in preventing attacks. Tricyclic antidepressants, especially Amitriptyline, have shown efficacy in reducing the frequency of attacks, particularly in patients with comorbid anxiety or depression but usually less preferred in pediatric age group.

Calcium channel blockers such as Verapamil are another option that may help in preventing episodes. Serotonin modulators such as Cyproheptadine, an antihistamine with serotonin-blocking properties, are particularly effective in children [33].

CGRP monoclonal antibodies such as Erenumab, Fremenazumab, and Galcanezumab are promising subcutaneous agents for migraine prophylaxis. An intravenous CGRP monoclonal antibody eptinezumab is another potential agent for pediatric age group although their placebo-controlled clinical trials have not been concluded yet [36].

7.8 Conclusion

Abdominal migraine is a debilitating condition of both children and adults that requires a comprehensive management approach. Since differential diagnosis is based on clinical findings and there is no biomarker or neuroimaging clue, it is very important to consider a wide range of both gastrointestinal and pain syndromes especially in pediatric age group. Treatment of this relatively rare condition resembles migraine treatment approach, including acute symptom relief and lifestyle modifications and prophylaxis. While pharmacologic interventions such as NSAIDs, triptans, and antiemetics provide symptomatic relief, prophylactic treatments play a crucial role in long-term management. Also, CGRP monoclonal antibodies are promising relatively new agents in this particular syndrome. Additionally, non-pharmacologic approaches such as cognitive-behavioral therapy, stress management, and dietary modifications significantly contribute to reducing episode frequency. Early diagnosis, patient education, and individualized treatment plans are essential to improving quality of life for individuals suffering from abdominal migraine. Ongoing research is necessary to further understand its pathophysiology and develop more targeted treatment modalities.

References

1. Olesen J, Headache Classification Committee of the International Headache Society (IHS). The International Classification of Headache Disorders, 3rd edition. Cephalalgia. 2018;38:1–211.
2. Tarantino S, Capuano A, Torriero R, Citti M, Vollono C, Gentile S, Vigevano F, Valeriani M. Migraine equivalents as part of migraine syndrome in childhood. Pediatr Neurol. 2014;51(5):645–9.
3. Russell G, Abu-Arafeh I, Symon DN. Abdominal migraine: evidence for existence and treatment options. Pediatr Drugs. 2002;4:1–8.
4. Kizhakkayil Tency N, Roy A, Krishnakumaran N, Thomas AM. Unraveling abdominal migraine in adults: a comprehensive narrative review. Cureus. 2023;15(8):e43760.
5. Mani J, Madani S. Pediatric abdominal migraine: current perspectives on a lesser-known entity. Pediatric Health Med Ther. 2018;9:47–58.

6. Headache Classification Subcommittee of the International Headache Society. The international classification of headache disorders: 2nd edition. Cephalalgia. 2004;24(1):9–160.
7. Napthali K, Koloski N, Talley NJ. Abdominal migraine. Cephalalgia. 2016;36(10):980–6.
8. Drossman DA, Corazziari E, Delvaux M, Spiller R, Talley NJ, Thompson WG, Whitehead WE. Rome III: The functional gastrointestinal disorders. 3rd ed. McLean: Degnon Associates; 2006.
9. Irwin S, Barmherzig R, Gelfand A. Recurrent gastrointestinal disturbance: abdominal migraine and cyclic vomiting syndrome. Curr Neurol Neurosci Rep. 2017;17(3):21.
10. Korterink J, Devanarayana NM, Rajindrajith S, Vlieger A, Benninga MA. Childhood functional abdominal pain: mechanisms and management. Nat Rev Gastroenterol Hepatol. 2015;12(3):159–71.
11. Bentley D, Katachburian A, Brostoff J. Abdominal migraine and food sensitivity in children. Clin Allergy. 1984;14(5):499–500.
12. Özge A, Öksüz N, Ayta S, Uluduz D, Yıldırım V, Toros F, Taşdelen B. Atopic disorders are more common in childhood migraine and correlated headache phenotype. Pediatr Int. 2014;56(6):868–72.
13. Egger J, Carter CM, Wilson J, Turner MW, Soothill JF. Is migraine food allergy? A double-blind controlled trial of oligoantigenic diet treatment. Lancet. 1983;322(8355):865–9.
14. Bentley D, Kehely A, al-Bayaty M, Michie CA. Abdominal migraine as a cause of vomiting in children: a clinician's view. J Pediatr Gastroenterol Nutr. 1995;21:S49–51.
15. Goadsby PJ. Pathophysiology of migraine. Ann Indian Acad Neurol. 2012;15:S15–22.
16. Loewendorf AI, Matynia A, Saribekyan H, Gross N, Csete M, Harrington M. Roads less traveled: sexual dimorphism and mast cell contributions to migraine pathology. Front Immunol. 2016;7:140.
17. D'Andrea G. Pathogenesis of chronic migraine: the role of neuromodulators. J Headache Pain. 2015;16(S1):A38.
18. Good PA. Neurologic investigations of childhood abdominal migraine: a combined electrophysiologic approach to diagnosis. J Pediatr Gastroenterol Nutr. 1995;21(Suppl 1):S44–8.
19. Tan V, Sahami AR, Peebles R, Shaw RJ. Abdominal migraine and treatment with intravenous valproic acid. Psychosomatics. 2006;47(4):353–5.
20. Jones AL, Roberts RC, Colvin DW, Rubin GL, Coughtrie MW. Reduced platelet phenolsulphotransferase activity towards dopamine and 5-hydroxytryptamine in migraine. Eur J Clin Pharmacol. 1995;49(1):109–14.
21. Gibb C, Glover V, Gilbertson NB, Bentley D, Sandler M. Platelet phenolsulphotransferase activity and 'abdominal migraine'. Arch Dis Child. 1988;63(12):1500–1.
22. McFerron BA, Waseem S. Chronic recurrent abdominal pain. Pediatr Rev. 2012;33(11):509–17.
23. Amin MA, Manna RM, Nahin S, Hawlader MDH. Abdominal migraine with acute watery diarrhea and dehydration: successful treatment with Valproic acid in a pediatric case. Clin Case Rep. 2024;12(3):e8703.
24. Drossman DA. Functional gastrointestinal disorders: history, pathophysiology, clinical features and Rome IV. Gastroenterology. 2016;150:1262–79.
25. Drossman DA, Hasler WL. Rome IV-functional GI disorders: disorders of gut-brain interaction. Gastroenterology. 2016;150(6):1257–61.
26. Roberts JE, deShazo RD. Abdominal migraine, another cause of abdominal pain in adults. Am J Med. 2012;125:1135–9.
27. Abu-Arafeh I, Russell G. Prevalence and clinical features of abdominal migraine compared with those of migraine headache. Arch Dis Child. 1995;72(5):413–7.
28. Mortimer MJ, Kay J, Jaron A. Clinical epidemiology of childhood abdominal migraine in an urban general practice. Dev Med Child Neurol. 1993;35(3):243–8.
29. Dignan F, Abu-Arafeh I, Russell G. The prognosis of childhood abdominal migraine. Arch Dis Child. 2001;84(5):415–8.

30. Kunishi Y, Iwata Y, Ota M, Matsubayashi M, Kanno M, Kuboi Y, Yoshie K, Kato Y. Abdominal migraine in a middle-aged woman. Intern Med. 2016;55(19):2793.
31. Hershey AD. Current approaches to the diagnosis and management of paediatric migraine. Lancet Neurol. 2010;9(2):190–204.
32. Baglioni V, Bozza F, Beatrice A, Cameli N, Colacino Cinnante EM, Lentini G, Faedda N, Natalucci G, Guidetti V. Non-pharmacological treatments in paediatric migraine. J Clin Med. 2024;13(5):1278.
33. Hershey AD. Pediatric headache. Continuum (Minneap Minn). 2015;21(4 Headache):1132–45.
34. Puledda F, de Boer I, Messina R, Garcia-Azorin D, Portes Souza MN, Al-Karagholi MA, de Dhaem OB, Tassorelli C, May A. Worldwide availability of medications for migraine and tension-type headache: a survey of the international headache society. Cephalalgia. 2024;44(11):3331024241297688.
35. Tsai M, Monkul Nery ES, Kerr L, Khanna R, Komori M, Dennehy EB, Wilbraham D, Winner P. Pharmacokinetics, safety, and tolerability of lasmiditan in pediatric patients with migraine. Clin Pharmacokinet. 2021;60(6):819–28.
36. Loh NR, Whitehouse WP, Howells R. What is new in migraine management in children and young people? Arch Dis Child. 2022;107(12):1067–72.

Chapter 8
Episodic Syndromes That May Be Associated with Migraine: Benign Paroxysmal Vertigo

Tiago Gomes De Paula and Thais Rodriges Villa

8.1 Introduction

Benign paroxysmal positional vertigo (BPPV) is one of the most common causes of episodic vertigo, and its relationship with vestibular migraine (VM) has generated increasing interest in clinical practice and research. VM, in turn, is one of the main causes of episodic vertigo, often underdiagnosed despite its high prevalence among migraine patients [1, 2]. The overlap between BPPV and VM creates a diagnostic challenge, as both share similar vestibular symptoms, such as dizziness and vertigo, complicating appropriate clinical management [1, 2]. In this chapter, we will discuss the pathophysiology, diagnosis, and treatment of BPPV in the context of VM, with an emphasis on practical approaches and controlling this condition.

8.2 Pathophysiology of Vestibular Migraine and BPPV

The pathophysiology of VM is not yet fully elucidated, but it is believed to involve a complex interaction between the trigeminal and vestibular systems. Studies show that the trigeminal nucleus has reciprocal connections with the vestibular nuclei, and this interaction can generate vestibular symptoms during migraine attacks [3, 4]. Additionally, the involvement of neurotransmitters such as serotonin and norepinephrine is proposed as one of the mechanisms contributing to vestibular dysregulation in migraine patients [3].

VM is characterized by episodes of vertigo associated with migraine, with vestibular symptoms that can last from minutes to hours, often accompanied by other symptoms such as photophobia, phonophobia, and nausea [1, 3]. BPPV, on the other

T. Gomes De Paula · T. R. Villa (✉)
Headache Center Brasil, São Paulo, Brazil

D. Uludüz et al. (eds.), *Rare Causes of Headache Disorders*, Headache,
https://doi.org/10.1007/978-3-032-10242-3_8

hand, is caused by the displacement of otoliths within the semicircular canals of the inner ear, resulting in short episodes of vertigo, typically triggered by changes in head position [2, 5]. BPPV is often associated with migraine, and the risk of recurrence is higher in patients who have both VM and BPPV [1, 6].

The overlap between VM and BPPV occurs because both conditions share similar vestibular mechanisms, such as hyperexcitability of the vestibular nuclei. This may explain why some patients present symptoms of both conditions simultaneously [4, 6]. It is important to remember that migraine patients exhibit greater vestibular sensitivity, contributing to the frequency and severity of vertigo episodes [3].

Studies suggest that VM may affect vestibular pathways at multiple levels, involving mechanisms such as activation of the vestibular nuclei by the trigeminal nucleus [3, 5]. In BPPV, activation of these same circuits may also trigger vertigo, leading to significant overlap between the two conditions [2, 5]. The interaction between the trigeminal and vestibular systems seems to be the convergence point between VM and BPPV, especially in patients with chronic migraine [5].

8.3 Case Study

A 36-year-old female patient sought care at Headache Center Brasil in São Paulo with a history of dizziness episodes that began at the age of 15, associated with nausea, aural fullness, and tinnitus. At 25, her symptoms worsened and became daily. Later, she developed headaches with photophobia, phonophobia, and visual aura.

At the age of 32, the patient was diagnosed with BPPV and VM after Dix-Hallpike maneuvers showed typical nystagmus and imaging exams revealed no abnormalities. Previous treatments with propranolol, flunarizine, amitriptyline, and venlafaxine were ineffective in controlling the disease. Treatments such as amitriptyline and venlafaxine initially led to a slight reduction in crises; however, this improvement was neither sustained nor progressive, and the crises remained frequent, significantly impacting her quality of life. At admission, the patient had a severe disability level (Migraine disability assessment schedule (MIDAS) IV, severe disability).

At the age of 36, she started treatment with botulinum toxin, showing significant improvement after the first cycle and progressive improvement in subsequent cycles. After eight cycles of botulinum toxin treatment, the patient experienced a marked reduction in the frequency and intensity of vertigo episodes, with progressive disease control. Her quality of life improved considerably, reflecting the success of the treatment.

In view of this case, we initiated treatment with botulinum toxin, which demonstrated significant improvement after the first cycle and progressive improvement in subsequent cycles. After eight cycles of treatment with botulinum toxin, the patient showed a marked reduction in the frequency and intensity of vertigo episodes, with progressive control of the disease. Her quality of life improved considerably, reflecting the success of the treatment.

8.4 Case Discussion

The case presented here highlights the complexity of the differential diagnosis between BPPV and VM. Both present with vestibular symptoms such as vertigo, which can lead to inaccurate or incomplete initial diagnoses. The patient experienced years of disabling symptoms until the coexistence of the two conditions was specified.

Diagnostic Key: The clinical history and careful listening to the patient about her migraine symptoms were crucial to confirm the combined diagnosis [2, 4, 7, 8].

Clinical Dilemma: The delay in recognizing VM in patients initially presented with BPPV alone reflects the need for greater vigilance and clearer protocols to differentiate the two conditions, especially in patients with a history of migraine [6, 8].

8.5 Clinical Management

This case demonstrates the efficacy of treatment with botulinum toxin in a patient refractory to conventional therapies, such as propranolol, flunarizine, amitriptyline, and venlafaxine.

First Line: Repositioning maneuvers in isolated cases of BPPV, with the Epley and Semont maneuvers, continue to be the mainstay of management.

Vestibular Migraine: Preventive treatment with beta-blockers and anticonvulsants is often used, but the lack of response in cases such as our patient's reinforces the importance of considering alternatives such as botulinum toxin and anti-CGRP (calcitonin gene-related peptide) monoclonal antibodies [9].

Vestibular Rehabilitation: A multimodal approach combining vestibular rehabilitation and drug prophylaxis can maximize outcomes [2, 7, 8, 10].

8.6 Clinical Aspects and Quality of Life

The delay in introducing effective treatments, such as botulinum toxin, questions current clinical practices. Why are proven therapies reserved for refractory cases, when they could benefit patients soon after initial therapy has failed? The significant improvement in patient quality of life after the introduction of botulinum toxin highlights its importance in the therapeutic armamentarium [8, 11].

8.7 Diagnosis

The diagnosis of BPPV in the context of vestibular migraine requires a thorough evaluation, as both conditions can present overlapping symptoms. For BPPV, the classic diagnosis involves performing repositioning maneuvers, such as the Dix-Hallpike maneuver, which induces characteristic nystagmus in patients with the canalicular form of BPPV [1, 3]. For VM, the diagnostic criteria established by the International Headache Society and the Bárány Society require that the patient presents vestibular symptoms of moderate to severe intensity, associated with migraine features such as headache, photophobia, phonophobia, and/or aura [5, 7, 10, 12].

In patients with VM, vestibular and audiometric tests are often normal, but may reveal abnormalities during vertigo episodes, making it essential to differentiate positional vertigo from spontaneous vertigo that occurs in VM [1]. The duration of episodes can range from a few minutes to several hours, and vestibular symptoms may precede, accompany, or follow the headache episode [1, 5]. Additionally, imaging tests, such as magnetic resonance imaging (MRI), are generally used to rule out other neurological conditions that may be associated [10]. Evaluation using questionnaires like the Dizziness Handicap Inventory can also help quantify the impact of dizziness and assist in the decision to intensify treatment [8].

One of the biggest challenges in the differential diagnosis between VM and BPPV is the similarity of vestibular symptoms, such as movement-triggered vertigo. In some cases, BPPV may be diagnosed initially, but over time, the development of migraine symptoms or refractoriness to treatment indicates the concomitant presence of VM [3, 4].

8.8 Treatment

The management of BPPV and VM depends on controlling vestibular symptoms and appropriate prophylaxis. BPPV is classically treated with repositioning maneuvers, such as the Epley and Semont maneuvers, which have a high success rate in repositioning otoliths [3, 6, 12, 13]. However, in patients with BPPV and VM, clinical approaches may be more complex, requiring a combination of prophylactic therapies for migraine and specific treatments for vestibular symptoms [2, 4, 7, 10].

In VM, prophylactic therapy includes the use of beta-blockers (such as propranolol), calcium channel blockers (such as flunarizine), anticonvulsants (such as topiramate and valproic acid), and tricyclic antidepressants (such as amitriptyline) [2, 3, 10, 12]. However, in refractory cases, botulinum toxin and anti-CGRPs have emerged as effective alternatives, significantly reducing the intensity of episodes and migraine-related disability [1, 4, 9].

Recently, monoclonal antibodies against CGRP (calcitonin gene-related peptide), such as galcanezumab, have shown efficacy in the prophylactic treatment of chronic migraine, including cases of vestibular migraine. Galcanezumab works by blocking the CGRP receptor [9].

In cases refractory to medications, botulinum toxin is an effective option. Studies have shown that patients who fail treatment with conventional medications, such as propranolol and topiramate, experience significant improvement with botulinum toxin, both in reducing headache crises and vestibular symptoms [8, 12]. Liu et al. highlighted that patients who failed first-line medication were more likely to benefit from botulinum toxin [8].

Vestibular rehabilitation is another valuable tool for improving balance and reducing vertigo symptoms in patients with VM and BPPV, improving patients' quality of life [3]. The multimodal approach, which combines vestibular rehabilitation with the use of prophylactic medications, has shown superior results in controlling symptoms [2, 7, 8, 10].

8.9 Conclusion

The overlap between BPPV and VM often coexists, challenging physicians and complicating proper diagnosis and management. Repositioning maneuvers are effective in BPPV, but in patients with concomitant VM, management requires a more comprehensive approach. Botulinum toxin has proven to be a valuable therapy in refractory cases, providing significant symptomatic relief. Early recognition of the severity of symptoms and intensification of treatment, when necessary, are crucial to improving patients' quality of life.

References

1. Yollu U, Uluduz DU, Yilmaz M, Yener HM, Akil F, Kuzu B, Kara E, Hayir D, Ceylan D, Korkut N. Vestibular migraine screening in a migraine-diagnosed patient population, and assessment of vestibulocochlear function. Clin Otolaryngol. 2017;42(2):225–33. https://doi.org/10.1111/coa.12699. Epub 2016 Aug 1.
2. Dieterich M, Obermann M, Celebisoy N. Vestibular migraine: the most frequent entity of episodic vertigo. J Neurol. 2016;263(Suppl 1):S82–9. https://doi.org/10.1007/s00415-015-7905-2. Epub 2016 Apr 15. PMID: 27083888; PMCID: PMC4833782.
3. Görür K, Gür H, İsmi O, Özcan C, Vayisoğlu Y. The effectiveness of propranolol, flunarizine, amitriptyline and botulinum toxin in vestibular migraine complaints and prophylaxis: a non-randomized controlled study. Braz J Otorhinolaryngol. 2022;88(6):975–81. https://doi.org/10.1016/j.bjorl.2021.02.005. Epub 2021 Mar 7. PMID: 33722518; PMCID: PMC9615515.
4. Benjamin T, Gillard D, Abouzari M, Djalilian HR, Sharon JD. Vestibular and auditory manifestations of migraine. Curr Opin Neurol. 2022;35(1):84–9. https://doi.org/10.1097/CO.0000000000001024. PMID: 34864754; PMCID: PMC8755616.
5. Barbosa F, Villa TR. Vestibular migraine: diagnosis challenges and need for targeted treatment. Arq Neuropsiquiatr. 2016;74(5):416–22. https://doi.org/10.1590/0004-282X20160037.

6. Mahrous MM. Vestibular migraine and benign paroxysmal positional vertigo, close presentation dilemma. Acta Otolaryngol. 2020;140(9):741–4. https://doi.org/10.1080/00016489.2020.1770857. Epub 2020 Jun 18.
7. Kim SK, Hong SM, Park IS, Choi HG. Association between migraine and benign paroxysmal positional vertigo among adults in South Korea. JAMA Otolaryngol Head Neck Surg. 2019;145(4):307–12. https://doi.org/10.1001/jamaoto.2018.4016. PMID: 30676633; PMCID: PMC6481427.
8. Liu YF, Macias D, Donaldson L, Dornhoffer JR, Rizk HG. Pharmacotherapy failure and progression to botulinum toxin injection in vestibular migraine. J Laryngol Otol. 2020;134(7):586–91. https://doi.org/10.1017/S002221512000095X. Epub 2020 Jul 27.
9. Sharon JD, Krauter R, Chae R, Gardi A, Hum M, Allen I, Levin M. A placebo controlled, randomized clinical trial of galcanezumab for vestibular migraine: the INVESTMENT study. Headache. 2024;64(10):1264–72. https://doi.org/10.1111/head.14835. Epub ahead of print.
10. Agessi LM, Villa TR. Vestibular migraine with visual aura and olfactory hallucination in children: two case reports. Neuropediatrics. 2018;49(6):414–6. https://doi.org/10.1055/s-0038-1673642. Epub 2018 Oct 10.
11. Surmeli R, Surmeli M, Yalcin AD, Sahin Yilmaz AA, Erden Habesoglu T, Gunay G. Vestibular migraine: Onabotulinum toxin effectivity, prospective-randomized study. Clin Neurol Neurosurg. 2025;254:108949. https://doi.org/10.1016/j.clineuro.2025.108949. Epub 2025 May 4.
12. Salmito MC, Duarte JA, Morganti LOG, Brandão PVC, Nakao BH, Villa TR, Ganança FF. Prophylactic treatment of vestibular migraine. Braz J Otorhinolaryngol. 2017;83(4):404–10. https://doi.org/10.1016/j.bjorl.2016.04.022. Epub 2016 Jun 2. PMID: 27320656; PMCID: PMC9442697.
13. Chen J, Zhang S, Cui K, Liu C. Risk factors for benign paroxysmal positional vertigo recurrence: a systematic review and meta-analysis. J Neurol. 2021;268(11):4117–27. https://doi.org/10.1007/s00415-020-10175-0. Epub 2020 Aug 24.

Part II
Trigeminal Autonomic Cephalalgias (TACs)

Chapter 9
Short-Lasting Unilateral Neuralgiform Headache Attacks with Conjunctival Injection and Tearing (SUNCT)

Utku Topbaş, Nevra Öksüz, and Aynur Özge

9.1 Introduction

Short-lasting unilateral neuralgiform headache attacks with conjunctival injection and tearing (SUNCT) is one of the rare headache syndromes included in the primary trigeminal autonomic cephalalgias group, according to the International Classification of Headache Disorders, 3rd edition[1] (ICHD-3) [1]. Its prevalence was found to be 6.6 per 100,000 [2]. The typical age of onset is between 40 and 60 years and cases between 3 and 88 years have been reported [3]. The prevalence of SUNCT between men and women is similar with recent case series [4].

The pathophysiology of SUNCT is not fully understood. The anatomical structures responsible for SUNCT are the hypothalamus, trigeminovascular complex (TCC), and the cranial autonomic system [5]. Afferent fibers are responsible for extracranial and intracranial pain synapse with the TCC. The second order neurons of the TCC synapse with the thalamus and pain matrix to produce pain. TCC is known to synapse with the ipsilateral superior salivatory nucleus (SSN). Therefore, it modulates the SSN during pain and is responsible for ipsilateral cranial autonomic symptoms via the sphenopalatine ganglion [6]. The hypothalamus is known to have a pain-modulating effect on the TCC. In the pathogenesis of SUNCT, pain occurs continuously at regular intervals due to the central disinhibition of the hypothalamus on the TCC [6].

U. Topbaş · N. Öksüz (✉) · A. Özge
Mersin State Hospital, Mersin, Turkey

D. Uludüz et al. (eds.), *Rare Causes of Headache Disorders*, Headache,
https://doi.org/10.1007/978-3-032-10242-3_9

9.2 Case Presentation

A 67-year-old male Hasan was admitted to our tertiary headache clinic for severe headaches. His headache was localized to the right temporal and periorbital regions, lasting around one minute. The pain was excruciatingly severe; he described it as if something had screwed into his right eye for one minute before stopping suddenly. When pain occurred, he felt a tingling sensation in his periorbital area, and his right eye was reddish. He complained of tears in his right eye. His headache was triggered by certain activities, such as eating, talking, and washing his face. When the pain starts, it occurs five to ten times an hour, most of the day, with attacks occurring daily or every other day for three years. When he came to the headache clinic, he seemed to accept his headache episodes. He said, "I believe that this pain came to my head because God wanted to punish me for the sins I committed." He had coronary artery disease and hypertension, and he was using acetylsalicylic acid, metoprolol, and ramipril for chronic diseases. There was no family history to explain this pain. Neurologic examinations were remarkable except for right eye ptosis. Both indomethacin and oxygen tests were negative. Diagnosis of short-lasting unilateral neuralgiform headache attacks with conjunctival injection and tearing (SUNCT) was made. Imaging with contrast-enhanced magnetic resonance imaging (MRI) and MR Angiography showed no vascular or structural abnormalities. We admitted the patient to the neurology unit and started treatment with intravenous (IV) lidocaine (infusion 1.5 mg/kg/h). The headache was completely resolved by the third day of treatment. We continued the treatment for an additional 24 hours to ensure the headaches did not return. After that, we sent the patient home and gradually started lamotrigine treatment, tapering it to 300 mg per day. During the first follow-up visit after six weeks, the patient still reported headaches, but they were relieved by about 50%. To improve the situation, we added topiramate to the treatment and gradually increased the dosage to 200 mg per day. After four weeks, the patient reported a 95% reduction in headache symptoms.

9.3 Headache Characteristics in SUNCT

Pain in SUNCT is almost always unilateral. The pain is of short duration (1–600 s) and is always accompanied by autonomic symptoms. If conjunctival injection and tears are present, it is called SUNCT. Pain is usually described by patients as shooting, stabbing electrical-shock like [3, 7]. Rarely it can be described as throbbing [3]. Pain intensity is severe or very severe. In most patients, pain is localized to the V1 branch of the trigeminal nerve, while pain tends to radiate to the V2 and V3 branches and even to the cervical branches. In some, the pain may also be in the neck, where cervical branches carry the pain [3, 8] (Fig. 9.1). While attacks occur mostly spontaneously, they are triggered by stimuli such as talking, eating, touching the face, and shaving, as in trigeminal neuralgia [7, 8]. While there is a refractory period

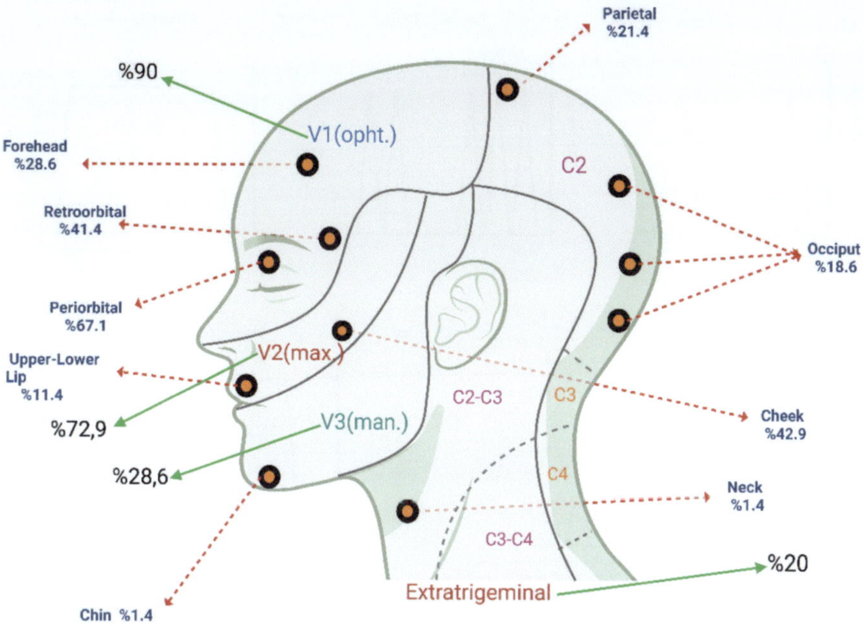

Fig. 9.1 Distribution of pain in SUNCT

between attacks in trigeminal neuralgia, this refractory period is absent in SUNCT [7]. Even immediately after the pain has ended, pain may be stimulated with triggers. Four different pain patterns are defined for SUNCT (Fig. 9.2).

1. Single or repetitive stabs: Each episode lasts on average 60 s (1–600 s). Attacks recur periodically throughout the day (average 20–30). There is no long refractory period between episodes [3].
2. Plateau like pattern: The pain peaks very quickly (max. 2–3 s) and continues at a constant intensity for 5–600 s and then abruptly stops [3].
3. Saw tooth pattern: It consists of stabbing pain superimposed on severe pain at the base. The stabbing comes in a regular pattern and is superimposed on the pain at the base. The duration of pain can last up to 20 minutes [7].
4. Plateau-like with exacerbations: A form of pain in which random, very short (1–2 s) spikes are added to the constant pain (5–300 s) [3].

Since the duration of pain can last up to 600 s, it can be misdiagnosed as paroxysmal hemicrania. In SUNCT, attacks are unresponsive to indomethacin, which is always responsive in paroxysmal hemicrania. During pain, patients usually have psychomotor agitation as in cluster headache. However, some patients with short-term pain and somatic triggers tend to wait until the pain subsides. They prefer to remain immobile to avoid triggers [3]. Attacks recur frequently during the day (1–200 times). The ICHD-3 diagnostic criteria for SUNCT are as follows (Table 9.1) [1].

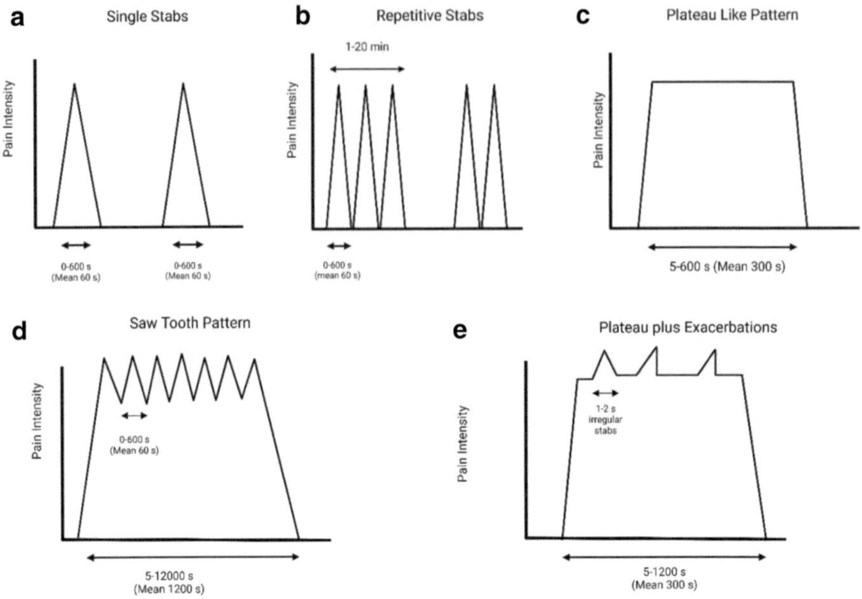

Fig. 9.2 Headache subtypes seen on SUNCT

Table 9.1 Diagnostic criteria for SUNCT

Diagnostic criteria for short-lasting unilateral neuralgiform headache
A. At least 20 attacks fulfilling criteria B through D
B. Moderate or severe unilateral head pain, with orbital, supra-orbital, temporal and/or other trigeminal distribution, lasting for 1–600 seconds and occurring as single stabs, a series of stabs, or in a sawtooth pattern
C. At least one of the following five cranial autonomic symptoms or signs, ipsilateral to the pain:
1. Conjunctival injection and/or lacrimation
2. Nasal congestion and/or rhinorrhea
3. Eyelid edema
4. Forehead and facial sweating
5. Miosis and/or ptosis
D. Attacks have a frequency of at least one a day
E. Not better accounted for by another ICHD-3 diagnosis
Diagnostic Criteria for SUNCT
A. Attacks fulfilling criteria for short-lasting unilateral neuralgiform headache attacks
B. Both conjunctival injection and lacrimation (tearing) ipsilateral to the pain
Episodic SUNCT: Attacks occurring in periods lasting from seven days to one year, separated by pain-free periods lasting at least three months
Chronic SUNCT: Attacks occurring without a remission period, or with remissions lasting less than three months, for at least one year.

9.4 Diagnosis Algorithm

When patient complains for one side locked severe headache with cranial autonomic symptoms:

Step 1: Ask for duration and number of attacks in one day. Notably, all trigeminal autonomic cephalgia headaches except cluster headache occur at least one per day. If more than ten attacks, then cluster headache is unlikely. If the patient complains severe headache more continuously than half hour, diagnosis of SUNCT/SUNA is unlikely.

Step 2: Ask for the prominence of cranial autonomic symptoms and the presence of refractory periods. Trigeminal neuralgia has a refractory period. If the pain doesn't have a refractory period, SUNCT/SUNA is likely.

Step 3: Make the indometacin test to rule out paroxysmal hemicrania. Give 100 mg of indomethacin IM. If the pain resolves, paroxysmal hemicrania is likely the diagnosis.

Step 4: When pain arises, give the patient 8–12 L/min oxygen with a mask. If the pain resolves or reduces in intensity, a diagnosis of cluster headache is likely.

Step 5: If the indomethacin and oxygen tests were negative, SUNCT or SUNA is most likely the diagnosis. If the pain is frequent and disabling, give the patient IV lidocaine. If the pain resolves or reduces, SUNCT/SUNA is most likely the diagnosis.

Step 6: Search for secondary causes, prefer imaging with MRI and MR Angiography for structural and vascular abnormalitics.

9.5 Secondary SUNCT

SUNCT is included in primary headaches, but its association with structural anomalies in the brain has been reported. Meningitis, trauma, posterior fossa lesions, and pituitary lesions can be counted among the secondary causes [8, 9]. Some of the secondary causes are listed in Table 9.2

9.6 Management

SUNCT pain can be very disabling for patients, especially when occurs frequently. It is a challenging situation for patients and some patients may consider suicide because of this pain. Therefore, once diagnosed, treatment should start as soon as possible. If the patient's attacks are persistent and we can see cranial autonomic findings in the patient examination, we should start acute pain treatment as soon as possible.

Table 9.2 : Secondary causes of SUNCT

Cerebellopontine arteriovenous malformation
Cavernous hemangioma
Brainstem infarction
Pilocytic astrocytoma expanding to the trigeminal root
Vascular loops compressing the trigeminal nerve
Parietal and parieto-occipital space occupying lesions
Pathologic white matter lesions in multiple sclerosis
Vertebral artery dissection
Neuromyelitis optica spectrum disorder
Cerebellopontine angle meningioma
Macroadenoma and microadenoma in pituitary

In acute pain, intravenous 2% lidocaine solution should be given as a continuous infusion at a dose of 1.5–3 mg/kg/h with monitoring [10]. Electrocardiogram (ECG), liver, and kidney function tests should be performed, and hypomagnesemia and hypokalemia should be corrected before starting the drug. It should never be used in the presence of atrioventricular (AV) block on ECG. Heart rate and blood pressure should be monitored every 5 minutes for the first 30 minutes, heart rate and blood pressure should be monitored every 15 minutes for the next 4 hours and every 2–4 hours thereafter, and lidocaine should be stopped in case of abnormality. Treatment can be extended for up to seven days until the patient's pain is relieved [10].

In patients without frequent and disabling attacks, preventive treatment should be initiated. We recommend lamotrigine at a dose of 100–400 mg/day in the first step [11]. The treatment goal should be reached by increasing the dose by 25 mg/day in the first two weeks, 50 mg/day in the third and fourth weeks, and 50 mg once a week after initiation. Generally, 200 mg/day is the maintenance dose for patients, but it may be necessary to increase the dose up to 400 mg/day to be considered lamotrigine-refractory. Since the success of alternative therapies may be low in lamotrigine-resistant patients, preventive treatment with lamotrigine should be insisted [11].

In patients who cannot tolerate lamotrigine or have refractory pain, gabapentin, oxcarbazepine, topiramate, carbamazepine, and duloxetine can be started [11]. They may also be considered as an adjunct to lamotrigine. Additional oral preventive therapies are summarized in Table 9.3.

If oral treatment fails or is not tolerated, occipital nerve blocks and botulinum toxin applications can be performed. Occipital nerve blockade is performed with 2% lidocaine and 8 mg dexamethasone in a 1:1 mixture and approximately 1/4 of

Table 9.3 Oral medical treatments used for the treatment of SUNCT [12]

Drug	Maintenance dose	Adverse effect	Comment
Lamotrigine	100–400 mg/day	Tremor, Stevens-Johnson syndrome, influenza-like illness, headache	Primary therapeutic agent, gradually adjust dosage
Oxcarbazepine	300–2400 mg/day	Hyponatremia, nausea, dizziness, anxiety, ataxia, depressed mood	Could demonstrate superior efficacy compared to carbamazepine
Gabapentin	600–3600 mg/day	Somnolence, tiredness, dizziness, fatigue, central nervous system (CNS) depressed mood, ataxia	Alternative treatment option for SUNCT
Topiramate	50–400 mg/day	Drowsiness, depressed mood, nephrolithiasis, anxiety, cognitive dysfunction, angle closure glaucoma	Consider supplementary treatment options improved therapeutic outcomes in SUNCT
Carbamazepine	200–1600 mg/day	Cognitive dysfunction, dizziness, ataxia, anxiety, depressed mood, nausea, hyponatremia	Titrate slowly Demonstrates reduced therapeutic efficacy relative to alternative medications

the cases respond [4, 11]. Botulinum toxin can be applied to the painful area at 1.5 cm intervals on the epidermis, 2.5–5 IU. This treatment, which is useful in patients with trigeminal neuralgia, may also be effective in patients with SUNCT [4, 12]. Calcitonin gene-related peptide (CGRP) antagonist therapies are beneficial in some patient groups [12].

9.7 Refractory SUNCT and Surgical Treatments

Patients who do not respond to oral therapies and other transitional therapies are considered refractory SUNCT. We use surgical treatment options for patients with refractory SUNCT. Microvascular decompression (MVD), occipital nerve stimulation (ONS), and deep brain stimulation (DBS) are among these surgical options. MVD is one of the options that can be used as a treatment, especially in the presence of an aberrant trigeminal vascular loop [13]. ONS aims at pain desensitization by continuous occipital nerve stimulation, resulting in increase in the traffic in the trigeminal pain pathway [14]. DBS treatment applied to the posterior hypothalamus and ventral tegmentum of the mesencephalon showed near-complete improvement in refractory SUNCT patients [15]. Although it is a very effective treatment, due to serious adverse effects (hemorrhage in the brain stem, vertigo, permanent diplopia), this treatment should be kept as a reserve for refractory patients.

9.8 Conclusion

SUNCT is a severe and disabling headache associated with unilateral cranial autonomic syndromes. It is crucial to accurately diagnose SUNCT and differentiate it from other types of autonomic headaches. Patients with severe and frequent headache attacks should be treated acutely to stop the pain. In the presence of SUNCT, structural and vascular anomalies should be ruled out, at least by neuroimaging. In the absence of response to prophylactic treatments, occipital nerve blockade and botulinum toxin applications can be tried. In refractory cases, appropriate surgical procedures may be performed.

References

1. Headache Classification Committee of the International Headache Society (IHS) The International Classification of Headache Disorders, 3rd ed. Cephalalgia. 2018;38(1):1–211. https://doi.org/10.1177/0333102417738202. PMID: 29368949.
2. Williams MH, Broadley SA. SUNCT and SUNA: clinical features and medical treatment. J Clin Neurosci. 2008;15(5):526–34. https://doi.org/10.1016/j.jocn.2006.09.006. Epub 2008 Mar 5. PMID: 18325769.
3. Lambru G, Rantell K, Levy A, Matharu MS. A prospective comparative study and analysis of predictors of SUNA and SUNCT. Neurology. 2019;93(12):e1127–37. https://doi.org/10.1212/WNL.0000000000008134. Epub 2019 Aug 19. PMID: 31427501.
4. Kang MK, Cho SJ. SUNCT, SUNA and short-lasting unilateral neuralgiform headache attacks: debates and an update. Cephalalgia. 2024;44(2):3331024241232256. https://doi.org/10.1177/03331024241232256. PMID: 38415675.
5. Cohen A. SUN: short-lasting unilateral neuralgiform headache attacks. Headache. 2017;57(6):1010–20. https://doi.org/10.1111/head.13088. Epub 2017 May 4. PMID: 28474431.
6. Burish MJ, Rozen TD. Trigeminal autonomic Cephalalgias. Neurol Clin. 2019;37(4):847–69. https://doi.org/10.1016/j.ncl.2019.07.001. Epub 2019 Aug 24. PMID: 31563236.7.
7. Pareja JA, Sjaastad O. SUNCT syndrome. A clinical review. Headache. 1997;37(4):195–202. https://doi.org/10.1046/j.1526-4610.1997.3704195.x. PMID: 9150613.
8. Cohen AS, Matharu MS, Goadsby PJ. Short-lasting unilateral neuralgiform headache attacks with conjunctival injection and tearing (SUNCT) or cranial autonomic features (SUNA)--a prospective clinical study of SUNCT and SUNA. Brain. 2006;129(Pt 10):2746–60. https://doi.org/10.1093/brain/awl202. Epub 2006 Aug 11. PMID: 16905753.
9. Cação G, Correia FD, Pereira-Monteiro J. SUNCT syndrome: a cohort of 15 Portuguese patients. Cephalalgia. 2016;36(10):1002–6. https://doi.org/10.1177/0333102415620252. Epub 2015 Nov 26. PMID: 26611683.
10. Baraldi C, Pellesi L, Guerzoni S, Cainazzo MM, Pini LA. Therapeutical approaches to paroxysmal hemicrania, hemicrania continua and short lasting unilateral neuralgiform headache attacks: a critical appraisal. J Headache Pain. 2017;18(1):71. https://doi.org/10.1186/s10194-017-0777-3. Epub 2017 Jul 20. PMID: 28730562; PMCID: PMC5519518.
11. Lambru G, Stubberud A, Rantell K, Lagrata S, Tronvik E, Matharu MS. Medical treatment of SUNCT and SUNA: a prospective open-label study including single-arm meta-analysis. J Neurol Neurosurg Psychiatry. 2021;92(3):233–41. https://doi.org/10.1136/jnnp-2020-323999. Epub 2020 Dec 24. PMID: 33361408; PMCID: PMC7892380.

12. Duggal AK, Chowdhury D. SUNCT and SUNA: An Update. Neurol India. 2021;69(Supplement):S144–59. https://doi.org/10.4103/0028-3886.315990. PMID: 34003160.
13. Sebastian S, Schweitzer D, Tan L, Broadley SA. Role of trigeminal microvascular decompression in the treatment of SUNCT and SUNA. Curr Pain Headache Rep. 2013;17(5):332. https://doi.org/10.1007/s11916-013-0332-0. PMID: 23564233.
14. Lambru G, Shanahan P, Watkins L, Matharu MS. Occipital nerve stimulation in the treatment of medically intractable SUNCT and SUNA. Pain Physician. 2014;17(1):29–41. PMID: 24452643.
15. Miller S, Akram H, Lagrata S, Hariz M, Zrinzo L, Matharu M. Ventral tegmental area deep brain stimulation in refractory short-lasting unilateral neuralgiform headache attacks. Brain. 2016;139(Pt 10):2631–40. https://doi.org/10.1093/brain/aww204. Epub 2016 Aug 14. PMID: 27524793.

Chapter 10
Short-Lasting Unilateral Neuralgiform Headache Attacks with Cranial Autonomic Symptoms (SUNA)

Gabriele Sebastianelli, Pubudu Amarasena, and Francesca Puledda

10.1 Introduction

Short-lasting unilateral neuralgiform headache attacks are a group of primary headache disorders classified under trigeminal autonomic cephalalgias (TACs). They share some clinical characteristics with TACs, including strictly unilateral head pain in the trigeminal territory and cranial autonomic symptoms (CAS). Their prevalence and frequency are uncertain. A recent meta-analysis revealed that they are present in approximately 0.32% of patients evaluated for headache or facial pain [1]. Additionally, a population-based nationwide registry in Norway reported a 1-year prevalence of 1.2 per 100,000 [2], representing the rarest headache disorders among the TACs.

The third edition of the International Classification of Headache Disorders (ICHD-3) [3] recognizes two different subtypes depending on the presence of the associated CAS: short-lasting unilateral neuralgiform headache attacks with conjunctival injection and tearing (SUNCT) and short-lasting unilateral neuralgiform headache attacks with cranial autonomic symptoms (SUNA). However, it is unclear whether these represent two separate entities or different manifestations of the same disease [1].

G. Sebastianelli
Sapienza University of Rome, Department of Medico-Surgical Sciences and Biotechnologies, Polo Pontino, Latina, Italy

P. Amarasena · F. Puledda (✉)
Headache Group, Wolfson Sensory, Pain and Regeneration Centre, King's College London, London, UK
e-mail: francesca.puledda@kcl.ac.uk

D. Uludüz et al. (eds.), *Rare Causes of Headache Disorders*, Headache,
https://doi.org/10.1007/978-3-032-10242-3_10

This chapter provides a comprehensive overview of the clinical characteristics and pathophysiological mechanisms of SUNA, aiming to improve the identification and distinction of this condition from other TACs and offer strategies for its management.

10.2 Pathophysiology

The exact pathophysiology of SUNA and its relationship to SUNCT remains unknown. Their pathophysiology involves a complex interaction between central and peripheral nervous structures, with the trigeminal autonomic reflex (TAR) playing a pivotal role in developing the prominent CAS that accompany the pain. TAR is composed of an afferent and an efferent limb, the trigeminal and the facial nerve, respectively. Various nociceptive triggers can activate the afferent limb, which transmits the stimulus to the second-order neurons into the trigeminocervical complex (TCC). The TCC has a reflex connection into the pons with the superior salivatory nucleus (SSN). The efferent pathway arises from the preganglionic parasympathetic fibers of the SSN, which through the greater superficial petrosal nerve are conveyed to the sphenopalatine ganglion (SPG), where postganglionic parasympathetic fibers arise and innervate nasal and lacrimal glands (Fig. 10.1) [4–6].

A peripheral neurovascular conflict with morphological changes is highly prevalent on the symptomatic side in patients with SUNA and SUNCT, and this could be responsible for the peripheral ignition of pain [7]. This suggests a possible shared pathophysiology with trigeminal neuralgia (TN), indicating a potential overlap between these conditions [7]. However, central permissive mechanisms, such as the disinhibition of the TAR, are needed for the development of prominent CAS and the reoccurrence of attacks without the refractory period [8, 9], which distinguishes SUNA from TN. The posterior hypothalamus was shown to activate during spontaneous SUNCT attacks [10, 11] and was hypothesized to be responsible for the central disinhibition of TAR [8, 9], playing a pivotal role in the pathophysiology of short-lasting unilateral neuralgiform headache attacks [10]. Indeed, the posterior hypothalamus is connected with the TCC by the trigeminohypothalamic and reticulohypothalamic tracts, by which it receives nociceptive signals from areas innervated by the trigeminal system (such as cranial skin, meninges, and intracranial blood vessels) [12, 13]. Through the secretion of orexin neuropeptides, the posterior hypothalamus can regulate autonomic functions and modulate the nociception activity of the TCC, including nociceptive processing of meningeal input [14]. Furthermore, several studies have demonstrated that hypothalamic deep brain stimulation reduces pain in patients with drug-resistant SUNA and SUNCT, confirming its central role in the pathophysiology of these conditions [15–17].

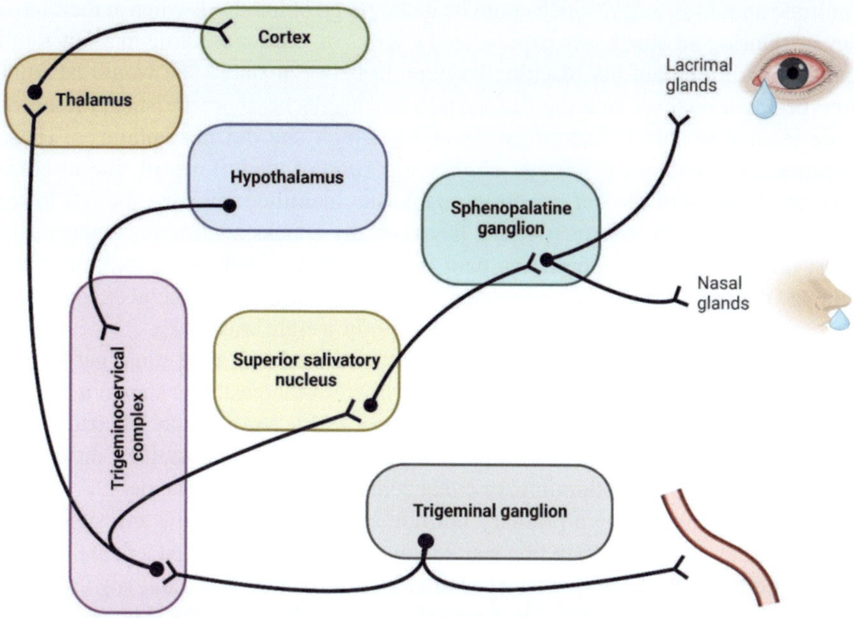

Fig. 10.1 Trigeminal autonomic reflex (TAR) and its connectionsThe trigeminal autonomic reflex (TAR) afferent limb is constituted by the nerve endings of the trigeminal nerve that innervate the intracranial blood vessels. These fibers have their cell bodies in the trigeminal ganglion and transmit the signals to the second order neurons into the trigeminocervical complex (TCC), which is directly modulated by the hypothalamus. The TCC has a reflex connection with the superior salivatory nucleus, from which originate the preganglionic parasympathetic fibers that form the efferent limb of the TAR. Through the greater superficial petrosal nerve, these fibers synapse into the sphenopalatine ganglion, where postganglionic parasympathetic fibers arise and innervate nasal and lacrimal glands. Additionally, pain signals reach the cortex by ascending from TCC to the third-order neurons in the thalamusCreated in BioRender. https://BioRender.com/f68r610

10.3 Case Presentation

Our patient is a 38-year-old teacher who presented to the emergency department due to worsening of her preexisting facial pain and was referred to the headache team. She had recently moved to the area and had been investigated and treated in several local services in her previous residence. She has responded poorly to various treatment options offered previously and was on gabapentin 300 mg three times a day, which had been partially beneficial. Over the week preceding her visit, the frequency and severity of her facial pain had significantly worsened. She had been unable to eat or drink and had to take leave from work due to the pain.

Her pain had started at the age of 32 years, and she did not recall having any significant headache prior to this. Her facial pain was characterized by frequent, sharp, electrical shock-like pain, mainly affecting the forehead, periorbital and maxillary region on the left side. Attacks last between 30 s to 2 min, and she described multiple attacks in a day, which could be in the range of hundreds when at their most severe. During an attack, she experienced a series of stabs presenting in a saw tooth pattern, with the pain not reaching baseline in between stabs. She would be pain-free between attacks. Delving further into her headache characteristics, the headache team was able to identify a few CAS which she did not volunteer. These included grittiness of the left eye, slight congestion of the left nostril, and discomfort and fullness of the left ear during pain. She identified touching the left lower eyelid and chewing food as triggers; however, the attacks occurred spontaneously most of the time. If triggered, the pain would continue without a break until she stopped the trigger itself (e.g., touching the face or eating). Her general examination and neurological examination were normal. Body weight was 76 kg.

A magnetic resonance imaging (MRI) scan of the head, trigeminal nerve, and internal acoustic meatus with contrast, performed in the past, had shown a loop of the left superior cerebellar artery near the root entry zone of the left trigeminal nerve. There was no signal abnormality at the root entry zone itself or distortion, displacement, abnormal thinning, or enhancement of the trigeminal nerve.

Blood tests, including a pituitary hormone panel, did not show any significant abnormalities. When the pain first started, our patient had consulted a dental practitioner and had treatment for a decayed upper left molar tooth without any improvement in the facial pain. Her local neurology team then saw her. She received a diagnosis of TN, and was treated with several medications including carbamazepine, oxcarbazepine, pregabalin, amitriptyline, and baclofen with minimal improvement. She had also undergone microvascular decompression of the left trigeminal nerve, which resulted in pain freedom for 3 weeks, followed by a return to her pre-surgery baseline.

TN and SUNA were considered the most likely explanations for her headache. Several characteristics supported SUNA over trigeminal neuralgia. These included the ipsilateral CAS and the lack of a refractory period. Additionally, the pain localization in the distribution of the ophthalmic and maxillary branches of the trigeminal nerve favored the SUNA diagnosis, as TN commonly involves the maxillary and mandibular branches and involvement of the ophthalmology branch is less common. It is interesting to note that the brain MRI scan showed a blood vessel in close proximity to the ipsilateral trigeminal nerve. However, there was no distortion or displacement of the trigeminal nerve. Also, she did not have a sustained, satisfactory response to microvascular decompression. These factors suggest that TN was less likely to be the cause of her facial pain.

Due to the significant impact in her quality-of-life short-term bridging therapies were considered as a first step. Greater occipital nerve injection was considered unsafe due to the previous history of microvascular decompression surgery and a decision was taken to start lidocaine infusion.

She was admitted to the critical care unit and baseline tests including an electrocardiogram (ECG), liver and renal function tests, electrolytes, and a pregnancy test were arranged, all of which were within expected ranges. She was started on intravenous lidocaine with continuous cardiac monitoring at rate of 1 mg/min further increased by 0.5 mg/min daily. She noticed an improvement in the severity and frequency of attacks at a dose of 3 mg/min. The infusion was continued at this rate for a total treatment duration of 7 days, at which her symptoms significantly improved. She was discharged on her the same dose of gabapentin.

About 4 weeks after leaving the hospital she noted a slight worsening of symptoms and lamotrigine was added to her preventive medications, which was titrated up to 100 mg twice a day and the combination resulted in a significant improvement of the frequency and severity of attacks.

10.4 Case Discussion

TACs are often misdiagnosed, leading to an average diagnostic delay of about 5 years [18, 19]. This not only delays appropriate treatment but also risks exposing patients to ineffective or potentially harmful therapies. Our case illustrates these pitfalls well. Indeed, it showed how delays can result in a significant negative impact on quality of life, which could have been minimized if the correct diagnosis had been made earlier.

A thorough history is paramount in evaluating headache disorders. Rather than passively listening to the patient, history-taking should be an active data-gathering process, allowing the clinician to identify key diagnostic clues. An example stemming from this case is the presence of cranial autonomic symptoms and refractory periods for triggers, which paved the way for a correct diagnosis of SUNA after a delay of 6 years. As Sir William Osler supposedly stated, "*Listen to your patient, he is telling you the diagnosis*" [20].

10.5 Clinical Characteristics

SUNA is characterized by unilateral head or facial pain occurring as either single or multiple stabs and associated with ipsilateral cranial autonomic symptoms. It differs from SUNCT by the presence of only one or neither between conjunctival injection and lacrimation (Headache Classification Committee of the International Headache Society (IHS) The International Classification of Headache Disorders, third edition [3].

The majority of patients with SUNA have a primary chronic form [1, 21–23]. While data regarding periodicity is scarce, a median of four bouts per year lasting 2 weeks was noted in those with episodic SUNA [22].

SUNA is typically unilateral, but side variability has been observed in a small proportion of patients [21, 22, 24, 25]. Pain is most often felt in trigeminal areas; however, other areas of the head supplied by the C2/C3 nerve roots through the occipital nerves can also be affected in around a third to a half of the patients [1, 21]. Of the trigeminal areas, pain is most often felt in the distribution of the ophthalmic branch of the trigeminal nerve, followed by maxillary branch and less often in the mandibular distribution [1, 21, 22, 24].

The pain in SUNA is moderate to severe, with a character most often described as stabbing, jabbing, electric shock-like, or shooting [1, 22, 23, 26]. Three distinct patterns a attacks have been described (Fig. 10.2): single stabs, group of stabs where the stabs occur back-to-back with the pain returning to the baseline after each stab, and saw-tooth pattern in which there are multiple stabs in which the pain does not return to the baseline in between attacks [1, 21, 26, 27]. The duration of an attack typically ranges between 1 and 600 s, and the frequency of attacks ranges between 1 and 100 with an average of around 20 attacks a day [1, 22].

Presence of cranial autonomic symptoms ipsilateral to the pain is essential for the diagnosis of short-lasting unilateral neuralgiform headache attacks and the presence of only one or neither of conjunctival injection and tearing differentiates SUNA from SUNCT (Headache Classification Committee of the International Headache Society (IHS) The International Classification of Headache Disorders, third edition 2018). Lacrimation, nasal symptoms, and ptosis are the most reported cranial autonomic symptom in SUNA [1, 21–23, 25].

Trigger factors are a well-recognized phenomenon in SUNA, and most patients experience both triggered and spontaneous attacks. While spontaneous attacks can be completely absent in a small percentage of patients, this is infrequent. Cutaneous triggers such as light touch and cold wind, and intraoral stimuli such as eating and brushing are the most frequently reported triggers.

Classically patients with SUNA would be pain free in between attacks; however, interictal background pain is not uncommon in clinical practice. In these patients,

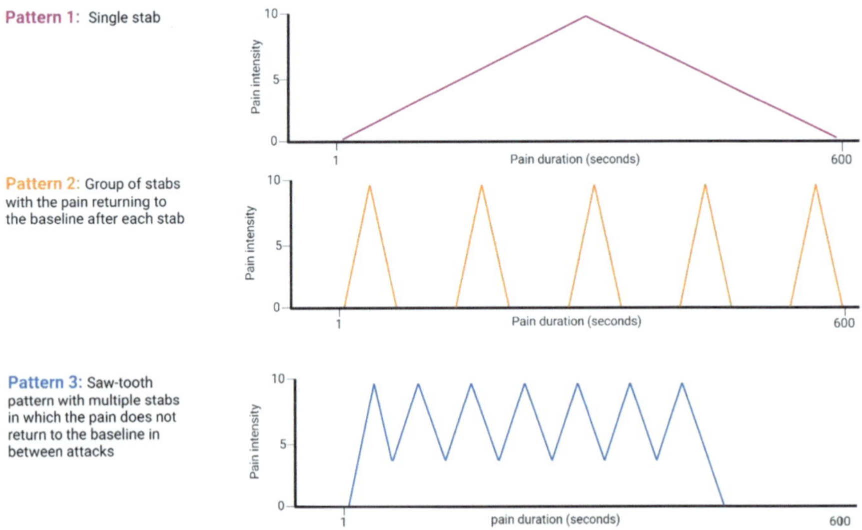

Fig. 10.2 Patterns of pain in short-lasting unilateral neuralgiform headache attacks with cranial autonomic symptoms (SUNA). (Created in BioRender. Sebastianelli, G. (2025) https://BioRender.com/h08m845)

the headache phenotype should be carefully evaluated to identify the presence of other primary headache disorders, such as migraine or hemicrania continua, as well as secondary headache disorders, particularly medication-overuse headache [21, 22].

Although neurological examination is generally normal in patients with SUNA, sensory abnormalities, such as reduced sensation or hyperesthesia, have been noted occasionally [21].

10.6 Diagnostic Algorithm

Differential diagnoses of SUNA include TN, primary stabbing headache (PSH), and other TACs, including SUNCT, paroxysmal hemicrania (PH), and cluster headache (CH). SUNA is a clinical diagnosis, and no tests exist to confirm it. Various clinical features can help narrow the differentials and guide the correct diagnosis. These include the types of associated CAS, pain duration, frequency, triggers, refractory periods, and treatment response.

The distinction between SUNA and SUNCT is mainly due to the obligatory occurrence of both conjunctival injection and tearing in SUNCT during the pain, while only one or neither of the symptoms could be present during SUNA attacks. Additionally, the triggering rate by cutaneous stimuli is reported to be lower in SUNA than in SUNCT [21].

TN remains the main and the most challenging differential diagnosis. Several similarities are shared between these diseases, including clinical features, such as quality, localization, and duration of pain, cutaneous triggers, and response to similar medications [8]. Indeed, in both TN and SUNA, the pain can involve the three branches of distribution of the trigeminal nerve [21, 28, 29], with neuralgiform features described as sharp, stabbing, burning, or electrical shock-like, lasting from a few seconds to a minute. However, SUNA has the presence of constant pain ipsilateral to the side of the attacks in approximately 50% of patients [21], which is, by definition, not possible in TN. Indeed, patients with TN with constant background pain meet the diagnosis of trigeminal neuralgia with concomitant continuous pain (Headache Classification Committee of the International Headache Society (IHS) The International Classification of Headache Disorders, third edition 2018) [3]. Additionally, both SUNA and TN can be triggered by similar cutaneous/intraoral triggers, including chewing, eating, nose blowing, touching the face, and brushing teeth [21, 30]. However, the rate of cutaneous stimuli in triggering attacks has a lower frequency in SUNA than in SUNCT [21] and is lower than in TN [31] and a refractory period, in which the attacks cannot be triggered or cannot start spontaneously for a few seconds to minutes immediately after an attack is typical of TN and rare in SUNA [1, 21, 22, 24, 26, 27, 32].

Both conditions respond to similar medications, including sodium channel blockers. However, lamotrigine is considered the first choice for the preventive treatment of SUNA, while oxcarbazepine and carbamazepine are considered second-line treatments for SUNA and first-line choices in TN [33].

One of the most important distinguishing features between TN and SUNA is the presence of prominent CAS in the latter. These include conjunctival injection or tearing, nasal congestion, rhinorrhea, eyelid oedema, facial sweating or flushing, aural fullness, miosis, and ptosis (Headache Classification Committee of the International Headache Society (IHS) The International Classification of Headache Disorders, third edition 2018) [3]. However, it is important to note that CAS symptoms can also be present in TN, including tearing [29, 30], but are mainly described as mild.

CH and PH are classified as TACs and share the strictly unilateral side of the pain and cranial autonomic symptoms with SUNA. The duration of pain is crucial in distinguishing SUNA from CH or PH. By definition, SUNA has the shortest duration, ranging from 1 to 600 s, while CH can last from 15 to 180 min and PH from 2 to 30 min. Then, PH can sometimes mimic SUNA in the shortest attacks. However, the key element in distinguishing between these two conditions is the response to indomethacin, which is absolute in PH while being absent in SUNA. Additionally, in contrast to SUNA, PH attacks are mainly spontaneous and are not caused by cutaneous facial triggers [34, 35].

PSH is characterized by localized stabs of pain in the head that last up to a few seconds (Headache Classification Committee of the International Headache Society (IHS) The International Classification of Headache Disorders, third edition 2018) [3]. Unlike SUNA, there are no cranial autonomic symptoms in PSH. In most cases, the pain is not triggerable and is located in extra trigeminal regions, primarily in the auricular, posterior parietal, occipital, and nuchal areas [36].

Finally, it is important to exclude secondary causes in patients with clinical features of SUNA, as different secondary causes that can mimic short-lasting unilateral neuralgiform headache attacks are reported in the literature [37]. These include vascular loops compressing the entry zone of the trigeminal root [37, 38] and pathologies involving the cerebellopontine angle [39], brainstem [40–42], or cavernous sinus. Additional investigations, such as neuroimaging, are required in all patients with a clinical presentation of SUNA.

Step 1: Clinical Suspicion.

- *Identify key symptoms:*
  - Moderate or severe strictly unilateral head pain, with trigeminal distribution.
  - Pain lasts for 1–600 s and occurs as single stabs, series of stabs, or in a saw-tooth pattern.
  - Presence of cranial autonomic symptoms ipsilateral to the pain.

Step 2: Narrow the Differentials and Differentiate from Other TACs:

- *Identify clinical differences*:
  - Response to indomethacin.
  - Pain features: location, radiation, and duration.
  - Triggers.
  - Refractory period.
  - Entity of cranial autonomic symptoms.
  - Other accompanying symptoms.

Step 3: Apply ICHD-3 Diagnostic Criteria for Short-Lasting Unilateral Neuralgiform Headache Attacks (2018).

A. At least 20 attacks fulfilling criteria B–D.
B. Moderate or severe unilateral head pain, with orbital, supraorbital, temporal, and/or other trigeminal distribution, lasting for 1–600 s and occurring as single stabs, series of stabs, or in a saw-tooth pattern.
C. At least one of the following five cranial autonomic symptoms or signs, ipsilateral to the pain:
   (a) Conjunctival injection and/or lacrimation.
   (b) Nasal congestion and/or rhinorrhea.
   (c) Eyelid oedema.
   (d) Forehead and facial sweating.
   (e) Forehead and facial flushing.
   (f) Sensation of fullness in the ear.
   (g) Miosis and/or ptosis.
D. Occurring with a frequency of at least one a day.
E. Not better accounted for by another ICHD-3 diagnosis.

Step 4: Distinguish SUNA from SUNCT.

- *Apply ICHD-3 diagnostic criteria for SUNA (2018)*:
  A. Attacks fulfilling criteria for 3.3 short-lasting unilateral neuralgiform headache attacks and criterion B below.
  B. Only one or neither of conjunctival injection and lacrimation (tearing).

Step 5: Distinguish episodic from chronic SUNA.

- *Investigate for pain-free periods lasting at least 3 months (2018)*:
  - Episodic: At least two bouts lasting from 7 days to 1 year (when untreated) and separated by pain-free remission periods of ≥3 months.
  - Chronic: Attacks occurring without a remission period or with remissions lasting <3 months, for at least 1 year.

Step 6: Exclude secondary causes and neurovascular compression:

- *Perform brain MRI*:
  - Dedicated views of the pituitary glands and the trigeminal nerves.

10.7 Management

Due to the short-lasting nature of the attacks, acute treatment options are unlikely to be of any benefit in SUNA. For patients with infrequent and non-debilitating attacks preventive medications can be considered, while those with frequent and debilitating attacks may benefit from short-term bridging treatments as a first step to improve the quality of life. Invasive surgical procedures have been used for patients refractory to conventional treatment options; however, these need further research to determine their effectiveness in the management of SUNA.

Intravenous lidocaine is considered as the first-line bridging treatment option for both SUNCT and SUNA. Intravenous lidocaine can lead to a significant improvement of symptoms in 80–90% of patients with SUNA and the benefit can last about 3 weeks on average [25, 27, 33]. Lidocaine is usually administered as an intravenous infusion at a rate of 1–4 mg/min up to 7 days and requires continuous cardiac monitoring during the infusion [43].

Greater occipital nerve blockade is another short-term treatment option which is used for most primary headache disorders. Although not as effective as lidocaine, a beneficial effect lasting about 40 days on average can be seen in around 40% of patients with SUNA.

Intravenous dihydroergotamine, sumatriptan, high-flow oxygen, corticosteroids. and intramuscular indomethacin injections have not shown consistent efficacy to be considered as short-term bridging treatments for SUNA [25, 44].

Lamotrigine is the most effective preventive treatment. A single-center, prospective, open-label study reported at least some degree of headache improvement in 72% of patients with SUNA, and at least 50% improvement in the number of attacks, attack severity, or duration in 58% of patients [33, 45].

Alternative medical treatment options that can be considered if lamotrigine is not tolerated or ineffective include oxcarbazepine, carbamazepine, gabapentin, pregabalin, and topiramate. Limited data suggest that duloxetine, lacosamide, and mexiletine can also be considered as treatment options. Topiramate has the highest rate of discontinuation (32%), followed by pregabalin, carbamazepine and oxcarbazepine [23, 25, 27, 33, 45].

Non-invasive vagal nerve stimulation (nVNS) has shown some efficacy in primary headache disorders including migraine, cluster headache, and indomethacin responsive headache disorders; however, data on the efficacy of nVNS in SUNA from a single case series with two patients have not been encouraging and needs further research [46, 47].

Several studies have demonstrated an increased prevalence of neurovascular contact on the ipsilateral trigeminal nerve in patients with short-lasting unilateral neuralgiform headache attacks [7, 27]. Based on this observation, microvascular decompression of the trigeminal nerve has been considered as a treatment option for patients with refractory SUNA. A series of 47 patients with short-lasting unilateral neuralgiform headache attacks which included 16 patients with SUNA reported a positive response to microvascular decompression in 62.5% of the SUNA cohort (mean follow-up of 57 months) [48]. Cerebrospinal fluid leak, neuropathic pain on the wound site, and facial numbness were the most frequent complications [48].

Occipital nerve stimulation has been used for the treatment of primary headache disorders and limited data suggests that this can be effective in about two-thirds of the patients with short-lasting unilateral neuralgiform headache attacks [49]. Lead-related problems and infections were the common causes of surgical revision in patients who had occipital nerve stimulation for headache disorders [50].

In a small case series, pulsed radiofrequency targeting the sphenopalatine ganglion was reported to be beneficial in seven out of nine patients for a median of 6 months [51]. Several studies have also reported beneficial effects of deep brain stimulation in patients with short-lasting unilateral neuralgiform headache attacks, targeting the hypothalamus or the ventral tegmental area [15, 16, 49]. Further studies are needed to confirm the efficacy of these treatment modalities in the treatment of SUNA.

Destructive procedures targeting the trigeminal nerve and the sphenopalatine ganglion including glycerol rhizotomy, radiofrequency thermocoagulation, and gamma knife radiosurgery have been used to treat short-lasting unilateral neuralgiform headache attacks [52–54]. However, symptoms recurrence after these procedures is not uncommon and caution is needed when considering these treatment options due to complications associated with these procedures such as anesthesia dolorosa and trigeminal sensory impairment [52, 53, 55].

10.8 Conclusion

SUNA is a rare and challenging primary headache disorder that is often misdiagnosed. Investigating subtle symptoms, such as the lack of refractory period, the presence of CAS, and the localization of pain, is crucial to distinguishing SUNA from other diseases with similar presentations. Additionally, it is mandatory to exclude secondary causes in all patients presenting with clinical features suggestive of SUNA.

This chapter has provided an overview of the pathophysiology, case presentation, diagnostic approach, and management strategies for SUNA, emphasizing the importance of detailed history-taking to identify key diagnostic clues. By improving the identification of this rare disease, clinicians can select the most appropriate treatment and reduce the burden of disability associated with it.

References

1. Larsen JG, Henningsen MJ, Karlsson WK, Christensen RH, Al-Khazali HM, Amin FM, Ashina H. Epidemiology and clinical features of short-lasting unilateral neuralgiform headache attacks: a systematic review and meta-analysis. Cephalalgia. 2024;44(8):03331024241271976. https://doi.org/10.1177/03331024241271976.
2. Hagen K. One-year prevalence of cluster headache, hemicrania continua, paroxysmal hemicrania and SUNCT in Norway: a population-based nationwide registry study. J Headache Pain. 2024;25(1):30. https://doi.org/10.1186/s10194-024-01738-x.
3. Headache Classification Committee of the International Headache Society (IHS). The international classification of headache disorders, 3rd edition. Cephalalgia. 2018;38(1):1–211. https://doi.org/10.1177/0333102417738202.
4. May A, Goadsby PJ. The trigeminovascular system in humans: pathophysiologic implications for primary headache syndromes. J Cereb Blood Flow Metab. 1999;19(2):115–27. https://doi.org/10.1097/00004647-199902000-00001.
5. Eller M, Goadsby P. Trigeminal autonomic cephalalgias. Oral Dis. 2016;22(1):1–8. https://doi.org/10.1111/odi.12263.
6. Coppola G, Abagnale C, Sebastianelli G, Goadsby PJ. Pathophysiology of cluster headache: from the trigeminovascular system to the cerebral networks. Cephalalgia. 2024;44(2):3331024231209317. https://doi.org/10.1177/03331024231209317.
7. Lambru G, Rantell K, O'Connor E, Levy A, Davagnanam I, Zrinzo L, Matharu M. Trigeminal neurovascular contact in SUNCT and SUNA: a cross-sectional magnetic resonance study. Brain. 2020;143(12):3619–28. https://doi.org/10.1093/brain/awaa331.
8. Lambru G, Matharu MS. SUNCT, SUNA and trigeminal neuralgia: different disorders or variants of the same disorder? Curr Opin Neurol. 2014;27(3):325. https://doi.org/10.1097/WCO.0000000000000090.
9. Leone M, Bussone G. Pathophysiology of trigeminal autonomic cephalalgias. Lancet Neurol. 2009;8(8):755–64. https://doi.org/10.1016/S1474-4422(09)70133-4.
10. May A, Bahra A, Büchel C, Turner R, Goadsby PJ. Functional magnetic resonance imaging in spontaneous attacks of SUNCT. Ann Neurol. 1999;46(5):791–4. https://doi.org/10.1002/1531-8249(199911)46:5<791::AID-ANA18>3.0.CO;2-8.
11. Sprenger T, Valet M, Platzer S, Pfaffenrath V, Steude U, Tölle TR. SUNCT: bilateral hypothalamic activation during headache attacks and resolving of symptoms after trigeminal decompression. Pain. 2005;113(3):422–6. https://doi.org/10.1016/j.pain.2004.09.021.
12. Malick A, Burstein R. Cells of origin of the trigeminohypothalamic tract in the rat. J Comp Neurol. 1998;400(1):125–44. https://doi.org/10.1002/(SICI)1096-9861(19981012)400:1<125::AID-CNE9>3.0.CO;2-B.
13. Malick A, Strassman RM, Burstein R. Trigeminohypothalamic and reticulohypothalamic tract neurons. J Neurophysiol. 2000;84(4):2078–112. https://doi.org/10.1152/jn.2000.84.4.2078.
14. Bartsch T, Levy MJ, Knight YE, Goadsby PJ. Differential modulation of nociceptive dural input to orexin receptors in the posterior hypothalamic area. Pain. 2004;109(3):367–78. https://doi.org/10.1016/j.pain.2004.02.005.
15. Leone M, Franzini A, D'Andrea G, Broggi G, Casucci G, Bussone G. Deep brain stimulation to relieve drug-resistant SUNCT. Ann Neurol. 2005;57(6):924–7. https://doi.org/10.1002/ana.20507.
16. Lyons MK, Dodick DW, Evidente VG. Responsiveness of SUNCT to hypothalamic deep brain stimulation. J Neurosurg. 2009;110(2):279–81. https://doi.org/10.3171/2008.4.17493.
17. Bartsch T, et al. Deep brain stimulation in intractable SUNCT. Cephalalgia. 2011;31(13):1405–8. https://doi.org/10.1177/0333102411409070.
18. Viana M, et al. Diagnostic and therapeutic errors in TACs and hemicrania continua: a systematic review. J Headache Pain. 2013;14(1):14. https://doi.org/10.1186/1129-2377-14-14.
19. Wei DY, Moreno-Ajona D, Renton T, Goadsby PJ. TACs presenting in an orofacial pain clinic. J Headache Pain. 2019;20(1):69. https://doi.org/10.1186/s10194-019-1019-7.

20. Aronson JK. When I use a word... Listening to the patient. BMJ. 2022;376:o646. https://doi.org/10.1136/bmj.o646.
21. Cohen AS, Matharu MS, Goadsby PJ. SUNCT and SUNA: a prospective clinical study. Brain. 2006;129(10):2746–60. https://doi.org/10.1093/brain/awl202.
22. Lambru G, Rantell K, Levy A, Matharu MS. A prospective comparative study of SUNA and SUNCT. Neurology. 2019;93(12):e1127–37. https://doi.org/10.1212/WNL.0000000000008134.
23. Prakash S, et al. Retrospective comparative study in patients with SUNA and SUNCT. Ann Indian Acad Neurol. 2023;26(5):672–7. https://doi.org/10.4103/aian.aian_502_23.
24. Zhang S, et al. SUNCT vs. SUNA: multicenter study. J Headache Pain. 2022;23(1):137. https://doi.org/10.1186/s10194-022-01509-6.
25. Weng HY, et al. Phenotypic and treatment outcome data on SUNCT and SUNA. Cephalalgia. 2018;38(9):1554–63. https://doi.org/10.1177/0333102417739304.
26. Wei DY, Yuan Ong JJ, Goadsby PJ. Overview of TACs: diagnosis and management. Ann Indian Acad Neurol. 2018;21(Suppl 1):S39–44. https://doi.org/10.4103/aian.AIAN_348_17.
27. Williams MH, Broadley SA. SUNCT and SUNA: clinical features and medical treatment. J Clin Neurosci. 2008;15(5):526–34. https://doi.org/10.1016/j.jocn.2006.09.006.
28. Katusic S, et al. Incidence and clinical features of trigeminal neuralgia. Ann Neurol. 1990;27(1):89–95. https://doi.org/10.1002/ana.410270114.
29. Simms HN, Honey CR. Autonomic symptoms in trigeminal neuralgia. J Neurosurg. 2011;115(2):210–6. https://doi.org/10.3171/2011.4.JNS101843.
30. Benoliel R, et al. From CTN to SUNHA. Headache. 2017;57(6):997–1009. https://doi.org/10.1111/head.13040.
31. Di Stefano G, et al. Triggering trigeminal neuralgia. Cephalalgia. 2018;38(6):1049–56. https://doi.org/10.1177/0333102417721677.
32. Kugelberg E, Lindblom U. Mechanism of pain in trigeminal neuralgia. J Neurol Neurosurg Psychiatry. 1959;22(1):36–43. https://doi.org/10.1136/jnnp.22.1.36.
33. Lambru G, et al. Medical treatment of SUNCT and SUNA. J Neurol Neurosurg Psychiatry. 2021;92(3):233–41. https://doi.org/10.1136/jnnp-2020-323999.
34. Sjaastad O. The fate of the first described cases. J Headache Pain. 2006;7(3):151–6. https://doi.org/10.1007/s10194-006-0303-5.
35. Cittadini E, Matharu MS, Goadsby PJ. Paroxysmal hemicrania: prospective study. Brain. 2008;131(4):1142–55. https://doi.org/10.1093/brain/awn010.
36. Fuh JL, Kuo KH, Wang SJ. Primary stabbing headache in a headache clinic. Cephalalgia. 2007;27(9):1005–9. https://doi.org/10.1111/j.1468-2982.2007.01365.x.
37. Arca KN, Halker Singh RB. SUNCT and SUNA: an update and review. Curr Pain Headache Rep. 2018;22(8):56. https://doi.org/10.1007/s11916-018-0707-3.
38. Köseoğlu E, et al. SUNCT syndrome and trigeminal nerve compression. Cephalalgia. 2005;25(6):473–5. https://doi.org/10.1111/j.1468-2982.2005.00875.x.
39. Talavera B, et al. SUNCT secondary to cerebellopontine angle meningioma. Pain Med. 2021;22(1):226–8. https://doi.org/10.1093/pm/pnaa105.
40. De Benedittis G. SUNCT associated with cavernous angioma. Cephalalgia. 1996;16(7):503–6. https://doi.org/10.1046/j.1468-2982.1996.1607503.x.
41. Jin D, et al. Secondary SUNCT due to medullary infarction. J Headache Pain. 2016;17(1):12. https://doi.org/10.1186/s10194-016-0604-2.
42. Lambru G, et al. Coexistent SUNCT and TN due to medullary infarction. Cephalalgia. 2017;37(5):486–90. https://doi.org/10.1177/0333102416652093.
43. Matharu MS, Cohen AS, Goadsby PJ. SUNCT responsive to lidocaine. Cephalalgia. 2004;24(11):985–92. https://doi.org/10.1111/j.1468-2982.2004.00886.x.
44. Lambru G, et al. SUNCT and SUNA exacerbation with IV DHE. Cephalalgia. 2015;35(12):1115–24. https://doi.org/10.1177/0333102415570495.
45. Baraldi C, et al. Therapeutical approaches to short-lasting neuralgiform headaches. J Headache Pain. 2017;18(1):71. https://doi.org/10.1186/s10194-017-0777-3.

46. Villar-Martinez MD, Goadsby PJ. Non-invasive vagal nerve stimulation. Front Pain Res. 2023;4:1062892. https://doi.org/10.3389/fpain.2023.1062892.
47. Trimboli M, et al. Non-invasive vagus nerve stimulation for refractory headaches. Cephalalgia. 2018;38(7):1276–85. https://doi.org/10.1177/0333102417731349.
48. Lambru G, et al. Trigeminal microvascular decompression for SUNCT/SUNA. Brain. 2022;145(8):2882–93. https://doi.org/10.1093/brain/awac109.
49. Miller S, Watkins L, Matharu M. Long-term follow-up with occipital nerve stimulation. Cephalalgia. 2018;38(5):933–42. https://doi.org/10.1177/0333102417721716.
50. Palmisani S, et al. Occipital nerve stimulation: a 6-year review. J Headache Pain. 2013;14(1):67. https://doi.org/10.1186/1129-2377-14-67.
51. Ornello R, et al. SPG radiofrequency for SUNCT/SUNA. Headache. 2020;60(5):938–45. https://doi.org/10.1111/head.13788.
52. Hannerz J, Linderoth B. Neurosurgical treatment of SUNCT. Br J Neurosurg. 2002;16(1):55–8. https://doi.org/10.1080/02688690275351260 0.
53. Black DF, Dodick DW. Intractable SUNCT cases. Cephalalgia. 2002;22(3):201–4. https://doi.org/10.1046/j.1468-2982.2002.00348.x.
54. Zaed I, et al. Gamma knife radiosurgery for SUNCT. World Neurosurg. 2020;133:167–71. https://doi.org/10.1016/j.wneu.2019.10.016.
55. Fujimaki T, et al. Glycerol injection for trigeminal neuralgia. J Neurosurg. 1990;73(2):212–6. https://doi.org/10.3171/jns.1990.73.2.0212.

Part III
Other Primary Headache Disorders

Chapter 11
Primary Cough Headache

PingKun Chen, Hung Yi Wu, and Shuu-Jiun Wang

11.1 Introduction

Primary cough headache (PCH) is a headache disorder characterized by sudden and intense pain triggered by coughing or other Valsalva maneuvers (e.g., sneezing, bending over, or straining) without evidence of intracranial lesions [1]. It typically manifests as a brief, sharp headache that can range from a few seconds to two hours in duration, and it is usually bilateral. The condition, while uncommon, is important to recognize, as it can sometimes be confused with other, more severe neurological conditions that require urgent treatment. This chapter reviews the pathophysiology, headache characteristics, diagnostic algorithm, and management strategies for primary cough headache, aiming to provide a comprehensive understanding of this distinctive headache disorder.Primary cough headache is considered a rare condition. Epidemiological studies suggest that the prevalence of PCH is relatively low, with estimates of its occurrence ranging between 0.4 and 1.2% of all headache

P. Chen
School of Medicine, China Medical University College of Medicine, Taichung, Taiwan

Bozhi Clinic, Taichung, Taiwan

H. Y. Wu
Zhijia Clinic, Taichung, Taiwan

S.-J. Wang (✉)
College of Medicine, National Yang Ming Chiao Tung University, Taipei, Taiwan

Department of Neurology, Neurological Institute, Taipei Veterans General Hospital, Taipei, Taiwan

Brain Research Center, National Yang Ming Chiao Tung University, Taipei, Taiwan
e-mail: sjwang@vghtpe.gov.tw

D. Uludüz et al. (eds.), *Rare Causes of Headache Disorders*, Headache, https://doi.org/10.1007/978-3-032-10242-3_11

clinic referrals [2, 3]. It primarily affects adults, particularly those between the ages of 40 and 60, and is more common in men than women, with a male-to-female ratio of approximately 3:1 [3, 4]. The onset of symptoms typically occurs after the age of 40 [5], and the condition is often observed in individuals who have a history of chronic coughing or heavy physical exertion.

11.2 Pathophysiology

The pathophysiology of PCH remains incompletely understood, with several hypotheses proposed to explain its occurrence. One of the most widely accepted theories is that PCH is triggered by an increase in intracranial pressure during Valsalva maneuvers such as coughing, sneezing, or straining. These actions can cause a sudden rise in pressure within the skull, which may affect sensitive intracranial structures, leading to headache. The sharp, intense pain associated with PCH is believed to result from this brief but significant increase in pressure, which can sensitize pain pathways in the brain. Several contributing factors may enhance this pressure increase, including increased central venous pressure, posterior fossa crowding, heightened venous pressure due to venous stenosis, and a relative increase in the pressure gradient between cisternal and lumbar cerebrospinal fluid (CSF). Additionally, receptor sensitization due to neuroinflammation or prior irritation may also play a role, making the cranial structures more responsive to pressure changes during Valsalva maneuvers [6].

A study by Raskin et al. evaluated 30 patients with PCH and offered them two treatment options: indomethacin or lumbar puncture (LP) [7]. Sixteen patients chose indomethacin, while fourteen opted for LP. The results revealed that the opening pressures and basic cellular counts were within normal limits for all patients, but six of the fourteen patients who underwent LP showed immediate improvement after the procedure. Based on these findings, the authors suggested that the increase in central venous pressure, particularly through the jugular venous system and epidural venous plexus, during the Valsalva maneuver plays a significant role in triggering the headache. The rise in intrathoracic and intra-abdominal pressure during coughing is believed to contribute to this phenomenon, ultimately resulting in the sharp headache characteristic of PCH.

Our study found that posterior fossa crowdedness may be another contributing factor to PCH. Using morphometric magnetic resonance imaging (MRI) analysis, we found that patients with PCH had a significantly smaller posterior cranial fossa (PCF) area compared to controls, leading to a higher hindbrain/PCF ratio [8]. This crowding may cause increased intracranial pressure during Valsalva maneuvers, contributing to the development of PCH. These anatomical abnormalities, including shorter clivus length and a lower position of the cerebellar tonsillar tip, indicate that structural factors may play a role in making the brain more vulnerable to pressure changes.

Another study found that heightened venous pressure due to venous stenosis may contribute to the development of PCH [9]. This theory posits that abnormalities in the venous system, particularly in the jugular or epidural veins, could lead to increased pressure in the cranial veins during Valsalva maneuvers. The elevated venous pressure could make the brain more sensitive to pressure changes, thereby triggering the headache. Venous congestion, possibly exacerbated by factors like venous stenosis, could thus be a key mechanism in the pathophysiology of PCH.

Another study regarding the pathophysiology of PCH suggests that the disorder may be linked to a relative increase in the pressure gradient between cisternal and lumbar cerebrospinal fluid (CSF) pressure, rather than a direct rise in intracranial pressure. In our prior small open-label trial, acetazolamide was successfully used to treat four out of five patients with PCH. We proposed that the increased pressure gradient, which affects the flow of CSF, could contribute to the onset of headaches during Valsalva maneuvers like coughing [10]. This theory emphasizes the role of pressure fluctuations in the CSF compartments rather than focusing solely on changes in intracranial pressure.

Another contributing factor involves receptor sensitization, which may be triggered by prior infections or other factors that lead to neuroinflammation [11]. The pain receptors in the cranial structures become more sensitive due to repeated irritation or inflammation. When the pressure in the cranial cavity increases during activities like coughing, the already sensitized receptors may overreact, resulting in the sharp, lancinating pain characteristic of PCH. This sensitization could make individuals more prone to experiencing headaches when exposed to triggers that might otherwise not cause such a response.

11.3 Case Presentation

A 33-year-old male engineer with no prior history of headache or other systemic illnesses presented with a sudden onset headache. He reported engaging in regular weight training and experienced an abrupt, severe, dull headache involving the entire head during a heavy lift while performing a Valsalva maneuver. The headache reached peak intensity rapidly and resolved spontaneously within approximately one minute. A similar headache recurred upon repeating the same maneuver. Over the subsequent days, he noted the recurrence of identical headaches triggered by coughing and sneezing.

There were no associated symptoms such as nausea, vomiting, photophobia, phonophobia, or cranial autonomic features (e.g., lacrimation, rhinorrhea). Physical and neurological examinations were unremarkable. Brain magnetic resonance imaging (MRI) revealed no significant abnormalities. The patient was started on indomethacin therapy, to which he responded excellently, with complete resolution of symptoms.

11.4 Case Discussion

This case illustrates a typical presentation of primary cough headache, a benign headache disorder characterized by brief, sudden-onset head pain triggered by activities that acutely increase intracranial pressure, such as coughing, sneezing, or performing a Valsalva maneuver. The patient reported transient, intense, diffuse headaches consistently provoked by these maneuvers, in the absence of associated symptoms or focal neurological deficits.

Although the clinical features strongly suggest a primary cough headache, it is essential to exclude secondary causes, including posterior fossa lesions (e.g., Chiari I malformation), vascular anomalies, or other structural abnormalities, as they can present with similar manifestations. In this case, neuroimaging with brain MRI demonstrated no abnormalities. The patient showed an excellent response to indomethacin, a finding that further supports the diagnosis of primary cough headache.

11.5 Clinical Characteristics

Primary cough headache is characterized by:

- *Sudden onset*: The pain typically begins abruptly and reaches its peak intensity within seconds to minutes of the triggering event (i.e., coughing or sneezing).
- *Intensity*: The headache is usually described as moderate to severe, sharp, and lancinating.
- *Duration*: It is generally a brief headache, lasting anywhere from a few seconds to several minutes. However, some cases may experience headaches that last longer, up to 2 h [2].
- *Bilateral pain*: The pain is usually bilateral, affecting both sides of the head, and may involve the occipital or temporal regions.
- *Absence of accompanying symptoms*: Unlike primary headaches such as migraine, cough headache is not typically associated with nausea, vomiting, or photophobia. However, some patients may report mild autonomic symptoms like tearing or nasal congestion.
- *Triggering factors*: The headache is most commonly triggered by coughing, but other Valsalva maneuvers (e.g., sneezing, bending over, straining during defecation, or lifting heavy objects) can also induce an episode. It is often exacerbated by physical activities that increase intracranial pressure.

11.6 Diagnostic Algorithm

To accurately diagnose PCH, it is important to differentiate it from other headache syndromes that may present with similar features. The differential diagnosis can be approached in two steps: a thorough patient history to identify key symptoms and appropriate neuroimaging to exclude secondary causes.

11.6.1 Step 1: Detailed Patient History

A detailed patient history is critical to identify key symptoms that will help differentiate PCH from other headache syndromes.

- *Primary Exercise Headache*: This headache often affects younger individuals and frequently presents with migrainous features, including nausea, photophobia, and phonophobia. The headache disorder is typically triggered by prolonged physical exercise rather than an acute event like coughing. Unlike PCH, which typically starts immediately after a cough or Valsalva maneuver, exercise-induced headaches do not begin at the onset of exercise and may take longer to develop. The duration of primary exercise headaches is also typically longer, often lasting up to several hours.
- *Idiopathic Intracranial Hypertension (IIH)*: This headache disorder is characterized by diffuse, constant headache that can be aggravated by coughing or Valsalva maneuvers. Patients with IIH often complain of pulsatile tinnitus, diplopia, and transient visual obscurations. Additionally, these patients may present with focal neurological deficits, including the VIth cranial nerve palsy, papilledema, enlarged blind spots, or visual field defects. In contrast to PCH, which is brief and sharp in nature, IIH headaches tend to be more chronic and diffuse. The clinical history, along with specific visual symptoms and examination findings, can help differentiate IIH from PCH.

11.6.2 Step 2: Neuroimaging to Exclude Secondary Causes

Since the clinical presentation can be identical in both primary and secondary cough headaches, neuroimaging should be considered for all newly diagnosed patients with cough headaches.

Various underlying conditions can mimic or cause secondary cough headaches, and these must be carefully evaluated. The most common etiology for secondary cough headache is Chiari type 1 malformation, accounting for more than 90% of patients [11]. Several other intracranial lesions were reported sporadically. A case report revealed that a 59-year-old man with spontaneous intracranial hypotension complicated by cerebral venous thrombosis presented with cough headaches, which were resolved following corticosteroid and anticoagulant treatment [12]. Additionally, a 40-year-old man with internal jugular vein valve incompetence was found to have cough headaches triggered by Valsalva maneuvers, which improved after treatment with indomethacin [13]. A 63-year-old woman experienced cough headaches caused by an intradiploic leptomeningeal cyst, confirmed via MRI [14]. A 23-year-old man with chronic renal failure developed cough headaches due to posterior reversible encephalopathy syndrome, with blood pressure management leading to symptom resolution [15]. Reversible cerebral vasoconstriction syndrome was diagnosed in a 52-year-old woman with recurrent cough headaches, which improved with blood pressure control and antiplatelet therapy [16]. A pediatric case of a 7-year-old boy with internal jugular phlebectasia showed that cough headaches resolved as the underlying cough from pertussis improved [17]. These cases underscore the importance of neuroimaging to rule out various secondary causes that may require different management strategies. By combining a detailed history with appropriate neuroimaging, healthcare providers can effectively differentiate primary cough headache from other headache disorders, ensuring that secondary causes are ruled out and proper treatment is provided.

11.7 International Classification of Headache Disorders, 3rd Edition (ICHD-3) Diagnostic Criteria for Primary Cough Headache

A. At least two headache episodes fulfilling criteria B-D
B. Brought on by and occurring only in association with coughing, straining and/or other Valsalva maneuver
C. Sudden onset
D. Lasting between 1 s and 2 h
E. Not better accounted for by another ICHD-3 diagnosis

11.8 Management

The management of PCH is aimed at both acute relief of symptoms and preventing future attacks. The primary treatment for acute episodes of PCH involves the use of indomethacin, which is considered first-line therapy due to its ability to reduce both the intensity and frequency of headaches [18]. Like other nonsteroidal anti-inflammatory drugs (NSAIDs), indomethacin works by inhibiting prostaglandin synthesis. However, the exact mechanism by which indomethacin is effective for PCH, unlike other NSAIDs, remains unclear. It is believed that the drug's efficacy may be related to its ability to reduce intracranial pressure and inflammation. The typical dose ranges from 50 to 200 mg per day, depending on the severity of the attack. One point worth mentioning is that responsiveness to indomethacin does not necessarily rule out the possibility of secondary cough headache. Our study demonstrated that indomethacin may also be effective in certain cases with secondary causes [2]. However, indomethacin is not without side effects, and its use is limited by gastrointestinal disturbances, including dyspepsia, ulcers, and gastritis. This makes it less suitable for patients with a history of gastroesophageal reflux disease, and in such cases, alternative therapies are considered.

For patients with frequent or disabling PCH attacks, preventive treatments may be necessary to reduce the frequency and severity of episodes.

1. *Beta-Blockers*: Medications like propranolol have been shown to prevent attacks of PCH in some patients [19]. Beta-blockers help by reducing intracranial pres-

sure fluctuations and by stabilizing vascular tone, which may prevent the onset of headaches triggered by Valsalva maneuvers, such as coughing or sneezing. Doses typically range from 40 to 120 mg per day [20].

2. *Acetazolamide and Topiramate*: Both acetazolamide, a carbonic anhydrase inhibitor, and topiramate, an anticonvulsant with carbonic anhydrase inhibitor function, have been suggested as preventive therapies. Acetazolamide works by reducing the production of CSF, thus decreasing intracranial pressure, which may be an important factor in the pathophysiology of PCH. A study found acetazolamide to be effective in reducing headache severity in some patients, although side effects such as numbness can occur. The typical dose is 250–2000 mg per day, depending on the patient's tolerance [10, 20]. Topiramate, like acetazolamide, helps lower intracranial pressure and has been shown to be effective in preventing PCH episodes, particularly when other treatments are insufficient. The dosage for topiramate typically ranges from 50 to 100 mg per day, depending on patient response [20, 21].
3. *Lumbar Puncture*: Some patients with PCH respond well to lumbar puncture (LP) as a preventive therapy. This procedure involves draining a small volume of CSF, which is thought to reduce intracranial pressure and relieve headache symptoms. A case study showed that therapeutic lumbar puncture (draining 40 cc of CSF) can provide long-term relief of symptoms [7]. This treatment is particularly useful for patients who have not responded to medications like indomethacin or acetazolamide.
4. *Non-invasive Vagus Nerve Stimulation*: Non-invasive vagus nerve stimulation (nVNS) has emerged as a promising alternative for treating PCH, especially in cases where indomethacin is contraindicated or poorly tolerated. nVNS works by modulating pain pathways through stimulation of the vagus nerve, which is involved in the trigeminal–autonomic reflex that plays a key role in primary headache disorders. Studies have shown that nVNS can reduce the frequency and severity of headaches, with one case report documenting a complete resolution of PCH after three months of treatment [22].

11.9 Conclusions

Primary cough headache is a rare but distinct form of headache that should be considered in patients with sudden, severe, and brief headaches triggered by coughing or other Valsalva maneuvers. While the exact pathophysiology remains unclear, management with indomethacin provides significant relief for most patients. However, indomethacin responsiveness does not exclude the possibility of secondary headache. Imaging studies are crucial for excluding secondary causes of headache, and preventive treatments may be required for individuals with frequent attacks. Despite its rarity, recognizing and appropriately managing primary cough headache can significantly improve the quality of life for affected individuals, and further research into its pathophysiology and optimal treatments is warranted.

References

1. Headache Classification Committee of the International Headache Society (IHS) The International Classification of Headache Disorders, 3rd edition. Cephalalgia. 2018;38(1):1–211. https://doi.org/10.1177/0333102417738202. PMID: 29368949.
2. Chen PK, Fuh JL, Wang SJ. Cough headache: a study of 83 consecutive patients. Cephalalgia Int J Headache. 2009;29(10):1079–85. https://doi.org/10.1111/j.1468-2982.2009.01844.x. PMID: 19438909.
3. Pascual J, Combarros O, Leno C, Polo JM, Rebollo M, Berciano J. Distribution of headache by diagnosis as the reason for neurologic consultation. Med Clin (Barc). 1995;104(5):161–4. PMID: 7877373.
4. Alvarez R, Ramón C, Pascual J. Clues in the differential diagnosis of primary vs secondary cough, exercise, and sexual headaches. Headache J Head Face Pain. 2014;54(9):1560–2. https://doi.org/10.1111/head.12449. PMID: 25298032.
5. Villar-Martínez MD, Moreno-Ajona D, Chan C, Goadsby PJ. Indomethacin-responsive headaches – a narrative review. Headache. 2021;61(5):700–14. https://doi.org/10.1111/head.14111. PMID: 34105154.
6. Nandyala A, Zhang N. Primary cough headache. Curr Pain Headache Rep. 2023;27(11):679–84. https://doi.org/10.1007/s11916-023-01171-w. PMID: 37747622.
7. Raskin NH. The cough headache syndrome: treatment. Neurology. 1995;45(9):1784. https://doi.org/10.1212/WNL.45.9.1784. PMID: 7675251.
8. Chen YY, Lirng JF, Fuh JL, Chang FC, Cheng HC, Wang SJ. Primary cough headache is associated with posterior fossa crowdedness: a morphometric MRI study. Cephalalgia. 2004;24(9):694–9. https://doi.org/10.1111/j.1468-2982.2004.00739.x. PMID: 15315524.
9. Donnet A, Valade D, Houdart E, Lanteri-Minet M, Raffaelli C, Demarquay G, Hermier M, Guegan-Massardier E, Gerardin E, Geraud G, Cognard C, Levrier O, Lehmann P. Primary cough headache, primary exertional headache, and primary headache associated with sexual activity: a clinical and radiological study. Neuroradiology. 2013;55(3):297–305. https://doi.org/10.1007/s00234-012-1110-0.
10. Wang SJ, Fuh JL, Lu SR. Benign cough headache is responsive to acetazolamide. Neurology. 2000;55(1):149–50. https://doi.org/10.1212/WNL.55.1.149. PMID: 10891932.
11. Pascual J. Primary cough headache. Curr Pain Headache Rep. 2005;9(4):272–6. https://doi.org/10.1007/s11916-005-0036-1. PMID: 16004844.
12. Ferrante T, Latte L, Abrignani G, Russo M, Manzoni GC, Torelli P. Cough headache secondary to spontaneous intracranial hypotension complicated by cerebral venous thrombosis. Neurol Sci. 2012;33(2):429–33. https://doi.org/10.1007/s10072-011-0757-3. PMID: 21904865.
13. Liu H, Cao X, Zhang M, He M, Li M, Song Y, Dong Z, Yu S. A case report of cough headache with transient elevation of intracranial pressure and bilateral internal jugular vein valve incompetence: a primary or secondary headache? Cephalalgia. 2018;38(3):600–3. https://doi.org/10.1177/0333102417703763.
14. Heijkoop TY, Hammer S, Koppen H. Cough headache in a patient with an intradiploic leptomeningeal cyst: a case report. Headache J Head Face Pain. 2019;59(4):590–2. https://doi.org/10.1111/head.13483. PMID: 30756374.
15. Maramattom BV. Cough headache as a presenting feature of posterior reversible encephalopathy syndrome (PRES). Clin Med. 2021;21(2):e237–8. https://doi.org/10.7861/clinmed.2020-1080. PMID: 33762394.
16. Kato Y, Hayashi T, Sano H, Kato R, Tanahashi N, Takao M. Cough headache presenting with reversible cerebral vasoconstriction syndrome. Intern Med. 2018;57(10):1459–61. https://doi.org/10.2169/internalmedicine.0061-17. PMID: 29321411.
17. Omata Y, Takahashi Y, Nakazawa T, Omata T. Paediatric primary cough headache with internal jugular phlebectasia. BMJ Case Rep. 2021;14(6):e242590. https://doi.org/10.1136/bcr-2021-242590. PMID: 34167982.

18. Mathew NT. Indomethacin responsive headache syndromes. Headache J Head Face Pain. 1981;21(4):147–50. https://doi.org/10.1111/j.1526-4610.1981.hed2104147.x. PMID: 7021474.
19. Sandoe CH, Kingston W. Exercise headache: a review. Curr Neurol Neurosci Rep. 2018;18(6):28. https://doi.org/10.1007/s11910-018-0840-8. PMID: 29675548.
20. Cordenier A, De Hertogh W, De Keyser J, Versijpt J. Headache associated with cough: a review. J Headache Pain. 2013;14(1):42. https://doi.org/10.1186/1129-2377-14-42. PMID: 23687906.
21. Medrano V, Mallada J, Sempere A, Fernández S, Piqueras L. Primary cough headache responsive to topiramate. Cephalalgia. 2005;25(8):627–8. https://doi.org/10.1111/j.1468-2982.2005.00903.x. PMID: 16033389.
22. Moreno-Ajona D, Villar-Martínez MD, Goadsby PJ, Hoffmann J. Primary cough headache treated with non-invasive vagal nerve stimulation. Neurology. 2020;95(13):593–4. https://doi.org/10.1212/WNL.0000000000010535. PMID: 32753438.

Chapter 12
Primary Exercise Headache

Arão Belitardo de Oliveira, Yohannes Woubishet Woldeamanuel, and Julio Pascual

12.1 Introduction

Primary exercise headache (PEH) is a rare, exertion-triggered headache disorder classified under the International Classification of Headache Disorders, 3rd edition (ICHD-3) [1]. Distinct from secondary causes like subarachnoid hemorrhage, PEH manifests during or after physical activity, impacting individuals ranging from casual exercisers to elite athletes. Its benign nature belies its potential to disrupt quality of life [1]. The emerging evidence of therapeutic effects for primary headache disorders from physical activity and prescribed exercise of different modalities has prompted clinicians and healthcare professionals to advise and prescribe exercises as a lifestyle pillar in clinical practice [3–7]. Nevertheless, PHE often leads patients to curtail exercise, which is a counterproductive outcome given exercise's broader health benefits, especially for those presenting with other preexisting major primary headache disorders (e.g., migraine).

This chapter employs a case-based approach, centered on a 32-year-old male marathon runner presenting with bilateral throbbing headaches during runs, resolving within hours. We explore PEH's diagnosis, epidemiology, physiopathology, and treatment, emphasizing pharmacological and behavioral strategies to manage symptoms without discouraging physical activity. Recent evidence highlights the

A. B. de Oliveira (✉)
Center for Clinical and Epidemiological Research, Hospital Universitário, Universidade de Sao Paulo, Sao Paulo, Brazil

Y. W. Woldeamanuel
Department of Neurology, Division of Headache, Mayo Clinic, Phoenix, AZ, USA

J. Pascual
University Hospital Marqués de Valdecilla, Universidad de Cantabria and IDIVAL, Santander, Spain

D. Uludüz et al. (eds.), *Rare Causes of Headache Disorders*, Headache,
https://doi.org/10.1007/978-3-032-10242-3_12

importance of tailored interventions to maintain exercise engagement, a priority for clinicians treating this rare headache disorder.

PEH's epidemiology varies considerably. Although primary exercise headache is considered rare in general, prevalence estimates range from 1.0% to 12.3% in the general adult population, rising to 19.8% among resistance training athletes and 30.4% in adolescents [8–12]. This disparity reflects a wide range of population studied and exercise exposure as a key determinant, evident in our marathon-running patient. Peak prevalence occurs in the 20s–30s, with conflicting data on sex predilection, though athletes (e.g., runners, weightlifters) predominate due to exertion exposure duration and intensity [8, 9, 12–14].

12.2 Pathophysiology

PEH's pathophysiology is still poorly understood and mostly elusive. PEH's mechanisms are likely to include musculoskeletal, cardiopulmonary, hemodynamic/cerebrovascular processes that directly or indirectly facilitate trigeminocervical activation through common biomarkers mediators (Fig. 12.1). The migraine-like

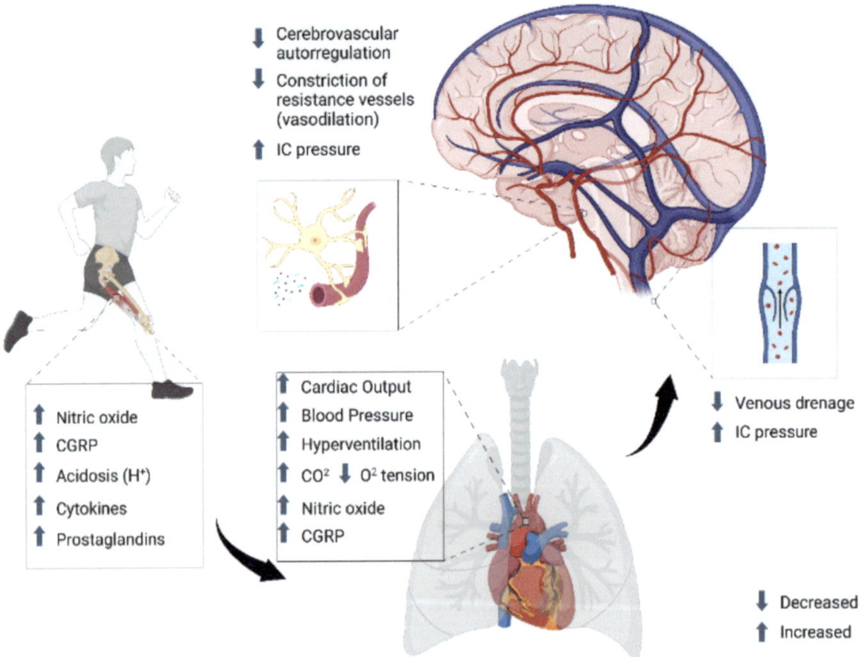

Fig. 12.1 Hypothetical pathophysiological mechanisms of PEH integrating musculoskeletal, cardiopulmonary, and cerebrovascular factors. Figure created using Biorender website platform (www.biorender.com). CGRP calcitonin gene-related peptide, H^+ Hydrogen ions, IC Intracranial

features of PEH and higher occurrence in people with previous or family history of migraine may suggest overlapping pathways or common molecular mediators [2, 8, 15, 16]. Our runner's headaches during marathons likely stem from some combinations of these multiple pathways.

Strenuous exercise induces the release of pro-inflammatory, nociceptive mediators from working muscles such as cytokines and prostaglandins, which are associated with major primary headache disorders [17–19]. The increase in cardiac output and shear-stress in the vasculature stimulate nitric oxide (NO) formation and release, a classical headache-provoking molecule [17]. A recent report showed an increase in the circulating levels of calcitonin gene-related peptide (CGRP) in 48 runners after a half-marathon event [20]. Besides, the metabolic stress and related respiratory decompensation (e.g., acidosis, hypoxia) are hallmark of intense exercise, and are also considered headache triggers [17, 21]. In susceptible individuals or in the context of Valsalva maneuvers, wherein incompetent venous vasculature is present, retrograde flow may result in a temporary rise in blood flow, elevating intracranial pressure and ultimately triggering head pain [22, 23]. Dysfunctional myogenic cerebrovascular autoregulation has been proposed [24]. In this scenario, the capacity to sustain stable tissue perfusion despite variations in pressure (i.e., increased cardiac output, blood pressure) and metabolic demands is disrupted, and the constriction of resistance cerebral blood vessels is not guaranteed, thus, resulting in vasodilation and head pain [2, 8, 24].

12.3 Case Presentation

A 32-year-old male professional marathon runner presented with a six-month history of bilateral throbbing headaches occurring exclusively during long-distance runs. The headaches typically began after 20–30 min of sustained exertion, described as pulsatile, moderate to severe in intensity, and occasionally associated with photophobia, but without nausea, vomiting, aura, or focal neurological symptoms. The episodes resolved spontaneously within two to four hours of cessation of activity, without the need for medication.

The patient reported no prior personal or familial history of migraine or aneurysm, no recent trauma, and no systemic symptoms. He denied any headache outside the context of exercise. He had not changed his training routines significantly, though he had recently increased the frequency of high-intensity interval sessions. There were no signs of dehydration or environmental triggers (e.g., heat, altitude) contributing to the symptoms.

Neurological examination was unremarkable. Blood pressure and fundoscopy were normal. Brain magnetic resonance imaging (MRI) and MR angiography revealed no abnormalities, excluding potential secondary causes such as exertional arterial dissection, subarachnoid hemorrhage, or structural malformations.

Given the exercise-precipitated nature of the headaches, lack of red flags, normal imaging, and fulfillment of the ICHD-3 criteria, a diagnosis of primary exercise headache (PEH) was established.

Initial management focused on behavioral strategies including structured warm-up protocols, diaphragmatic breathing training, hydration optimization, and posture correction. The patient was educated on avoiding Valsalva maneuvers and encouraged to maintain physical activity with modifications. Despite improvements, occasional headache recurrences prompted the addition of 25 mg indomethacin, taken 30–60 min before runs exceeding 15 km, resulting in complete resolution of symptoms.

Over a three-month follow-up, the patient reported resuming full marathon training and competition without further headache episodes. He continued adherence to non-pharmacological strategies and required indomethacin only during high-intensity sessions. The case illustrates a prototypical presentation of PEH and underscores the importance of preserving physical activity through a tailored, stepwise treatment approach.

12.4 Case Discussion

The runner's history lacks trauma, systemic symptoms, or familial aneurysm risk, lowering suspicion of sinister mimics like reversible cerebral vasoconstriction syndrome (RCVS) or cardiac cephalgia. Normal physical exam (blood pressure, fundoscopy) and MRI/MRA results reinforce PEH over secondary causes. Diagnostic rigor is critical, as exertion-related headaches may signal vascular pathology, necessitating imaging in atypical cases (e.g., sudden onset, age >50) [1, 2, 8].

12.5 Diagnostic Approach and Algorithm

History-taking confirms exercise specificity and duration, with red flags prompting urgent evaluation. Our patient's gradual onset and resolution, absent comorbidities, align with PEH, validated by imaging exclusion of mimics. Table 12.1 encapsulates this framework, guiding clinicians through case-based differentiation.

Accurate diagnosis of PEH relies on ICHD-3 criteria (Table 12.1), requiring exclusion of secondary etiologies—a process illustrated by our case. The patient reports headaches exclusively during marathon running, lasting 2–4 h, with no neurological deficits, fitting ICHD-3's definition: exercise-precipitated, <48 h duration, and not attributable to another cause [1].

Table 12.1 ICHD-3 diagnostic criteria for primary exercise headache

Primary exercise headache	Probable primary exercise headache
A. At least two headache episodes fulfilling criteria B–D; B. Brought on by and occurring only during or after strenuous physical exercise; C. Lasting <48 h; D. Not better accounted for by another ICHD-3 diagnosis (e.g., secondary headache)	A. At least two headache episodes fulfilling criteria B–D; 1. A single headache episode fulfilling criteria B and C; 2. At least two headache episodes fulfilling criterion B but not criterion C; B. Brought on by and occurring only during or after strenuous physical exercise C. Lasting <48 h D. Not better accounted for by another ICHD-3 diagnosis (e.g., secondary headache)

Notes: Exclusion of secondary causes (e.g., subarachnoid hemorrhage, arterial dissection) is mandatory [1]

12.6 Treatment

Treating PEH aims to prevent attacks and alleviate symptoms without deterring exercise, a critical consideration for our marathon runner. As there is no consensus and treatment are based on case series, case reports, and expert opinion only, management blends pharmacological and robust behavioral strategies to adjust exercise regimes, as well as to guarantee physical activity practice as an essential health behavior.

Behavioral Management: Discouraging exercise risks undermining patients' physical and mental well-being, so interventions prioritize adaptation over avoidance.

Key strategies include:

Graduated Exercise Protocols: Gradual intensity escalation reduces hemodynamic spikes. Adoption of 10–15-min dynamic warm-ups (e.g., light jogging, stretching) is highly recommended [15, 16, 25]. Our patient adopted this, cutting episodes from monthly to rare occurrences. Clinicians can tailor protocols (e.g., 5% weekly intensity increases) to individual thresholds, monitored via headache diaries.

Breathing Techniques: Avoiding Valsalva maneuvers mitigates intracranial pressure surges. Controlled diaphragmatic breathing during exertion, taught via biofeedback or coaching, is encouraged [2, 8, 11, 15]. Our runner's adoption of rhythmic breathing during runs proved effective, preserving marathon participation.

Hydration and Environmental Adjustments: Dehydration exacerbates vascular stress; maintaining euhydration (e.g., 500 mL water pre-exercise) might lower PEH risk [11]. Avoiding hot, humid conditions—common triggers—further supports exercise continuation, as our patient adjusted training to cooler mornings [8, 15].

Posture and Muscle Relaxation: Cervical strain contributes to PEH, so posture correction (e.g., neutral spine alignment) and post-exercise stretching (e.g., trapezius release) reduce muscular referral [2, 16]. Our patient's twice-weekly yoga sessions decreased headache frequency, reinforcing exercise compatibility.

Behavioral Reinforcement: Framing exercise as beneficial, not harmful, counters fear-avoidance. Cognitive-behavioral techniques—for example, reframing PEH as manageable via preparation—boost adherence. Our patient's motivation to maintain running improved with clinician encouragement and a structured plan, avoiding discouragement.

These strategies, requiring minimal resources, empower patients to self-manage PEH while exercising safely. Regular follow-ups assess efficacy, and adjust plans as needed (e.g., increasing warm-up duration if breakthroughs occur).

Pharmacological Options: When behavioral measures suffice partially, preemptive treatment complements them. Indomethacin remains first-line, effective in over 80% of cases, most likely by blocking prostaglandin/NO-mediated vasodilation [26]. Dose can vary (25–150 mg per day) and acute therapy immediately before exercise is a reasonable option (e.g., 25–50 mg, 30–60 min pre-exercise) [2, 15, 26]. Our patient used 25 mg before long runs, eliminating headaches without altering training. Other medications such as some non-steroidal anti-inflammatory drugs, paracetamol, ergotamine, and triptans have been studied, the latter being specifically indicated for moderate-to-severe intensity attacks [2, 15, 26, 27].

Emerging Therapies: CGRP antagonists (e.g., gepants) as an off-label pretreatment strategy have shown effectiveness [26].

12.7 Conclusion

Primary exercise headache exemplifies a rare disorder, in which precise diagnosis and management preserve patients' active lifestyles. Our 32-year-old runner's case—exercise-triggered, self-resolving headaches—highlights ICHD-3-guided differentiation (Table 12.1) from secondary mimics, confirmed by imaging. Epidemiologically, PEH's niche prevalence among exercisers underscores its relevance, while physiopathology (Fig. 12.1) probably integrates potential vascular, muscular, and molecular trigeminovascular triggers.

Treatment, enriched with behavioral strategies, ensures exercise continuation rather than cessation. Graduated protocols, breathing techniques, and posture adjustments, alongside indomethacin, enabled our patient to sustain marathons—a model for clinicians. Future research should refine global prevalence and test CGRP therapies, but current evidence empowers a proactive, exercise-friendly approach, enhancing patient outcomes in this rare headache disorder.

References

1. Headache Classification Committee of the International Headache Society. The International Classification of Headache Disorders, 3rd edition. Cephalalgia. 2018;38(1):1–211. https://doi.org/10.1177/0333102413485658.
2. González-Quintanilla V, Madera J, Pascual J. Update on headaches associated with physical exertion. Cephalalgia. 2023;43(3). https://doi.org/10.1177/03331024221146989.
3. La Touche R, Oliveira AB, Paris-Alemany A, Reina-Varona A. Incorporating therapeutic education and exercise in migraine management: a biobehavioral approach. J Clin Med. 2024;13(20):6273. https://doi.org/10.3390/jcm13206273.
4. Oliveira AB, Mercante JPP, Peres MFP, et al. Physical inactivity and headache disorders: a cross-sectional analysis in the Brazilian Longitudinal Study of Adult Health (ELSA-Brasil). Cephalalgia. 2021;41(14):1467–85. https://doi.org/10.1177/03331024211029217.
5. Oliveira AB, Fernando M, Peres P, et al. Physical activity pattern and migraine according to aura symptoms in the Brazilian Longitudinal Study of Adult Health (ELSA-Brasil) cohort: a cross-sectional study. Headache. 2022;62(8):977–88. https://doi.org/10.1111/head.14380.
6. Hagen K, Åsberg AN, Stovner L, et al. Lifestyle factors and risk of migraine and tension-type headache. Follow-up data from the Nord-Trøndelag Health Surveys 1995–1997 and 2006–2008. Cephalalgia. 2018;38(13):1919–26. https://doi.org/10.1177/0333102418764888.
7. Woldeamanuel YW, Oliveira ABD. What is the efficacy of aerobic exercise versus strength training in the treatment of migraine? A systematic review and network meta-analysis of clinical trials. J Headache Pain. 2022;23:1–12. https://doi.org/10.1186/s10194-022-01503-y.
8. Upadhyaya P, Nandyala A, Ailani J. Primary exercise headache. Curr Neurol Neurosci Rep. 2020;20(5):7–10. https://doi.org/10.1007/s11910-020-01028-4.
9. Rabiee B, Mohammadinejad P, Kordi R, Yunesian M. The epidemiology of exertional headache in the general population of Tehran, Iran. Headache. 2015;55(9). https://doi.org/10.1111/head.12610.
10. Sjaastad O, Bakketeig LS, Exertional headache. I. Vågå study of headache epidemiology. Cephalalgia. 2002;22(10). https://doi.org/10.1046/j.1468-2982.2002.00466.x.
11. González-Quintanilla V, Pascual J. Other primary headaches: an update. Neurol Clin. 2019;37(4). https://doi.org/10.1016/j.ncl.2019.07.010.
12. Chen SP, Fuh JL, Lu SR, Wang SJ. Exertional headache – a survey of 1963 adolescents. Cephalalgia. 2009;29(4):401–7. https://doi.org/10.1111/j.1468-2982.2008.01744.x.
13. Evans RW. Sports and headaches. Headache. 2018;58:3. https://doi.org/10.1111/head.13263.
14. Noormohammadpour P, Shafiei M, Shahi MHP, et al. Incidence of primary exercise headache in resistance trained athletes. Asian J Sports Med. 2017;8(4). https://doi.org/10.5812/asjsm.59489.
15. Dodick DW, Pascual J. Primary stabbing, cough, exertional, and thunderclap headaches. In: Olesen J, Goadsby PJ, Ramadan NM, Tfelt-Hansen P, Welch KMA, editors. The headaches. 3rd ed. Lippincott: Williams & Wilkins; 2006. p. 831–40.
16. Halker RB, Vargas BB. Primary exertional headache: updates in the literature. Curr Pain Headache Rep. 2013;17(6). https://doi.org/10.1007/s11916-013-0337-8.
17. Ashina M, Hansen JM, Dunga Á, BO, Olesen J. Human models of migraine-short-term pain for long-term gain. Nat Rev Neurol. 2017;13(12):713–24. https://doi.org/10.1038/nrneurol.2017.137.
18. Bø SH, Davidsen EM, Gulbrandsen P, et al. Cerebrospinal fluid cytokine levels in migraine, tension-type headache and cervicogenic headache. Cephalalgia. 2009;29(3):365–72. https://doi.org/10.1111/j.1468-2982.2008.01727.x.
19. Thuraiaiyah J, Erritzøe-Jervild M, Al-Khazali HM, Schytz HW, Younis S. The role of cytokines in migraine: a systematic review. Cephalalgia. 2022;42(14):1565–88. https://doi.org/10.1177/03331024221118924.

20. Tarperi C, Sanchis-Gomar F, Montagnana M, et al. Effects of endurance exercise on serum concentration of calcitonin gene-related peptide (CGRP): a potential link between exercise intensity and headache. Clin Chem Lab Med (CCLM). 2020;58(10):1707–12.
21. Gross EC, Lisicki M, Fischer D, Sándor PS, Schoenen J. The metabolic face of migraine—from pathophysiology to treatment. Nat Rev Neurol. 2019;15(11):627–43. https://doi.org/10.1038/s41582-019-0255-4.
22. Doepp F, Valdueza JM, Schreiber SJ. Incompetence of internal jugular valve in patients with primary exertional headache: a risk factor? Cephalalgia. 2008;28(2). https://doi.org/10.1111/j.1468-2982.2007.01484.x.
23. Lisicki M, Ferreira LP. Internal jugular vein valve incompetence: a key consideration in patients with exercise-induced headache. Cephalalgia. 2024;44(11):0-1. https://doi.org/10.1177/03331024241297831.
24. Heckmann JG, Hilz MJ, Muck-Weymann M, Neundorfer B. Benign exertional headache/benign sexual headache: a disorder of myogenic cerebrovascular autoregulation? Headache. 1997;37(9):597–8. https://doi.org/10.1046/j.1526-4610.1997.3709597.x.
25. Lambert RW, Jr; Burnet D. Prevention of exercise induced migraine by quantitative warm-up. Headache. 1985;25(6):317–9.
26. Villar-Martínez MD, Moreno-Ajona D, Chan C, Goadsby PJ. Indomethacin-responsive headaches—a narrative review. Headache. 2021;61(5):700–14. https://doi.org/10.1111/head.14111.
27. Chen SP, Pascual J, Wang SJ. Exertional and sex headache. In: Ferrari MD, Haan J, Charles A, Dodick DW, Sakai F, editors. Oxford textbook of headache syndromes. 1st ed. Oxford University Press; 2020. p. 226–9. https://doi.org/10.1093/med/9780199659869.001.0001.

Chapter 13
Primary Headache Associated with Sexual Activity

Füsun Mayda Domaç

13.1 Introduction

Primary headache associated with sexual activity (HAS) is classified within the fourth group of primary headaches in International Classification of Headache Disorders-3 [1]. HAS, being a benign headache, has been previously named as coital, preorgasmic, orgasmic, intercourse or sexual headache or cephalalgia, and nomenclature has changed to primary headache associated with sexual activity [2–4]. In International Classification of Headache Disorders, 1st edition (ICHD-1), three subtypes were identified: 1-dull and intensifying, 2-explosive at orgasm and 3-postural and post-coital [5], whereas in ICHD-2, two subtypes have remained: 1. pre-orgasmic and 2. orgasmic headache [6]. Subtypes have been removed in ICHD-3 beta and ICHD-3 classifications. Still, in diagnostic criteria, characteristics of pain have been remarked either as progressively increasing with sexual excitement or as suddenly appearing during or before orgasm [1, 7]. In ICHD-3, HAS has been regarded as a single entity with variable presentation [1]. An underlying intracranial pathology may also be present with headache during sexual activity; therefore, detailed examination for differential diagnosis must be applied before the diagnosis of this benign primary headache [8]. In this chapter, the clinical features, diagnosis and management strategies of HAS will be discussed to increase awareness of HAS among specialists.

Although the exact lifetime prevalence of HAS is not known [9], research has indicated that it ranges from 0.9% to 1.6% [10–12]. According to our previously published article, HAS was identified in 2% of the patients who were followed up at our headache outpatient clinic. We have suggested that the low ratio of HAS

F. M. Domaç (✉)
University of Health Sciences, Hamidiye Medical Faculty, Neurology Department, Erenköy Mental Health and Nervous Diseases Training and Research Hospital, İstanbul, Türkiye
e-mail: fusundomac@yahoo.cım.tr

D. Uludüz et al. (eds.), *Rare Causes of Headache Disorders*, Headache,
https://doi.org/10.1007/978-3-032-10242-3_13

diagnosis may be due to patients' unwillingness or embarrassment in describing the occurrence of their headaches [13].

HAS can occur at any sexually active age, but is mostly seen in the third or fourth decades in both females and males. Male to female ratio ranges from 1.2 to 3:1, and in males with obesity and hypertension, the ratio can be higher [1, 9, 14]. In our published case series, the mean age of the patients was 37.07 ± 7 67 with a male predominance [13].

13.2 Pathophysiology

Although several mechanisms have been proposed, the exact mechanism of HAS remains unknown. Headaches occurring during the preorgasmic phase have been linked to excessively contracted jaw and neck muscles during sexual activity. Evers et al. have reported that a sudden increase in both heart rate and blood pressure might cause headaches during orgasm [15]. Vasospasm was also considered a potential factor in the pathophysiology, but it does not appear to be a reasonable explanation [4, 16]. HAS has also been regarded as a variant of migrainous headache, as many patients have a history of migraine; therefore, the cause of HAS was suggested to result from haemodynamic changes during orgasm [2, 17]. Calcitonin gene-related peptide (CGRP) was also thought to be an essential mediator facilitating HAS attacks [18]. Genetic inheritance was also suspected, as HAS has been identified among members of families [3, 19].

13.3 Case Presentation

EA, a 30-year-old newlywed woman, presented with a severe throbbing headache that commenced during orgasm. In the previous week, she had two attacks of headache during sexual intercourse, which developed abruptly during orgasm with high intensity (8 out of 10 on the visual analogue scale). The headaches were bilateral and localised at the occipital areas, gradually diminishing within half an hour but lasting for approximately two hours. Neither photophobia nor phonophobia, nausea or vomiting accompanied the headaches. After the third headache attack associated with sexual activity the night before, she was admitted to the neurology outpatient clinic.

Additionally, she has had a history of migraine without aura for three years. The frequency of unilateral migraine headaches was two or three times a month, localised at the frontotemporal region. The intensity of attacks was moderate and mainly responded to analgesic treatment. Triggers included hunger and stress, and during these attacks, she also experienced photophobia, phonophobia and nausea. She did not report any other illnesses or a history of drug treatment, smoking or alcohol consumption.

On her physical examination, her temperature was 36.5 °C, and her systolic and diastolic blood pressures were 120/78 mm Hg, with a heart rate of 82 per minute. Her body mass index was 23.2. Electrocardiography showed sinus rhythm. Neurological examination and fundoscopy were unremarkable. A cranial computed tomography (CT) was performed, revealing no intracranial or subarachnoid haemorrhage. Routine blood tests also fell within normal ranges. To assess for reversible vasoconstriction syndrome, cerebral arteriopathies, dissection, aneurysm, cranial venous sinus thrombosis, mass, or other intracranial pathologies, cranial magnetic resonance imaging (MRI), MR angiography and MR venography were conducted. None of these investigations revealed pathological findings related to HAS. She was started on indomethacin and advised to take it 30 min before sexual activity. During follow-up, she reported two additional attacks during orgasm in a month, with moderate intensity (5 out of 10 on the visual analogue scale) and lasting half an hour. She also experienced two migraine attacks unrelated to HAS. Propranolol was prescribed, and at her follow-up after two months, it was found to be effective for both migraine and sexual activity-related headaches.

13.4 Case Discussion

Headache during sexual activity may result from a life-threatening condition; early diagnosis is crucial for appropriate treatment. EA's headaches highlight the importance of ruling out intracranial pathologies and vascular abnormalities. Her headache characteristics, being associated with orgasm during sexual intercourse, and the exclusion of secondary headache causes, were key in considering a primary headache related to sexual activity.

13.5 Clinical Characteristics

Headache occurring during sexual excitement is usually dull and increases with rising excitement. The occurrence of a headache is unpredictable [20]. Although headaches are mainly associated with intercourse, they can also be related to masturbation [21]. Severe headaches mostly occur during orgasm, and the intensity diminishes within 5–15 min [15]. The duration of mild headaches can last from 24 to 72 h, while severe headaches may last from minutes up to 24 h. Headaches may be throbbing, pressing, explosive or stabbing; they may be unilateral or bilateral (at least 60%) and are mainly located in the occipital area or can be diffuse [1, 13, 22, 23]. Nausea, vomiting, photophobia or phonophobia is rare, and autonomic symptoms are not typically present [4, 24].

For the accurate diagnosis of HAS, at least two attacks that are not better explained by another diagnosis are required. If there is only one attack, the diagnosis remains as probable HAS [1]. Lin et al. have suggested an algorithm to identify the causes of headaches associated with sexual activity [20, 23]. To exclude most common underlying causes such as subarachnoid or intracranial haemorrhage, reversible vasoconstriction syndrome, arterial dissection, cerebral venous sinus thrombosis or space-occupying lesions, initial assessment with non-contrast cranial CT is recommended, followed by cranial MRI, CT or MR angiography and venography [4, 8, 20, 23]. Frese et al. proposed that episodic and chronic forms of HAS exist, based on their follow-up of patients for at least 12 months. They identified episodic HAS in 75% of their patients, the chronic form in 25% [25]. Lin et al. have reported that patients with HAS had a greater chance of evolving to a chronic type in ≥1 year [23].

In several months, remissions may occur, but in some patients, attacks may recur or transform into a chronic form [8]. Frese et al. have reported that even in patients with chronic HAS, the outcome seems to be favourable. After three years of follow-up, 69% of patients experienced remissions [25]. In our reported case series, we have followed up with our patients for two years, and none of them experienced recurrence or progression to a chronic course [13]. In some studies, it was observed that patients with HAS also experience migraine headaches [12, 13]. Frese et al. investigated cognitive processing in HAS patients by visual event-related potentials. They did not observe a loss of cognitive habituation and concluded that this finding was similar to those observed in migrainous patients in previous studies [26]. In a case report, after orgasm, a female patient with a history of migraine with aura experienced a visual aura followed by a throbbing unilateral headache [27]. In another case report, two patients experienced auras (one with brainstem aura, one with visual aura and vertigo) associated with orgasm without accompanying headaches and with evidence of underlying cranial pathologies [28]. Tension-type headache, hypnic headache and primary exercise headache may also co-occur in patients with HAS [4].

13.6 Diagnostic Algorithm

Step 1: Clinical Suspicion

- *Identify Key Symptoms*:
  - Bilateral, sudden onset, throbbing pain associated with orgasm and gradually diminished, lasting for 3 h

Step 2: Initial Diagnostic Workup

- *Perform*

  Cranial CT

  - Evaluate for intracranial or subarachnoid haemorrhage

  Cranial MRI

- Assess for mass or other intracranial pathologies

Cranial and MR Angiography

- Assess for reversible vasoconstriction syndrome
- Assess for cerebral arteriopathies, dissection or aneurysm

Step 3: Additional Diagnostic Evaluations

MR Venography

- Assess for cerebral sinus thrombosis

Electrocardiography

- Exclude referred pain of cardiac ischaemia

Step 4: Apply ICHD-3 Diagnostic Criteria [1]

A. At least two episodes of pain in the head and/or neck fulfilling criteria B–D
B. Brought on by and occurring only during sexual activity
C. Either or both of the following:
   1. Increasing in intensity with increasing sexual excitement
   2. Abrupt explosive intensity just before or with orgasm
D. Lasting from 1 min to 24 h with severe intensity and/or up to 72 h with mild intensity
E. Not better accounted for by another ICHD-3 diagnosis

Step 5: Confirm Diagnosis

The diagnosis of primary headache associated with sexual activity is based on differential diagnosis and excluding underlying vascular and structural cranial pathologies and pharmacological causes of abrupt, severe and throbbing headaches.

13.7 Management

Nonpharmacological treatments include patient education about the existing headache. Abstaining from sexual activity if the beginnings of a headache develop or taking a more passive role in sexual activity can also be advised. Still, these may not be acceptable for all patients [4]. Pharmacological treatment of HAS is based on case series and experience. Being an infrequent headache disorder, there are no randomised controlled studies for both acute and prophylactic treatments [22]. Symptomatic acute treatment includes triptans, nonsteroidal anti-inflammatory drugs (NSAIDs) and antiemetic drugs (whether in combination or alone). Naproxen (500 mg orally), metoclopramide (10 mg intravenous [IV]), prochlorperazine

(10 mg IV or intramuscular [IM]), zolmitriptan intranasal spray (5 mg) and sumatriptan (3, 4 and 6 mg subcutaneous injections) can be therapeutic options [29].

Preventive therapies can be either pre-emptive (before sexual activity) or daily treatments. Diclofenac, acetaminophen, acetylsalicylic acid, ergotamine and benzodiazepines have been used before sexual activity, but their beneficial effects seem to be limited [17]. Indomethacin, taken 30 min before sexual activity, appeared to be successful in most patients [13, 25, 30, 31]. Naratriptan (2.5 mg) has been noted to be of value before sexual intercourse [32], but Frese et al. have observed that only half of the patients responded to triptans [33].

If headaches recur, contraindications exist or symptoms persist, daily preventive therapy may be recommended. Oral indomethacin (25 mg/day up to 225 mg/day) or beta-blockers such as propranolol (40 mg daily up to 240 mg daily) [13, 25], as well as metoprolol, nadolol, bisoprolol and nebivolol [18, 25], have been reported to be effective. Calcium channel blockers, including nimodipine [23, 34] and diltiazem [35, 36], have shown benefits in case reports. Propranolol and indomethacin are beneficial in 80–90% of patients in case series [2, 3, 13, 20, 25, 29, 33, 37, 38].

If there are contraindications to these treatments or symptoms persist, antiseizure drugs such as topiramate (50–100 mg/day) [23, 32, 39–41] or CGRP-targeted therapies can be considered [18, 31]. Erenumab (70 mg) is effective in a patient experiencing frequent HAS and migraine attacks [18]. The greater occipital nerve blockade procedure was applied to a patient with HAS, using a local anaesthetic and steroid combination at the symptomatic site, resulting in a complete resolution of the pain [42].

13.8 Conclusion

Headache during sexual activity may develop due to life-threatening conditions, and early diagnosis is essential for adequate treatment. Excluding aetiologies for secondary headaches is pivotal in considering HAS. Understanding the pathophysiological mechanism of HAS will lead to new therapeutic targets and the utilisation of new treatment options. Awareness about headaches associated with sexual activity should be raised among specialists, and patients must be educated about their existing headaches and encouraged to seek treatment.

References

1. Headache Classification Committee of the International Headache Society (IHS). The International Classification of Headache Disorders, 3rd edition. Cephalalgia. 2018;38(1):1–211.
2. Porter M, Jankovic J. Benign coital cephalagia. Differential diagnosis and treatment. Arch Neurol. 1981;38:710.
3. Johns DR. Benign sexual headache within a family. Arch Neurol. 1986;43:1158.

4. Maynard P, Pace A. Primary headache associated with sexual activity: a review of the literature. Curr Pain Headache Rep. 2024;28(7):627–32.
5. Classification and diagnostic criteria for headache disorders, cranial neuralgias and facial pain. Headache Classification Committee of the International Headache Society. Cephalalgia. 1988;8 Suppl 7:1–96.
6. Headache Classification Subcommittee of the International Headache Society. The International Classification of Headache Disorders: 2nd edition. Cephalalgia. 2004;24 Suppl 1:9–160.
7. Headache Classification Committee of the International Headache Society (IHS). The International Classification of Headache Disorders, 3rd edition (beta version). Cephalalgia. 2013;33(9):629–808.
8. Starling AJ. Unusual headache disorders. Continuum (Minneapolis, Minnesota). 2018;24(4, Headache):1192–208.
9. Frese A, Eikermann A, Frese K, Schwaag S, Husstedt IW, Evers S. Headache associated with sexual activity: demography, clinical features, and comorbidity. Neurology. 2003;61(6):796.
10. Rasmussen BK, Olesen J. Symptomatic and nonsymptomatic headaches in a general population. Neurology. 1992;42(6)
11. Biehl K, Evers S, Frese A. Comorbidity of migraine and headache associated with sexual activity. Cephalalgia. 2007;27(11):1271–3.
12. Tunç T, Üçler S, Okuyucu E, Coşkun Ö, Emre U, İnan LE. Features of stabbing, cough, exertional and sexual headaches in a Turkish population of headache patients. J Clin Neurosci. 2008;15(7):774–7.
13. Arı BC, Mayda Domac F, Ulutas S. Primary headache associated with sexual activity: a case series of 13 patients. J Clin Neurosci. 2020;79(51):3.
14. Ks A, Dhikav V. Primary headache associated with sexual activity. Singapore Med J. 2009;50(5)
15. Evers S, Lance JW. Primary headache attributed to sexual activity. In The headaches, 3rd ed.; Olesen J, Goadsby PJ, Ramadan MN, Tfelt-Hansen P, Welch, KMA, Eds.; Lippincott Williams and Wilkins: Philadelphia 2006; pp. 841–845
16. Donnet A, Valade D, Houdart E, Lanteri-Minet M, Raffaelli C, Demarquay G, Hermier M, Guegan-Massardier E, Gerardin E, Geraud G, Cognard C, Levrier O, Lehmann P. Primary cough headache, primary exertional headache, and primary headache associated with sexual activity: a clinical and radiological study. Neuroradiology. 2013;55(3):297–305. https://doi.org/10.1007/s00234-012-1110-0.
17. Pascual J, González-Mandly A, Oterino A, Martín R. Primary cough headache, primary exertional headache, and primary headache associated with sexual activity. Handb Clin Neurol. 2010;97:459–68.
18. Makarevičius G, Ryliškienė K. Successful treatment of primary headache associated with sexual activity using erenumab: case report. Cephalalgia. 2022;42(7):680–3.
19. Vergallo A, Baldacci F, Rossi C, Lucchesi C, Gori S. Sexual headache: two familiar orgasmic headache cases and review of the literature. Acta Neurol Belg. 2015;115(4):757–8.
20. Sanda GH, Newman L, Lipton R. Cough, exertional, and other miscellaneous headaches. Med Clin North Am. 1991;75:733.
21. Lin PT, Chen SP, Wang SJ. Update on primary headache associated with sexual activity and primary thunderclap headache. Cephalalgia. 2023;43(3):3331024221148657.
22. Ściślicki P, Sztuba K, Klimkowicz-Mrowiec A, Gorzkowska A. Headache associated with sexual activity-a narrative review of literature. Medicina (Kaunas). 2021;57(8):735.
23. Lin PT, Wang YF, Fuh JL, Lirng JF, Ling YH, Chen SP, Wang SJ. Diagnosis and classification of headache associated with sexual activity using a composite algorithm: a cohort study. Cephalalgia. 2021;41(14):1447–57.
24. Allena M, Rossi P, Tassorelli C, Ferrante E, Lisotto C, Nappi G. Focus on therapy of the Chapter IV headaches provoked by exertional factors: primary cough headache, primary exertional headache and primary headache associated with sexual activity. J. Headache Pain. 2010;11:525–30.

25. Frese A, Rahmann A, Gregor N, Biehl K, Husstedt IW, Evers S. Headache associated with sexual activity: prognosis and treatment options. Cephalalgia. 2007;27(11):1265–70.
26. Frese A, Frese K, Ringelstein EB, Husstedt IW, Evers S. Cognitive processing in headache associated with sexual activity. Cephalalgia. 2003;23(7):545–51.
27. D'Andrea G, Granella F, Verdelli F. Migraine with aura triggered by orgasm. Cephalalgia. 2002;22(6):485–6.
28. Angus-Leppan H, Caulfield A. Orgasmic migraine aura: report of two cases. Cephalalgia. 2019;39:153–6.
29. Anand KS, Dhikav V. Primary headache associated with sexual activity. Singapore Med J. 2009;50(5):e176–7.
30. Yeh YC, Fuh JL, Chen SP, Wang SJ. Clinical features, imaging findings and outcomes of headache associated with sexual activity. Cephalalgia. 2010;30(11):1329–35.
31. Utku U. Primary headache associated with sexual activity: case report. Med Princ Pract. 2013;22(6):588–9.
32. Evans RW, Pascual J. Orgasmic headaches: clinical features, diagnosis and management. Headache. 2000;40:491–4.
33. Frese A, Gantenbein A, Marziniak M, Husstedt IW, Goadsby PJ, Evers S. Triptans in orgasmic headache. Cephalalgia. 2006;26(12):1458–61. https://doi.org/10.1111/j.1468-2982.2006.01224.x.
34. Lee JW, Ha YS, Park SC, Seo IY, Lee HS. Orgasmic headache treated with nimodipine. J Sex Med. 2013;10(7):1893–6.
35. Akpunou BE, Ahrens J. Sexual headaches: case report, review and treatment with calcium blocker. Headache. 1991;31(3):141–5.
36. Villar-Martinez MD, Moreno-Ajona D, Chan C, Goadsby PJ. Indomethacin-responsive headaches- a narrative review. Headache. 2021;61(5):700–14.
37. Paulson GW, Klawans HL Jr. Benign orgasmic cephalgia. Headache. 1974;13(4):181–7.
38. Raskin NH. Short-lived headaches. Neurol Clin. 1997;15(1):143–52.
39. Arikanoglu A, Uzar E. Primary headaches associated with sexual activity respond to topiramate therapy: a case report. Acta Neurol Belg. 2011;111(3):222–4.
40. Bandini F, Arena E, Mauro G. Pre-orgasmic sexual headache responsive to topiramate: a case report. Cephalalgia. 2012;32(10):797–8.
41. Goadsby P, Lipton R. Primary and secondary headache disorders. In: Ed L, Mayer SA, editors. Merrit's neurology. Wolters Kluwer Health; 2021. p. 521–37.
42. Selekler M, Kutlu A, Dundar G. Orgasmic headache responsive to greater occipital nerve blockade. Headache. 2009;49(1):130–1.

Chapter 14
Cold-Stimulus Headache

Daniella Araújo de Oliveira and Marcelo Valença

14.1 Introduction

The cold-stimulus headache is described as a headache induced by a cold stimulus applied externally to the head, ingested, or inhaled [1]. When triggered by exposure to cold environments, such as immersion in icy water or exposure to low outdoor temperatures, it is classified as subtype 4.5.1: Headache attributed to the external application of a cold stimulus. The other subtype, commonly known as "brain freeze" or ice cream headache (4.5.2: Headache attributed to ingestion or inhalation of a cold stimulus), is a benign condition characterized by sudden and transient head pain induced by the consumption of cold foods or beverages [1].

In the latest international classification of headaches, a new subtype, 4.5.3 Probable Cold-stimulus Headache, was described. Its diagnostic criteria differ from those of other subtypes, as it considers only a single episode of headache that occurs exclusively during or immediately after exposure to a cold stimulus applied externally to the head, or ingested or inhaled. Unlike other headaches, cold-stimulus headaches are not disabling and appear to occur in susceptible individuals (International Classification of Headache Disorders, 3rd edition [ICHD-3]) [1].

In the clinical context, understanding the underlying mechanisms of the cold-stimulus headache deepens the comprehension of the activation of the trigeminovascular pathway and the role of cold in the pathogenesis of migraine. This chapter

D. A. de Oliveira (✉)
Federal University of Pernambuco, Recife, Pernambuco, Brazil
e-mail: daniella.aoliveira@ufpe.br

M. Valença
Federal University of Pernambuco, Recife, Pernambuco, Brazil

Center of Excellence in the Treatment of Migraine and Other Headache Disorders, Hospital Esperança, Recife, Pernambuco, Brazil

D. Uludüz et al. (eds.), *Rare Causes of Headache Disorders*, Headache,
https://doi.org/10.1007/978-3-032-10242-3_14

focuses on the clinical, diagnostic, and therapeutic aspects of this condition, integrating scientific evidence and case examples to provide practical insights for its management. The primary goal is to explore in detail the headache attributed to ingestion or inhalation of cold stimuli, expanding knowledge about its pathophysiology and association with migraine.

Regarding headache attributed to ingestion or inhalation of a cold stimulus, the prevalence varies widely, ranging from 8% to 79%, even when using the criteria established by the International Headache Society [2–12]. This variation is likely influenced by the methods used to evaluate or induce pain, as well as by the age range of the studied population. Several studies have assessed the prevalence of this headache using questionnaires [2, 4, 7, 9, 11]. In contrast, others employ experimental stimulation [3, 5, 6, 8, 10, 13], which may include the ingestion of cold water, ice cream, or even palate stimulation with ice cubes.

When analyzing prevalence by age group, it is evident that in adult populations, prevalence was 8 [5, 9], 15 [14], 37 [12], and 60% [8]. In adolescent populations, prevalence rates ranged from 23 [4], 41 [6], 60% [11], to as high as 79% [7]. Considering studies conducted experimentally, the prevalence of headache attributed to ingestion or inhalation of a cold stimulus was 41% [6] among adolescents, while in adults, the prevalence was 60 [8], 37 [5, 10], and 44% [3].

Studies have shown a higher incidence of headache attributed to ingestion or inhalation of a cold stimulus in individuals with a history of migraine, suggesting a possible interaction between cold sensitivity and a predisposition to migraine. Both experimental studies and questionnaire-based studies indicate that individuals with migraines reported cold-stimulus headaches more frequently than those with other types of headaches or no headaches at all [2, 4, 5, 7, 8, 10].

In questionnaire-based studies, the prevalence of headache attributed to ingestion or inhalation of a cold stimulus ranged from 33 [4] to 55.2% [7] and up to 93% [2] in patients with migraine.

14.2 Pathophysiology

Although the exact pathophysiology of headache attributed to the ingestion or inhalation of a cold stimulus is not fully understood, several factors are believed to play important roles, including the activation of the trigeminal nerve, cerebral vasoconstriction and vasodilation, the trigeminovascular reflex, and individual sensitivity to cold [12, 15–17].

It is suggested that transient activation of sensory mechanisms in the trigeminal region, frequently triggered by cold exposure, partially contributes to the onset of pain. Additionally, the pain threshold may be a significant factor, as well as possible local vasoconstriction, reduced blood flow, or stimulation of nociceptors [12, 17, 18].

Exposure to cold, especially in areas like the palate or pharynx, activates local thermoreceptors that stimulate the afferent fibers of the trigeminal nerve. This activation is transmitted to the trigeminal nucleus in the brainstem, resulting in a referred pain sensation in the head. It is speculated that the participation of Transient Receptor Potential Melastatin 8 (TRPM8) is crucial in this process, as this cold-sensitive receptor, expressed in primary afferent neurons of the trigeminal ganglia or dorsal root, plays a role in neuronal sensitization, mediating responses to thermal stimuli and contributing to pain transmission [19, 20].

Additionally, cold can trigger a rapid vascular response in the cranial region, starting with vasoconstriction followed by compensatory dilation of the blood vessels [12]. These fluctuations can exacerbate the onset of pain, especially in individuals with migraine, as the underlying mechanism of transitioning from vasoconstriction to vasodilation of cranial arteries, often associated with the pathophysiology of migraine, can be observed in cold-stimulus headache attributed to ingestion or inhalation of cold stimuli [17, 18]. It is possible that TRPM8, by regulating the activation of cold-related nerve fibers, plays a crucial role in these vascular responses, directly influencing the perception of pain by increasing sensitivity to cold stimuli [21].

Finally, the trigeminovascular reflex plays a key role in various primary headaches, including cold-stimulus headache, which is attributed to the ingestion or inhalation of cold stimuli. Activation of this system can lead to the release of inflammatory neuropeptides, such as calcitonin gene-related peptide (CGRP), which amplifies pain perception. Moreover, cold sensitivity is influenced by genetic and neurophysiological factors, with individuals who have a history of migraine showing a greater predisposition to respond intensely to cold stimuli [18, 19].

14.3 Case Presentation

We will describe the clinical case of two volunteers who experienced a migraine headache after being stimulated with ice. To induce pain, a standardized ice cube measuring 15 × 20 mm was placed on the palate. The volunteers were instructed to close their mouths and keep the lower jaw immobile during the test. The ice contact time on the palate was set at 90 s. Both volunteers reported a prior history of headache attributed to the ingestion or inhalation of cold stimuli and were able to tolerate the ice stimulation for the full 90 s. They also stated that they avoided consuming cold foods to prevent the unpleasant sensation, and when consuming, they preferred to eat in a slower, more gradual manner at lower temperatures as alternatives to avoid triggering the pain.

The study was approved by the Ethics in Research Committee of the Health Science Center of the Federal University in Pernambuco, Brazil, under protocol number 089/2008 in accordance with resolution 196/96 of the National Health Council and in line with the principles of the Declaration of Helsinki.

14.3.1 *Clinical Case 1*

A 19-year-old healthy woman with a diagnosis of migraine for approximately 10 years. The frequency of migraine attacks was, on average, two episodes per week, with a pain intensity of 8 on the numeric visual scale. She reported not using any prophylactic treatment for headaches, relying instead on analgesics to abort the attacks. During ice stimulation, the pain was described as an intense stabbing sensation of short duration (13 s), with a pain intensity of 9 on the numeric visual scale, occurring bilaterally in the temporal region, spontaneously resolving within 2 min after removal of the cold stimulus. Approximately one hour after ice stimulation, the patient experienced a migraine attack lasting an average of six hours, accompanied by other associated symptoms such as nausea and photophobia.

14.3.2 *Clinical Case 2*

A 38-year-old healthy woman with a diagnosis of migraine for five years. She reported frequent migraine attacks, approximately three episodes per week, with a pain intensity of 10 on the numeric visual scale. She had not been under specialized medical care for headache management for the past three years and relied on analgesics to abort attacks. During ice stimulation, the pain was described as an intense stabbing sensation, short in duration (25 s), with an intensity of 8 on the numeric visual scale, occurring unilaterally in the temporal region (the side associated with her habitual migraine). The pain spontaneously resolved within 2 min after removal of the cold stimulus. The volunteer then began a migraine episode approximately three hours after the ice test, lasting an average of twelve hours, accompanied by nausea, vomiting, osmophobia, photophobia, and phonophobia. In both cases, the volunteers reported using medication for pain relief but did not achieve success.

14.4 Case Discussion

These cases demonstrate the complexity of cold-stimulus headache in patients with a previous diagnosis of migraine. Both patients experienced a cold-induced headache during the ice stimulation protocol, characterized by a short-lasting, intense stabbing pain localized to the temporal region. Notably, the pain resolved spontaneously within two minutes after removal of the cold stimulus in both cases.

In the first case, a 19-year-old woman with a long-standing history of migraine experienced an attack approximately one hour after cold exposure, accompanied by classic migrainous symptoms. In the second case, a 38-year-old woman developed a migraine episode about three hours after the ice stimulation, which lasted for approximately twelve hours.

The temporal relationship between the cold stimulus and the onset of migraine episodes in both patients raises the possibility of a triggering role of cold exposure in susceptible individuals. Neither patient had been under prophylactic treatment, and both relied solely on abortive analgesics, which proved insufficient in managing their symptoms. This highlights the importance of considering preventive strategies, particularly in patients with frequent and disabling attacks, and in whom cold exposure may act as a potential trigger.

Although CSH typically presents as a brief, self-limited pain, its ability to trigger full-blown migraine attacks in individuals with migraine predisposition suggests a potential pathophysiological overlap or sensitization. Further, the variable latency between the stimulus and the onset of migraine, as well as the different profiles of associated symptoms, reflects the heterogeneity of responses in migraine patients.

14.5 Clinical Characteristics

Headache attributed to ingestion or inhalation of cold stimuli is characterized by sharp, short-lasting pain, typically described as pulsating or stabbing, occurring after the consumption of cold food or beverages or inhalation of cold air. It is commonly referred to as the frontal or temporal region, and more frequently bilateral (though it can be lateralized to the side of habitual migrainosus headache in individuals experiencing unilateral headache). The pain spontaneously resolves upon removal of the cold stimulus. Although not incapacitating, its presentation can be uncomfortable, with intensity ranging from moderate-to-intense but transient [1]. Rarely do individuals with this condition seek medical attention, as it is an avoidable condition.

The primary trigger of headache attributed to ingestion or inhalation of cold stimuli is the consumption of icy foods or beverages, such as ice cream or cold water [1]. For this reason, individuals with this type of headache often avoid consuming such foods [22]. Studies indicate that about half of migraine patients take specific precautions when consuming cold foods, aiming to minimize the risk of triggering painful episodes [2, 11].

Individuals with a history of migraine are more predisposed to headache attributed to ingestion or inhalation of cold stimulus, likely due to hyperexcitability of the trigeminovascular system [2, 4, 5, 7, 8, 10, 17]. This heightened sensitivity to cold stimuli suggests a shared pathophysiological link between the two conditions, involving the amplification of pain perception mediated by inflammatory neuropeptides and sensory neural pathways [18]. These factors highlight the importance of considering a migraine history in the evaluation of patients with headache induced by cold stimuli.

14.6 Diagnostic Algorithm for Cold-Stimulus Headache

The diagnosis of headache attributed to ingestion or inhalation of cold stimulus is predominantly clinical, based on a detailed patient history and the identification of typical triggers, according to the criteria proposed by the International Classification of Headache Disorders [1].

Step 1: Clinical Suspicion

- *Identify Key Symptoms*:
  - Sudden-onset, sharp or stabbing head pain triggered by direct exposure to cold stimuli (e.g., ice packs, cold wind, swimming in cold water, ingestion of cold food or drinks).
  - Pain is typically short in duration (seconds to minutes), localized to the forehead, temples, or occipital region.
  - In some cases, particularly in individuals with migraine, the cold stimulus may trigger a delayed migraine attack (minutes to hours later).
  - No underlying structural abnormalities on neuroimaging.

Step 2: Rule Out Secondary Causes

- *Clinical History and Examination*:
  - Exclude other causes of cold-induced pain, such as trigeminal neuralgia, sinus pathology, or Raynaud's phenomenon.
  - Evaluate for signs of systemic illness or neurological deficit.

Step 3: Evaluate for Comorbid Migraine

- *Assess Headache History*:
  - Determine the presence of an underlying primary headache disorder, especially migraine.
  - Identify if cold-stimulus acts as a consistent trigger for migraine episodes;
  - Consider the frequency, intensity, and duration of subsequent migraine attacks.

Step 4: Apply ICHD-3 Diagnostic Criteria (Table 14.1)

- *Use the criteria from ICHD-3 (2018) to classify*:
  - 4.5.1: External application of cold stimulus.
  - 4.5.2: Ingestion or inhalation of cold stimulus.
  - 4.5.3: Probable Cold-stimulus Headache (when criteria are almost, but not fully, met).

Table 14.1 Diagnostic criteria for headaches according to the third edition of the International Classification of Headache Disorders [1]

4.5 Cold-stimulus headache
Description: Headache brought on by a cold stimulus applied externally to the head or ingested or inhaled.
4.5.1 Headache attributed to the external application of a cold stimulus
Description: Headache following exposure of the unprotected head to a very low environmental temperature.
Diagnostic criteria:
A. At least two acute headache episodes fulfilling criteria B and C
B. Brought on by and occurring only during application of an external cold stimulus to the head.
C. Resolving within 30 min after removal of the cold stimulus
D. Not better accounted for by another ICHD-3 diagnosis.
4.5.2 Headache attributed to ingestion or inhalation of a cold stimulus
Description: Short-lasting frontal or temporal pain, which may be intense, is induced in susceptible people by the passage of cold material (solid, liquid, or gaseous) over the palate and/or posterior pharyngeal wall.
Diagnostic criteria:
A. At least two episodes of acute frontal or temporal headache fulfilling criteria B and C
B. Brought on by and occurring immediately after a cold stimulus to the palate and/or posterior pharyngeal wall from ingestion of cold food or drink or inhalation of cold air
C. Resolving within 10 min after removal of the cold stimulus
D. Not better accounted for by another ICHD-3 diagnosis.
4.5.3 Probable cold-stimulus headache
Diagnostic criteria:
A. A single headache episode fulfilling criteria B and C
B. Brought on by and occurring only during or immediately after a cold stimulus applied externally to the head or ingested or inhaled.
C. Resolving within 10 min after removal of the cold stimulus
D. Not fulfilling ICHD-3 criteria for any other headache disorder.
E. Not better accounted for by another ICHD-3 Diagnosis
Comment: Codable subforms are 4.5.3.1 Headache, probably attributed to external application of a cold stimulus, and 4.5.3.2 Headache, probably attributed to ingestion or inhalation of a cold stimulus.

14.7 Treatment/Management

Management of cold-stimulus headache primarily involves educating patients about potential triggers, such as exposure to low ambient temperatures or the consumption of cold foods and beverages. Preventive strategies are limited to the avoidance of these stimuli, as there is currently no evidence-based prophylactic treatment recommended for this type of headache.

- *Avoidance Strategies*:

  Educate the patient to avoid known cold triggers (e.g., sudden cold drinks, unprotected exposure to cold air or water).

- *Immediate Removal of the Cold Stimulus*:

  Patients should be instructed to stop or terminate exposure to the triggering cold stimulus immediately. This may involve avoiding cold foods or beverages, staying out of cold environments, or covering exposed skin when in contact with cold temperatures. Immediate cessation of the stimulus is usually sufficient to quickly relieve symptoms, as the headache typically resolves within seconds to minutes after the trigger is removed.

14.8 Conclusion

The report of these two cases, in which an ice stimulus applied to the oral cavity triggered not only immediate pain (i.e., cold-stimulus headache) but also pain occurring one and three hours after the cold stimulus, a full-blown migraine attack lasting for hours, demonstrates that ice-induced headache can act as a trigger for a migraine episode. This observation highlights another connection between these two types of headaches, not only in their occurrence in susceptible migraine patients but also in the potential role of cold-stimulus headache as a trigger for a migraine episode a few hours after the cold stimulus.

Although not debilitating, a headache attributed to ingestion or inhalation of cold stimulus raises important questions about the underlying mechanisms of cold-induced pain and its interactions with other primary headaches, such as migraine. It is speculated that these two conditions share similar pathophysiological mechanisms, such as neuronal hyperexcitability and the activation of the trigeminovascular system [18].

In this context, it is speculated that the TRPM8 receptor, a cold-sensitive ion channel activated by low temperatures (<28 °C) and cooling compounds like menthol, may have implications as a central mediator in cold-stimulus headache. Its activation, located in peripheral thermoreceptors, particularly in the oral cavity and pharynx, triggers a cascade of neural signals that propagate through the trigeminal nerve to the central nervous system [19, 21]. Thus, it is possible that TRPM8 acts as a modulator of neuronal excitation in cold conditions, contributing to the perception of pain. Increased expression or heightened sensitivity may explain why some individuals are more susceptible to headache attributed to the ingestion or inhalation of cold stimuli [20, 21].

Furthermore, the fundamental role of the trigeminovascular reflex in the observed pathophysiology is highlighted [17]. In the two clinical cases presented, the activation of this system likely led to the release of inflammatory neuropeptides, such as CGRP (calcitonin gene-related peptide). This release may have played a key role in sensitizing the trigeminovascular neurons, contributing to the onset of the migraine attacks observed in the volunteers [3, 18].

The headache attributed to ingestion or inhalation of cold stimulus is a common clinical condition that clearly illustrates the complex interplay between environmental, physiological, and neurological factors in the genesis of pain. Despite its non-disabling nature, understanding its mechanisms, such as possible activation of the trigeminal nerve, cerebral vasoconstriction, vasodilation, the trigeminovascular reflex, and the role of the TRPM8 receptor, not only improves clinical management but also paves the way for new research in primary headaches and the mechanisms of pain in general.

The typical presentation, characterized by acute, short-duration pain triggered by cold stimuli, facilitates the clinical diagnosis but requires careful consideration to rule out secondary conditions in atypical presentations. Simple preventive strategies, combined with patient education, are often sufficient to manage most cases, while advancements in molecular neuroscience, such as the study of TRPM8, offer promising prospects for future treatments. By recognizing and exploring this condition, healthcare professionals and researchers can not only alleviate patient discomfort but also contribute to a broader understanding of headache mechanisms.

References

1. Headache Classification Committee of the International Headache Society (IHS) The International Classification of Headache Disorders, 3rd edition. Cephalalgia. 2018;38(1):1–211.
2. Raskin NH, Knittle SC. Ice cream headache and orthostatic symptoms in patients with migraine. Headache. 1976;16(5):222–5.
3. Bird N, MacGregor EA, Wilkinson MI. Ice cream headache—site, duration, and relationship to migraine. Headache. 1992;32(1):35–8.
4. Aromaa M, Sillanpää ML, Rautava P, Helenius H. Childhood headache at school entry: a controlled clinical study. Neurology. 1998;50(6):1729–36.
5. Mattsson P. Headache caused by drinking cold water is common and related to active migraine. Cephalalgia. 2001;21(3):230–5.
6. Kaczorowski M, Kaczorowski J, headaches Ice. Ice cream evoked headaches (ICE-H) study: randomised trial of accelerated versus cautious ice cream eating regimen. BMJ. 2002;325(7378):1445–6.
7. Fuh JL, Wang SJ, Lu SR, Juang KD. Ice-cream headache—a large survey of 8359 adolescents. Cephalalgia. 2003;23(10):977–81.
8. Selekler HM, Erdogan MS, Budak F. Prevalence and clinical characteristics of an experimental model of 'ice-cream headache' in migraine and episodic tension-type headache patients. Cephalalgia. 2004;24(4):293–7.
9. Sjaastad O, Bakketeig LS. Hydrogen sulphide headache and other rare, global headaches: Vågå study. Cephalalgia. 2006;26(4):466–76.
10. de Oliveira DA, Valença MM. The characteristics of head pain in response to an experimental cold stimulus to the palate: an observational study of 414 volunteers. Cephalalgia. 2012;32(15):1123–30.
11. Zierz AM, Mehl T, Kraya T, Wienke A, Zierz S. Ice cream headache in students and family history of headache: a cross-sectional epidemiological study. J Neurol. 2016;263(6):1106–10.

12. Drummond PD, Lance JW. Neurovascular disturbances in headache patients. Clin Exp Neurol. 1984;20:93–9.
13. Mages S, Hensel O, Zierz AM, Kraya T, Zierz S. Experimental provocation of 'ice-cream headache' by ice cubes and ice water. Cephalalgia. 2017;37(5):464–9.
14. Rasmussen BK, Olesen J. Symptomatic and nonsymptomatic headaches in a general population. Neurology. 1992;42(6):1225–31.
15. Sleigh JW. Ice cream headache. Cerebral vasoconstriction causing decrease in arterial flow may have role. BMJ. 1997;315(7108):609.
16. Hensel O, Burow P, Mages S, Wienke A, Kraya T, Zierz S. Increased blood flow velocity in middle cerebral artery and headache upon ingestion of ice water. Front Neurol. 2019;10:677.
17. Lance JW. Fifty years of migraine research. Aust N Z J Med. 1988;18(3):311–7.
18. Chebini A, Dilli E. Cold stimulus headache. Curr Neurol Neurosci Rep. 2019;19(7):46.
19. Knowlton WM, Palkar R, Lippoldt EK, McCoy DD, Baluch F, Chen J, et al. A sensory-labeled line for cold: TRPM8-expressing sensory neurons define the cellular basis for cold, cold pain, and cooling-mediated analgesia. J Neurosci. 2013;33(7):2837–48.
20. McKemy DD, Neuhausser WM, Julius D. Identification of a cold receptor reveals a general role for TRP channels in thermosensation. Nature. 2002;416(6876):52–8.
21. Takashima Y, Daniels RL, Knowlton W, Teng J, Liman ER, McKemy DD. Diversity in the neural circuitry of cold sensing revealed by genetic axonal labeling of transient receptor potential melastatin 8 neurons. J Neurosci. 2007;27(51):14147–57.
22. Hulihan J. Ice cream headache. BMJ. 1997;314(7091):1364.

Chapter 15
External-Pressure Headache

Erlene Roberta Ribeiro dos Santos, Juliana Ramos de Andrade, and Welber Sousa Oliveira

15.1 Introduction

External-pressure headaches (EPH) are a distinct group of primary headache disorders caused by sustained mechanical forces applied to the scalp [1]. Previously classified as cranial neuralgias in the International Classification of Headache Disorders, second edition (ICHD-2), they have been redefined as primary headaches in ICHD-3, reflecting a better understanding of their pathophysiology. EPH includes three subtypes: external-compression headaches (ECH), typically caused by tight headgear such as helmets or personal protective equipment (PPE), and external-traction headaches (ETH), associated with hairstyles or accessories exerting pulling forces. These subtypes are distinguished by their causative mechanisms, with diagnostic criteria emphasizing the transient and reversible nature of these headaches. The onset of pain is directly linked to the application of external force, and resolution occurs rapidly after the removal of the trigger [1].

The significance of EPH has been highlighted in specific occupational and environmental contexts. During the coronavirus disease 2019 (COVID-19) pandemic, healthcare workers reported bilateral headaches linked to the prolonged use of N95 masks and goggles, underscoring the condition's prevalence in high-stress settings

E. R. R. dos Santos (✉)
Department of Physical Education, Federal University of Pernambuco, Recife, PE, Brazil

Coordinator of the Public Policy and Advocacy Committee of the Brazilian Headache Society, Recife, PE, Brazil

J. R. de Andrade
Danish Headache Center, Translational Research Centre, Rigshospitalet, Copenhagen of University, Denmark Brazilian Headache Society – Experimental and Clinical Research Committee, Copenhagen, Denmark

W. S. Oliveira
Centro Especializado em Hipermobilidade e Dor, Brasília, Federal District, Brazil

D. Uludüz et al. (eds.), *Rare Causes of Headache Disorders*, Headache,
https://doi.org/10.1007/978-3-032-10242-3_15

[2]. Similar patterns have been observed in military and occupational settings where helmets and other equipment are mandatory.

Although typically mild and transient, EPH can become severe and persist in individuals with pre-existing headache disorders, affecting their quality of life and productivity. Understanding its definition, classification, and epidemiology is essential for accurate diagnosis and management. This includes ergonomic adaptations, preventive strategies, and prompt symptom relief to minimize its impact, particularly in settings where headgear or similar accessories are unavoidable.

15.2 Case Presentation

A 53-year-old woman presented with a long-standing history of headaches that began at menarche, predominantly occurring during perimenstrual periods. These headaches were described as frontal, constant, and moderate to severe in intensity, often accompanied by photophobia and phonophobia, though she denied nausea or osmophobia. The headaches were aggravated by routine physical activity and occurred approximately two to three days per month. More recently, following the onset of amenorrhea, the intensity of her headaches diminished. The episodes were often preceded by cervical pain, and she reported no auras. Over-the-counter analgesics were typically effective in managing her symptoms.

The patient also noted sensitivity to other headgear, such as glasses and headbands, which needed to be lightweight and soft to avoid triggering headaches.

Approximately one year ago (in 2024), she began participating in water-based exercise (hydro-gymnastics) and experienced headaches directly related to the use of a swim cap. When wearing a fabric swim cap with an elastic band, she experienced mild, localized discomfort at the points of contact with the elastic. This discomfort resolved immediately upon removing the cap and did not require the use of analgesics. However, after switching to a silicone swim cap, her headaches became more severe and diffuse, described as holocranial with a pressing quality. These headaches were accompanied by photophobia and phonophobia, significantly affecting her ability to concentrate during exercise sessions. Unlike the headaches caused by the fabric swim cap, these episodes persisted even after removing the silicone cap and occasionally required the use of common analgesics. Due to the worsening of her symptoms, she eventually discontinued hydro-gymnastics.

15.3 Case Discussion

This case presents a female patient with a pre-existing history of headaches that meet the criteria for episodic migraine without aura and menstrual related migraine without aura. Her history of avoiding head accessories, such as glasses and headbands, due to pain, already suggested a previous diagnosis of external-pressure headache (EPH). This condition became even more evident when she began water-based exercise, which required the use of a swim cap. Studies indicate that patients with pre-existing headache disorders are three times more likely to develop de novo accessory-associated headaches [2].

Her experience with two different cap materials provides valuable insights and supports the diagnosis of external-pressure headache. When using a fabric swim cap with an elastic band, her pain was localized to the contact points with the elastic, without diffuse holocranial involvement, and resolved entirely upon removal. In contrast, the silicone swim cap, which applied more intense and diffuse compression, triggered holocranial pain. This pain persisted for more than an hour after removing the cap and was accompanied by migrainous features such as photophobia, phonophobia, difficulty concentrating, and an inability to continue exercising. Prolonged exposure to compressive stimuli can lead to sensitization, exacerbating migrainous headaches in predisposed individuals [3].

This case underscores the importance of patient education on selecting appropriate headgear and implementing strategies to minimize pericranial pressure. For healthcare providers, recognizing EPH as a distinct headache subtype is essential for tailoring management plans and improving patients' quality of life. Beyond encouraging physical activity, these observations can also benefit individuals in occupational settings, such as healthcare professionals using personal protective equipment (PPE), who may experience similar headaches. Addressing these issues has the potential to enhance both comfort and productivity in such environments.

15.4 Diagnostic Algorithm

In the ICHD 3, this headache type is classified under Group 4: Other primary headaches. This category includes headache disorders considered primary because they result from physiological, non-damaging stimuli [1].

The classification of EPH encompasses headache disorders caused by external forces applied to the scalp, either through compression or traction, without significant underlying tissue damage. The International Classification of Headache Disorders (ICHD-3) defines three subtypes within this group: 4.6.1 External-compression headache, 4.6.2 External-traction headache, and 4.6.3 Probable external pressure headache (Table 15.1). These subtypes are distinguished by their causative mechanisms. The diagnostic criteria emphasize the transient and reversible nature of these headaches. The onset of pain is directly linked to the application of external force, and the resolution occurs rapidly after the removal of the trigger [1]. These features distinguish these headaches from conditions such as occipital neuralgia, which involves neuropathic pain, and tension-type headache, which is diffuse and unrelated to external stimuli.

The ECH subtype is typically associated with prolonged pressure on the scalp or forehead caused by external objects such as helmets, goggles, or tight headbands. These headaches are often seen in occupational or recreational settings [1]. The

Table 15.1 Diagnostic criteria for external-pressure headache subtypes according to the ICHD-3 [1]

Headache type	Diagnostic criteria
External-pressure headache (4.6)	Headache resulting from sustained compression of or traction upon pericranial soft tissues. Comment: 4.6 External-pressure headache is a primary headache disorder because compression and traction are too subtle to cause damage to the scalp; in other words, they are physiological stimuli.
External-compression headache (4.6.1)	A. At least two episodes fulfilling criteria B–D B. Provoked by and occurring within one hour of sustained external compression C. Maximal pain at the site of compression D. Resolves within 1 h after compression relief E. Not better explained by another ICHD-3 diagnosis.
External-traction headache (4.6.2)	A. At least two episodes fulfilling criteria B–D B. Provoked by and occurring during sustained external traction C. Maximal pain at the site of traction D. Resolves within 1 h after traction relief E. Not better explained by another ICHD-3 diagnosis.
Probable external-compression headache (4.6.3)	A. Either of the following: 1. A single episode of headache fulfilling criteria B and D 2. At least two episodes of headache fulfilling criterion B and either but not both of criteria C and D B. Brought on by and occurring only during sustained external compression of or traction on the forehead and/or scalp C. Maximal at the compression or traction site D. Resolving within 1 h after compression or traction is relieved E. Not fulfilling ICHD-3 criteria for any other headache disorder F. Not better accounted for by another ICHD-3 diagnosis. Comment: Codable subforms are 4.6.3.1 Probable external-compression headache and 4.6.3.2 Probable external traction headache.

COVID-19 pandemic significantly increased the prevalence of this subtype due to the widespread and prolonged use of personal protective equipment (PPE), such as N95 masks and face shields, among healthcare workers. The repetitive pressure on the pericranial soft tissues, especially from tight-fitting PPE, has been cited in numerous studies as a significant trigger for this condition [4].

In contrast, ETH results from continuous pulling forces exerted on the scalp. Common triggers include hairstyles such as tight ponytails, braids, or hijabs [5, 6]. This subtype is more likely to occur in individuals with pre-existing scalp sensitivity or tenderness. The pain is typically localized to the area of traction, but may radiate if the force persists for a prolonged period [1].

15.5 Pathophysiology

The distinction between intracranial and extracranial headache origins is crucial for understanding and managing EPH. Intracranial headaches, such as those caused by meningitis, subarachnoid hemorrhage, or migraine, arise from internal brain structures. In contrast, extracranial headaches, including ECH and ETH, originate from superficial tissues such as the skin, subcutaneous layers, muscle fascia, and cutaneous nerves, particularly branches of the trigeminal and occipital nerves [5].

The ECH are believed to result from the compression of cutaneous nerves, especially branches of the trigeminal and occipital nerves [3]. Bands or accessories applied around the head, such as goggles (e.g., swimming goggles), tight hats, professional helmets, or PPE like face shields, masks, and goggles, can exert pressure on areas such as the occipitofrontal and temporalis muscles (Fig. 15.1) [3, 7]. This localized mechanical stress may irritate superficial sensory nerves, induce peripheral sensitization, and activate the trigeminocervical complex, potentially triggering headaches. Additionally, compression-induced neuralgia and cervical tension can further contribute to headache development [8]. During the COVID-19 pandemic, prolonged PPE use was frequently reported to trigger or exacerbate headaches, particularly in healthcare workers with pre-existing headache disorders [7]. Similarly,

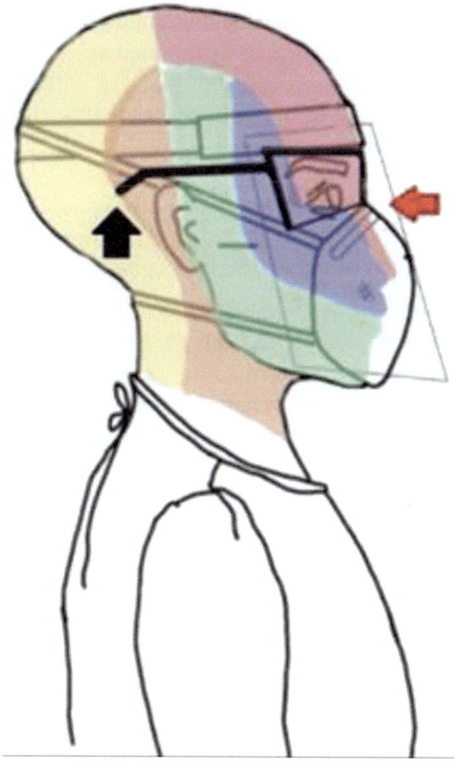

Fig 15.1 Relationship between the straps of the PPE and the cutaneous nerves of the head, branches of the trigeminal nerve, and cervical spinal nerve. The black arrow indicates the overlap of straps and rods in regions innervated by branches of the cervical spinal nerves. The red arrow points to the upper nasal region affected by the adjustment of the N95 mask's metal clip and the bridge of the glasses

the traction caused by tightly tied ponytails, headbands, or similar accessories demonstrates how mechanical forces can produce extracranial headache symptoms, with relief achieved by loosening or removing the source of pressure [5].

The influence of prolonged external stimuli is particularly significant in individuals predisposed to headaches, such as those with migraines or tension-type headaches. Compression of superficial sensory nerves—whether caused by PPE or other external sources—increases the likelihood of headache onset or intensifies pre-existing headache disorders. The literature highlights that these effects are especially pronounced in individuals with underlying headache risk factors, emphasizing the need for tailored preventive strategies and further investigation into these mechanisms [2, 9].

15.6 Clinical Presentation

15.6.1 External-Compression Headache (ECH)

The ECH is characterized by moderate pain that does not typically impede routine activities. The pain often intensifies gradually over minutes and is described as mild to moderate on the visual analog scale (VAS), with an average intensity of 4/10 [3, 10].

The pain is usually constant and non-pulsatile, localized to the area under pressure [3]. It is commonly reported as a sensation of pressure or heaviness, present in 87.5% of cases, while throbbing or pulling pain was noted in 11.7% of participants [2]. In healthcare workers using PPE, headaches were bilateral and occurred at points of contact with masks, goggles, or elastic straps [2]. Similarly, helmet-induced headaches were diffuse, with a pressing pain reported as the predominant type, alongside pulsating and sharp pain in fewer cases [11].

The source of compression strongly influences the location of pain. The frontal region is most frequently affected, although headaches related to helmets often extend diffusely to other areas of the head [11]. Pain onset typically occurs within 60 min of applying the compressive source and resolves spontaneously within 30 min to 1 h after its removal [10]. However, in some cases, continued use could lead to habituation and eventual remission of symptoms [11].

While ECH is generally not accompanied by associated symptoms [3], 23.4% of healthcare workers reported mild symptoms, including nausea, photophobia, phonophobia, neck discomfort, or movement sensitivity [2]. However, these symptoms were more likely in individuals with pre-existing primary headache disorders, such as migraines or tension-type headaches [2]. Notably, prolonged use of N95 masks and protective eyewear, especially when exceeding four hours per day, significantly increases the risk of headaches [2]. Rigid helmets with non-distensible materials and poorly adjustable bands were also identified as primary triggers [10].

In some cases, the persistence of the compressive stimulus exacerbated headache severity, particularly in individuals predisposed to migraines. Among affected individuals, 13.4% reported progression to unilateral, pulsating headaches with nausea and photophobia. For these individuals, removing the compressive accessory was insufficient to alleviate the pain, requiring symptomatic treatment with medications and rest. Interestingly, medications effective for their previous headache types were not consistently effective for ECH [10].

Prolonged exposure to compressive stimuli can lead to sensitization, causing more severe migrainous headaches in predisposed individuals [3]. Healthcare workers with pre-existing headache disorders were three times more likely to develop de novo PPE-associated headaches, particularly those working in high-stress environments such as emergency departments. Despite this, 68.8% of participants with PPE-related headaches did not require analgesics, and most who did used over-the-counter medications like paracetamol or non-steroidal anti-inflammatory drugs [2].

15.6.2 External-Traction Headache (ETH)

The ETH have a clinical presentation that is often influenced by the specific external stimulus. Ponytail headache, for example, is a well-recognized extracranial headache associated with hair being tied tightly in a ponytail. In a previous study, 50 out of 93 women reported experiencing headaches caused by this hairstyle. Pain was localized to the site of the hair tie in some cases, while in others it extended to areas such as the vertex, forehead, parietal region, or neck. The onset of pain occurred during or shortly after tying the hair, and loosening the ponytail provided immediate or gradual relief, typically within an hour. The headache was described as mild to moderate and purely extracranial, without accompanying autonomic or migrainous symptoms [5].

Similarly, hijab headache has been identified as an extracranial headache syndrome among women wearing a hijab. In another study, five cases involving women aged 20–63 years. All reported experiencing headaches directly related to donning the hijab. Four of these women had no prior history of headaches, while the fifth noted an increase in the severity and frequency of pre-existing tension-type headaches. The pain was typically mild or moderate, bilateral, and throbbing, localized to the vertex or parietal areas, with one individual describing pain involving the entire head. Symptom onset occurred within 30 min to 4 h of wearing the hijab, and relief was achieved within an hour of removing it. Notably, modifications to the hijab style, such as repositioning pins or using different fabrics, provided some relief for a subset of these women. One patient reported reduced symptoms during a two-year hiatus from wearing the hijab, further supporting the direct link between the headscarf and headache onset [6].

Both syndromes highlight the predictable clinical pattern of external-pressure headaches: pain localized to areas under mechanical stress, a clear temporal relationship between the application of the stimulus and the onset of symptoms, and rapid resolution upon removing or loosening the source of pressure. Although mild and self-limiting, these headaches can significantly impact individuals' daily comfort and activities, particularly when external pressure is prolonged or unavoidable due to cultural or occupational practices.

15.7 Management

Management and prevention of EPH primarily focus on addressing the underlying mechanical triggers and minimizing the impact of prolonged external pressure. Strategies include non-pharmacological approaches, pharmacological treatments, and patient education, tailored to individual cases and occupational needs.

15.7.1 Nonpharmacological Strategies

The cornerstone of managing EPH is the removal or adjustment of pressure-causing devices. Patients are advised to either avoid headgear or ensure it fits properly and comfortably. Trying different sizes or styles of helmets or adjusting internal components, such as leather bands, can help alleviate discomfort [3]. Frequent removal of the headgear during use to relieve pressure can also prevent the progression of pain [10].

Ergonomic modifications are particularly effective for individuals who cannot avoid wearing headgear, such as healthcare workers or military personnel. Suggestions include loosening ponytails or adopting alternative hijab styles to reduce tension and pressure on sensitive areas. When PPE is required, ensuring a proper fit and alternating between different designs may reduce the risk of EPH [3].

15.7.2 Pharmacological Strategies

Most EPH cases do not require pharmacological treatment. Studies show that up to 68.8% of participants with PPE-associated headaches did not use analgesics during episodes. When necessary, over-the-counter medications such as paracetamol or non-steroidal anti-inflammatory drugs are the most commonly used options for acute pain relief [2]. Similarly, among military personnel experiencing helmet-induced headaches, 28% occasionally used over-the-counter analgesics to alleviate symptoms [11].

For patients with underlying migraine or other primary headache disorders, prolonged exposure to external compression can trigger severe migrainous episodes. In these cases, removing the causative stimulus alone is insufficient, and standard migraine-specific medications, such as triptans or preventive treatments, may be necessary to control the symptoms [10]. However, the efficacy of these treatments for compression-related headaches remains inconsistent and often requires further individualized management strategies.

15.7.3 *Patient Education and Awareness*

Raising awareness about EPH among at-risk populations is crucial for prevention. Educational materials can inform patients and workers about the importance of proper headgear fit and the potential risks associated with prolonged compression. Emphasizing the importance of trying different headgear designs to find the most comfortable options and taking regular breaks to relieve pressure can help reduce the frequency and intensity of headaches [3]. For healthcare workers, awareness programs about the risk of PPE-associated headaches and practical strategies for minimizing their occurrence can enhance comfort and productivity, particularly in high-stress environments such as emergency departments [2].

15.8 Conclusion

The EPH represent a distinct group of primary headache disorders, often triggered by mechanical forces such as compression or traction applied to the scalp. These headaches, while typically mild and transient, can significantly affect individuals' quality of life, particularly in occupational or cultural contexts where the use of headgear or specific hairstyles is unavoidable. This chapter has explored the classification, pathophysiology, clinical presentation, and management strategies for EPH, emphasizing its growing relevance during the COVID-19 pandemic and in high-risk occupational settings.

The pathophysiology of EPH involves localized mechanical stress on cutaneous nerves, leading to peripheral sensitization and activation of pain pathways. Accurate diagnosis relies on recognizing the characteristic temporal relationship between symptom onset and the application of external pressure, as well as the rapid resolution of symptoms upon removing the stimulus. Effective management focuses on non-pharmacological strategies, including ergonomic modifications and patient education, while pharmacological interventions are reserved for more severe or persistent cases, particularly in individuals with a predisposition.

Despite advances in understanding EPH, significant knowledge gaps remain. Future research should address the long-term impact of repetitive external compression, the role of individual susceptibility factors, and the development of optimized prevention and management strategies. Increased awareness and tailored interventions can mitigate the burden of EPH, enhancing comfort and functionality in both occupational and daily settings.

References

1. Headache Classification Committee of the International Headache Society (IHS). The International Classification of Headache Disorders, 3rd edition. Cephalalgia, 2018. 38(1): p. 1–211.

2. Ong JJY, et al. Headaches associated with personal protective equipment – a cross-sectional study among frontline healthcare workers during COVID-19. Headache. 2020;60(5):864–77.
3. Krymchantowski AV. Headaches due to external compression. Curr Pain Headache Rep. 2010;14(4):321–4.
4. Ribeiro ERR, Lal A, Tardieux FM, Ribeiro ECO, Fortes HMS, Valença MM. Cefaleia por pressão externa: uma entidade frequente e menos reconhecida. In: Valença MM, editor. Cefaleia, vol. 1. Advances in Science; 2022. p. 223–33.
5. Blau JN. Ponytail headache: a pure extracranial headache. Headache. 2004;44(5):411–3.
6. Ansari HN, Solomon GD. Hijab (headscarf) headache. Headache. 2015;55(3):437–8.
7. Ong JJY, et al. Headache Related to PPE Use during the COVID-19 Pandemic. Curr Pain Headache Rep. 2021;25(8):53.
8. Barmherzig R, Kingston W. Occipital neuralgia and Cervicogenic headache: diagnosis and management. Curr Neurol Neurosci Rep. 2019;19(5):20.
9. dos Santos ERR, Lal A, Tardieux FM, Fortes HMS, Valença MM. External compression headache during Covid-19 pandemic: a neglected entity. Headache Medicine. 2023;14(2):77–82.
10. Krymchantowski A, et al. Helmet-related, external compression headache among police officers in Rio de Janeiro. MedGenMed. 2004;6(2):45.
11. Rahmani Z, et al. Helmet-induced headache among Danish military personnel. Scand J Public Health. 2017;45(8):818–23.

Chapter 16
Epicrania Fugax

Gonçalo Diniz Pinho and Raquel Gil Gouveia

16.1 Introduction

Epicrania Fugax (EF) is a rare primary headache disorder characterized by brief, intense paroxysms of stabbing or shock-like unilateral pain localized to the scalp that start in specific points and follow a fast trajectory usually in postero-anterior direction, though antero-posterior, coronal, diagonal, or multidirectional patterns of radiation have also been reported [1–5]. These trajectories do not conform to specific nerve territories and may even involve the face [6]. At the end of attacks, ipsilateral autonomic signs such as lacrimation, conjunctival injection, and/or rhinorrhea may occur [7].

Epicrania Fugax is listed in the appendix of the *International Classification of Headache Disorders* (ICHD) [7]. Still, shares features with other epicranial pain syndromes categorized under primary headaches, such as nummular headache and primary stabbing headache. Similar to nummular headache, EF typically originates from a well-defined circular area or a broader linear band located in the frontal, temporal, parietal, or occipital regions of the scalp. However, unlike nummular headache, EF is distinguished by the rapid and transient migration of pain to other neurocranial areas. Primary stabbing headache is characterized by brief, sharp, unilateral pain typically lasting around one second and occurring in diverse sites on the cranial surface, including extra-trigeminal areas. However, it may be fixed in up to a third of patients. Attacks may be associated with sudden head or body movements

G. D. Pinho
Neurology Department, Hospital da Luz Lisboa, Lisboa, Portugal

R. G. Gouveia (✉)
Neurology Department, Hospital da Luz Lisboa, Lisboa, Portugal

Center for Interdisciplinary Research in Health, Universidade Católica Portuguesa, Lisboa, Portugal

D. Uludüz et al. (eds.), *Rare Causes of Headache Disorders*, Headache, https://doi.org/10.1007/978-3-032-10242-3_16

(jolts), and their frequency can vary widely, ranging from a single attack per year to up to 50 attacks per day, with no consistent temporal pattern.

These epicranial primary headaches can be mistaken for headaches secondary to pericranial neuralgias, particularly those involving the trigeminal nerve, most notably the first branch (V1), auriculotemporal neuralgia [8] as well as the intermediate branch of the facial nerve (cranial nerve VII), the glossopharyngeal nerve (cranial nerve IX), or cervical nerve root compression. The key distinguishing feature lies in their variable onset and radiation patterns, which often do not follow classical dermatomal distribution [9–11]. Additionally, the differential diagnosis may include trigeminal autonomic cephalalgias, such as Short-lasting Unilateral Neuralgiform Headache with Conjuntival Injection and Tearing (SUNCT) or Short-lasting Unilateral Neuralgiform Headache attacks with Cranial Autonomic Symptoms (SUNA), especially when mild autonomic symptoms are present [9].

Secondary forms of EF have been described in association with ipsilateral structural lesions, most notably involving the posterior fossa, such as intracranial tumors, abscesses, or ischemic stroke, as well as peripheral abnormalities, including post-surgical or traumatic scalp scars [12–15], thus justifying a broad etiological assessment, particularly in older patients.

Most reported cases involve female patients, with a female-to-male ratio of approximately 1.6:1 and a mean age of 45 years. However, the age at onset varies widely, ranging from 19 to 84 years. The time from symptom onset to diagnosis is also highly variable, spanning from 2 days to 38 years. Some studies have suggested a possible association with specific personality traits and the presence of anxiety or depressive symptoms [16, 17]. No pediatric cases have been documented to date [9].

Given the absence of population-based studies and the fact that all reported cases originate from headache clinics, the available epidemiological data are likely subject to selection bias. The frequent comorbidity with other primary headache disorders, such as migraine, tension-type headache, trigeminal neuralgia, cluster headache, and auriculotemporal neuralgia, further supports this. It is plausible that patients presenting with EF were identified primarily due to these associated headache conditions, which brought them to medical care and increased the likelihood of referral to specialized neurological attention [9].

16.2 Pathophysiology

The pathophysiology of EF remains incompletely understood but is believed to involve both peripheral and central mechanisms. This dual involvement is supported by reports of secondary EF-like cases linked to lesions at either level, including surgical epicranial scars, trigeminal root lesions, and brainstem infarctions [9].

Current hypotheses propose a multifactorial interplay involving focal neuropathy of terminal cranial sensory fibers, anomalous or redundant anastomoses between these fibers, either congenital or acquired (e.g., via aberrant reinnervation), and central trigeminal sensitization, which may occur independently or in the context of a central nervous system lesion [5, 18].

The pain's non-dermatomal distribution and directional propagation suggest mechanisms such as ephaptic transmission between neighboring nerve endings or trans diploic signal conduction [19, 20]. A potential role for pathology affecting the proximal cervical nerve roots (before their distal branching) has also been proposed [3]; in such cases, however, coexisting cervical or other headache syndromes should be carefully ruled out.

Involvement of the trigemino-cervical complex is likely, as it integrates nociceptive input from both the trigeminal and upper cervical spinal nerves. This convergence may underlie the characteristic linear, strictly unilateral trajectory of pain in EF, which can be accompanied by ipsilateral autonomic symptoms [9]. Additional central subcortical mechanisms in the brainstem or spinal cord may contribute to the extracranial radiation patterns observed in some patients [21]. However, unlike migraine or other primary headache disorders, EF pain is typically dynamic and sharply localized, rather than static or diffuse.

This challenges the extent to which higher-order central sensitization (such as thalamo-cortical involvement) contributes to its clinical presentation, and suggests a distinct pathophysiological profile compared to other central pain syndromes, such as migraine or other primary headache disorders with allodynia [9].

The observation that anxiety and depressive symptoms are more frequently reported in EF patients than in those with other headache disorders [9] could also suggest a more prominent central component to pain processing. However, paradoxically, patients with low-frequency EF episodes have been found to exhibit higher levels of anxiety, which argues against a direct correlation with central modulation of pain. This inconsistency may be better explained by referral bias as individuals with higher levels of anxiety may be more likely to seek medical care [22].

16.3 Case Presentation

A 61-year-old woman presented to the neurology clinic with a two-year history of brief, recurring episodes of dull pain, occasionally accompanied by tenderness, localized to the right scalp. Her past medical history included low-frequency episodic tension-type headache starting back in her 40s, as well as arterial hypertension and anxiety. She recalled a previous episode of blunt parietal trauma in her youth, requiring observation in the hospital for a few hours. Yet, she denied posttraumatic headache and did not relate the site of pain origin to the trauma location. She also denied having had any precipitating event of skin lesions at the time of symptom onset. Her daily medication included escitalopram 10 mg id and losartan 100 mg id.

She described a sharp, intense (8/10 VAS) pain as occurring in a horizontal bar-like area extending from the occipital to frontal scalp regions, moving rapidly in a linear fashion. Each episode lasted fewer than 10 s and occurred 10–20 times per day, sometimes persisting daily, for up to two weeks, without seasonal predominance. Sometimes, a dull discomfort persisted in the same area, between paroxysms. There were periods of pain freedom that lasted days, up to one month. There were no identifiable triggers, nor were there associated migraine or cranial autonomic symptoms during attacks.

General and neurological examinations were unremarkable. Notably, cranial artery palpation was normal, with no trophic skin changes or sensory abnormalities in trigeminal or cervical dermatomes. There was no craniofacial or cervical tenderness on palpation or maneuvering, and deep tendon reflexes were preserved.

Laboratory investigations, including erythrocyte sedimentation rate, C-reactive protein, serum electrolytes, calcium, albumin, magnesium, phosphorus, lactate dehydrogenase, alkaline phosphatase, Herpes Zoster serology, and vitamin B complex, were all within normal limits. Cranial magnetic resonance imaging (MRI) and Doppler ultrasound of the superficial temporal arteries revealed no abnormalities. Cervical spine MRI showed uncovertebral arthrosis from C5 to C7, with mild bilateral foraminal stenosis but no significant spinal canal narrowing or cord compression.

Rescue treatment with paracetamol and ibuprofen provided only occasional mild relief and was used less than once per week. A therapeutic trial with indomethacin was ineffective. Switching escitalopram with duloxetine yielded modest improvement at two months. She was subsequently referred to the headache clinic, where gabapentin was started and titrated to 1200 mg/day, resulting in a good and sustained clinical response at the six-month follow-up.

16.4 Case Discussion

This case raised several red flags, including the new onset of headache after the age of 60, with a phenotype consistent with a rare primary headache disorder. The differential diagnosis of secondary headaches in this patient included posterior fossa structural lesions, giant cell arteritis, zoster sine herpete, and high cervical nerve root compression, all of which were ruled out through an extensive diagnostic workup. Initial treatment strategies, including nonsteroidal anti-inflammatory drugs, indomethacin, and duloxetine, were ineffective. However, initiation of antiepileptic therapy resulted in significant and sustained symptom relief, supporting a neuropathic pain.

16.5 Characteristics of Epicrania Fugax and Differential Diagnosis

EF is most commonly perceived in the sensory territories of the upper trigeminal (particularly V1) and occipital nerves. However, the pain does not strictly follow anatomical boundaries and is almost invariably unilateral [3, 21, 23]. Notably, in a few reported cases, the pain trajectory has crossed the sagittal plane [4, 9].

Patients typically describe EF as brief, sharply localized paroxysms lasting less than 10 seconds. These episodes are characterized by a rapid, linear (occasionally irregular and zigzagging) pain that travels across the scalp on one side of the head, a presentation considered pathognomonic for this condition [24]. Although one or both hemicrania may be affected, the pain projection pattern is nearly always ipsilateral to its point of origin. The pain typically moves in a postero-anterior (forward) direction, while retrograde (backwards) radiation is less frequently reported. In very rare cases, pain has been observed to alternate sides between episodes or radiate beyond the head to other regions such as the lower face, thorax, abdomen, or limbs [6, 9, 11, 25, 26], maintaining the same fast, progressive, and orderly propagation pattern characteristic of EF.

The pain in EF is typically neuralgic in nature (commonly described as electric shock-like or stabbing) but may also present as burning, sharp, or oppressive, and is generally of moderate to severe intensity. In up to one-third of patients, EF may be accompanied by ipsilateral autonomic symptoms such as conjunctival injection, tearing, or rhinorrhea, suggesting activation of the trigemino-autonomic reflex [3, 24]. The headache's topography and the temporal pattern of attacks are useful to differentiate it from trigeminal autonomic cephalalgias (TACs).

EF episodes are characteristically very brief, usually lasting less than 15 s and never exceeding one minute. Unlike TACs, EF does not follow a consistent circadian or seasonal pattern. The frequency of attacks varies widely; episodes may occur sporadically, only a few times per year, or several times daily. Attacks can appear as isolated events, in clusters of pain paroxysms, or both. Notably, EF attacks have not been reported during sleep. While most patients experience daily attacks for prolonged periods, others may report more infrequent episodes with spontaneous or treatment-induced remissions. No seasonal predominance has been observed [9].

Paroxysms may be triggered by pressure or touch at the site of pain onset, neck movements, stress, eye movements, or Valsalva maneuvers [9]. Persistent local allodynia may persist after attacks [20], requiring differentiation from trigeminal or other cranial neuralgias.

The brief, stabbing nature of EF also necessitates differentiation from primary stabbing (ice-pick) headache. In some patients, a longer-lasting, duller pain may persist at the site of origin between paroxysms, mimicking nummular headache [19, 21, 27]. Additionally, EF may resemble linear headache (a variant of nummular headache) where the painful and dysesthetic area is linear rather than round or coin-shaped. In both conditions, the affected area may cross several terminal nerve territories. However, a key distinction is that EF pain is migratory, traveling across the scalp, whereas linear headache pain typically remains stationary [9].

16.6 Diagnostic Algorithm

Step 1: Clinical Suspicion

- *Identify Key Symptoms*:

  Clinical Presentation: Recurrent, short-lasting, unilateral, superficial, shock-like pain with a dynamic trajectory, most commonly postero-anterior, but occasionally antero-posterior, coronal, or diagonal in direction.

The pain typically follows a linear, zigzag, or back-and-forth path across mixed trigeminal and occipital sensory nerve distributions.
Clinical Evaluation: Assessment should include careful documentation of associated symptoms (e.g., autonomic features) and the temporal pattern of pain paroxysms, including frequency, duration, and triggering factors.
Physical Examination: Thorough evaluation should focus on the area of pain onset, with detailed inspection and palpation of the cranium, epicranial skin, muscles, and arteries. A complete neurological examination is essential, along with general physical assessment, to exclude secondary causes and identify possible contributing factors.

Step 2: Diagnostic Workup

- *Blood Tests*:
  - Exclude systemic inflammation or vasculitis, particularly giant cell arteritis, depending on the patient's age.
  - Screen for nutritional or metabolic causes of neuropathy (e.g., vitamin deficiencies, diabetes).
  - Assess for potential inflammatory or toxic neuropathies; include zoster serology if clinical suspicion exists.
  - Evaluate for metabolic bone diseases, such as Paget's disease.
- *Neuroimaging: Brain and cervical spine MRI to investigate*:
  - Lesions affecting the trigeminal sensory nerve root, brainstem, or cervical spinal cord.
  - Mass-occupying lesions or compressive abnormalities (e.g., pontocerebellar angle tumors, aneurysms).
  - Structural changes due to bone remodeling (e.g., Paget's disease).
  - Trophic or infiltrative lesions affecting superficial sensory nerve fibers or overlying skin.
- *Additional Diagnostic Workup (age-dependent and based on clinical suspicion)*:
  - *Temporal artery Doppler ultrasound* to rule out giant cell arteritis.
  - *Electroneuromyography (ENMG)* for evaluation of peripheral nerve dysfunction.
  - *Somatosensory evoked potentials (SSEPs)* to assess central sensory pathways, including the brainstem and cervical spinal cord.
  - *Electroencephalography (EEG)* in cases with possible sensory focal seizures presenting as paroxysmal pain [21].

Step 3: Apply ICHD-3 Diagnostic Criteria [24]

A. Recurrent stabbing head pain attacks lasting 1–10 s and fulfilling criterion B

B. Pain moving with a linear or zigzag trajectory across the surface of one hemicranium, commencing and terminating in the distributions of different nerves
C. Not better accounted by another ICHD-3 diagnosis

16.7 Management

Management of EF primarily focuses on symptomatic relief and patient reassurance. Preventive daily anticonvulsant medications are considered the most effective treatment, with gabapentin and lamotrigine being the most commonly used. However, other options such as pregabalin, carbamazepine, oxcarbazepine, eslicarbazepine, lacosamide, levetiracetam, and valproic acid are also utilized, titrated to the most effective non-toxic doses [5, 9, 28].

Other medications such as amitriptyline, duloxetine, and indomethacin have shown some success in some instances. For patients with limited response or poor tolerability to these agents, local anesthetics (e.g., lidocaine, bupivacaine) with or without corticosteroids, and subcutaneous onabotulinum toxin A injections have been tried with favorable outcomes [9, 29, 30].

The prognosis for most patients is generally good, with many experiencing improvements with treatment or spontaneous remission. In patients who respond well to treatment, a gradual withdrawal of medication may be considered, although there is no established consensus or protocol for this approach. Some patients with infrequent attacks may choose not to initiate treatment, as symptom exacerbation without intervention is rare.

16.8 Conclusion

Epicrania Fugax was first defined in 2008 [20], and to date, over 100 cases have been described in the literature, making it a rare headache disorder. However, given the brief nature of the attacks, it is likely that many more patients exist who remain undiagnosed. These individuals may not seek medical attention due to the transient nature of the pain, or primary care physicians may not be aware of the condition, leading to missed diagnoses and a lack of referrals. Even within neurology clinics, this rare primary headache may be underdiagnosed due to the overlap of some of its characteristics with other primary headache disorders. The atypical pain patterns, such as the zigzag trajectory, shifts in direction, and radiation to other parts of the body, are often mistakenly attributed to anxiety, depression, or functional neurological disorders. While EF is frequently comorbid with mental health conditions, the increasing recognition of its unique manifestations and pathophysiological mechanisms has improved patient care and treatment options. A correct diagnosis is critical for encouraging patients and promoting better outcomes.

References

1. Mulero P, Guerrero AL, Herrero-Velázquez S, Cortijo E, Pedraza M, Peñas ML, Miranda S, Rojo E, Fernández R. Epicrania fugax with backward radiation: clinical characteristics of nine new cases. J Headache Pain. 2011;12(5):535–9. https://doi.org/10.1007/s10194-011-0353-1.
2. Pareja JA, Álvarez M, Montojo T. Epicrania fugax with backward radiation. J Headache Pain. 2012;13(2):175.
3. Man YH, Qi JJ, Yu TM, Yao G. Epicrania fugax with a novel sign: pain paroxysms with parallel forward or backward trajectories. Pain Med. 2020;21(4):873–5. https://doi.org/10.1093/pm/pnz239.
4. Cuadrado ML, Aledo-Serrano A, Di Capua D, Pareja JA. A multidirectional epicrania fugax. Cephalalgia. 2015;35(9):835–6. https://doi.org/10.1177/0333102414564893.
5. Barón-Sánchez J, Gutiérrez-Viedma Á, Ruiz-Piñero M, Pérez-Pérez A, Guerrero ÁL, Cuadrado ML. Epicrania fugax combining forward and backward paroxysms in the same patient: the first four cases. J Pain Res. 2017;10:1453–6. https://doi.org/10.2147/JPR.S135810.
6. Cuadrado ML, Aledo-Serrano Á, Jiménez-Almonacid J, De Lera M, Guerrero ÁL. Facial pain radiating upwards: could the pain of Epicrania fugax start in the lower face? Headache. 2015;55(5):690–5.
7. (IHS) C of the IHS. Headache Classification The International Classification of Headache Disorders, 3rd edition. Cephalalgia [Internet]. 2018 [cited 2019 Nov 15];38(1):1–211. Available from: www.uk.sagepub.com.
8. Navarrete JJ, Ruiz M, Juanatey A, Barón J, Cuadrado ML, Guerrero AL. The Relationship of Auriculotemporal Neuralgia and Epicrania Fugax. Pain Med. 2018;19(3):635–636. https://doi.org/10.1093/pm/pnx158.
9. Cuadrado ML. Epicranial headaches part 2: nummular headache and epicrania fugax. Cephalalgia. 2023;43(4):3331024221146976. https://doi.org/10.1177/03331024221146976.
10. Navarrete JJ, Ruiz M, Juanatey A, Barón J, Cuadrado ML, Guerrero AL. The relationship of auriculotemporal neuralgia and epicrania fugax. Pain Med. 2018;19(3):635–6. https://doi.org/10.1093/pm/pnx158.
11. Wang Y, Kan P-L, Tao Y-F, Li X-Y, Yang X-J, Liang G-L. A case of prethoracic pain radiating upward and initiating nervus intermedius neuralgia and migraine headache: could epicrania fugax pain start in the upper body? J Oral Facial Pain Headache. 2017;31(4):398–401.
12. García-Azorín D, Dotor García-Soto J, Martínez-Pías E, Guerrero-Peral AL. Epicrania fugax as the presenting symptom of a cerebellar abscess. Cephalalgia. 2019;39(9):1200–3.
13. Fernández-Matarrubia M, Gutiérrez-Viedma Á, Cuadrado ML. Case report: epicranial pain after radiotherapy for skull base meningioma – the first symptomatic epicrania fugax? Cephalalgia. 2016;36(14):1389–91.
14. Jaimes A, García-Sáez R, Gutiérrez-Viedma Á, Cuadrado ML. Case report: Wallenberg's syndrome, a possible cause of symptomatic epicrania fugax. Cephalalgia. 2018;38(6):1203–6.
15. Cuadrado ML, González-García N, Porta-Etessam J. Epicrania fugax originating from a surgical scar of the scalp. Pain Pract. 2022;22(6):600–1. https://doi.org/10.1111/papr.13109.
16. Rammohan K, Shyma MM, Das S, Shaji CV. Clinical features and psychiatric comorbidity of epicrania fugax. J Neurosci Rural Pract. 2018;9(1):143–8.
17. López-López A, González JL, Guerrero ÁL, Ordás CM, Muñoz I, Cuadrado ML. Stress, coping, and personality in patients with Epicrania fugax, and their relation to the clinical characteristics of pain. Pain Med (United States). 2017;18(1):152–60.
18. Gutiérrez-Viedma Á, González-García N, Yus M, Jorquera M, Porta-Etessam J, García-Moreno H, et al. Facial epicrania fugax: a prospective series of eight new cases. Cephalalgia. 2017;37(12):1145–51.
19. Herrero-Velázquez S, Guerrero AL, Pedraza MI, Mulero P, Ayllón B, Ruiz-Piñero M, et al. Nummular headache and epicrania fugax: possible association of epicranias in eight patients. Pain Med (United States). 2013;14(3):358–61.

20. Pareja JA, Cuadrado ML, Fernández-De-Las-Peñas C, Caminero AB, Nieto C, Sánchez C, et al. Epicrania fugax: an ultrabrief paroxysmal epicranial pain. Cephalalgia. 2008;28(3):257–63.
21. Gutiérrez-Sánchez M, García-Azorín D, Gutiérrez-Viedma Á, González-García N, Horga A, Martín S, et al. Paroxysmal headache with extracephalic irradiation: proposal for a new variant of epicrania fugax in a series of five patients. Cephalalgia. 2020;40(9):959–65.
22. Horenstein A, Heimberg RG. Anxiety disorders and healthcare utilization: a systematic review. Clin Psychol Rev. 2020;81:101894. https://doi.org/10.1016/j.cpr.2020.101894.
23. Guerrero AL, Cuadrado ML, Porta-Etessam J, García-Ramos R, Gómez-Vicente L, Herrero S, et al. Epicrania fugax: ten new cases and therapeutic results. Headache. 2010;50(3):451–8.
24. Cuadrado ML, Ordás CM, Sánchez-Lizcano M, Casas-Limón J, Matías-Guiu JA, García-García ME, et al. Epicrania fugax: 19 cases of an emerging headache. Headache. 2013;53(5):764–74.
25. Cuadrado ML, Guerrero AL, Pareja JA. Epicrania Fugax. Curr Pain Headache Rep. 2016;20(4):21. https://doi.org/10.1007/s11916-016-0557-9.
26. Gómez-Mayordomo V, García-Sáez R, Gallego-Gallego M, González-García N, Cuadrado ML. Cranial and facial epicrania fugax: combination of both clinical pictures in the same patients. Headache. 2020;60(3):621–3.
27. Wang Y, Pan QQ, Lu YN, Tian MM, Wang XH. Linear interictal pain in Epicrania Fugax: a reply. J Headache Pain. 2015;16(1):23.
28. Wang L, Pan JF, Lu YY, Hu LH, Lu YN, Pan QQ, et al. A recurrent headache circumscribed in a coronal line-shaped area around the head: a coronal linear headache. Springerplus. 2016;5(1):315.
29. Alberola-Amores FJ, Moral-Rubio J. Drug-resistant epicrania fugax: responding to onabotulinumtoxinA. Headache. 2023;63(6):839–42.
30. Cuadrado ML, Aledo-Serrano Á, Ruiz-Álvarez L. Eslicarbazepine acetate for a patient with highly resistant epicrania fugax. Pain Pract. 2015;15(1):E27. https://doi.org/10.1111/papr.12261.

Chapter 17
Nummular Headache

Tülay Yılmaz and Betül Baykan

17.1 Introduction

First described in 2002 by Pareja et al. [1] and previously referred to as "coin-shaped headache", nummular headache (NH) is recognized as a primary headache disorder in the International Classification of Headache Disorders-3 (ICHD-3) [2]. It is characterized by persistent, intermittent, or chronic pain confined to a specific, circumscribed region of the scalp, in the absence of any underlying structural or lesional cause. The painful region can be located anywhere on the scalp, but it is most commonly found in the parietal area. In rare instances, NH may present as bi- or multifocal complaints, with each affected region maintaining all the defining features of the condition. Pain intensity is typically mild to moderate, but it can occasionally become severe. In addition to the baseline discomfort, spontaneous or triggered exacerbations may occur. The duration is highly variable; up to 75% of the reported cases have shown a chronic pattern (lasting longer than three months), though episodes lasting seconds, minutes, hours, or days have also been reported [2]. Symptoms such as allodynia, dysesthesia, paresthesia, or hypoesthesia may accompany episodes of pain [3].

Although large-scale epidemiological studies are lacking, the annual incidence rate is estimated to be approximately 9 cases per 100,000 individuals. NH is more common in women (1.8:1) and typically begins in the fourth decade of life, although it has a wide age range of onset (4-79 years) [4]. In a recent hospital-based,

---

T. Yılmaz
Ümraniye Training and Research Hospital, University of Health Sciences, Istanbul, Turkey

B. Baykan (✉)
Neurology and Clinical Neurophysiology, EMAR Medical Center, Istanbul, Turkey

D. Uludüz et al. (eds.), *Rare Causes of Headache Disorders*, Headache,
https://doi.org/10.1007/978-3-032-10242-3_17

multicenter study, Head-MENA-A (Middle East, North Africa, Asia), which included a large cohort from Türkiye, the prevalence of NH among patients presenting with headaches was reported to be 0.3% [5].

17.2 Pathophysiology

The pathogenesis of NH remains unclear and has yet to be fully elucidated. Two primary theories have been proposed: one emphasizing a peripheral origin and the other focusing on central mechanisms. Initially, NH was described as a form of localized neuralgia arising from epicranial structures, particularly the terminal branches of cutaneous nerves. This hypothesis is supported by the fact that the pain is confined to a specific area and by the presence of sensory alterations, such as hypoesthesia, hyperesthesia, or paresthesia, in some patients. Additionally, some cases have reported trophic changes, such as hair heterochromia, within the affected area [6]. As stated, the origin of NH may involve a local lesion or dysfunction in the terminal branches of the pericranial nerves. Still, it may also be associated with a deeper level of localization. The presence of nerve fibers traversing the skull through emissary channels and fissures has been identified using fluorescence microscopy and electron microscopy [7]. The diffuse hypersensitivity of pericranial structures, characteristic of migraine and tension-type headaches, appears to be absent in NH [8]. Pressure algometry has revealed that pain thresholds are reduced specifically at the symptomatic site, while the remainder of the scalp shows no significant change, which is intriguing [7, 9]. On the other hand, NH does not align precisely with the distribution of peripheral innervation territories and does not consistently respond to local anesthetic injections [6]. Some patients exhibit triggers and symptoms resembling those seen in migraine, suggesting that central mechanisms may play a prominent role [10, 11]. In some cases, algometric assessments have revealed a generally reduced pain threshold, which supports the hypothesis of central sensitization [11]. Some patients with NH experience pain that crosses the midline of the scalp or occurs in multiple areas, which also suggests a central mechanism [6].

Although NH is classified as a primary headache, cases with secondary etiologies have also been reported. These cases are associated with underlying structural lesions or other causes such as meningioma, arachnoid cysts, fusiform aneurysms, prior local neurosurgery, varicella-zoster rash, cranial bone pathologies, or some benign cranial lesions. Almost all the cases described showed a close anatomical relationship between the pain and the underlying lesion. There are also reported cases following head trauma and cranial surgery. These observations suggest the existence of a secondary form of NH. Therefore, secondary causes should be carefully considered and excluded during the differential diagnosis [6, 12]. In some patients with NH, autoimmune markers have been detected, and it has been suggested that immunological mechanisms may trigger the pain in these patients. The presence of antinuclear antibodies (ANA) was the most frequently observed finding in the blood tests of these patients [13].

17.3 Case Presentation

This case report presents a 47-year-old female patient, S*, who has been experiencing unilateral, throbbing headache attacks for approximately 10 years. These headaches, which occur alternately on the right and left sides, originate from the occipital region and extend to one half of the head, often involving the eye. The attacks are accompanied by photophobia, phonophobia, nausea, and occasionally vomiting, typically lasting around eight hours. The frequency of the attacks has been reported as one to two times per month. The patient was previously diagnosed with migraine without aura. It was noted that her symptoms subsided with the use of eletriptan 40 mg during attack periods. However, in the past three months, the patient became concerned about a newly developed pain pattern that was distinct from her typical migraine attacks. She described a burning, numbness, and tingling sensation localized to a circular area of approximately 6 cm in diameter in the right parietal region. She stated that these new symptoms developed independently of her migraine episodes, were unrelated to stress, and lasted from one to three days. The patient noted that her symptoms completely resolved with the use of flurbiprofen.

The patient consulted her family physician due to this headache that, although not very severe, was noticeably different from her previous side-changing migraine attacks and consistently located at the same spot, causing concern. The family physician, sharing the patient's concern, recommended a referral to neurology to rule out any underlying conditions. Neurological examination revealed no abnormalities, and the pain was localized to a well-defined circular area in the right parietal region without any associated skin lesions. Laboratory tests and brain magnetic resonance imaging (MRI) showed no pathological findings.

Based on these findings, the patient was diagnosed with NH. She was informed that NH is a benign condition, and symptomatic treatment would be sufficient unless it significantly affected her quality of life. The treatment plan included NSAIDs for symptom relief on an as-needed basis, and gabapentin can be recommended in case of persistent or chronic symptoms.

During the follow-up period, no significant worsening of the patient's symptoms was observed, and the symptoms were well controlled with NSAID use.

17.4 Case Discussion

This case highlights the possibility that NH may coexist with other primary headache disorders, such as migraine [5, 14, 15], emphasizing the need for careful clinical differentiation. The key characteristic of NH is its localized circular nature, confined to a specific area of the scalp, which helps differentiate it from other headache types [1]. However, secondary causes such as meningioma, cranial lesions, head trauma, vascular anomalies, or infections such as varicella-zoster must be thoroughly ruled out [16, 17]. Therefore, a comprehensive medical history, neurological examination, and appropriate blood tests and neuro-imaging studies, preferably MRI with contrast enhancement, are crucial in the diagnostic process.

This case is significant as it highlights that both family physicians and patients may not adequately recognize this type of primary headache, leading to high concern. Studies have shown that primary care physicians often encounter patients with headache complaints but may lack sufficient knowledge in this area, underscoring the need for regular educational programs.

In this case, the patient's long-standing history of migraine suggests that NH may coexist with migraine, as reported in studies dealing with other primary headaches. Their high rate of co-existence with migraine may indicate shared predisposing factors, hinting at a "eadache continuum" concept for primary headaches [5].

The resolution of her symptoms with NSAIDs supports that symptomatic treatment may be sufficient in mild cases. However, if the symptoms are refractory to NSAIDs and become chronic, gabapentin, which is commonly used in the treatment of neuropathic pain, could be considered [18].

17.5 Clinical Characteristics

Pain is typically localized to a distinct cranial area, clearly outlined by the patient, and is most commonly round (80%) or oval-shaped (20%) (Fig. 17.1). The diameter of the painful region, as per diagnostic criteria, generally ranges between 1 and 6 cm [12]. However, cases with larger areas (up to 10 cm in diameter) have been reported [15]. Notably, the shape and size of the painful area remain consistent over time [12].

Pain is most frequently localized to the parietal region (44%) and less commonly to the occipital region (22%), with involvement of other regions being rare. It typically presents as a single focus, with bifocal cases being rare and multifocal presentations extremely rare. The pain is described as pressing, stabbing, burning, or throbbing [6]. Abnormal sensations, such as allodynia, dysesthesia, paresthesia, and hypoesthesia, may accompany pain episodes in the affected area. Pain intensity is typically mild to moderate; however, severe pain was reported in 25% of cases and very severe pain in 2%, highlighting that high-intensity pain is not uncommon. In a cohort of 102 patients, the mean score on the visual analog scale (VAS), used to assess pain intensity, was 5 [6]. In the Head-MENA-A study on other primary headache disorders, the mean VAS score for NH was found to be 6.6 (4–8) [5]. Typically, there were no associated symptoms, such as photophobia, phonophobia, or nausea. However, it has been reported that these symptoms are associated with some cases [5, 11].

The temporal pattern of NH is heterogeneous. NH consists of continuous pain with periods of exacerbations or remissions. Approximately three-quarters of the patients experience pain on more than half of the days in a month, while one-quarter

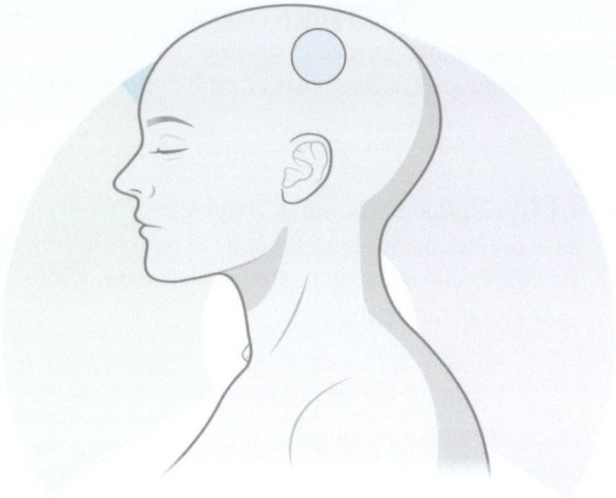

Fig 17.1 Nummular headache is most commonly localized in the parietal region. The pain is typically described within well-defined, round or oval-shaped areas

report pain on fewer than 15 days per month. On symptomatic days, the pain may be continuous or intermittent, with durations ranging from seconds to minutes, hours, or even days [2, 19].

17.6 Diagnosis

According to the ICHD-3 classification, NH is categorized under "The Primary Headaches" within the section of "4. Other Primary Headache Disorders" as *4.8 Nummular Headache* and *4.8.1 Probable Nummular Headache*. NH diagnosis is established according to the well-defined ICHD-3 criteria [2] listed below:

4.8 Nummular Headache

A: Continuous or intermittent head pain fulfilling criterion B

B: Felt exclusively in an area of the scalp with all of the following four characteristics:

1. Sharply contoured,
2. Fixed in size and shape,
3. Round or elliptical,
4. 1–6 cm in diameter

C: Not better accounted for by another ICHD-3 diagnosis

If only three of the B criteria are fulfilled, and it does not fulfill the ICHD-3 criteria for any other headache disorder and is not better accounted for by another ICHD-3 diagnosis, a diagnosis of probable NH can be made [2].

4.8.1 Probable Nummular Headache

A. Continuous or intermittent head pain fulfilling criterion B
B. Felt exclusively in an area of the scalp, with three only of the following four characteristics:
   1. Sharply contoured
   2. Fixed in size and shape
   3. Round or elliptical
   4. 1–6 cm in diameter
C. Not fulfilling ICHD-3 criteria for any other headache disorder
D. Not better accounted for by another ICHD-3 diagnosis

Other causes, particularly structural and dermatologic lesions, should have been ruled out through a thorough patient history, physical examination (including examination of the scalp, pericranial muscles, nerves, and arteries), and cranial MRI or computed tomography (CT) scan. Laboratory tests that may be conducted include a complete blood count, evaluations of metabolic and liver functions, thyroid function analysis, erythrocyte sedimentation rate, alkaline phosphatase levels, and screenings for antinuclear antibodies, rheumatoid factor, and other individualized tests [3, 20].

17.7 Differential Diagnosis

Linear headache (LH) is a newly described type of headache in recent years, characterized by persistent pain along a fixed linear trajectory and presenting in either episodic or chronic form. This headache type shares some features with NH, but significant differences also exist. Whether LH represents a variant of NH or a distinct headache type remains a topic of debate. Both types of headaches can exhibit symptoms of sensory dysfunction in the painful area. In both LH and NH, the pain is localized to a specific region, and its location remains fixed. While NH is typically confined to a circular or oval area, LH is characterized by a fixed, linear pathway, which distinguishes it from NH [21].

In the context of differential diagnosis, ruling out secondary cases is crucial, as indicated above. To exclude the presence of systemic or structural diseases, a thorough examination of the scalp and skull, as well as systemic and neurological assessments, neuroimaging, and blood screening, is essential. The differential diagnosis should carefully investigate potential causes such as intracranial lesions, vascular abnormalities, infections, and other secondary conditions [4].

Psychogenic headaches should also be considered in the differential diagnosis of NH. Initially, some authors hypothesized a psychogenic origin for NH, but current evidence does not support this view. A recent study comparing NH patients and healthy controls found no significant differences in depression or anxiety levels between the two groups. Additionally, depression and anxiety were not associated with key pain parameters such as intensity, exacerbations, pain area size, or frequency [22]. These findings indicate that NH occurs independently of anxiety and depression, distinguishing it clearly from psychogenic headaches.

17.8 Treatment

When no underlying cause is identified, primary NH typically follows a benign course. In such cases, reassuring patients about the non-serious nature of their condition often suffices, and additional treatment may not be necessary [4, 18]. Spontaneous remissions, either temporary or permanent, have been reported in the natural course of NH in up to 19.4% of patients [23]. However, for those experiencing severe or refractory pain that does not respond to analgesics, prophylactic treatment may be warranted.

Currently, no standardized treatment guidelines exist for NH; however, a limited number of drugs have been utilized in its management, with treatment suggestions primarily derived from clinical experience and observations [4, 18].

The managements used for NH management include NSAIDs, gabapentin, carbamazepine, botulinum toxin type A (BoNT-A), triptans, tricyclic antidepressants (TCA), and nerve block techniques. NSAIDs have been a mainstay in medium-term and acute exacerbation therapies, with variable effectiveness reported across studies, ranging from no response to partial or excellent results. Overall, analgesics and NSAIDs have been effective in over 60% of cases. Therefore, their as-needed use can be considered for patients with mild continuous pain, intermittent pain requiring occasional treatment, or as an add-on to preventive therapies [4].

Gabapentin was identified as the most commonly used treatment for NH, with a response rate of 67% [18]. It is recommended at a dose of 800 mg/day for its efficacy and tolerability [23]. Although there are no controlled clinical trials, various case reports and series have demonstrated that BoNT-A injections are highly effective and well-tolerated, with minimal side effects [4, 18, 24]. In the extensive series of 53 patients by García-Azorín et al., patients were administered 25 U of BoNT-A, distributed across one central and four peripheral points within the painful area. It was shown to reduce the monthly headache frequency significantly between weeks 8–12 and 20–24. Additionally, it decreased the number of intense headache days and acute medication days during the same periods. Approximately two-thirds of the patients achieved a 50% response rate, while half of them achieved a 75%

response rate [24]. In the study by Zhu et al., it was suggested that NH can be effectively treated with acupuncture or a combination of amitriptyline with indomethacin, ibuprofen, or carbamazepine [25]. At the case level, triptans have demonstrated effectiveness in patients with migrainous features [11, 26].

Subcutaneous anesthetic injections have been attempted in several patients; however, they have generally shown little to no therapeutic effect, with only rare instances of partial or temporary relief reported [12]. Dach et al. demonstrated that blocking the greater occipital nerve provided pain relief in their NH cases [27]. The combination of topiramate and palmitoylethanolamide has been reported as effective at the case level [28].

In secondary NH patients, symptom relief has been reported with specific treatments targeting the cause. For example, in a case related to varicella-zoster infection, antiviral therapy was effective; in a case associated with meningioma, surgical intervention was performed; and in cases related to superficial aneurysm and Langerhans histiocytosis, symptoms improved following surgical excision [4].

17.9 Conclusion

NH is a benign primary headache disorder that can coexist with other primary headache types. A thorough diagnostic approach is essential to exclude secondary causes. NSAIDs can be an effective treatment option, while prophylactic treatment may be required in refractory cases.

References

1. Pareja JA, Caminero AB, Serra J, et al. Nummular headache: a coin-shaped cephalgia. Neurology. 2002;58:1678–9. https://doi.org/10.1212/wnl.58.11.1678.
2. Olesen J. Headache Classification Committee of the International Headache Society (IHS) The International Classification of Headache Disorders, 3rd edition. Cephalalgia. 2018;38:1–211. https://doi.org/10.1177/0333102417738202.
3. Grosberg BM, Solomon S, Lipton RB. Nummular headache. Curr Pain Headache Rep. 2007;11:310–2. https://doi.org/10.1007/s11916-007-0209-1.
4. Cuadrado ML, López-Ruiz P, Guerrero ÁL. Nummular headache: an update and future prospects. Expert Rev Neurother. 2018;18:9–19. https://doi.org/10.1080/14737175.2018.1401925.
5. Atalar A, Genç H, Ur Özçelik E, et al. Other primary headache disorders: data from the HEAD-MENA-A study in Africa, Asia, and the Middle East. Clin Neurol Neurosurg. 2024;236:108112. https://doi.org/10.1016/j.clineuro.2023.108112.
6. Dai W, Yu S, Liang J, Zhang M. Nummular headache: peripheral or central? One case with reappearance of nummular headache after focal scalp was removed, and literature review. Cephalalgia. 2013;33:390–7. https://doi.org/10.1177/0333102412474504.
7. Cuadrado ML, Valle B, Fernández-de-las-Peñas C, et al. Pressure pain sensitivity of the scalp in patients with nummular headache: a cartographic study. Cephalalgia. 2010;30:200–6. https://doi.org/10.1111/j.1468-2982.2009.01895.x.
8. Fernández-de-las-Peñas C, Cuadrado ML, Barriga FJ, et al. Pericranial tenderness is not related to nummular headache. Cephalalgia. 2007;27:182–6. https://doi.org/10.1111/j.1468-2982.2007.01253.x.

9. Fernández-de-las-Peñas C, Cuadrado ML, Barriga FJ, et al. Local decrease of pressure pain threshold in nummular headache. Headache. 2006;46:1195–8. https://doi.org/10.1111/j.1526-4610.2006.00511.x.
10. Robbins MS, Grosberg BM. Menstrual-related nummular headache. Cephalalgia. 2010;30:507–8. https://doi.org/10.1111/j.1468-2982.2009.01947.x.
11. Barón J, Rodríguez C, Ruiz M, et al. Atypical nummular headache or circumscribed migraine: the utility of pressure algometry. Pain Res Manag. 2015;20:60–2. https://doi.org/10.1155/2015/567072.
12. Cuadrado ML. Epicranial headaches part 2: Nummular headache and epicrania fugax. Cephalalgia. 2023;43 https://doi.org/10.1177/03331024221146976.
13. Chen WH, Chen YT, Lin CS, et al. A high prevalence of autoimmune indices and disorders in primary nummular headache. J Neurol Sci. 2012;320:127–30. https://doi.org/10.1016/j.jns.2012.07.029.
14. Álvaro LC, García JM, Areitio E. Nummular headache: a series with symptomatic and primary cases. Cephalalgia. 2009;29:379–83. https://doi.org/10.1111/j.1468-2982.2008.01722.x.
15. Moon J, Ahmed K, Garza I. Case series of sixteen patients with nummular headache. Cephalalgia. 2010;30:1527–30. https://doi.org/10.1177/0333102410368445.
16. Chen WH, Li TH, Lee LH, Huang CC. Varicella-zoster virus infection and nummular headache: a possible association with epicranial neuralgia. Intern Med. 2012;51:2439–41. https://doi.org/10.2169/internalmedicine.51.7998.
17. Sánchez-Soblechero A, Luque-Buzo E, Lozano-Ros A, et al. Secondary nummular headache: are they more common than we thought? Headache. 2024; https://doi.org/10.1111/head.14879.
18. Patel UK, Saleem S, Anwar A, et al. Characteristics and treatment effectiveness of the nummular headache: a systematic review and analysis of 110 cases. BMJ Neurol Open. 2020;2. https://doi.org/10.1136/bmjno-2020-000049.
19. Ruscheweyh R, Buchheister A, Gregor N, et al. Nummular headache: six new cases and lancinating pain attacks as possible manifestation. Cephalalgia. 2010;30:249–53. https://doi.org/10.1111/j.1468-2982.2009.01893.x.
20. Garciá-Iglesias C, Martínez-Badillo C, García-Azorín D, et al. Secondary nummular headache: a new case series and review of the literature. Pain Med. 2021;22:2718–27. https://doi.org/10.1093/pm/pnab174.
21. Chavarría-Miranda A, Guerrero ÁL, Talavera B, et al. Linear headache: a novel entity or a variant of nummular headache? Clinical characteristics and treatment response in a series of 16 patients. Pain Med. 2021;22:1158–66. https://doi.org/10.1093/pm/pnaa436.
22. Fernández-de-las-Peñas C, Peñacoba-Puente C, López-López A, Valle B, Cuadrado ML, Barriga FJ, Pareja JA. Depression and anxiety are not related to nummular headache The Journal of Headache and Pain. 2009;10(6)441–5. https://doi.org/10.1007/s10194-009-0161-z.
23. Trigo J, García-Azorín D, Martinez Pias E, et al. Clinical characteristics of nummular headache and differentiation between spontaneous and posttraumatic variant: an observational study. J Headache Pain. 2019;20. https://doi.org/10.1186/s10194-019-0981-4.
24. García-Azorín D, Trigo-López J, Sierra Á, et al. Observational, open-label, non-randomized study on the efficacy of onabotulinumtoxinA in the treatment of nummular headache: the pre-numabot study. Cephalalgia. 2019;39:1818–26. https://doi.org/10.1177/0333102419863023.
25. Zhu KY, Huang Y, Zhong SS, et al. Nummular headache: 21 new cases and therapeutic results. Zhonghua Yi Xue Za Zhi. 2008;88:2935–7.
26. López-Ruiz P, Cuadrado ML, Aledo-Serrano A, et al. Superficial artery aneurysms underlying nummular headache—2 cases and proposed diagnostic work-up. Headache. 2014;54:1217–21. https://doi.org/10.1111/head.12398.
27. Dach F, Éckeli ÁL, Ferreira KDS, et al. Nerve block for the treatment of headaches and cranial neuralgias – a practical approach. Headache. 2015;55(Suppl 1):59–71. https://doi.org/10.1111/head.12516.
28. Chirchiglia D, Della Torre A, Signorelli F, et al. Administration of palmitoylethanolamide in combination with topiramate in the preventive treatment of nummular headache. Int Med Case Rep J. 2016;9:193–5. https://doi.org/10.2147/imcrj.s106323.

Part IV
Headache Attributed to Cranial or Cervical Vascular Disorder

Chapter 18
Headache Attributed to Arteriovenous Malformation

Cláudio Manoel Brito, Elder Machado Sarmento, and Leonardo Sarmento

18.1 Introduction

Headache is a common complaint, and it is most frequently classified as a primary headache, such as migraine or tension-type headache. However, headaches can also be secondary to a variety of underlying conditions, including cranial or cervical vascular disorders. One such condition is arteriovenous malformation (AVM), an abnormal connection between arteries and veins in the brain or spinal cord. AVMs are characterized by a tangle of abnormal vessels, where arteries connect directly to veins without the intervention of capillaries, which can lead to various neurological complications. The presence of an AVM can alter cerebral hemodynamics, predisposing to events such as hemorrhage, seizures, headache, and neurological deficits [1, 2]. Unfortunately, due to the gravity of AVM rupture and cerebral hemorrhage, research on headaches associated with brain AVMs is still scarce [3].

AVMs are rare vascular lesions, with an incidence rate of approximately 1.12 to 1.42 cases per 100,000 person-years [1, 4]. The estimated prevalence is 1 in 10,000 individuals [2]. Although AVMs can become symptomatic at any age, the most common presentation occurs in the third or fourth decade of life [4]. The prevalence of headache in patients with AVMs varies widely, with estimates ranging from 6 to 52% [5]. This variation may reflect different diagnostic criteria and patient populations studied. A study of 1289 patients with AVMs found that 14% presented with chronic headache [5]. A review of 51 patients with IVM (intracranial vascular malformations) found that 47% suffered from migraine-type headaches [6].

C. M. Brito (✉) · E. M. Sarmento
Headache, Sociedade Brasileira de Cefaleia, Barra Mansa, Brazil

L. Sarmento
Internal Medicine, Institution: Santa Casa de Barra Mansa, Barra Mansa, Brazil

D. Uludüz et al. (eds.), *Rare Causes of Headache Disorders*, Headache,
https://doi.org/10.1007/978-3-032-10242-3_18

18.2 Pathophysiology

The underlying mechanisms of headache in patients with AVMs are not fully understood. However, several theories have been proposed:

1. Increased intracranial pressure: AVMs can increase intracranial blood volume, leading to increased intracranial pressure and, consequently, headache.
2. Steal phenomenon: The high arteriovenous flow in AVMs can divert blood flow from adjacent brain areas, causing ischemia and headache [7].
3. Activation of the trigeminovascular system: AVMs can activate the trigeminovascular system, a neural pathway involved in the pathogenesis of migraine, resulting in headache [7].
4. Inflammation: Inflammation of blood vessels and surrounding tissues may contribute to headache.
5. Cortical spreading depression (CSD): CSD, an electrophysiological phenomenon underlying migraine aura, can be triggered by cortical ischemia or irritation [8].
6. Hemodynamic alterations: In rare cases, headache may be related to hemodynamic alterations, such as flow inversion in the internal jugular vein, which can lead to cerebral venous congestion [9].
7. Cortical lesions or microembolization: Symptomatic migraine with aura (MWA) may occur due to cortical lesions or microembolization from carotid pathologies [8].

18.3 Case Presentation

A 15-year-old boy, presented with a history of headaches that started at the age of 13. His headache was initially infrequent (occurring less than once a month), throbbing, and of moderate intensity. The pain was always restricted to the right frontoparietal region and mainly brought about by physical activities, such as playing soccer or running. Sometimes the headache was associated with nausea and dizziness. He reported relief with rest and/or sleep. In the last months, the pain became more frequent and more intense, preventing the patient from going to school on many occasions. Initially, he was treated with abortive medication, but lately, preventive medications were started (flunarizine and propranolol). So far, no neurological symptoms have been reported. There was no familial history of headache. In March 2024, he had dysesthesia in the left side of the body, during a headache crisis. A computed tomography (CT) of the head without contrast showed a right frontoparietal AVM. Digital subtraction angiography (DSA) confirmed it to be a Spetzler-Martin grade IV AVM [10] (Fig. 18.1). The patient was started on sodium divalproex of extended release, which controlled the dysesthesias and, partially, the headache (decreasing the frequency and intensity). The patient was offered interventional

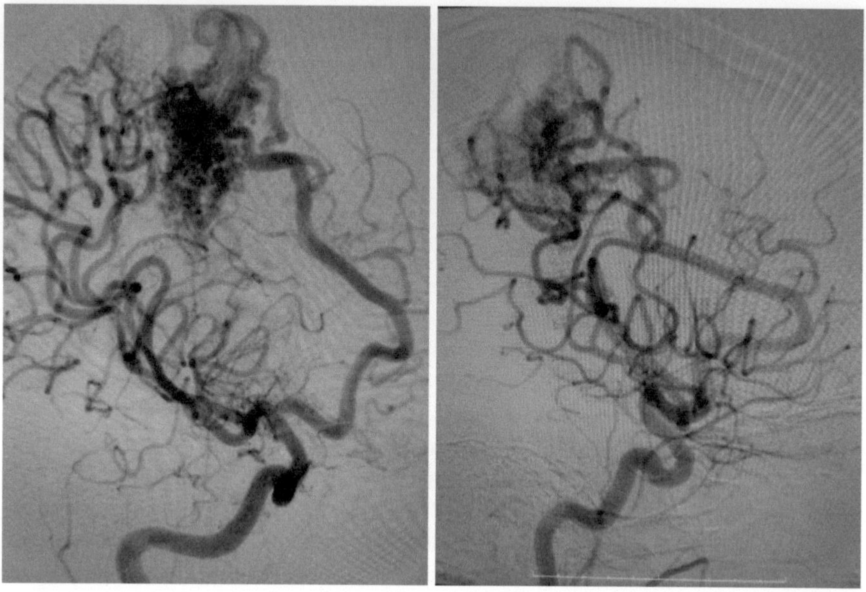

Fig. 18.1 DAS: Right frontoparietal AVM

treatment, but after a lengthy discussion of the risks and advantages of treatment, the parents opted for conservative treatment.

18.4 Case Discussion

The present case illustrates how a secondary headache can be mistaken for a primary headache, initially presenting as episodic, throbbing, and triggered by physical exertion, with relief upon rest or sleep. Some factors should raise suspicion of a secondary headache: the locked side, the progressive nature, and, finally, the focal sensitive crises on the left side of the body. The head CT suggested an arteriovenous malformation, later confirmed by magnetic resonance imaging (MRI) angiography. The sodium divalproate controlled the crises and helped prevent the headaches. Unfortunately, the family declined the proposed interventional treatment. The patient has been followed up for a year now, with no alterations in the neurological status.

18.5 Clinical Presentation

Headache attributed to AVMs can manifest in various forms, making diagnosis challenging. Presentations include hemorrhage (50% of cases), seizures (30% of cases), and headache (5–14% of cases) [1]. Some common characteristics of the headache include: The headache is usually ipsilateral to the AVM, although it may be bilateral in some cases. In some studies, headache was found to be ipsilateral to the AVM in all cases of migraine [11]. One study found a strong positive correlation (88.8%) between the side of the AVM and the side of pain [6].

The headache may be described as throbbing, pulsatile, or dull. The intensity of the headache can vary from mild to severe. Other neurological symptoms, such as seizures, focal neurological deficits, and visual changes, may accompany the headache. Patients with occipital AVMs frequently present with visual symptoms, such as scintillating scotomas and hemianopsia [12]. It is important to note that headaches attributed to AVMs can mimic primary headaches, such as migraine, making differential diagnosis essential. Headache associated with AVMs may present characteristics similar to those of migraine, including pulsatile quality and the presence of autonomic symptoms. Some studies have observed that a significant proportion of patients with AVMs had a history of migraine [13]. A history of previous migraine may complicate the diagnosis, necessitating consideration of the possibility of secondary headache due to AVM.

In a recent study, the risk factors associated with headaches in 946 patients with brain AVMs include female sex, supply artery dilation, and occipital lobe topography [3].

18.6 Diagnosis

The diagnosis of headache attributed to AVMs requires a systematic approach. It should follow the criteria established by the International Classification of Headache Disorders, 3rd edition (ICHD-3) (Headache Classification Committee of the International Headache Society, 2018) [14]:

A detailed history of the headache, including its characteristics, frequency, duration, and associated symptoms, is essential. A complete neurological examination should be performed to identify any neurological deficits.

Diagnostic criteria: According to ICHD-3, the diagnostic criteria for headache attributed to AVMs (code 6.3.2) are:

A. Any new headache fulfilling criterion C
B. An arteriovenous malformation (AVM) has been diagnosed
C. Evidence of causation demonstrated by at least two of the following:

   1. The headache has developed in close temporal relation to other symptoms and/or clinical signs of AVM, or has led to its discovery

2. Either or both of the following:
   (a) The headache has significantly worsened in parallel with the worsening of the AVM
   (b) The headache has significantly improved or resolved after effective treatment of the AVM
3. The headache is localized to the site of the AVM

D. Not better accounted for by another ICHD-3 diagnosis

Thomsen et al. (2021) proposed criteria for "symptomatic migraine," requiring evidence of a causal relationship between the underlying cause and migraine symptoms.

ICHD-3 emphasizes the importance of observing the evolution of headache over time, especially in relation to the diagnosis and treatment of AVM. Although not part of the formal diagnostic criteria, ICHD-3 notes that headache attributed to AVM is often described as pulsating and may be accompanied by other focal neurological signs. ICHD-3 recognizes that, in rare cases, AVM may cause cluster headache, emphasizing the importance of considering secondary causes even in typical presentations of primary headaches.

18.7 Differential Diagnosis

It is essential to consider other causes of headache, including primary headaches such as migraine, which may coexist or be mimicked by headache attributed to AVM. Neuroimaging is crucial for confirming the presence of an AVM and excluding other causes of headache. CT of the head is performed mainly when intracranial bleeding is suspected, which can be followed by CT angiography to diagnose the underlying arteriovenous malformation. Magnetic resonance imaging (MRI) with magnetic resonance angiography (MRA) is generally the preferred initial imaging examination. Catheter cerebral angiography is the gold standard for evaluating AVM anatomy and planning treatment. Cerebral angiography remains essential for surgical planning and detailed evaluation of the AVM [15].

18.8 Treatment

The treatment of headache attributed to arteriovenous malformations (AVMs) focuses on both alleviating pain and preventing serious complications, such as intracranial hemorrhage. Pain relief can be achieved through the use of analgesics, including nonsteroidal anti-inflammatory drugs (NSAIDs) and, when necessary, opioids—though the latter should be used cautiously due to the risk of dependency. In some instances, prophylactic medications such as beta-blockers, tricyclic antidepressants, or anticonvulsants may be prescribed to reduce the frequency and severity of headache episodes. Management of the underlying AVM is guided by a careful assessment of the hemorrhagic risk versus the procedural risks associated with intervention [1]. Treatment strategies may include microsurgical resection, stereotactic radiosurgery (SRS), endovascular embolization, or a combination of these approaches. The selection of the most appropriate modality depends on multiple factors, including the AVM's size, location, and vascular architecture, as well as the patient's age and overall health condition.

Microsurgery is generally indicated for superficial, small- to medium-sized AVMs in non-eloquent areas of the brain [16].

Advantages Complete and immediate removal of the AVM, high cure rate (95–99% in selected cases); immediate elimination of hemorrhage risk; relief of intracranial pressure in cases of associated hematomas.

Disadvantages Possibility of postoperative neurological deficits. In cases of giant occipital AVMs with frequent migraine-type headaches, surgical removal of the AVM may lead to headache resolution, allowing the patient to return to a normal life without the need for assistance [17]. A recent review and meta-analysis of 21 studies comprising 5452 patients with unruptured arteriovenous malformations showed the highest rate of obliteration with microsurgery [18]. Another review and meta-analysis about morbidity and mortality pointed out that studies with more than 50% of arteriovenous malformations Spetzler-Martin grades 1–2 exhibited significantly lower mortality rates compared to those with less than 50% cases of Spetzler-Martin grade 1–2.

Radiosurgery is often used for small (<3 cm), deep, or AVMs in eloquent areas of the brain [19].

Advantages Non-invasive treatment and lower risk of immediate complications. It is effective for AVMs in surgically difficult-to-access locations.

Disadvantages Gradual obliteration of the AVM (2–3 years for complete effect) and persistent risk of hemorrhage until complete obliteration, as well as the possibility of late radiation side effects. Limited efficacy for AVMs larger than 3 cm. Endovascular embolization has proven to be an effective technique for reducing AVM size and decreasing the risk of hemorrhage [20]. Can be used as an adjuvant treatment before microsurgery or radiosurgery to reduce AVM size and facilitate definitive treatment.

Multimodal treatment, combining embolization, microsurgery, and radiosurgery, has gained popularity in recent years, especially for complex AVMs [21].

Advantages: Allows treatment of complex and large AVMs, reduces risks associated with each modality, and can improve complete obliteration rates. Typical approach: Initial embolization to reduce AVM size and flow, followed by microsurgery for removal of the majority of the lesion; radiosurgery to treat any residual remnant.

18.9 Conclusion

Headache attributed to AVMs is a complex condition that requires a careful diagnostic and therapeutic approach. Although a headache can be debilitating, successful treatment of the AVM can lead to the resolution or significant improvement of the headache. Healthcare professionals must be aware of this entity to ensure proper diagnosis and treatment. The choice of treatment modality should be individualized, considering the characteristics of the AVM, clinical presentation, treatment team experience, and patient preferences. Multidisciplinary management, involving neurologists, neurosurgeons, and interventional radiologists, is crucial for optimizing clinical outcomes.

References

1. Abecassis IJ, Xu DS, Batjer HH, Bendok BR. Natural history of brain arteriovenous malformations: a systematic review. Neurosurg Focus. 2014;37(3):E7.
2. Dasenbrock HH, Du R. Presentation of cerebral arteriovenous malformations. World Neurosurg. 2015.
3. Zhang H, Han H, Ma L, Li R, Li Z, Li A, Yuan K, Zhu Q, Wang C, Zhang Y, Zhang H, Gao D, Guo G, Kang S, Ye X, Li Y, Sun S, Wang H, Hao Q, Chen Y, Wang R, Chen X, Zhao Y; Registry of Multimodality Treatment for Brain Arteriovenous Malformation in Mainland China (MATCH). A comprehensive analysis of patients with cerebral arteriovenous malformation with headache: assessment of risk factors and treatment effectiveness. J Headache Pain. 2024;25(1):72. https://doi.org/10.1186/s10194-024-01774-7. PMID: 38714978; PMCID: PMC11075233
4. Laakso A, Hernesniemi J. Arteriovenous malformations: epidemiology and clinical presentation. Neurosurg Clin N Am. 2012;23(1):1–6.
5. Hofmeister C, et al. Demographic, morphological, and clinical characteristics of 1289 patients with brain arteriovenous malformation. Stroke. 2000;31:1307–10.
6. Pereira Monteiro JM, Rosas MJ, Correia AP, Vaz AR. Migraine and intracranial vascular malformations. Headache. 1993;33:563–5.
7. Ellis JA, et al. Arteriovenous malformations and headache. J Clin Neurosci. 2016;23:38–43.
8. Thomsen AV, Sørensen MT, Ashina M, Hougaard A. Symptomatic migraine: a systematic review to establish a clinically important diagnostic entity. Headache. 2021:1–14.
9. Pereira L, Costa EC, Nunes T, Saraiva P, Ferreira J, Cruz P, Rodrigues M. Dynamics of a haemodynamic headache: a case report and literature review of headache secondary to flow inversion of the internal jugular vein. Cephalalgia. 2016;36(14):1370–8.
10. Spetzler RF, Martin NA. A proposed grading system for arteriovenous malformations. J Neurosurg. 1986;65(4):476–83. https://doi.org/10.3171/jns.1986.65.4.0476. PMID: 3760956.
11. Galletti F, et al. Occipital arteriovenous malformations and migraine. Cephalalgia. 2011;31:1320–4.
12. Kupersmith MJ, et al. Occipital arteriovenous malformations: visual disturbances and presentation. Neurology. 1996;46:953–7.
13. Waltimo O, Hokkanen E, Pirskanen R. Intracranial arteriovenous malformations and headache. Headache. 1975;15:133–5.
14. Headache Classification Committee of the International Headache Society (IHS). The International Classification of Headache Disorders, 3rd edition. Cephalalgia. 2018;38(1):1–211.

15. Lawton MT, Rutledge WC, Kim H, Stapf C, Whitehead KJ, Li DY, Krings T, terBrugge K, Kondziolka D, Morgan MK, Moon K, Spetzler RF. Brain arteriovenous malformations. Nat Rev Dis Primers. 2015;1:15008. https://doi.org/10.1038/nrdp.2015.8. PMID: 27188382.
16. Bradac O, Charvat F, Benes V. Treatment for brain arteriovenous malformation in the 1998-2011 period and review of the literature. Acta Neurochir. 2014;155(2):199–209.
17. Nagata S, Morioka T, Natori Y, Sasaki T. Surgical treatment of non-ruptured Giant occipital arteriovenous malformations with frequent migraine-like headache—two case reports. Neurol Med Chir. 2006;46(9):441–5.
18. Liu R, Zhan Y, Piao J, Yang Z, Wei Y, Liu P, Chen X, Jiang Y. Treatments of unruptured brain arteriovenous malformations: a systematic review and meta-analysis. Medicine (Baltimore). 2021;100(25):e26352. https://doi.org/10.1097/MD.0000000000026352. PMID: 34160402; PMCID: PMC8238300.
19. Ding D, Yen CP, Xu Z, Starke RM, Sheehan JP. Radiosurgery for patients with unruptured intracranial arteriovenous malformations. J Neurosurg. 2013;118(5):958–66.
20. Weber W, Kis B, Ruefenacht D, Dietrich PY. Endovascular management of brain arteriovenous malformations: experience of 15 years. J Neurol. 2008;255(8):1179–89.
21. Javadpour M, Al-Mahfoudh R, Mitchell PS, Kirollos R. Outcome of microsurgical excision of unruptured brain arteriovenous malformations in Aruba-eligible patients. Br J Neurosurg. 2012;26(6):925–7.

Chapter 19
Dural Arteriovenous Fistula (DAVF) Attributed Headache

Ece Yanık and Doğa Vurallı

19.1 Introduction

Dural arteriovenous fistulas (DAVFs) are rare vascular malformations characterized by pathological anastomoses between dural arteries and dural venous sinuses or cortical veins. These fistulas often arise in the dura surrounding a venous sinus, characteristically at the transverse-sigmoid junction. However, they can also occur in the cavernous sinus, superior sagittal sinus, anterior fossa, tentorium, and other locations [1]. DAVFs may be completely asymptomatic. Symptoms may range from mild symptoms to fatal hemorrhage. One of the most common clinical symptoms is headache. Headache may be the first or only presenting complaint [2].

In this chapter, we aim to define headache phenotypes and develop early diagnosis and treatment algorithms for DAVFs-related headache for future research by understanding the relationship between headache and DAVFs and establishing a high index of suspicion.

E. Yanık
Department of Neurology and Algology, Neuropsychiatry Center, Gazi University Faculty of Medicine, Ankara, Türkiye

D. Vurallı (✉)
Department of Neurology and Algology, Neuroscience and Neurotechnology Center of Excellence (NÖROM), Neuropsychiatry Center, Gazi University Faculty of Medicine, Ankara, Türkiye

D. Uludüz et al. (eds.), *Rare Causes of Headache Disorders*, Headache,
https://doi.org/10.1007/978-3-032-10242-3_19

19.2 Pathophysiology

Many mechanisms are involved in the pathophysiology of headache associated with DAVFs. These include venous hypertension, changes in intracranial pressure, and cortical and dural inflammation [3].

- *Venous Hypertension:* Impaired venous drainage leads to intracranial hypertension, causing diffuse or pressure-like headaches.
- *Cortical Venous Reflux:* When arterialized blood flows retrograde into cortical veins, it can cause seizures, focal neurological deficits, or hemorrhage, often preceded by headaches.
- *Dural and Perivascular Inflammation:* Inflammatory changes near the dura may activate pain-sensitive structures, contributing to headache syndromes.

As a result, stimulation of pain-related structures in the dura, increased intracranial pressure, venous ischemia, or hemorrhage may result in severe thunderclap headache. Venous drainage is a critical determinant of the clinical presentation and risk profile.

19.3 Case Presentation

A 64-year-old male patient presented with a history of new-onset headache. The headache was unilateral, consistently localized to the right side, and progressively worsened over several months. He had no prior history of headaches with similar characteristics or severity. The visual analog scale (VAS) score for pain intensity was 8/10. The headache was throbbing, sometimes pulsatile, predominantly occipital, and worsened at night. Additionally, the patient reported unilateral pulsatile tinnitus on the right side for over a year.

Blood tests, as well as neurological and general clinical examinations, were unremarkable. Given the new-onset headache, accompanying symptoms, and the patient's elderly age, further imaging was necessary. A cranial computed tomography (CT) scan, cranial magnetic resonance imaging (MRI), and magnetic resonance angiography (MRA) were performed that revealed diffuse, tubular, dilated venous vascular structures in the frontobasal and middle cranial fossa, extending toward the sinuses within the cisternal region of the posterior fossa. These findings raised the suspicion of an arteriovenous fistula, and digital subtraction angiography (DSA) was recommended for further evaluation.

Cerebral DSA confirmed the presence of a right-sided dural arteriovenous fistula, characterized by early arterial phase blood supply from all branches of the external carotid artery and early venous drainage into the sigmoid sinus and jugular vein. Imaging obtained during the early venous and late arterial phases is presented in Fig. 19.1a–c. The patient underwent endovascular embolization, resulting in complete occlusion of the fistula. At the two-month follow-up, he had no headache after the DAVF embolization.

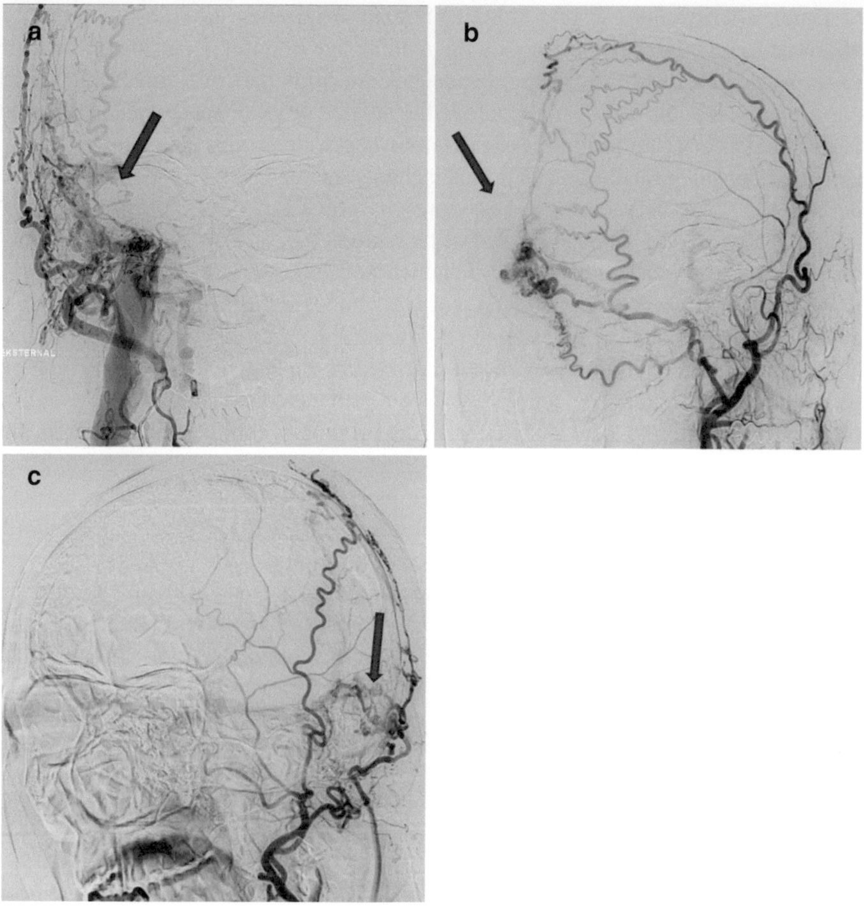

Fig. 19.1 (**a** and **b**) Fistulized vessels in the late arterial phase. (**c**) Fistulized vessels in the early venous phase

19.4 Case Discussion

This case highlights the importance of thorough evaluation in elderly patients presenting with new-onset, progressive headaches, as such symptoms may indicate underlying vascular pathologies [1]. Recognizing red flag signs in headache history is crucial for early diagnosis. Pulsatile tinnitus, while nonspecific, is a frequently reported symptom in patients with DAVFs [4]. This case underscores the significance of early identification and comprehensive management of DAVFs to prevent potential complications.

Dural arteriovenous fistula (DAVF)-related headaches are most commonly observed in middle-aged adults, with the median age of onset occurring in the fifth to sixth decades of life [5]. These headaches are often part of a more aggressive clinical presentation, which may include the sudden onset of severe headache, seizures, and various forms of intracranial hemorrhage, such as intraparenchymal, subarachnoid, or subdural bleeding. The headaches associated with DAVFs are typically described as extremely severe and may present with a variety of patterns [6]. They are often localized to the occipital or frontal regions but can also be diffuse. A thunderclap headache, characterized by a sudden and intense onset, may mimic subarachnoid hemorrhage and can signal cortical venous reflux—necessitating urgent evaluation. Pulsating headaches are also common and may be accompanied by an audible bruit, reflecting turbulent blood flow within the fistula. Unilateral orbital or retroorbital headache is frequently associated with cavernous sinus DAVFs and is often accompanied by ocular signs, such as proptosis, conjunctival injection, or cranial nerve palsies. In some patients, headaches may worsen with changes in head position, indicating a disruption in venous drainage. Additionally, headaches associated with pulsatile tinnitus—especially in cases involving the transverse or sigmoid sinuses—are a hallmark of DAVFs. Some cases may mimic chronic tension-type or migraine-like headaches, which can lead to misdiagnosis and delays in appropriate treatment. Notably, ocular symptoms in the context of nonmigrainous headache may suggest a carotid-cavernous fistula, whereas migrainous features may point toward other DAVF locations. Pulsatile tinnitus and symptoms of increased dural sinus flow are particularly characteristic of fistulas located in the transverse and sigmoid sinuses [7, 8].

19.5 Diagnostic Approach

The most common symptoms of DAVFs, including headache and tinnitus, are nonspecific, making the diagnosis challenging [8]. Red flags that may suggest DAVFs-related headache are: New onset or progressive headaches in middle-aged or older adults, headache with cranial nerve palsies or other focal neurologic findings, headache associated with pulsatile tinnitus, headache aggravated by Valsalva manoeuvers or changes in head position [4].

The International Headache Society (IHS) has established criteria for classifying the headache attributed to DAVF (6.3.3), considering the following factors: (i) temporal relation to other symptoms/signs of DAVF; (ii) parallel prognosis between DAVF and headache (headache worsening concurrently with other symptoms or clinical/radiological signs of the DAVF and improving or resolving after the effective treatment of the DAVF); (iii) association with other signs/symptoms (such as pulsatile tinnitus and ophthalmoplegia) and its clinical course (progressive, worse in the morning or worse due to a Valsalva's maneuver, during coughing and/or bending over); (iv) exact localization of headache and site of DAVF [9]. Intracerebral hemorrhage and cerebral venous thrombosis should be excluded before the diagnosis of headache attributed to DAVF [9]. Additional imaging is essential. Unexplained subarachnoid or lobar hemorrhages should prompt consideration of a DAVF in the differential diagnosis [10].

Magnetic resonance imaging (MRI) helps define the anatomy of DAVF. It can show dural thickening, thrombosis, stenosed venous sinuses, and hypertrophic arteries. In addition, complications such as diffuse white matter edema, dilated pial veins, infarction, and hemorrhage due to venous congestion are also seen [2]. Typical findings include cortical or deep venous dilatation, cerebral edema, and fistula-related microbleeds. Contrast-enhanced T1-weighted images may show dilated leptomeningeal and medullary vessels, venous ectasia, parenchymal enhancement, and venous sinus occlusion or thrombosis [1].

Magnetic resonance angiography (MRA), including time-of-flight (TOF) and contrast-enhanced techniques, is commonly used for noninvasive evaluation of vascular structures. TOF MRA is capable of visualizing arterialized veins, while dynamic contrast-enhanced MRA can reveal arteriovenous shunting and venous drainage patterns [11]. However, a notable limitation of MRA is its relatively lower spatial resolution compared to conventional angiography [12]. Computed tomography (CT), on the other hand, plays a key role in identifying complications such as intracranial or subarachnoid hemorrhage, hydrocephalus, and vasogenic edema [1]. CT may also reveal nonspecific findings such as asymmetry in the dural venous sinuses or mild dilatation of the cavernous sinus or superior ophthalmic vein; however, it is generally insufficient for detecting intracranial dural arteriovenous fistulas (DAVFs) on its own [12]. Computed tomography angiography (CTA) is a more effective modality for detecting DAVFs, as it can demonstrate arterialized veins, abnormal venous drainage patterns, and dilated venous sinuses [13]. Despite CTA's improved spatial resolution over MRA, digital subtraction angiography (DSA) remains the gold standard for definitive diagnosis and classification. DSA provides comprehensive information about the presence, location, and hemodynamic features of DAVFs, including identification of arterial feeders, venous drainage direction, venous ectasia, stenosis, arteriovenous shunts, cortical venous collaterals, calcifications, and involvement of pial and dural branches [2].

19.6 Management

Management of DAVF-related headache depends on the severity of symptoms, the presence of cortical venous reflux, and associated comorbidities [3, 8, 10].

- Conservative management: Asymptomatic or low-risk DAVFs can be monitored with regular imaging and symptomatic headache management.
- Endovascular treatment: The primary treatment modality for symptomatic or high-risk DAVFs is endovascular treatment using transarterial or transvenous embolization.

- Surgical Intervention: It is indicated in cases in which endovascular treatment is not feasible and involves microsurgical interruption of the fistula connection.
- Headache management: Analgesics may be helpful. In addition, treatment of secondary factors such as intracranial hypertension is effective in management.

19.7 Conclusion

These rare vascular malformations are essential causes of secondary headaches because of their potential complications. Headaches due to DAVFs can often be mistaken for primary headaches. Understanding the relationship between headaches and DAVFs, along with a high index of suspicion, is essential for early diagnosis and effective management. Appropriate imaging and multidisciplinary management are required. Future research should focus on identifying headache phenotypes and refining treatment algorithms for DAVF-associated headaches.

Acknowledgement We would like to sincerely thank Prof. Dr. Bijen Nazlıel for her counselling on the case.

References

1. Reynolds MR, Lanzino G, Zipfel GJ. Intracranial dural arteriovenous fistulae. Stroke. 2017;48(5):1424–31. https://doi.org/10.1161/STROKEAHA.116.012784.
2. Gupta A, Periakaruppan A. Intracranial dural arteriovenous fistulas: a review. Indian J Radiol Imaging. 2009;19(1):43–8. https://doi.org/10.4103/0971-3026.45344. PMID:19774139
3. Corbelli I, De Maria F, Eusebi P, Romoli M, Cardaioli G, Hamam M, Floridi P, Cupini LM, Sarchielli P, Calabresi P. Dural arteriovenous fistulas and headache features: an observational study. J Headache Pain. 2020;21(1):6. https://doi.org/10.1186/s10194-020-1073-1.
4. Padilha IG, Pacheco FT, Araujo AIR, Nunes RH, Baccin CE, Conti MLM, Maia ACM Jr, Rocha AJD. Tips and tricks in the diagnosis of intracranial dural arteriovenous fistulas: a pictorial review. J Neuroradiol. 2020;47(5):369–81. https://doi.org/10.1016/j.neurad.2019.06.004.
5. Brown RD Jr, Wiebers DO, Nichols DA. Intracranial dural arteriovenous fistulae: angiographic predictors of intracranial hemorrhage and clinical outcome in nonsurgical patients. J Neurosurg. 1994;81(4):531–8. https://doi.org/10.3171/jns.1994.81.4.0531.
6. van Rooij WJ, Sluzewski M, Beute GN. Dural arteriovenous fistulas with cortical venous drainage: incidence, clinical presentation, and treatment. AJNR Am J Neuroradiol. 2007;28(4):651–5.

7. Kim MS, Han DH, Kwon OK, Oh CW, Han MH. Clinical characteristics of dural arteriovenous fistula. J Clin Neurosci. 2002;9(2):147–55. https://doi.org/10.1054/jocn.2001.1029.
8. Miller TR, Gandhi D. Intracranial dural arteriovenous fistulae: clinical presentation and management strategies. Stroke. 2015;46(7):2017–25. https://doi.org/10.1161/STROKEAHA.115.008228.
9. Headache Classification Committee of the International Headache Society (IHS). The international classification of headache disorders, 3rd edition. Cephalalgia. 2018;38(1):1–211. https://doi.org/10.1177/0333102417738202.
10. Gandhi D, Chen J, Pearl M, Huang J, Gemmete JJ, Kathuria S. Intracranial dural arteriovenous fistulas: classification, imaging findings, and treatment. AJNR Am J Neuroradiol. 2012;33(6):1007–13. https://doi.org/10.3174/ajnr.A2798.
11. Noguchi K, Melhem ER, Kanazawa T, Kubo M, Kuwayama N, Seto H. Intracranial dural arteriovenous fistulas: evaluation with combined 3D time-of-flight MR angiography and MR digital subtraction angiography. AJR Am J Roentgenol. 2004;182(1):183–90. https://doi.org/10.2214/ajr.182.1.1820183.
12. Alatakis S, Koulouris G, Stuckey S. CT-demonstrated transcalvarial channels diagnostic of dural arteriovenous fistula. AJNR Am J Neuroradiol. 2005;26(9):2393–6.
13. Alkhaibary A, Alnefaie N, Alharbi A, Alammar H, Arishy AM, Alshaya W, Khairy S. Intracranial dural arteriovenous fistula: a comprehensive review of the history, management, and future prospective. Acta Neurol Belg. 2023;123(2):359–66. https://doi.org/10.1007/s13760-022-02133-6.

Chapter 20
Headache Attributed to Cavernous Angioma

Marcelo Valença and Luiz Severo Bem Junior

20.1 Introduction

Secondary headaches pose a significant diagnostic challenge, particularly when they mimic common primary headache patterns or are initially attributed to functional or psychiatric causes. Among these, headache attributed to a cavernous angioma (also known as a cerebral cavernous malformation [CCM]) is rare but clinically significant [1, 2]. It is classified under code 6.3.4 in the International Classification of Headache Disorders, third edition (ICHD-3). Although cavernous angiomas are frequently asymptomatic and detected incidentally on brain imaging, they can occasionally manifest with focal neurological symptoms, epileptic seizures, and, less commonly, headache.

The causal association between cavernous angiomas and headache remains a subject of debate, due to the limited number of systematic clinical studies and the potential overlap with seizures or minor hemorrhagic events. However, when there is a clear temporal relationship between headache onset and lesion detection, significant improvement following surgical resection, and an anatomically consistent location, the headache may be directly attributed to the cavernous angioma, in line with ICHD-3 diagnostic criteria.

In this chapter, we present and discuss a clinical case of a young male patient with a new-onset headache of an unusual pattern, initially misinterpreted as a

M. Valença
Federal University of Pernambuco, Recife, Pernambuco, Brazil

Center of Excellence in the Treatment of Migraine and Other Headache Disorders, Hospital Esperança, Recife, Pernambuco, Brazil

L. S. B. Junior (✉)
Neuroequillibrium-neuromodulation center, Recife, Pernambuco, Brazil

Paraiba Pain Center, Campina Grande, Paraiba, Brazil

D. Uludüz et al. (eds.), *Rare Causes of Headache Disorders*, Headache,
https://doi.org/10.1007/978-3-032-10242-3_20

manifestation of panic disorder. The subsequent diagnosis of a left temporal lobe cavernous angioma explained both his headache and seizure-like episodes. This case highlights the importance of neuroimaging in evaluating new-onset headaches. It illustrates the practical application of ICHD-3 criteria, emphasizing the need to differentiate between primary headache disorders, epileptic events, and headaches caused by structural brain lesions.

20.2 Pathophysiology of Headache in Cavernous Angioma

Headache associated with cerebral cavernous angiomas is a multifactorial phenomenon, often reflecting the complex interplay between structural, vascular, inflammatory, and epileptogenic mechanisms. These low-flow vascular malformations can provoke headache through several pathways. One key contributor is recurrent microhemorrhage, which is common in cavernous angiomas and can result in local hemosiderin deposition, reactive gliosis, and perilesional inflammation—factors that sensitize surrounding neural tissue and may trigger nociceptive pathways. Additionally, vasogenic edema due to the inflammatory response around the lesion can cause increased local intracranial pressure and further stimulate pain-sensitive structures.

In the present case, a relatively large cavernous angioma located in the left temporal lobe exemplifies the convergence of these mechanisms. The mass effect exerted by the lesion may stretch or compress adjacent cortical areas, further contributing to pain generation. Moreover, temporal lobe cavernomas are frequently associated with epileptic activity, and seizures themselves—or the peri-ictal state—may present with or be followed by headache. Therefore, in such patients, headache may represent not only a primary symptom of the lesion itself but also a secondary manifestation of seizure activity or local cortical irritation.

Taken together, headache in patients with cavernous angiomas, particularly when located in eloquent regions such as the temporal lobe, should be evaluated in the broader context of microbleeds, inflammation, epileptogenic potential, and mass effect. Understanding these overlapping mechanisms is essential for guiding both diagnostic workup and therapeutic strategies.

20.3 Case Report

A man, 32 years old, presented to the emergency department three times over the past 30 days with continuous, dull, occasionally pulsatile left frontotemporal headache, with intermittent exacerbations. The pain improved with common analgesics such as dipyrone and tramadol.

He worked in elevator repair and maintenance, reporting high levels of stress. He had been evaluated by neurologists and was thought to be experiencing panic attacks while inside elevators, with headache exacerbations attributed to stress and possible panic disorder. No neuroimaging was initially requested.

On his most recent emergency visit, an otorhinolaryngology consultation was requested. A computed tomography (CT) scan of the paranasal sinuses was performed, and a temporal lesion was incidentally revealed. The patient denied any history of headaches in the past 30 days.

Subsequent brain magnetic resonance imaging (MRI) revealed a lesion consistent with a cavernous angioma in the left temporal lobe. The axial T2-weighted MRI demonstrates a well-defined, heterogeneous lesion in the left temporal lobe (2.2 × 2.3 × 2.2 cm) located near the mesial region. The lesion exhibits the classic "popcorn" or "mulberry" appearance typical of a cavernous angioma (cavernoma), with a mixed signal intensity core reflecting blood products at different stages of degradation and a hypointense rim consistent with hemosiderin deposition. There is no evident surrounding edema or mass effect, suggesting a chronic lesion without recent hemorrhage. The hypointense rim suggests hemosiderin deposition, indicating prior microhemorrhages. The lesion is adjacent to the hippocampus and parahippocampal structures, consistent with mesial temporal involvement (Fig. 20.1), which may explain the patient's seizure-like episodes and headache.

The patient underwent surgical resection of the lesion with complete removal (Fig. 20.2). Postoperatively, he had no neurological deficits and reported complete resolution of the headaches.

The presumed panic attacks were later interpreted as epileptic seizures, consistent with mesial temporal lobe epilepsy. He was started on carbamazepine (200 mg every 8 hours) and continues treatment.

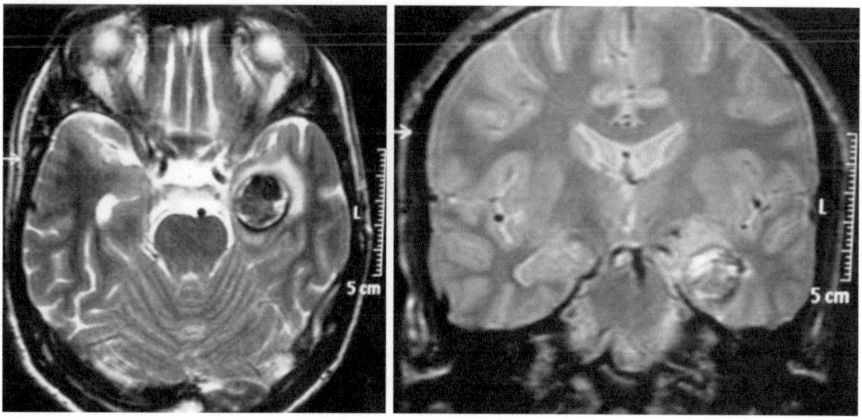

Fig. 20.1 MRI findings. Typical magnetic resonance imaging appearance of a cavernous angioma located in the left temporal lobe, near the mesial border of the temporal lobe, shown in the axial (left panel) and coronal (right panel) views

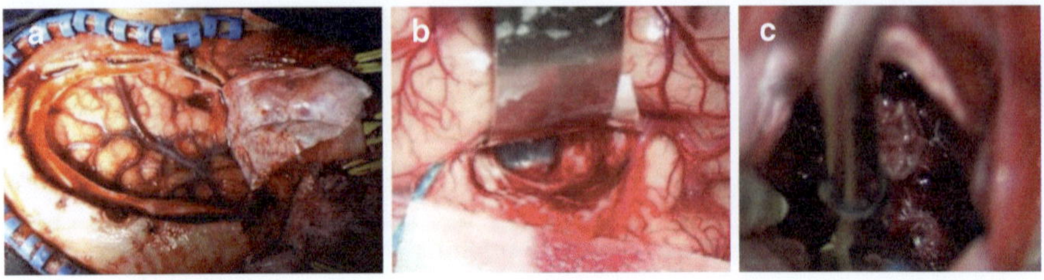

Fig. 20.2 Microsurgical procedure. (**a**) Left temporal craniotomy showing the lateral surface of the left temporal lobe with a corticotomy over the middle temporal gyrus. (**b**) With the aid of a temporal retractor, the dark-colored cavernoma is visualized. (**c**) The cavernoma is being removed using a surgical aspirator

20.4 Case Discussion

20.4.1 ICHD-3 Diagnostic Criteria—6.3.4 Headache Attributed to Cavernous Angioma

A. Any new headache fulfilling criterion C
B. A cavernous angioma has been diagnosed
C. Evidence of causation demonstrated by at least two of the following:

   1. The headache has developed in close temporal relation to other symptoms and/or clinical signs of the cavernous angioma, or led to its discovery.
   2. One or both of the following:

      - The headache has significantly worsened in parallel with other symptoms or clinical or radiological signs of growth of the cavernous angioma.
      - The headache has significantly improved or resolved after removal of the cavernous angioma.

   3. The headache is localized to the site of the cavernous angioma

D. The headache is not better accounted for by another ICHD-3 diagnosis

Note: Intracerebral hemorrhage has been excluded by appropriate investigations.

20.5 Commentary on the Presented Clinical Case

Criterion A—New headache:

The patient presented with a new, continuous headache that began approximately 30 days prior, thus fulfilling criterion A.

Criterion B—Diagnosis of cavernous angioma:

MRI revealed a lesion consistent with a cavernous angioma in the left temporal lobe.

Criterion C—Evidence of causality (at least two must be fulfilled):

- C1 (present): The headache led to the discovery of the cavernous angioma after imaging was requested by an otorhinolaryngologist.
- C2b (present): There was complete resolution of the headache following surgical removal of the lesion.
- C3 (present): The pain was localized to a region compatible with the lesion's location (left temporal lobe → left frontotemporal headache).
- Therefore, criterion C is fully satisfied.

Criterion D—Exclusion of other diagnoses:

The initial diagnostic hypothesis of panic disorder did not account for the persistent headache. After further investigation and definitive treatment of the lesion, the headache resolved completely, excluding other more likely alternative diagnoses. Furthermore, no hemorrhage was documented.

20.6 Clinical Presentation

Although the ICHD-3 notes that primary headache directly attributed to cavernous angiomas is rare—headache being more commonly secondary to seizures or hemorrhage—in this case there is strong temporal, anatomical, and therapeutic correlation. Thus, the most appropriate diagnosis is 6.3.4 Headache attributed to cavernous angioma.

However, since the patient presented with symptoms initially interpreted as panic attacks, which were retrospectively understood as epileptic seizures (mesial temporal lobe syndrome), it is also reasonable to consider coding part of the headache episode as 7.6 Headache attributed to epileptic seizure, particularly if the headache followed episodes of emotional discomfort (interpreted as epileptic equivalents).

20.7 Diagnostic Algorithm

1. Clinical Presentation

- Focal seizures (especially temporal lobe)
- Headache (persistent or intermittent)
- Focal neurological deficits
- Incidental finding on neuroimaging
- Family history of cerebral cavernous malformations (CCMs)

2. Initial Imaging
   - MRI of the brain with and without contrast is the imaging modality of choice
     - Preferred sequences: T2, T1, T2-FLAIR (fluid-attenuated inversion recovery), *Gradient Echo (T2)** or susceptibility-weighted imaging (SWI)
     - Findings:
       - "Popcorn" or "mulberry-like" appearance
       - Mixed signal core due to hemorrhagic products
       - Peripheral hypointense rim (hemosiderin)
3. Exclusion of Other Pathologies
   - Rule out arteriovenous malformations (AVMs) with MR angiography (MRA) or digital subtraction angiography (DSA) if atypical features are present
   - Differentiate from tumors, hemorrhagic metastases, or vascular malformations
4. Advanced Imaging (if needed)
   - Functional MRI: for lesions near eloquent cortex (motor, speech, etc.)
   - Perfusion MRI: to assess surrounding tissue edema or hemodynamic changes
   - CT scan: limited value but may show calcifications or acute hemorrhage
5. Genetic Testing (if indicated)
   - For patients with:
     - Multiple cavernomas
     - Family history of cavernomas
     - Early-onset or progressive lesions
   - Genetic panel for KRIT1 (CCM1), CCM2, and PDCD10 (CCM3) mutations
6. Electroencephalography (EEG)
   - If seizures are present or suspected
   - Localizes seizure focus; useful for pre-surgical evaluation
7. Neurosurgical/Neurological Evaluation
   - Assessment of surgical risk vs. benefit based on:
     - Location (e.g., brainstem, eloquent cortex)
     - Symptoms (seizures, hemorrhage, neurologic deficits)
     - Lesion size and growth
     - Hemorrhagic history

20.8 Conclusion

We found few reports in the literature describing cases of cavernomas associated with headache. One rare case involved an 18-year-old female presenting with severe headaches localized to the left temporal and facial regions. Imaging revealed a small dural-based parietal convexity mass, initially suggestive of a meningioma due to homogeneous enhancement and the presence of a "dural tail sign" on MRI [3]. Surgical resection, however, confirmed the lesion to be a cavernous angioma without evidence of prior hemorrhage. Postoperatively, the patient experienced complete resolution of her facial pain. Another report described an adolescent with atypical facial and head pain caused by a preexisting cerebellar cavernous angioma; both symptoms resolved following surgical excision of the lesion [4].

Additionally, a case of a brainstem cavernoma inducing migraine-like attacks has been documented [1]. There is also a report of a patient exhibiting a complex focal seizure accompanied by migraine-like headache, both attributable to a small cavernoma in the frontal lobe [5]. Furthermore, migraine-like headache was described in a patient with a frontal lesion [6]. An intriguing case involved a patient with an acute symptomatic migraine attack and chronic occipital neuralgia, both resulting from hemorrhage of a bulbocervical cavernoma [7].

This clinical case fulfills all ICHD-3 criteria for headache attributed to cavernous angioma (6.3.4), with an additional possibility of coding as headache attributed to epileptic seizure (7.6). The complete remission of the headache after resection of the lesion strongly supports a causal relationship with the cavernous angioma.

References

1. Malik S, Young W. Midbrain cavernous malformation causing migraine-like headache. Cephalalgia. 2006;26:1016–9. https://doi.org/10.1111/j.1468-2982.2006.01124.x.
2. Stellmann J-P, Kuhn M, Töpper R. Therapieresistenter Gesichtsschmerz durch ein Hirnstammkavernom. Fortschritte Der Neurologie · Psychiatrie. 2007;75:552–4. https://doi.org/10.1055/s-2007-980088.
3. Shen W, Chenn C, Hsue C, Lin T. Dural cavernous angioma mimicking a meningioma and causing facial pain. J Neuroimaging. 2000;10:183–5. https://doi.org/10.1111/jon2000103183.
4. Epstein MA, Berman PH, Schut L. Cavernous angioma presenting as atypical facial and head pain. J Child Neurol. 1990;5:27–30. https://doi.org/10.1177/088307389000500105.
5. Adhikari P, Nepali A, Shah A, Paudel S, Bhandari P, Nepali P. A small frontal lobe cavernoma presenting with headache mimicking migraine and complex focal seizure: a case report. Clin Case Rep. 2024;12 https://doi.org/10.1002/ccr3.8472.
6. Chirchiglia D, Della Torre A, Murrone D, Chirchiglia P, Marotta R. An unusual association of headache, epilepsy, and late-onset Kleist's pseudodepression syndrome in frontal lobe cavernoma of the cerebral left hemisphere. Int Med Case Rep J. 2017;10:163–6. https://doi.org/10.2147/IMCRJ.S133465.
7. Bruti G, Mostardini C, Pierallini A, Villani V, Modini C, Cerbo R. Neurovascular headache and occipital neuralgia secondary to bleeding of Bulbocervical Cavernoma. Cephalalgia. 2007;27:1074–9. https://doi.org/10.1111/j.1468-2982.2007.01363.x.

Chapter 21
Headache Attributed to Angiitis of the Central Nervous System: Giant Cell Arteritis

Luiz Paulo Queiroz and Andressa Miozzo Soares

21.1 Introduction

Giant cell arteritis (GCA) is a chronic granulomatous inflammatory vasculitis that affects predominantly large- and medium-sized arteries in individuals older than 50. GCA is the most common vasculitis in this age population [1].

There are three phenotypes of GCA: (1) cranial, (2) extracranial (large vessel), and (3) mixed. The mixed phenotype may occur in up to 80% of cases. Cranial GCA patients are at higher risk of visual and neurological complications; extracranial GCA includes the development of stenosis and aneurysms of the aorta and its branches, especially in the upper limbs (axillary arteries) [2]. There is also an association of GCA with polymyalgia rheumatica (PMR). Nearly 30–60% of patients with GCA have concomitant PMR; and up to 25% of patients with PMR may have subclinical GCA [1–3].

The incidence of GCA is approximately 20 new cases per 100,000 individuals above 50 years of age. The incidence is higher in Northern Europe and lower in Africa, Asia, and Arabic countries. It is more common in females than males (F2–3:1 M). Incidence increases with age, peaking in the 70's (70–79 years old) [4–7].

GCA is a medical emergency; if not diagnosed, it can lead to serious consequences for patients. The risk of permanent sight loss ranges from 8% to 30% [4]. The most affected cranial arteries are the temporal, ophthalmic, and posterior ciliary arteries. Rarely are the vertebral and carotid arteries involved. Aortic involvement is

L. P. Queiroz (✉)
Neurology Department, Universidade Federal de Santa Catarina, Florianópolis, Brazil
e-mail: lpqueiroz@floripa.com.br

A. M. Soares
Rheumatology Department, Universidade Federal de Santa Catarina, Florianópolis, Brazil

D. Uludüz et al. (eds.), *Rare Causes of Headache Disorders*, Headache,
https://doi.org/10.1007/978-3-032-10242-3_21

frequently missed due to the paucity of clinical manifestations, but it can be present in up to 65% of GCA patients at the time of diagnosis [4].

21.2 Case Presentation

This is a 72-year-old female patient, Heloisa. She was referred to rheumatology by her neurologist due to a new daily persistent headache, which started 2 months before. She reported intense throbbing pain in the temporoparietal region, sometimes on the right and sometimes on the left. The pain was constant and progressive, with no relieving or worsening factors. She had no nausea, no phonophobia or photophobia. In addition to the pain, she reported significant sensitivity in her scalp, which made it difficult for her to comb her hair. According to her report, the sensitivity seemed to be worsening in the last few weeks, causing allodynia, which was preventing her from sleeping. Her neurologist requested initial tests that indicated inflammatory changes, prompting the referral. The patient denied any visual disturbances, jaw claudication, pain, or stiffness in the pelvic and shoulder girdles.

In the first evaluation, the patient brought a magnetic resonance imaging (MRI) scan of the brain that showed only minimal foci of gliosis and a slight diffuse reduction in volume, compatible with the patient's age. Rheumatoid factor and antinuclear factor were negative, C-reactive protein (CRP) was 50.08 mg/L, and erythrocyte sedimentation rate (ESR) was 109 mm/hr. Suspicion of giant cell arteritis (GCA) was then raised, and Doppler ultrasound of the temporal, carotid, and vertebral arteries was requested, in addition to magnetic resonance angiography of the thoracic and abdominal aorta and their main branches.

None of the requested tests showed images suggestive of GCA. Meanwhile, the patient complained of progression of allodynia and, in addition to the imaging tests, had a new CRP of 57 mg/L and ESR of 117 mm/hr. Procalcitonin was negative.

It was decided to request an ^{18}F-fluorodeoxyglucose positron tomography (^{18}F-FDG-PET) of the whole body, due to high suspicion of GCA and the result is shown in Fig. 21.1a and b. After diagnosis, treatment with prednisone was started at a dose of 60 mg for 15 days, followed by 40 mg thereafter. Methotrexate was also started at a dose of 15 mg per week, combined with folic acid (5 mg) on the day after taking methotrexate. Tocilizumab 162 mg subcutaneous (SC) was requested weekly. After 30 days, the patient returned reporting resolution of the headache and scalp allo dynia. She also reported a significant reduction in fatigue, which she had not previously associated with the case. She brought tests, now with a CRP of 7.43 mg/L and ESR of 39 mm/hr.

A few weeks later, the patient had access to tocilizumab, which was initiated. Methotrexate was then suspended, and the dose of prednisone was reduced until it was discontinued. The patient achieved complete remission on tocilizumab monotherapy, as perceived both clinically and laboratory and by imaging (Fig. 21.1c and d).

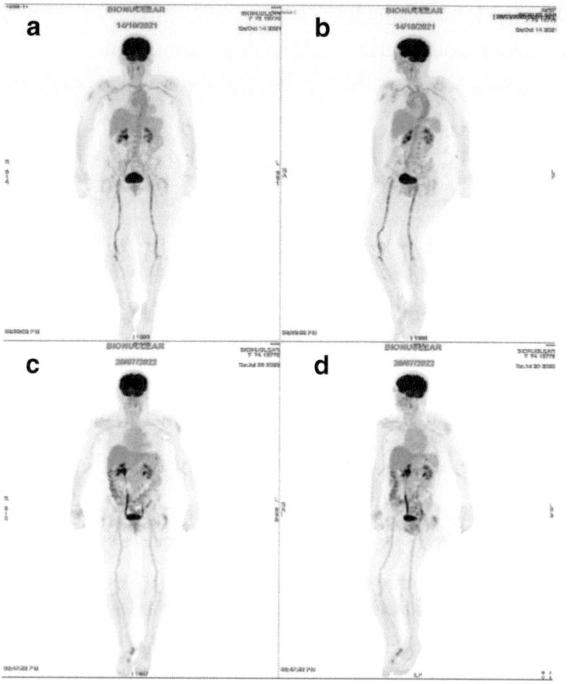

Fig. 21.1 ^{18}F-FDG-PET-CT performed longitudinally in a patient with large vessel giant cell arteritis. (**a** and **b**) scan at diagnosis (October 2021) showing pathological ^{18}F-FDG uptake (higher than the liver) in the walls of the abdominal aorta, thoracic aorta, supra-aortic branches, femoral arteries, popliteal arteries, and tibiofibular trunk. (**c** and **d**) Scan during clinical remission after starting Tocilizumab (July 2021) showing reduction in ^{18}F-FDG uptake (lower than the liver)

21.3 Clinical Characteristics

The most common premonitory and cardinal symptom of GCA is a new-onset headache or an uncommon headache (a change in the characteristics of a previous headache) in a patient over 50 years of age. It is a complaint in more than 70% of the cases [8]. Headache can be the only symptom of GCA, but this is only a modest discriminator when trying to predict the likelihood of GCA. The report of a temporal headache, however, does not significantly increase the probability of a diagnosis of GCA [2, 4]. Headaches are also common when there is a relapse.

Although the headache is usually described as temporal, it may be frontal, occipital, hemicranial, or holocranial (generalized). It can be continuous (occurring daily or almost daily in 60%) or paroxysmal (occurring in 40% of cases). The intensity can be from mild to severe, with fluctuations in severity [4]. Occasionally, the headache can mimic the characteristics of a migraine, with pulsating pain, nausea, phonophobia, and/or photophobia [9].

Most patients complain of unilateral headaches, but Moudrous et al. [5] reported that bilateral headaches were a positive predictive factor for a positive temporal artery biopsy (TAB), especially when associated with weight loss, thrombocytosis, and a positive halo sign on color Doppler ultrasound.

The diagnostic criteria of the International Classification of Headache Disorders—third edition (ICHD-3) [10] for headache attributed to GCA are:

A. Any new headache fulfilling criterion C.
B. Giant cell arteritis (GCA) has been diagnosed.
C. Evidence of causation demonstrated by at least two of the following:
    1. A headache has developed in close temporal relation to other symptoms and/or clinical or biological signs of onset of GCA, or has led to the diagnosis of GCA.
    2. Either or both of the following:
        (a) The headache has significantly worsened in parallel with the worsening of GCA.
        (b) The headache has significantly improved or resolved within 3 days of high-dose steroid treatment.
    3. Headache is associated with scalp tenderness and/or jaw claudication.
D. Not better accounted for by another ICHD-3 diagnosis.

In general, there is no association between headache characteristics and the presence of GCA [11]. The headache phenotype in these patients in terms of frequency, severity, and other associated symptoms is not yet well characterized.

Other cranial signs and symptoms (Fig. 21.2): Temporal cutaneous hyperalgesia, jaw claudication (up to 50% of cases), abnormalities of the temporal artery on examination (prominent, beaded or irregular artery, with a decreased pulse), tongue claudication, scalp or tongue necrosis, and rarely ischemic stroke. Tongue pain is rare, but if present, it increases the chance of a GCA [4].

Between 20% and 30% of patients develop ophthalmic signs and symptoms: transient monocular visual loss (Amaurosis fugax) or permanent loss of vision (5%) [2, 7]. Amaurosis fugax usually occurs within 8.5 days before permanent visual loss. It is the initial symptom of GCA in about 18% of the cases [7]. Of those with permanent visual loss or blurred vision at the time of the diagnosis, 44% had an amaurosis fugax previously. Some patients may present with Charles Bonnet syndrome [1].

These permanent losses of vision are due to arteritic anterior ischemic optic neuropathy (AAION), central retinal artery occlusion, branch retinal artery occlusion, posterior ischemic optic neuropathy, or choroidal infarction.

Other visual symptoms include transient or permanent diplopia, secondary to extraocular muscle ischemia or ocular cranial nerve palsies. Systemic symptoms are fever, myalgia, fatigue, night sweats, anorexia, unintentional weight loss, mood changes, arthralgias, stiffness of shoulders, and pelvic joints [1, 12]. Large vessel manifestations include aortitis, limb claudication, thoracic and abdominal aortic aneurysms, and myocardial infarction [12]. Pain and stiffness in the shoulders and the pelvic girdle, predominantly in the morning, may mean the associated presence of polymyalgia rheumatica [13].

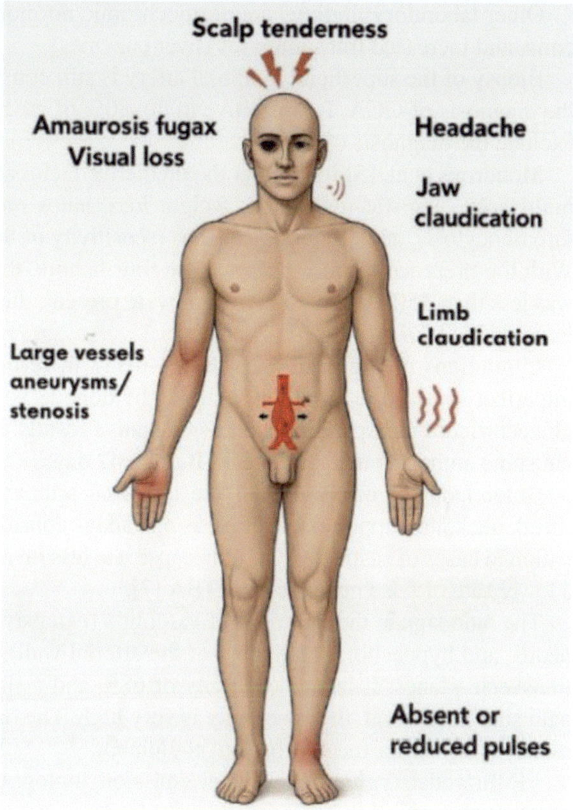

Fig. 21.2 Clinical manifestations in GCA

21.4 Diagnosis

The diagnosis of GCA will depend on an extensive clinical history that generates suspicion through characteristic symptoms and a detailed physical examination. This should be associated with inflammatory laboratory changes and the presence of vasculitis in imaging tests or biopsy [12].

Criteria for diagnosing GCA were established in 1990 by the American College of Rheumatology (ACR) [14], and a revision was proposed in 2021 [15]. In 2022, the ACR and the European Alliance of Associations for Rheumatology (EULAR) released guidelines for the classification of GCA, which is more useful for research purposes [16].

There are no currently specific blood biomarkers that can diagnose GCA. Elevated acute phase reactants: Erythrocyte sedimentation rate (ESR)—≥50 mm/h; C-reactive protein (CRP)—>10 or 20 mg/L; thrombocytosis—platelets >300,000; increased fibrinogen. Only 4% of GCA patients have normal ESR and CRP. CRP is a more sensitive marker for inflammation, as ESR levels can increase with age, anemia, chronic kidney disease, and hypergammaglobulinemia [1].

Other laboratory findings are normochromic normocytic anemia, hypoalbuminemia, and increased transaminases (liver enzymes).

Biopsy of the superficial temporal artery is still considered the gold standard for the diagnosis of GCA. It is positive in 50–80% of cases. A negative TAB does not exclude the diagnosis of GCA.

Moudrous et al. [5] found that the predictive factors for positive TAB were, after multivariate logistic regression: weight loss, halos on color Doppler ultrasound, thrombocytosis, and bilateral headache (sensitivity of 89% and specificity of 91%). With the presence of only one of these four factors, the chance of a positive TAB was less than 35%; when three or four were present, the chance of a positive biopsy increased to 97.9–99.9%.

Limitations of the TAB include the delay in results, its invasive nature, and imperfect sensitivity. The biopsy should be done as soon as possible after starting glucocorticoid therapy, to avoid false-negative results. The ideal is within 14 days, but some authors found positive TAB up to 42 days.

Color Doppler ultrasound of the temporal arteries and supra-aortic branches (head, neck, and upper extremities) is nowadays considered as the first-line examination in cases of suspected GCA, because it is less invasive, less expensive, and has a lower rate of false negative than TBA [7].

The halo sign is the hallmark of vasculitis (extensive, circumferential, homogeneous, and hypoechoic thickening of the arterial wall), visible on longitudinal and transverse planes. It has a sensitivity of 68% and a specificity of 81%. When the halo sign is bilateral, the specificity is very high. The halo sign disappears approximately 5 days after the appropriate equipment.

^{18}F-fluorodeoxyglucose positron emission tomography (^{18}F-FDG-PET) of the whole body is used to be indicated only for large vessel GCA. Still, recently, with new technology and protocols, it has been helpful also for the diagnosis of cranial disease [6, 12].

Computed tomography (CT) angiography and MRI angiography of aorta and its branches are both used to look for vasculitis mainly in aorta and its branches. The presence of circumferential and homogeneous arterial wall thickening and/or contrast enhancement of the arterial wall is suggestive of vasculitis [3, 12].

For typical presentations of GCA, there are almost no differential diagnoses. For atypical cranial GCA, there are a few: Anti-neutrophil cytoplasmic antibodies (ANCA)-associated vasculitis, temporal arteritis due to varicella zoster virus, atherosclerotic disease, uremic calcifying arteriopathy, posttraumatic arteriovenous fistulas or pseudoaneurysms, nonarteritic anterior ischemic optic neuropathy, and immunoglobulin 4 (IgG4)-related disease [12, 17].

21.5 Treatment

Whenever there is a high clinical suspicion of GCA, a high dose of glucocorticoid (40–60 mg/day) should be immediately started [18].

For patients with visual symptoms, pulses of IV methylprednisolone (250–1000 mg/day, for 3 days) may be considered, followed by oral prednisone, but its benefit has not been proven [12, 18, 19].

Currently, both the ACR and PANLAR (Pan American League of Associations for Rheumatology) recommend starting an immunosuppressant together with the use of corticosteroids at the diagnosis of GCA [18, 19]. Thanks to the giant cell arteritis actemra trial (GiACTA) study [20] that produced evidence in favor of the use of tocilizumab (a humanized monoclonal antibody to the interleukin-6 [IL-6] receptor) in GCA, this has been the recommended first-line immunosuppressant [18, 19]. If there is difficulty in accessing the use of this medication or contraindication, the use of methotrexate associated with glucocorticoid may be an alternative [19].

The isolated use of glucocorticoids is associated with high rates of relapse and complications related to the drug itself [18]. The duration of glucocorticoid therapy, when associated with immunosuppressants, is not well established, but it is suggested to progressively reduce the dose until its withdrawal, when possible, in 6 months. The duration of treatment with immunosuppressants is also not well established in the literature [12, 18, 19].

In patients with severe carotid and vertebral involvement, the use of aspirin associated with immunosuppressive treatment has been conditionally recommended [18, 19].

References

1. Ameer MA, Vaqar S, Khazaeni B. Giant cell arteritis (temporal arteritis). In: StatPearls [internet]. Treasure Island (FL): StatPearls Publishing; 2025.
2. Szekeres D, Al Othman B. Current developments in the diagnosis and treatment of giant cell arteritis. Front Med (Lausanne). 2022;9:1066503. https://doi.org/10.3389/fmed.2022.1066503.
3. Van der Geest KSM, Sandovici M, Brouwer E, et al. Large vessel giant cell arteritis. Lancet Rheumatol. 2024;6(6):e397–408. ISSN 2665-9913
4. Mollan SP, Lee AG, Davies B, et al. European Headache Federation recommendations for neurologists managing giant cell arteritis. J Headache Pain. 2020;21(1):28. Published March 17, 2020. ISSN 1129-2369
5. Moudrous W, Visser LH, Yilmaz T, H Wieringa M, Alleman T, Rovers J, Houben MPWA, Janssen PM, J B Janssen J, L Rensma P, J F Brekelmans G. A new prediction model for giant cell arteritis in patients with new onset headache and/or visual loss. Ann Med. 2022;54(1):2770–6. https://doi.org/10.1080/07853890.2022.2130971.
6. Wang D, Liu Z, Guo H, Yang L, Zhang X, Peng L, Cheng M, Jiang H. Headache attributed to giant cell arteritis complicated with rheumatic polymyalgia diagnosed with F18-fluorodeoxyglucose positron emission tomography and computed tomography: a case report. Front Neurol. 2023;14:1241676. https://doi.org/10.3389/fneur.2023.1241676.

7. Dinkin M, Johnson E. One giant step for giant cell arteritis: updates in diagnosis and treatment. Curr Treat Options Neurol. 2021;23(2):6. https://doi.org/10.1007/s11940-020-00660-2.
8. Öztaş M, Özgül H, Seyahi E, Uğurlu S. Presentation characteristics and clinical outcome of patients with giant cell arteritis followed by a single center. Turk J Med Sci. 2022;52(4):917–25. https://doi.org/10.55730/1300-0144.5391.
9. Devi S, Dash A, Purkait S, Sahoo B. Giant cell arteritis masquerading as migraine: a case report. Cureus. 2023;15(8):e44107. https://doi.org/10.7759/cureus.44107.
10. Headache Classification Committee of the International Headache Society (IHS). The international classification of headache disorders, 3rd edition. Cephalalgia. 2018;38(1):1–211. https://doi.org/10.1177/0333102417738202.
11. Shimohama S, Imai N, Tsubata T, Shinohara K, Moriya A, Yagi N, Konishi T, Serizawa M, Tashiro K. Headache-related characteristics of biopsy-confirmed giant cell arteritis and the relationship of transmural inflammation with artery tenderness and chordal thickening. Cureus. 2024;16(3):e56843. https://doi.org/10.7759/cureus.56843.
12. de Boysson H, Devauchelle-Pensec V, Agard C, André M, Bienvenu B, Bonnotte B, Carvajal Alegria G, Espitia O, Hachulla E, Heron E, Lambert M, Lega JC, Ly KH, Mekinian A, Morel J, Regent A, Richez C, Sailler L, Seror R, Tournadre A, Samson M, Collaborators. French protocol for the diagnosis and management of giant cell arteritis. Rev Med Interne. 2025;46(1):12–31. https://doi.org/10.1016/j.revmed.2024.10.011.
13. Espígol-Frigolé G, Dejaco C, Mackie SL, Salvarani C, Matteson EL, Cid MC. Polymyalgia rheumatica. Lancet. 2023;402(10411):1459–72. https://doi.org/10.1016/S0140-6736(23)01310-7.
14. Wolfe F, Smythe HA, Yunus MB, Bennett RM, Bombardier C, Goldenberg DL, Tugwell P, Campbell SM, Abeles M, Clark P, et al. The American College of Rheumatology 1990 criteria for the classification of fibromyalgia. Report of the multicenter criteria committee. Arthritis Rheum. 1990;33(2):160–72. https://doi.org/10.1002/art.1780330203.
15. Wiberg F, Naderi N, Mohammad AJ, Turesson C. Evaluation of revised classification criteria for giant cell arteritis and its clinical phenotypes. Rheumatology (Oxford). 2021;61(1):383–7. https://doi.org/10.1093/rheumatology/keab353.
16. Ponte C, Grayson PC, Robson JC, Suppiah R, Gribbons KB, Judge A, Craven A, Khalid S, Hutchings A, Watts RA, Merkel PA, Luqmani RA, DCVAS Study Group. 2022 American College of Rheumatology/EULAR classification criteria for giant cell arteritis. Ann Rheum Dis. 2022;81(12):1647–53. https://doi.org/10.1136/ard-2022-223480.
17. Greigert H, Ramon A, Tarris G, Martin L, Bonnotte B, Samson M. Temporal artery vascular diseases. J Clin Med. 2022;11(1):275. https://doi.org/10.3390/jcm11010275.
18. Scolnik M, Brance ML, Fernández-Ávila DG, Inoue Sato E, de Souza AWS, Magri SJ, Saldarriaga-Rivera LM, Ugarte-Gil MF, Flores-Suarez LF, Babini A, Zamora NV, Acosta Felquer ML, Vergara F, Carlevaris L, Scarafia S, Soriano Guppy ER, Unizony S, Pan American League of Associations for Rheumatology (PANLAR). Pan American League of Associations for Rheumatology guidelines for the treatment of giant cell arteritis. Lancet Rheumatol. 2022;4(12):e864–72. https://doi.org/10.1016/S2665-9913(22)00260-0.
19. Maz M, Chung SA, Abril A, Langford CA, Gorelik M, Guyatt G, Archer AM, Conn DL, Full KA, Grayson PC, Ibarra MF, Imundo LF, Kim S, Merkel PA, Rhee RL, Seo P, Stone JH, Sule S, Sundel RP, Vitobaldi OI, Warner A, Byram K, Dua AB, Husainat N, James KE, Kalot MA, Lin YC, Springer JM, Turgunbaev M, Villa-Forte A, Turner AS, Mustafa RA. 2021 American College of Rheumatology/Vasculitis Foundation Guideline for the Management of Giant Cell Arteritis and Takayasu Arteritis. Arthritis Rheumatol. 2021;73(8):1349–65. https://doi.org/10.1002/art.41774.
20. Stone JH, Tuckwell K, Dimonaco S, Klearman M, Aringer M, Blockmans D, Brouwer E, Cid MC, Dasgupta B, Rech J, Salvarani C, Schett G, Schulze-Koops H, Spiera R, Unizony SH, Collinson N. Trial of Tocilizumab in giant-cell arteritis. N Engl J Med. 2017;377(4):317–28. https://doi.org/10.1056/NEJMoa1613849.

Chapter 22
Headache or Facial or Neck Pain Attributed to Cervical Carotid or Vertebral Artery Dissection

Ş. Ozan Dörtkol and Esme Ekizoğlu

22.1 Introduction

C. Miller Fisher first described arterial dissection. It refers to the tear of the arterial wall and is classified according to the location of the dissection [1]. Cervical artery dissections (CAD), which refer to cervical carotid and vertebral artery dissections, are not uncommon and constitute the etiology behind a variety of neurological symptoms. The most common symptoms of dissections on the cervical segments of carotid or vertebral arteries are headache, facial, or neck pain [2]. Other common symptoms result from ischemia related to an ischemic stroke or to a transient ischemic attack. Cervicocerebral artery dissection is one of the important causes of stroke seen in the young population [3]. Dissections may also be complicated with dissecting aneurysms or subarachnoid hemorrhage (SAH).

The recorded incidence of CAD has been estimated to be 2.6–2.9 per 100,000 per year based on previous studies in the United States and France [4, 5]. Cervical artery dissection is likely underestimated in routine practice because cases with few or no clinical signs may be underdiagnosed or misdiagnosed [6]. However, CAD is the cause of approximately 24% of the strokes in young patients [7]. North American studies have found a higher incidence in women [4, 8], and European studies have found a higher incidence in men [9, 10]. One study reported that CAD occurred more frequently in cold months in association with increased brachial pulse pressure [11, 12]. Headache is reported as the most common symptom and also the most common initial symptom. Although isolated headache is rarely experienced, this may also occur as a symptom of extracranial dissection [13].

Ş. O. Dörtkol
Neurology Clinic, Istanbul Physical Medicine and Rehabilitation Training and Research Hospital, Istanbul, Turkey

E. Ekizoğlu (✉)
Department of Neurology, Istanbul Faculty of Medicine, Istanbul University, Istanbul, Turkey

D. Uludüz et al. (eds.), *Rare Causes of Headache Disorders*, Headache,
https://doi.org/10.1007/978-3-032-10242-3_22

22.2 Pathophysiology and Risk Factors

Arterial dissections develop as a result of a tear in the media and intima layers of the arterial wall. This condition becomes complex when blood enters the vascular wall, which leads to the formation of a thrombus [14]. Dissections are called "spontaneous" when there is no traumatic event, since they may result from major or minor trauma. A headache or neck congestion is likely due to the rupture in the vessel wall. The tear in the vessel wall likely leads to a cascade of events that also result in the release of several pro-inflammatory neurotransmitters from the blood vessels near nerve terminals. This may result in the onset of pain in the regions of dissection [15].

The genetic predisposition in the development of cervical dissections has been shown in patients with collagen vascular disorders [16]. Some studies reported that this condition was associated with a mutation in MTHFR C677T and deficiency of alpha-1 antitrypsin as genetic factors predisposing this condition [4].

However, most of the CADs occur as a result of minor neck trauma or manipulation, indicating the role of environmental factors [17]. Previous studies have also reported an association between CAD and acute or subacute infections [17]. No definitive data have been reported on CAD occurrence and vascular risk factors. However, low body mass index, hypertension, and low cholesterol level appear to increase the risk of arterial dissection. Furthermore, some previous studies have reported a possible association between CAD and migraine [18].

22.3 Case Presentation 1

A 34-year-old woman was admitted to the emergency department with a sudden onset of headache on the left side spreading to the forehead while cleaning the upper surface of a tall cabinet with neck hyperextension. She described that the pain was throbbing, accompanied by nausea, without any symptoms such as photophobia, phonophobia, and osmophobia. She also experienced blurred vision, which began at the same time as a headache and lasted for 15 min. She benefited from a painkiller, and her headache entirely resolved in 3 h. The same headache recurred 2 days later when carrying a heavy object and lasted for 15 min.

She was diagnosed with episodic migraine for 20 years, reporting two to three attacks per month. Her physical and neurological examinations were unremarkable. She was neither a smoker nor an alcohol user.

Brain magnetic resonance imaging (MRI) showed small acute infarcts in the left cerebellum. MRA revealed a left vertebral artery (VA) dissection leading to a 2 cm stenosis in the distal part of the V3 segment. Other etiological workup for stroke was normal. She was started on dual antiplatelet therapy and did not need further painkiller use during her hospital stay.

22.4 Case Discussion

This case illustrates that secondary headaches should be considered in a patient with a prior primary headache condition when the patient describes a sudden onset of a new headache. Detailed history taking may provide clues for diagnosis. This patient reported that the headache started while hyperextending her neck, which is a typical posture causing minor neck trauma. This case also highlights the importance of MRA (or computed tomography angiography [CTA]) in addition to brain imaging in patients suspected of having an arterial dissection-related headache.

22.5 Case Presentation 2

A 60-year-old male patient presented with a severe progressive headache on the left temporal region of his head that started 5 days before admission. He described the pain as throbbing and not accompanied by nausea and vomiting. He had no history of previous headaches or other diseases and did not report a recent head trauma or other suspicious condition. He found some relief from painkillers without complete recovery. Neurological examination was notable for miosis and ptosis on the left eye (Horner's syndrome), and mild right hemiparesis.

Brain MRI revealed an acute infarct in the left putamen and hyperintense flow void in the distal cervical and petrosal segments of the left internal carotid artery (ICA) on fluid-attenuated inversion recovery (FLAIR) sequences. CTA disclosed a left ICA dissection causing severe stenosis and intramural thrombus. The patient started on dual antiplatelet therapy, and analgesic drugs were administered. His headache resolved during hospital admission in 4 days, and the neurological findings recovered. Repeated CTAs showed complete resolution of the thrombus and stenosis; the patient reported being headache-free since discharge at the 3-month follow-up visit.

22.6 Case Discussion 2

This case illustrates the importance of a detailed, systematic, and neurological examination when evaluating patients admitted with headache to exclude secondary headaches. In this case, the headache was progressive and experienced for the first time. These are important clinical features that suggest a secondary headache disorder and require further diagnostic investigations. Moreover, neurological examination revealed Horner's syndrome on the left, suggesting carotid dissection in the differential diagnosis, together with the presence of headache. The pain was severe and unilateral to the affected cervical artery, lasted several days and resolved during follow-up within less than 1 month. All these features fulfilled third edition of the International Classification of Headache Disorders (ICHD-3) diagnostic criteria for *acute headache or facial or neck pain attributed to cervical carotid or vertebral artery dissection.*

22.7 Clinical Characteristics

The third edition of the International Classification of Headache Disorders (ICHD-3) established specific criteria to make the diagnosis of headache or facial or neck pain associated with cervical artery or vertebral artery dissection. These diagnostic criteria were given in Table 22.1 [19].

Factors influencing the development of headaches associated with CAD were reported to be female gender, dissection affecting posterior circulation, prior history of headaches, and low-density lipoprotein levels [20]. Acute onset headache was observed in 53% of the patients, and 35% of these patients experienced headache as the initial symptom. Therefore, artery dissections should also be assessed in the differential diagnosis of thunderclap headache [21].

The pain was reported to be throbbing pain in one third (35%) of the patients and localized usually on one side of the head or neck (71.7%) [22]. In carotid artery dissections, pain was most frequently localized in the temporal region (46%), followed by the frontal region (19.2%). In contrast, in vertebrobasilar artery dissections, the

Table 22.1 ICHD-3 diagnostic criteria for acute headache or facial or neck pain attributed to cervical carotid or vertebral artery dissection

A. Any new headache and/or facial or neck pain fulfilling criteria C and D
B. Cervical carotid or vertebral dissection has been diagnosed
C. Evidence of causation demonstrated by at least two of the following:
1. Pain has developed in close temporal relation to other local signs of the cervical artery dissection, or has led to its diagnosis 2. Either or both of the following: (a) Pain has significantly worsened in parallel with other signs of the cervical artery dissection (b) Pain has significantly improved or resolved within 1 month of its onset 3. Either or both of the following (a) Pain is severe and continuous for days or longer (b) Pain precedes signs of acute retinal and/or cerebral ischemia 4. Pain is unilateral and ipsilateral to the affected cervical artery
D. Either of the following:
1. The headache has revolved within 3 months 2. The headache has not yet resolved, but 3 months have not yet passed
E. Not better accounted for by another ICHD-3 diagnosis

occipital region and the nape of the neck stood out as the locations where the pain was most frequently observed (79.7%) [22]. The severity of the headache may vary depending on age. A previous study compared the clinical features of dissections in the young population and the elderly and observed that both neck pain and headaches were more frequently experienced by young people than the elderly [23].

In a recently published review that evaluates the clinical characteristics of patients with CAD, it has been reported that headache was a more prevalent symptom in cases of vertebral artery dissection than in those of carotid artery dissection [22]. Furthermore, Uludüz et al. observed that patients with vertebral artery dissection experienced more frequent headaches with higher rates of photophobia and phonophobia in comparison to patients with carotid artery dissection [24]. Another report has also described a case of vertebral artery dissection with migraine-like headache accompanied by photophobia and nausea [25]. The higher rates of headache, photophobia, and phonophobia in patients with vertebral artery dissection are thought to be associated with trigeminovascular system activation [26]. However, another study evaluating 51 patients with vertebral artery dissection reported that only 4% of the patients reported photophobia at the time of diagnosis [27]. In a survey conducted by Mayer-Suess et al., headaches occurred frequently with a sudden onset in patients with arterial dissection. The character of the pain in vertebral artery dissection was often described as a pulling sensation, whereas in carotid artery dissection, it was typically characterized as dull and throbbing. Furthermore, among patients with vertebral artery dissection, it was noted that the duration of headaches was significantly longer than in carotid artery dissection [28]. A recent study reported that headaches associated with CAD were more severe, more often unilateral, and more frequent than those associated with large artery occlusion. It was also found that headaches were frequently throbbing in patients with dissection, but pulsating in those with occlusion [29].

The relationship between migraine and CAD has also been reported in some reports, although the sample sizes were usually limited to small groups. While an association between migraine with aura and CAD has been reported [29], a cohort study investigating 2485 ischemic stroke patients showed that the prevalence of CAD was higher in patients with migraine without aura compared with migraine with aura [19].

It should also be noted that clinical presentations in CAD may vary depending on the localization and the surrounding structures of the dissected segment as well. *Horner's syndrome* is mostly seen in carotid dissections because pericarotid sympathetic fibers are frequently affected. However, vertebrobasilar dissections cause symptoms associated with brainstem ischemia, such as vertigo, ataxia, and nausea [30, 31]. One of the most common presentations in patients is cerebral ischemia, which occurs in two-thirds of patients [4]. Symptoms are consistent with the ischemic area in these patients. Rarely seen presentations include retinal infarctions leading to monocular vision loss or ischemic optic neuropathy [32, 33].

22.8 Diagnostic Workup

Several neuroimaging tests are helpful in the diagnosis of arterial dissection. Computed tomographic angiography (CTA) has half the spatial resolution of digital subtraction angiography (DSA) and twice the spatial resolution of magnetic resonance angiography (MRA) [34]. Rapid image acquisition and widespread availability make CTA the most frequently preferred diagnostic method. The specificity (67–100%), sensitivity (64–100%), negative (70–100%), and positive predictive (65–100%) values of CTA for the detection of cervical or cephalic arterial dissection are comparable to those of DSA [35–37]. An asymmetrical and irregular vessel wall appearance is the most common finding. Intramural hematoma is seen as a crescent-shaped hyperdensity in addition to the thickening of the vessel wall [38]. CTA can also easily demonstrate intimal flaps and pseudoaneurysms, which is a common consequence of extracranial dissection and occur in 13–49% of patients with CAD [39]. Although well-tolerated and relatively safe and less invasive than DSA, CTA involves exposure to iodinated contrast and radiation, which may be harmful for patients with impaired renal function or allergies to contrast material. CTA is a neuroimaging test that is relatively contraindicated during pregnancy and in childhood [40].

The combination of axial T1-weighted cervical MRI examination with fat suppression is used for a noninvasive imaging modality to detect dissection. It is more sensitive to detect small intramural hematomas than CT imaging [41]. The characteristic MRI finding is the hyperintense crescent sign observed on T1-weighted and FLAIR sequences that results from intramural leaking of the blood, causing the intramural hematoma that appears in the shape of a half-moon spiral [41–43]. Recent studies have also demonstrated the effectiveness and reliability of susceptibility-weighted imaging (SWI) in detecting intramural hematoma [44]. Other abnormalities that can be identified through magnetic resonance imaging (MRI) include vessel diameter enlargement and hyperintense signal abnormality on the entire vessel, compromise of the vessel lumen by the adjacent tissue with an abnormally increased signal, and poor to no visualization of the vessel [45].

Digital subtraction angiography is accepted as the gold standard test to identify and reveal the features of dissected segments. This procedure allows dynamic characterization of the blood flow across the lesion. However, it carries risks of stroke, retroperitoneal hemorrhage, vascular perforation, and contrast-induced nephropathy [46].

22.9 Treatment

Although there is a limited number of studies on the treatment of dissections, the most important treatment step is the acute treatment to prevent possible complications such as ischemic stroke or subarachnoid hemorrhage. The primary therapeutic management strategy is therefore to start antiplatelets or anticoagulants as soon as possible for stroke prevention in CAD [47]. Acute treatment with intravenous thrombolysis and/or mechanical thrombectomy is also recommended in selected cases [41]. However, other symptoms, such as headaches, may also require treatment. It has been observed that headaches secondary to dissections may improve with antimigraine medications [41]. Medical management is based on both empirical and clinical observations. Nevertheless, a previous study showed that headaches associated with CAD had a better prognosis than headaches caused by other vascular causes [48].

22.10 Prognosis

There are very few studies evaluating the long-term prognosis of headaches associated with CAD. Evaluations of the clinical course of internal carotid artery dissections have noted that headaches resolved within a short time frame in a significant portion of patients [49]. As headaches improve typically shortly after the diagnosis, prolonged headaches are rarely reported in the literature. Analgesics are administered to the majority of patients and are beneficial in the majority of the reported cases. Only one case has been documented in which the headache resolved after a short course of steroid treatment [50]. Infrequently, arterial dissections with dissecting aneurysms can lead to subarachnoid hemorrhage. A poorer prognosis was observed in these cases where dissecting aneurysms occur [51]. Recurrence of dissections has a low rate of approximately 1% during at least 1 year of follow-up [9].

References

1. Fisher CM, Ojemann RG, Roberson GH. Spontaneous dissection of cervico-cerebral arteries. Can J Neurol Sci. 1978;5(1):9–19.
2. Fisher CM. The headache and pain of spontaneous carotid dissection. Headache. 1982;22(2):60–5. https://doi.org/10.1111/j.1526-4610.1982.hed2202060.x.
3. Putaala J, Metso AJ, Metso TM, Konkola N, Kraemer Y, Haapaniemi E, Kaste M, Tatlisumak T. Analysis of 1008 consecutive patients aged 15 to 49 with first-ever ischemic stroke: the Helsinki young stroke registry. Stroke. 2009;40(4):1195–203. https://doi.org/10.1161/STROKEAHA.108.529883. Epub 2009 Feb 26
4. Lee VH, Brown RD Jr, Mandrekar JN, Mokri B. Incidence and outcome of cervical artery dissection: a population-based study. Neurology. 2006;67(10):1809–12. https://doi.org/10.1212/01.wnl.0000244486.30455.71.
5. Béjot Y, Daubail B, Debette S, Durier J, Giroud M. Incidence and outcome of cerebrovascular events related to cervical artery dissection: the Dijon Stroke Registry. Int J Stroke. 2014;9(7):879–82. https://doi.org/10.1111/ijs.12154. Epub 2013 Oct 22
6. Salehi OS. Cervical artery dissection. Continuum (Minneap Minn). 2023;29(2):540–65. https://doi.org/10.1212/CON.0000000000001233.

7. Nedeltchev K, der Maur TA, Georgiadis D, Arnold M, Caso V, Mattle HP, Schroth G, Remonda L, Sturzenegger M, Fischer U, Baumgartner RW. Ischaemic stroke in young adults: predictors of outcome and recurrence. J Neurol Neurosurg Psychiatry. 2005;76(2):191–5. https://doi.org/10.1136/jnnp.2004.040543.
8. Schievink WI, Mokri B, O'Fallon WM. Recurrent spontaneous cervical-artery dissection. N Engl J Med. 1994;330(6):393–7. https://doi.org/10.1056/NEJM199402103300604.
9. Touzé E, Gauvrit JY, Moulin T, Meder JF, Bracard S, Mas JL, Multicenter Survey on Natural History of Cervical Artery Dissection. Risk of stroke and recurrent dissection after a cervical artery dissection: a multicenter study. Neurology. 2003;61(10):1347–51. https://doi.org/10.1212/01.wnl.0000094325.95097.86.
10. Arnold M, Kappeler L, Georgiadis D, Berthet K, Keserue B, Bousser MG, Baumgartner RW. Gender differences in spontaneous cervical artery dissection. Neurology. 2006;67(6):1050–2. https://doi.org/10.1212/01.wnl.0000237341.30854.6a.
11. Kloss M, Metso A, Pezzini A, Leys D, Giroud M, Metso TM, Tatlisumak T, Lichy C, Bersano A, Abboud S, Grau A, Lyrer PA, Debette S, Dallongeville J, Martin J, Caso V, Grond-Ginsbach C, Engelter ST. Towards understanding seasonal variability in cervical artery dissection (CeAD). J Neurol. 2012;259(8):1662–7. https://doi.org/10.1007/s00415-011-6395-0.
12. Mizutani T. Natural course of intracranial arterial dissections. J Neurosurg. 2011;114(4):1037–44. https://doi.org/10.3171/2010.9.JNS10668. Epub 2010 Oct 15
13. Debette S, Compter A, Labeyrie MA, Uyttenboogaart M, Metso TM, Majersik JJ, Goeggel-Simonetti B, Engelter ST, Pezzini A, Bijlenga P, Southerland AM, Naggara O, Béjot Y, Cole JW, Ducros A, Giacalone G, Schilling S, Reiner P, Sarikaya H, Welleweerd JC, Kappelle LJ, de Borst GJ, Bonati LH, Jung S, Thijs V, Martin JJ, Brandt T, Grond-Ginsbach C, Kloss M, Mizutani T, Minematsu K, Meschia JF, Pereira VM, Bersano A, Touzé E, Lyrer PA, Leys D, Chabriat H, Markus HS, Worrall BB, Chabrier S, Baumgartner R, Stapf C, Tatlisumak T, Arnold M, Bousser MG. Epidemiology, pathophysiology, diagnosis, and management of intracranial artery dissection. Lancet Neurol. 2015;14(6):640–54. https://doi.org/10.1016/S1474-4422(15)00009-5.
14. Fusco MR, Harrigan MR. Cerebrovascular dissections—a review, Part I: spontaneous dissections. Neurosurgery. 2011;68(1):242–57; discussion 257. https://doi.org/10.1227/NEU.0b013e3182012323.
15. Reeves AG, Swenson RS. Disorders of the nervous system; 2008.
16. Kloss M, Wiest T, Hyrenbach S, Werner I, Arnold ML, Lichy C, Grond-Ginsbach C. MTHFR 677TT genotype increases the risk for cervical artery dissections. J Neurol Neurosurg Psychiatry. 2006;77(8):951–2. https://doi.org/10.1136/jnnp.2006.089730.
17. Guillon B, Berthet K, Benslamia L, Bertrand M, Bousser MG, Tzourio C. Infection and the risk of spontaneous cervical artery dissection: a case-control study. Stroke. 2003;34(7):e79–81. https://doi.org/10.1161/01.STR.0000078309.56307.5C. Epub 2003 Jun 12
18. De Giuli V, Grassi M, Lodigiani C, Patella R, Zedde M, Gandolfo C, Zini A, DeLodovici ML, Paciaroni M, Del Sette M, Azzini C, Toriello A, Musolino R, Calabrò RS, Bovi P, Sessa M, Adami A, Silvestrelli G, Cavallini A, Marcheselli S, Bonifati DM, Checcarelli N, Tancredi L, Chiti A, Lotti EM, Del Zotto E, Tomelleri G, Spalloni A, Giorli E, Costa P, Poli L, Morotti A, Caria F, Lanari A, Giacalone G, Ferrazzi P, Giossi A, Piras V, Massucco D, D'Amore C, Di Lisi F, Casetta I, Cucurachi L, Cotroneo M, De Vito A, Coloberti E, Rasura M, Simone AM, Gamba M, Cerrato P, Micieli G, Malferrari G, Melis M, Iacoviello L, Padovani A, Pezzini A, Italian Project on Stroke in Young Adults Investigators. Association between migraine and cervical artery dissection: the Italian project on stroke in young adults. JAMA Neurol. 2017;74(5):512–8. https://doi.org/10.1001/jamaneurol.2016.5704.
19. Headache Classification Committee of the International Headache Society (IHS). The international classification of headache disorders, 3rd edition. Cephalalgia. 2018;38(1):1–211. https://doi.org/10.1177/0333102417738202.

20. Wang Y, Cheng W, Lian Y, Zhang J, Zheng Y, Hu Y, Chen Y, Wu S, Huang Z, Shi Y. Characteristics and relative factors of headache caused by cervicocerebral artery dissection. J Neurol. 2019;266(2):298–305. https://doi.org/10.1007/s00415-018-9111-5. Epub 2018 Dec 12
21. Silbert PL, Mokri B, Schievink WI. Headache and neck pain in spontaneous internal carotid and vertebral artery dissections. Neurology. 1995;45(8):1517–22. https://doi.org/10.1212/wnl.45.8.1517.
22. Vidale S. Headache in cervicocerebral artery dissection. Neurol Sci. 2020;41(Suppl 2):395–9. https://doi.org/10.1007/s10072-020-04651-8.
23. Traenka C, Dougoud D, Simonetti BG, Metso TM, Debette S, Pezzini A, Kloss M, Grond-Ginsbach C, Majersik JJ, Worrall BB, Leys D, Baumgartner R, Caso V, Béjot Y, Compter A, Reiner P, Thijs V, Southerland AM, Bersano A, Brandt T, Gensicke H, Touzé E, Martin JJ, Chabriat H, Tatlisumak T, Lyrer P, Arnold M, Engelter ST, CADISP-Plus Study Group. Cervical artery dissection in patients ≥60 years: often painless, few mechanical triggers. Neurology. 2017;88(14):1313–20. https://doi.org/10.1212/WNL.0000000000003788. Epub 2017 Mar 3
24. Uludüz D, Mastanzade T, Demirci S, Midi İ, Göksan B. Headache characteristics and frequency of migraine in patients with cervical artery dissections. Acta Neurol Belg. 2021;121(5):1173–8. https://doi.org/10.1007/s13760-021-01674-6. Epub 2021 Apr 23
25. Jatuzis D, Valaikiene J. Migraine-like presentation of vertebral artery dissection after cervical manipulative therapy. Pers Med. 2012;1:452–4. https://doi.org/10.1016/j.permed.2012.03.010.
26. Teodoro T, Ferreira J, Franco A, Almeida V, Casimiro C, Coelho M, Ferro JM, Albuquerque L. Vertebral artery dissection mimicking status migrainosus. Am J Emerg Med. 2013;31(12):1721.e3–5. https://doi.org/10.1016/j.ajem.2013.07.025. Epub 2013 Sep 21
27. Hicks PA, Leavitt JA, Mokri B. Ophthalmic manifestations of vertebral artery dissection. Patients seen at the Mayo Clinic from 1976 to 1992. Ophthalmology. 1994;101(11):1786–92.
28. Mayer-Suess L, Frank F, Töll T, Boehme C, Gizewski ER, Ratzinger G, Broessner G, Kiechl S, Knoflach M. Head/neck pain characteristics after spontaneous cervical artery dissection in the acute phase and on a long-run. Cephalalgia. 2022;42(9):872–8. https://doi.org/10.1177/03331024221079298. Epub 2022 Mar 18
29. Wang Y, Cheng W, Lian Y. The headache and neck pain in ischemic stroke patients caused by cervicocerebral artery dissection. A case-control study. J Stroke Cerebrovasc Dis. 2019;28(3):557–61. https://doi.org/10.1016/j.jstrokecerebrovasdis.2018.10.034. Epub 2018 Nov 16
30. Hart RG, Easton JD. Dissections of cervical and cerebral arteries. Neurol Clin. 1983;1(1):155–82.
31. Hosoya T, Adachi M, Yamaguchi K, Haku T, Kayama T, Kato T. Clinical and neuroradiological features of intracranial vertebrobasilar artery dissection. Stroke. 1999;30(5):1083–90. https://doi.org/10.1161/01.str.30.5.1083.
32. Biousse V, Touboul PJ, D'Anglejan-Chatillon J, Lévy C, Schaison M, Bousser MG. Ophthalmologic manifestations of internal carotid artery dissection. Am J Ophthalmol. 1998;126(4):565–77. https://doi.org/10.1016/s0002-9394(98)00136-6.
33. Baumgartner RW, Arnold M, Baumgartner I, Mosso M, Gönner F, Studer A, Schroth G, Schuknecht B, Sturzenegger M. Carotid dissection with and without ischemic events: local symptoms and cerebral artery findings. Neurology. 2001;57(5):827–32. https://doi.org/10.1212/wnl.57.5.827.
34. Bushberg JM. Introduction to medical imaging. In: Bushberg JT, Seibert JA, Leidholdt Jr EM, Boone JM, editors. The essential physics of medical imaging. 2nd ed. Philadelphia: Lippincott Williams & Wilkins; 2002. p. 15.

35. Elijovich L, Kazmi K, Gauvrit JY, Law M. The emerging role of multidetector row CT angiography in the diagnosis of cervical arterial dissection: preliminary study. Neuroradiology. 2006;48(9):606–12. https://doi.org/10.1007/s00234-006-0100-5. Epub 2006 Jun 3
36. Chen CJ, Tseng YC, Lee TH, Hsu HL, See LC. Multisection CT angiography compared with catheter angiography in diagnosing vertebral artery dissection. AJNR Am J Neuroradiol. 2004;25(5):769–74.
37. Vertinsky AT, Schwartz NE, Fischbein NJ, Rosenberg J, Albers GW, Zaharchuk G. Comparison of multidetector CT angiography and MR imaging of cervical artery dissection. AJNR Am J Neuroradiol. 2008;29(9):1753–60. https://doi.org/10.3174/ajnr.A1189. Epub 2008 Jul 17
38. Shakir HJ, Davies JM, Shallwani H, Siddiqui AH, Levy EI. Carotid and vertebral dissection imaging. Curr Pain Headache Rep. 2016;20(12):68. https://doi.org/10.1007/s11916-016-0593-5.
39. Larsson SC, King A, Madigan J, Levi C, Norris JW, Markus HS. Prognosis of carotid dissecting aneurysms: results from CADISS and a systematic review. Neurology. 2017;88(7):646–52. https://doi.org/10.1212/WNL.0000000000003617. Epub 2017 Jan 13
40. Hakimi R, Sivakumar S. Imaging of carotid dissection. Curr Pain Headache Rep. 2019;23(1):2. https://doi.org/10.1007/s11916-019-0741-9.
41. Schievink WI. Spontaneous dissection of the carotid and vertebral arteries. N Engl J Med. 2001;344(12):898–906. https://doi.org/10.1056/NEJM200103223441206.
42. Kirsch E, Kaim A, Engelter S, Lyrer P, Stock KW, Bongartz G, Radü EW. MR angiography in internal carotid artery dissection: improvement of diagnosis by selective demonstration of the intramural haematoma. Neuroradiology. 1998;40(11):704–9. https://doi.org/10.1007/s002340050668.
43. Provenzale JM. Dissection of the internal carotid and vertebral arteries: imaging features. AJR Am J Roentgenol. 1995;165(5):1099–104. https://doi.org/10.2214/ajr.165.5.7572483.
44. Gao PH, Yang L, Wang G, Guo L, Liu X, Zhao B. Symptomatic unruptured isolated middle cerebral artery dissection: clinical and magnetic resonance imaging features. Clin Neuroradiol. 2016;26(1):81–91. https://doi.org/10.1007/s00062-014-0337-z. Epub 2014 Sep 6
45. Bagh I, Olin JW, Froehlich JB, Kline-Rogers E, Gray B, Kim ESH, Sharma A, Weinberg I, Wells BJ, Gu X, Gornik HL. Association of multifocal fibromuscular dysplasia in elderly patients with a more benign clinical phenotype: data from the US registry for fibromuscular dysplasia. JAMA Cardiol. 2018;3(8):756–60. https://doi.org/10.1001/jamacardio.2018.1638.
46. Brott TG, Hobson RW 2nd, Howard G, Roubin GS, Clark WM, Brooks W, Mackey A, Hill MD, Leimgruber PP, Sheffet AJ, Howard VJ, Moore WS, Voeks JH, Hopkins LN, Cutlip DE, Cohen DJ, Popma JJ, Ferguson RD, Cohen SN, Blackshear JL, Silver FL, Mohr JP, Lal BK, Meschia JF, CREST Investigators. Stenting versus endarterectomy for treatment of carotid-artery stenosis. N Engl J Med. 2010;363(1):11–23. https://doi.org/10.1056/NEJMoa0912321. Epub 2010 May 26. Erratum in: N Engl J Med. 2010;363(5):498. Erratum in: N Engl J Med. 2010;363(2):198
47. CADISS trial investigators, Markus HS, Hayter E, Levi C, Feldman A, Venables G, Norris J. Antiplatelet treatment compared with anticoagulation treatment for cervical artery dissection (CADISS): a randomised trial. Lancet Neurol. 2015;14(4):361–7. https://doi.org/10.1016/S1474-4422(15)70018-9. Epub 2015 Feb 12. Erratum in: Lancet Neurol. 2015;14(6):566. 10.1016/S1474-4422(15)00045-9.
48. De Giuli V, Graziano F, Zini A, Zedde M, Patella R, Lodigiani C, Marcheselli S, DeLodovici ML, Paciaroni M, Casetta I, Giorli E, Adami A, Braga M, Casella C, Giossi A, Silvestrelli G, Tancredi L, Lotti EM, Poli L, Caria F, Piras V, Cucurachi L, Gamba M, Grassi M, Padovani A, Pezzini A, Italian Project on Stroke in Young Adults (IPSYS) Investigators. Migraine improvement after spontaneous cervical artery dissection the Italian Project on Stroke in Young Adults

(IPSYS). Neurol Sci. 2019;40(1):59–66. https://doi.org/10.1007/s10072-018-3578-9. Epub 2018 Sep 21
49. Rao AS, Makaroun MS, Marone LK, Cho JS, Rhee R, Chaer RA. Long-term outcomes of internal carotid artery dissection. J Vasc Surg. 2011;54(2):370–4; discussion 375. doi: https://doi.org/10.1016/j.jvs.2011.02.059. Epub 2011 May 28.
50. Kuhn J, Mueller W, Harzheim A, Bewermeyer H. Anhaltender, therapierefraktärer Kopfschmerz nach beidseitiger Dissektion der A. carotis interna [Long-lasting, refractory headache after bilateral dissection of the internal carotid artery]. Schmerz. 2006;20(6):527–30. German. https://doi.org/10.1007/s00482-005-0463-2.
51. Metso TM, Metso AJ, Helenius J, Haapaniemi E, Salonen O, Porras M, Hernesniemi J, Kaste M, Tatlisumak T. Prognosis and safety of anticoagulation in intracranial artery dissections in adults. Stroke. 2007;38(6):1837–42. https://doi.org/10.1161/STROKEAHA.106.479501. Epub 2007 May 10

Chapter 23
Post-endarterectomy Headache

Paulo Sergio Faro Santos

23.1 Introduction

Endarterectomy is the treatment of choice for the prevention of stroke in patients with symptomatic carotid stenosis [1]. Although this procedure is generally safe and effective, postoperative headache is a recognized but often underestimated complication [1–4]. The objective of this chapter is to present and analyze in depth a clinical case of post-endarterectomy headache with its characteristics and management.

23.2 Pathophysiology

The pathophysiology of post-endarterectomy headache is not yet fully understood, but some hypotheses may help in understanding the mechanism of this headache, namely:

- *Oculosympathetic autonomic dysfunction*: In a case series of post-endarterectomy headache, a group of patients who developed cluster headache phenotype had significantly decreased oculosympathetic activity compared with the control group without headache. The authors suggest that damage to the sympathetic plexus resulting from the surgical procedure may be involved in the development of postoperative headache.
- *Cerebral hemodynamic abnormalities*: Björne et al. described the case of a patient with chronic cluster headache who had been in remission for over 20 years and who, the day after carotid endarterectomy, returned to experience attacks identical to his previous headache. It is known that pharmacologically

P. S. Faro Santos (✉)
Faro Institute, Curitiba, PR, Brazil

D. Uludüz et al. (eds.), *Rare Causes of Headache Disorders*, Headache,
https://doi.org/10.1007/978-3-032-10242-3_23

induced vasodilation can trigger an attack in a susceptible individual during a period of cluster headache. This knowledge led them to suspect that the state of cerebral hyperperfusion caused by the restoration of blood flow after the surgical procedure had reactivated the headache in this patient [5, 6]. In addition, cerebral hyperperfusion syndrome, a rare complication characterized by headache, focal neurological deficits and seizures in the absence of cerebral ischemia, is well described and is also believed to be related to failure of cerebral blood autoregulation [7].

- *Activation of the Trigeminovascular System*: Surgical manipulation of vascular and nervous structures during the procedure can activate the trigeminovascular system and cause the release of several chemical mediators, including calcitonin gene related peptide (CGRP) and substance P, leading to vasodilation and sensitization of pain pathways, contributing to the manifestation of headache [5, 8].

23.3 Case Presentation

A 64-year-old man was diagnosed with a transient ischemic attack due to recurrent episodes of left hemiparesis lasting up to 30 min. The patient had a past medical history of hypercholesterolemia and a sedentary lifestyle. He denied any history of recurrent headaches. Neurological examination revealed no focal deficits. Brain magnetic resonance imaging (MRI) showed no signs of acute ischemia, but only white matter hyperintensities on fluid-attenuated inversion recovery (FLAIR) (Fazekas 2), with no other significant changes. Cervical arterial computed tomography (CT) angiography revealed substantial carotid stenosis (>70%) of the right internal carotid artery, for which he underwent carotid endarterectomy.

From the fifth postoperative day onwards, he developed a moderate-intensity right-sided fronto-orbitotemporal headache, which occurred in attacks lasting between 20 and 40 min, once a day, and was associated with conjunctival hyperemia, lacrimation, and rhinorrhea ipsilateral to the pain. His blood pressure was within normal limits.

Due to the pattern of symptoms, the patient was treated acutely with oxygen, obtaining a good therapeutic response. A new cervical arterial magnetic resonance imaging and angioresonance were performed, but they did not show ischemic or hemorrhagic lesions, nor arterial stenosis or dissection. As the headache attacks continued daily for more than 1 week, verapamil was started, and the headache regressed approximately 40 days later.

23.4 Case Discussion

This case illustrates a typical situation of post-endarterectomy headache. Symptoms appeared within the first week after the procedure, and their characteristics were cluster headache-like, according to the 3rd edition of the International Classification of Headache Disorders (ICHD-3) [9]. Complementary tests were performed to rule out complications such as cerebral hemorrhage or ischemia, arterial stenosis, or dissection; all of which were normal. According to the phenotype, treatment was successful with oxygen and verapamil.

23.5 Headache Characteristics of Post-endarterectomy

The ICHD-3 describes three post-endarterectomy headache phenotypes: tension-like, cluster-like, and severe headache [9].

The first type was described in detail by Tehindrazanarivelo et al., and, in this sample, approximately 60% of patients developed a headache after surgery. Most individuals presented a headache that appeared in the first 5 days after surgery (mainly in the first 2 days), which could be a continuous episode or several episodes per day, lasting from a few minutes to several hours (5 min to 12 h), and its average duration was 3 days. Other characteristics of the headache are mainly bilateral location (72%), frontal (55%), of mild to moderate intensity (78%), pressure or heaviness (77%), without associated symptoms and without requiring treatment (77%) [4].

Some authors [3, 6, 10] have reported cases of cluster-like headache after endarterectomy. Still, it was De Marinis et al. [5] who showed the particularities of the second type of headache, which occurred in 30% of individuals. The headache began, on average, 48 h after the procedure, with each attack lasting 2–3 h, and occurring once or twice a day, during all the days it was active, which was generally about 2 weeks. Only two cases that lasted 3–4 months were described. The pain had a continuous-pulsating or pulsating characteristic of moderate-to-severe intensity, in the frontal, retroocular, periocular, and temporoparietal regions, always ipsilateral to the surgery. It may or may not be associated with local autonomic manifestations (conjunctival hyperemia, lacrimation, nasal congestion, and rhinorrhea—25%) and Horner's syndrome (25%) [5].

The third form of headache presentation is part of cerebral hyperperfusion syndrome, which is a well-known complication that affects 1–3% of patients after endarterectomy. It's a condition characterized by numerous symptoms and findings that include headache, seizures, hypertension, focal neurological deficits, and intracerebral hemorrhage [7, 11]. Headache is usually one of the first symptoms of the syndrome and begins 3 days after surgery, abruptly or not, it can be unilateral (ipsilateral to the procedure) or bilateral, pulsatile, of severe intensity, associated or not with nausea, occurring in episodes over weeks to months [12–14].

23.6 Diagnostic Algorithm

Step 1: Clinical Suspicion

- *Identify Key Symptoms*:
  - Headache initiating after carotid endarterectomy

Step 2: Clinical and Neurological Examination

- *Identify complications signs*:
  - Arterial hypertension
  - Focal neurological deficits

Step 3: Diagnostic Workup

- *Brain Computed Tomography Scan*:
  - Assess for intracranial hemorrhage
- *Brain Magnetic Resonance Imaging*:
  - Look for signs of ischemic infarct
- *Carotid artery duplex*:
  - Assess for restenosis or dissection.
- *Transcranial Doppler*:
  - Assess cerebral hemodynamic disturbances

Step 4: Apply ICHD-3 Diagnostic Criteria

A. Any new headache fulfilling criterion C
B. Carotid endarterectomy has been performed
C. Evidence of causation demonstrated by at least two of the following:
   1. A headache develops within 1 week of the carotid endarterectomy
   2. The headache resolves within 1 month after the carotid endarterectomy
   3. Both of the following:
      (a) The headache is unilateral, on the side of the carotid endarterectomy
      (b) A headache has one of the following three distinct characteristics:
         - Diffuse mild pain
         - Cluster headache-like pain occurring once or twice a day in attacks lasting 2–3 h
         - Pulsating severe pain

D. Not better accounted for by another ICHD-3 diagnosis.

23.7 Management

Headache management should be based on its subtype, as each type probably has a different underlying pathophysiological mechanism. Another way to establish treatment is according to the headache phenotype.

A headache that begins early and has tension-like characteristics can be treated with analgesics and anti-inflammatories alone, since it is usually mild and self-limiting. For the control of cluster-like headache, some authors have described a good therapeutic response to conventional drugs (oxygen, verapamil, and lithium) for the management of primary cluster headache [6, 10]. In addition, there is a report of a good therapeutic response to sumatriptan in a patient with cluster headache secondary to carotid artery dissection [15].

Meanwhile, treatment of the third headache subtype is mainly preventive, since cerebral hyperperfusion syndrome, the underlying cause of this headache, is a potentially serious complication [7]. Lee et al. [11] observed that patients who developed post-endarterectomy headache had greater intraoperative variability in blood pressure and suggested strict control of intraoperative blood pressure parameters and limiting their variability to decrease the incidence of not only headache but also cerebral hyperperfusion syndrome. Furthermore, Dolan and Mushlin [12] described a case in which there was a dramatic improvement in post-endarterectomy headache and arterial hypertension after the use of prazosin, which inhibits postsynaptic $\alpha 1$-adrenoceptors.

23.8 Conclusion

Headache secondary to carotid endarterectomy is common but underestimated. It is essential to recognize its existence and understand its presentation so that proper investigation and treatment can be carried out, since it varies according to its phenotype. Furthermore, it can precede serious complications, in the case of cerebral hyperperfusion syndrome, and its recognition can help in the management of this condition.

References

1. Abbott AL. Extra-cranial carotid artery stenosis: an objective analysis of the available evidence. Front Neurol. 2022;13:739999. https://doi.org/10.3389/fneur.2022.739999.
2. Leung YYR, Bera K, Urriza Rodriguez D, Dardik A, Mas JL, Simonte G, Rerkasem K, Howard DPJ. Safety of carotid endarterectomy for symptomatic stenosis by age: meta-analysis with individual patient data. Stroke. 2023;54(2):457–67. https://doi.org/10.1161/StrokeAHA.122.040819.

3. Messert B, Black JA. Cluster headache, hemicrania, and other head pains: morbidity of carotid endarterectomy. Stroke. 1978;9(6):559–62. https://doi.org/10.1161/01.str.9.6.559.
4. Tehindrazanarivelo AD, Lutz G, PetitJean C, Bousser MG. Headache following carotid endarterectomy: a prospective study. Cephalalgia. 1992;12(6):380–2. https://doi.org/10.1111/j.1468-2982.1992.00380.x.
5. De Marinis M, Zaccaria A, Faraglia V, Fiorani P, Maira G, Agnoli A. Post-endarterectomy headache and the role of the oculosympathetic system. J Neurol Neurosurg Psychiatry. 1991;54(4):314–7. https://doi.org/10.1136/jnnp.54.4.314.
6. Björne A, Hindfelt B, Havelius U. Recurrence of cluster headache after carotid thrombendarterectomy. Headache. 1994;34(4):230–3. https://doi.org/10.1111/j.1526-4610.1994.hed3404230.x.
7. Lin Y-H, Liu H-M. Update on cerebral hyperperfusion syndrome. J NeuroIntervent Surg. 2020;12:788–93. https://doi.org/10.1136/neurintsurg-2019-015621.
8. Ashina M, Hansen JM, Do TP, Melo-Carrillo A, Burstein R, Moskowitz MA. Migraine and the trigeminovascular system-40 years and counting. Lancet Neurol. 2019;18(8):795–804. https://doi.org/10.1016/S1474-4422(19)30185-1.
9. Headache Classification Committee of the International Headache Society (IHS). The International Classification of Headache Disorders, 3rd edition. Cephalalgia. 2018;38(1):1–211. https://doi.org/10.1177/0333102417738202.
10. Dirkx THT, Koehler PJ. Post-operative cluster headache following carotid endarterectomy. Eur Neurol. 2017;77(3–4):175–9. https://doi.org/10.1159/000456004.
11. Lee D, Batista PM, McMackin KK, Ha A, Trani J, Carpenter JP, Lombardi JV. Intraoperative blood pressure lability carries a higher risk of headache after carotid endarterectomy. J Vasc Surg. 2022;75(2):592–598.e1. https://doi.org/10.1016/j.jvs.2021.08.070.
12. Dolan JG, Mushlin AI. Hypertension, vascular headaches, and seizures after carotid endarterectomy. Case report and therapeutic considerations. Arch Intern Med. 1984;144(7):1489–91.
13. Pearce J. Headache after carotid endarterectomy. Br Med J. 1976;2:85–6. PMID: 1276821. PMCID: PMC1687795. https://doi.org/10.1136/bmj.2.6027.85.
14. Leviton A, Caplan L, Salzman E. Severe headache after carotid endarterectomy. Headache. 1975;15(3):207–10. https://doi.org/10.1111/j.1526-4610.1975.hed1503207.x.
15. Leira EC, Cruz-Flores S, Leacock RO, Abdulrauf SI. Sumatriptan can alleviate headaches due to carotid artery dissection. Headache. 2001;41(6):590–1. https://doi.org/10.1046/j.1526-4610.2001.041006590.x.

Chapter 24
Headache Attributed to Cerebral Venous Thrombosis (CVT)

Derya Uluduz and Aynur Özge

24.1 Introduction

Cerebral venous thrombosis (CVT) is a complex and potentially life-threatening condition characterized by the formation of a blood clot in the dural venous sinuses or cerebral veins, leading to increased intracranial pressure (ICP) and potential venous infarction [1–3]. This results in significant morbidity and mortality if not promptly diagnosed and treated. CVT can affect both the superficial and deep venous systems of the brain, leading to a variety of clinical manifestations, including venous infarction and cerebral edema. CVT is relatively rare compared to arterial strokes, with an estimated annual incidence of about 3–4 per million people. However, it can be more common in specific populations such as young women and those with prothrombotic conditions.

Headache is a primary symptom of CVT, occurring in up to 90% of cases, and can sometimes present as the sole symptom, complicating its diagnosis [1–4]. The headache associated with CVT can be diverse, ranging from subacute onset to thunderclap headache patterns, often with diffuse or bilateral characteristics [5, 6]. This variability, combined with the absence of specific diagnostic markers, makes early detection crucial yet challenging. The lack of a typical headache pattern and the potential for isolated headache presentation without other neurological signs further complicate the diagnosis, leading to delays in treatment initiation [4, 5]. The epidemiology of CVT-related headaches underscores their diagnostic challenge, with headache being the sole presentation in approximately 15% of patients [4, 7].

D. Uluduz (✉)
Medical Faculty, Neurology Department, Istanbul University Cerrahpasa, Samatya, Türkiye

A. Özge
Mersin State Hospital, Mersin, Turkey

D. Uludüz et al. (eds.), *Rare Causes of Headache Disorders*, Headache,
https://doi.org/10.1007/978-3-032-10242-3_24

Understanding the relationship between CVT and headache is essential for improving diagnostic accuracy and patient outcomes.

24.2 Case Presentation

A 24-year-old primigravida female presented to the emergency department with a generalized tonic–clonic seizure 2 weeks postpartum following an uneventful vaginal delivery. The seizure lasted approximately 3 min, and she remained unconscious for 20 min afterwards. In the preceding 3 days, she had been experiencing an excruciating headache that began insidiously but progressively worsened. The pain was predominantly occipital, radiating down to her neck and extending towards the vertex. She described it as a relentless, throbbing sensation, akin to an intense pressure building inside her skull. The headache was resistant to simple analgesics and was exacerbated by movement, particularly when she changed positions or attempted to stand. She also reported a sense of heaviness in her head, making it difficult for her to concentrate or engage in routine activities. Throughout this period, she developed associated symptoms of nausea and vomiting, which became more pronounced as the headache intensified. Bright lights and loud noises aggravated her discomfort, forcing her to retreat into a dark and quiet room. Despite her worsening symptoms, she attributed them to postpartum fatigue and dehydration, delaying medical attention until the convulsive episode occurred.

Upon arrival, the patient appeared drowsy, with fluctuating consciousness. Her vital signs were stable, with a temperature of 36.6 °C, a heart rate of 70 bpm, blood pressure of 110/60 mmHg, a respiratory rate of 22 breaths per minute, and an oxygen saturation of 99% on room air. A general physical examination revealed no abnormalities. Neurological evaluation and fundoscopic examination were unremarkable. Her medical and family history, including thromboembolic conditions, were unremarkable, and she had no history of drug use or hormonal therapy. Given her young age and lack of significant past medical history, neuroimaging was performed to rule out vascular pathologies.

A non-contrast computed tomography (CT) scan revealed hyperdensity in the superior sagittal sinus, suggestive of a dense clot sign, with no evidence of parenchymal hemorrhage (Picture 24.1). Magnetic resonance imaging (MRI) with T2-FLAIR (fluid-attenuated inversion recovery) sequences demonstrated hyperintense signals in the cortical and deep venous structures, indicative of venous congestion, without signs of infarction or hemorrhagic transformation (Picture 24.2). MR venography (MRV) confirmed the absence of flow voids in the superior sagittal sinus and transverse sinus, indicative of venous occlusion, without any arteriovenous malformation or aneurysmal dilation (Picture 24.3). Laboratory investigations, including a complete blood count, biochemical screening, coagulation profile, inflammatory markers, and a thrombophilia panel, yielded normal results. Specific tests for autoimmune and inherited thrombophilic conditions, such as

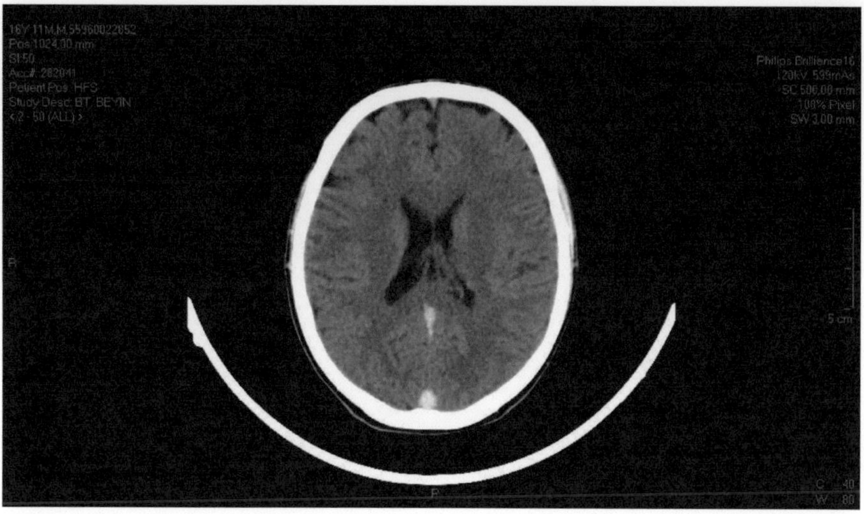

Picture 24.1 Cranial CT demonstrates hyperdensity within the superior sagittal sinus, consistent with the dense sinus sign

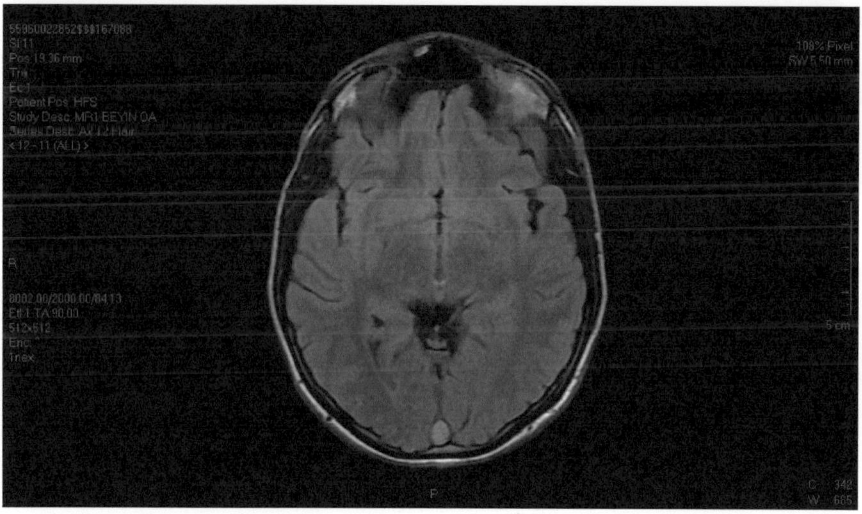

Picture 24.2 Axial T2-FLAIR images; hyperintensity along the internal cerebral veins and vein of Galen, consistent with impaired venous drainage

antiphospholipid antibodies, Factor V Leiden mutation, protein C/S deficiency, and lupus anticoagulant, were negative.

The diagnosis of postpartum cerebral venous sinus thrombosis (CVT) was established, and anticoagulation therapy with heparin was initiated, later transitioning to therapeutic oral warfarin. On the fourth day of hospitalization, she experienced

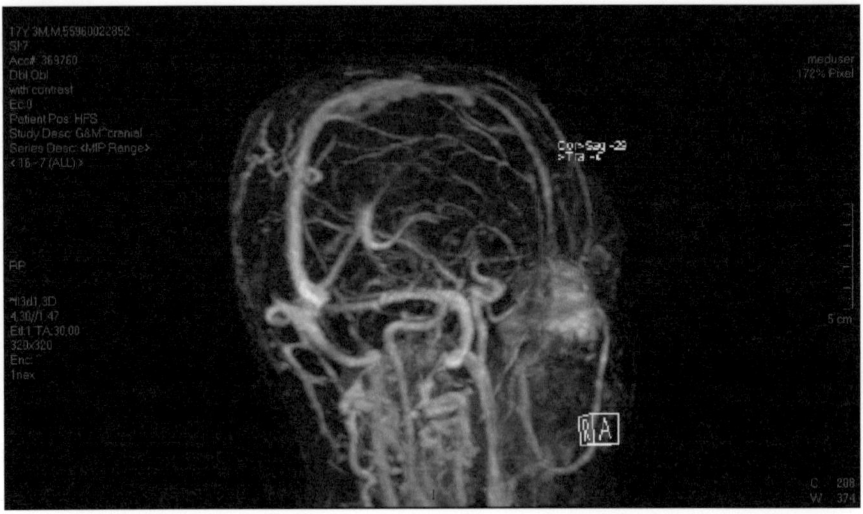

Picture 24.3 MR venography; reduced or absent flow in the right transverse and sigmoid sinuses, and interrupted flow in the superior sagittal sinus

another generalized tonic–clonic seizure lasting 2 min, prompting the initiation of levetiracetam at a dose of 1000 mg per day. She was discharged with full neurological recovery and was advised to continue oral anticoagulation therapy.

24.3 Case Discussion

Cerebral venous sinus thrombosis is a rare but serious postpartum complication, often presenting with seizures, headaches, and focal neurological deficits. Pregnancy and the puerperium increase the risk due to hypercoagulability and endothelial changes. The diagnosis relies on a high degree of clinical suspicion and confirmatory imaging, with MR venography being the gold standard for detecting venous occlusions. In this case, the patient presented with postpartum headache, seizure, and focal neurological deficits, necessitating urgent neuroimaging. The CT scan revealed a dense clot sign, while MRI and MR venography confirmed sinus thrombosis. The absence of identifiable thrombophilic risk factors suggested that puerperium was the primary contributing factor.

Early anticoagulation is the cornerstone of treatment, preventing thrombus propagation and promoting recanalization. Seizures are common in CVT patients, requiring antiepileptic therapy in cases of recurrent episodes. The patient's favorable outcome highlights the importance of early recognition and timely intervention. This case underscores the need for heightened awareness of CVT in postpartum patients presenting with new-onset headaches, seizures, or neurological deficits.

Prompt diagnosis and appropriate management are crucial in preventing complications and ensuring a good prognosis.

24.4 Pathophysiology

The primary mechanisms underlying cerebral venous thrombosis (CVT)-related headaches involve venous outflow obstruction, increased intracranial pressure (ICP), cortical vein infarction, cerebral edema, and venous hemorrhage. Each of these mechanisms contributes to the complex headache profile associated with CVT, making diagnosis and management challenging (Fig. 24.1).

Venous Outflow Obstruction and Increased Intracranial Pressure (ICP) When a venous sinus or cerebral vein becomes occluded, normal venous drainage is disrupted, leading to venous congestion. This congestion results in a secondary increase in ICP due to impaired cerebrospinal fluid (CSF) absorption at the arachnoid granulations. The pressure buildup within the cranial vault can exert direct mechanical stress on pain-sensitive structures, including the dura mater and meningeal vessels, which are richly innervated by nociceptive fibers originating from the trigeminovascular system. The elevated ICP manifests clinically as a headache that is often

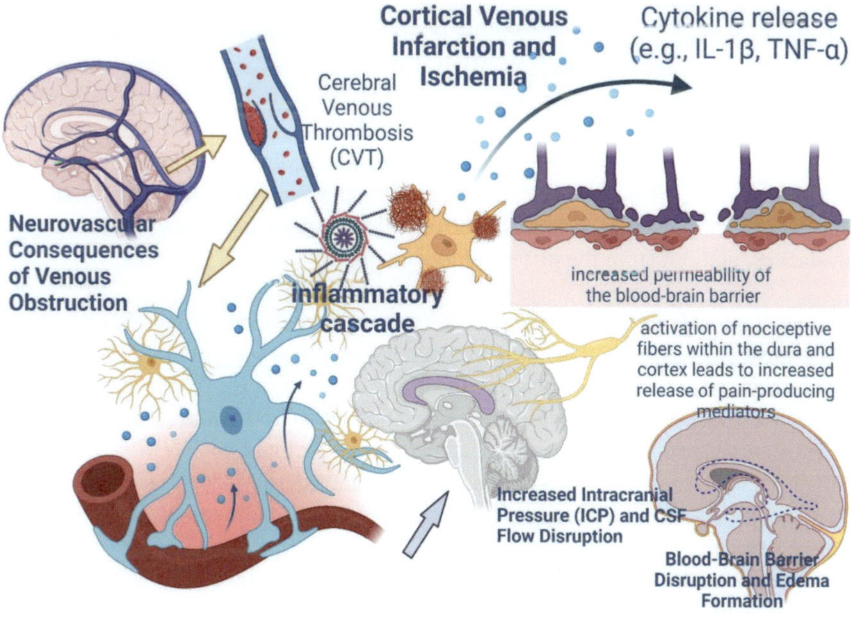

Fig. 24.1 Venous obstruction triggers inflammation, blood–brain barrier disruption, increased intracranial pressure, and nociceptive activation, ultimately leading to cortical infarction, edema, and headache

described as severe, progressive, and diffuse. It is frequently exacerbated by Valsalva maneuvers, such as coughing, straining, or positional changes, due to transient increases in venous pressure that further compromise cerebral venous drainage [8–10]. Additionally, elevated ICP can lead to papilledema, which may contribute to visual disturbances and worsen the headache through secondary optic nerve involvement [11].

Cortical Vein Infarction and Neuroinflammation In addition to venous congestion, CVT can lead to cortical vein infarction, a consequence of sustained venous hypertension and hypoxia [4, 8]. The resultant ischemic injury triggers an inflammatory cascade involving microglial activation, cytokine release (e.g., interleukin-1β (IL-1β), tumor necrosis factor alpha [TNF-α]), and increased permeability of the blood–brain barrier (BBB) [12].

This inflammatory response plays a pivotal role in sensitizing pain pathways. The activation of nociceptive fibers within the dura and cortex leads to increased release of pain-producing mediators such as substance P, calcitonin gene-related peptide (CGRP), and bradykinin [13]. These molecules amplify pain transmission by lowering the activation threshold of trigeminovascular afferents, making the headache more persistent and refractory to conventional analgesics [14].

Cerebral Edema and Its Contribution to Headache Pathophysiology Cerebral edema is another significant contributor to CVT-related headaches and can be classified into cytotoxic and vasogenic edema. Cytotoxic edema results from cellular energy failure due to ischemia, leading to intracellular water accumulation. In contrast, vasogenic edema arises from BBB disruption, allowing plasma proteins and fluids to enter the extracellular space [8, 9, 15]. Both forms of edema exacerbate ICP elevation and contribute to worsening headache symptoms. The expansion of brain tissue within the fixed cranial vault intensifies meningeal and vascular stretch, further activating pain-sensitive structures. This can lead to diffuse, non-localized headaches that mimic primary headache disorders such as migraines or tension-type headaches, complicating the differential diagnosis.

Venous Hemorrhage and Meningeal Irritation Venous hemorrhage is a potential consequence of severe venous hypertension leading to vessel rupture. The extravasation of blood into cerebral tissue can irritate the meninges, further exacerbating headache severity. Hemorrhagic transformation of venous infarcts adds another layer of complexity by increasing localized mass effect and potentiating secondary inflammatory responses [15]. The presence of hemosiderin–laden macrophages and blood degradation products can induce oxidative stress, leading to prolonged activation of nociceptive pathways. This results in a persistent, throbbing headache that may resemble a thunderclap headache or other secondary headache disorders such as subarachnoid hemorrhage.

24.5 Pain Pathways Involved in CVT-Related Headaches

The pain mechanisms underlying CVT-related headaches are multifaceted, involving both peripheral and central sensitization. The activation of the trigeminovascular system, combined with secondary inflammatory and vascular changes, leads to increased excitability of central pain-processing networks in the brainstem and thalamus. This central sensitization contributes to headache chronicity and may explain why some CVT patients develop prolonged post-thrombotic headaches even after recanalization [16].

Given the complex interplay of venous congestion, neuroinflammation, cerebral edema, and hemorrhagic transformation, CVT-related headaches require a tailored treatment approach [17]. Management strategies should focus on anticoagulation to prevent thrombosis progression, symptomatic relief with analgesics, and measures to reduce ICP, such as acetazolamide or therapeutic lumbar punctures (LPs) in select cases. Early recognition and intervention are crucial to mitigate long-term neurological complications and improve patient outcomes.

24.6 Clinical Characteristics

Cerebral venous thrombosis (CVT) is a complex condition that often presents with headache as a primary symptom, occurring in up to 90% of cases [1]. The headache associated with CVT can exhibit diverse characteristics, making its diagnosis challenging [18]. CVT-related headaches typically have a subacute or progressive onset, though some cases may present with a thunderclap headache pattern, which is sudden and severe, reaching its peak within minutes [1, 19, 20]. Thunderclap headaches in CVT can be particularly concerning, as they may mimic subarachnoid hemorrhage [7, 21]. The headache can be diffuse or localized, sometimes described as throbbing or band-like [19, 22]. Diffuse headaches are common, affecting the whole head, while localized headaches may involve specific regions such as the frontal, temporal, or occipital areas [21]. CVT-related headaches are often accompanied by nausea, photophobia, and focal neurological signs such as seizures, motor weakness, or visual disturbances [1]. These symptoms can vary widely among patients and may not always be present.

Comparison with Other Secondary Headaches CVT-related headaches can be confused with other secondary headache disorders due to overlapping symptoms. For example, idiopathic intracranial hypertension (IIH) also presents with headache and increased intracranial pressure, but typically includes visual disturbances like papilledema [6]. Meningitis may also cause headache, but is usually accompanied by fever and neck stiffness [23]. Stroke can present with a sudden-onset headache, but is typically associated with focal neurological deficits [23].

Red flags for CVT include the sudden onset of severe headache, seizures, or focal neurological deficits such as weakness or visual disturbances [1, 2, 24]. These symptoms necessitate prompt imaging and diagnosis to prevent complications and improve outcomes.

24.7 Diagnosis of CVT-Related Headache

Diagnosing cerebral venous thrombosis (CVT)-related headaches involves a combination of clinical suspicion and differential diagnosis, as the symptoms can mimic other conditions such as idiopathic intracranial hypertension or subarachnoid hemorrhage [25, 26]. The headache associated with CVT often presents with nonspecific features, making it crucial to consider CVT in the differential diagnosis of patients with headache, especially when accompanied by signs of increased intracranial pressure or focal neurological deficits [25].

Clinical Presentation and Pathophysiology The headache associated with CVT is highly variable and can range from a diffuse, pressure-like pain to a thunderclap headache suggestive of subarachnoid hemorrhage. The underlying mechanism is related to impaired venous drainage, leading to increased intracranial pressure (ICP), cerebral congestion, and potential venous infarction [26]. The increased ICP results from obstructed cerebrospinal fluid (CSF) absorption at the arachnoid granulations due to venous hypertension, contributing to persistent headaches, often exacerbated by Valsalva maneuvers, coughing or postural changes.

Focal neurological deficits such as hemiparesis, aphasia, or seizures may arise from localized venous infarcts due to thrombosis-induced ischemia. The presence of papilledema on fundoscopic examination can further support the diagnosis of raised ICP secondary to CVT. In some cases, patients may also present with altered mental status or encephalopathy, particularly if there is significant cerebral edema or hemorrhagic transformation [25].

Neuroimaging Approaches Neuroimaging plays a pivotal role in the diagnosis of CVT. The gold standard imaging modality is magnetic resonance imaging (MRI) combined with magnetic resonance venography (MRV), which provides high sensitivity and specificity in detecting thrombosed cerebral veins or dural sinuses [1]. MRI sequences such as susceptibility-weighted imaging (SWI) and T2* gradient echo can help visualize the thrombus by detecting deoxygenated blood products. In contrast, contrast-enhanced MRV can delineate the extent of venous obstruction. Computed tomography (CT) and CT venography (CTV) can serve as alternatives, particularly in emergency settings where MRI may not be immediately available. A hyperdense appearance of the thrombosed sinus on non-contrast CT (commonly observed in the superior sagittal sinus) or the "empty delta sign" on contrast-enhanced CT suggests CVT [26]. However, CT imaging alone may miss early or partial thrombosis, necessitating further confirmation with MRV. In ambiguous cases, digital subtraction angiography (DSA) may be considered as a confirmatory tool to visualize venous outflow patterns and detect subtle occlusions not delineated by MRV or CTV [27].

Lumbar Puncture and CSF Analysis in CVT While lumbar puncture (LP) is not a primary diagnostic tool for CVT, it can provide supportive evidence by revealing elevated opening pressure, which indicates increased ICP [25]. Elevated protein levels and mild pleocytosis in the CSF may suggest secondary inflammatory or ischemic processes. However, normal CSF findings do not exclude CVT, and LP should be performed cautiously in the presence of significant intracranial hypertension to prevent brain herniation.

Biomarkers and Laboratory Tests for Prothrombotic States Since CVT often occurs in the setting of an underlying hypercoagulable state, laboratory investigations are essential to identify potential risk factors. Prothrombotic screening should include testing for inherited and acquired thrombophilic disorders such as: Factor V Leiden mutation (leading to activated protein C resistance), prothrombin gene mutation (G20210A), antithrombin III, protein C, and protein S deficiencies (impairing anticoagulant pathways), antiphospholipid syndrome (testing for lupus anticoagulant, anticardiolipin, and β2-glycoprotein-I antibodies), elevated homocysteine levels, which can predispose to endothelial dysfunction and thrombosis [26]. Additional inflammatory markers, such as D-dimer, can assist in early screening, as elevated levels indicate ongoing fibrinolysis in the presence of a thrombus. However, D-dimer levels may be normal in isolated cortical vein thrombosis or subacute CVT, necessitating further imaging confirmation [26].

24.8 Treatment Approaches

The cornerstone of CVT treatment is anticoagulation therapy, which aims to prevent clot propagation, facilitate recanalization, and reduce venous congestion. Unfractionated heparin (UFH) is used in the acute phase, particularly in critically ill patients, as it offers the advantage of rapid reversal in cases of hemorrhagic complications. UFH is administered intravenously and requires dose adjustments based on activated partial thromboplastin time (aPTT) values [27, 28]. Low-molecular weight heparin (LMWH) is preferred over UFH due to its more predictable pharmacokinetics, lower risk of heparin-induced thrombocytopenia, and reduced need for monitoring. LMWH has been shown to have better efficacy and safety compared to UFH in CVT treatment [9]. Warfarin is initiated after the acute phase, usually as a bridging therapy following heparin, targeting an international normalized ratio (INR) of 2–3. Warfarin has traditionally been used for long-term anticoagulation in CVT [9]. Direct oral anticoagulants (DOACs) are increasingly considered as alternatives to warfarin due to their ease of use, fixed dosing, and lower bleeding risk. Recent studies suggest comparable efficacy of DOACs in CVT treatment, but more extensive trials are needed for definitive guidelines [29]. Notably, anticoagulation is recommended even in the presence of intracranial hemorrhage, as CVT-induced bleeding often results from venous congestion rather than primary vessel rupture. The rationale for continued anticoagulation is to reduce venous hypertension, thereby preventing further hemorrhage and facilitating clot resolution.

In cases where anticoagulation therapy fails or neurological deterioration progresses despite optimal medical management, endovascular treatment may be considered. These interventions include mechanical thrombectomy, like catheter-based techniques that physically remove thrombi from the occluded venous sinuses, restoring venous drainage and reducing ICP [30]. Catheter-directed thrombolysis involves direct administration of thrombolytic agents (e.g., recombinant tissue plasminogen activator, rtPA) into the thrombus to accelerate clot dissolution [31]. Angioplasty with stenting is rarely performed, but is considered in cases with persistent venous sinus stenosis contributing to ongoing venous hypertension [26, 32, 33]. Endovascular interventions remain reserved for severe cases where conventional anticoagulation fails, particularly in the setting of extensive cerebral edema or coma. In severe cases with significant neurological deterioration, endovascular interventions such as mechanical thrombectomy or thrombolysis may be considered to restore venous outflow and alleviate intracranial hypertension [26, 32].

Management of Increased Intracranial Pressure (ICP) Elevated ICP is a major contributor to CVT-related headaches and may lead to secondary neurological deterioration if not effectively controlled. Acetazolamide, a carbonic anhydrase inhibitor, reduces cerebrospinal fluid (CSF) production, thereby lowering ICP. It is commonly used in patients with signs of intracranial hypertension, such as papilledema. Acetazolamide has been shown to have an acceptable safety profile at dosages up to 4 g/d in treating idiopathic intracranial hypertension, though it is associated with side effects like paresthesia and dysgeusia [34, 35]. Agents such as mannitol and hypertonic saline can be administered to reduce cerebral edema in acute settings. Both agents are effective in reducing ICP, but hypertonic saline may offer a greater and longer-lasting effect compared to mannitol. Corticosteroids are not routinely recommended unless there is an associated inflammatory component, such as vasculitis or autoimmune thrombosis. Corticosteroids have shown minimal benefit in reducing ICP in conditions like traumatic brain injury and ischemic stroke. Still, they may be beneficial in bacterial meningitis by reducing complications like sensorineural hearing loss [36]. In cases of refractory increased ICP with impending brain herniation, decompressive craniectomy or ventriculostomy may be required to relieve pressure and prevent fatal outcomes. Decompressive craniectomy has been shown to improve survival and functional outcomes in patients with malignant cerebral infarctions by effectively controlling ICP [37].

Analgesics and anti-inflammatory drugs are used for the symptomatic relief of headaches. However, prolonged use of nonsteroidal anti-inflammatory drugs (NSAIDs) should be avoided due to bleeding risks when combined with anticoagulation [10–13]. The use of corticosteroids is controversial and generally not recommended unless there are specific indications, such as significant inflammation. In some cases, CVT-related headaches may mimic migraines, and similar treatment strategies may be employed.

Some patients may experience persistent or recurrent headaches post-CVT, which can evolve into chronic daily headache or post-thrombotic headache syndromes [13]. The risk of developing chronic headache conditions is a concern, necessitating long-term follow-up and management [13]. CVT can lead to cognitive impairments and neuropsychological issues, which require rehabilitation efforts to improve quality of life [8]. Patients should be advised on lifestyle modifications to prevent future episodes, including management of prothrombotic conditions and avoiding triggers for headache exacerbation.

24.9 Future Directions and Research Gaps

Despite significant advances in the understanding and management of cerebral venous sinus thrombosis (CVT) and its associated headaches, several gaps remain that warrant further research and clinical innovation. The identification of reliable biomarkers could facilitate earlier diagnosis of CVT, reducing delays in treatment initiation. Research into inflammatory markers, coagulation profiles, and endothelial dysfunction could provide valuable insights into CVT pathophysiology and aid in risk stratification. CVT-related headaches exhibit substantial heterogeneity, ranging from migraine-like to tension-type or thunderclap headaches. Tailoring treatment strategies based on individual headache phenotypes could enhance symptom control and improve patient quality of life. While acute treatment is well-established, there is a need for structured long-term follow-up protocols to monitor recurrence risk, persistent headaches, and cognitive or psychological sequelae in CVT survivors. Future studies should explore optimal surveillance intervals and preventive strategies.

24.10 Conclusion

Cerebral venous sinus thrombosis remains a complex and potentially life-threatening condition, often presenting with persistent and debilitating headaches. Early recognition and accurate diagnosis are crucial to initiating timely anticoagulation therapy and managing intracranial hypertension effectively.

This review highlights the importance of neuroimaging as the cornerstone of CVT diagnosis, the role of anticoagulation in preventing disease progression, and the need for personalized approaches in headache management. The long-term burden of CVT-related headaches underscores the necessity for continued research into biomarkers, neuroimaging techniques, and individualized treatment protocols. Given the multifaceted nature of CVT, an interdisciplinary approach involving neurologists, hematologists, radiologists, and other specialists is essential to optimize patient outcomes. Future studies should focus on refining diagnostic tools, improving therapeutic strategies, and developing comprehensive long-term care models to enhance the quality of life for CVT survivors.

References

1. Duman T, Uluduz D, Midi I, Bektas H, Kablan Y, Goksel BK, Milanlioglu A, Necioglu Orken D, Aluclu U, VENOST Study Group. A multicenter study of 1144 patients with cerebral venous thrombosis: the VENOST study. J Stroke Cerebrovasc Dis. 2017;26(8):1848–57. https://doi.org/10.1016/j.jstrokecerebrovasdis.2017.04.020.
2. García-Azorín D, Monje MHG, González-García N, Guerrero ÁL, Porta-Etessam J. Presence of red flags in patients with cerebral venous sinus thrombosis admitted to the emergency department because of headache: a STROBE compliant cohort-study. Medicine (Baltimore). 2020;99(29):e20900. https://doi.org/10.1097/MD.0000000000020900.
3. Riva N, Squizzato A. Stroke: patients with CVT urgently need high-quality evidence. Nat Rev Neurol. 2017;13(11):644–6. https://doi.org/10.1038/nrneurol.2017.143.
4. Duman T, Çınar N, Uludüz D, Domaç FM, Öztürk S, Yayla V, Karahan AY, Afşar N, Sungur MA, Göksu EÖ, Yürekli VA, Genç H, Utku U, Şahin Ş, Tekeli H, Tokuç FE, Uzuner N, Şenol MG, Yılmaz A, Gökçe M, Demirci S, Küsbeci ÖY, Uzuner GT, Batur Çağlayan HZ, Açıkgöz M, Kurucu H, Özdağ MF, Baybaş S, Ekmekçi H, Çabalar M, Yaman M, Bektaş H, Kaplan Y, Göksel BK, Milanlioğlu A, Örken DN, Aluclu MU, Çolakoğlu S, Tüfekçi A, Bakar M, Nazliel B, Tasçılar N, Göksan B, Kozak HH, Mısırlı CH, Küçükoğlu H, Midi İ, Mengüllüoğlu N, Aytaç E, Yeşilot N, İnce B, Yalın OÖ, Güneş T, Oruç S, Demir S. Headache as the sole presenting symptom of cerebral venous sinuses thrombosis: Subgroup analysis of data from the VENOST study. Agri. 2021;33(1):7–14. English. https://doi.org/10.14744/Agri.2020.77698.
5. Timóteo Â, Inácio N, Machado S, Pinto AA, Parreira E. Headache as the sole presentation of cerebral venous thrombosis: a prospective study. J Headache Pain. 2012;13(6):487–90. https://doi.org/10.1007/s10194-012-0456-3.
6. Cumurciuc R, Crassard I, Sarov M, Valade D, Bousser MG. Headache as the only neurological sign of cerebral venous thrombosis: a series of 17 cases. J Neurol Neurosurg Psychiatry. 2005;76(8):1084–7. https://doi.org/10.1136/jnnp.2004.056275.
7. Sparaco M, Feleppa M, Bigal ME. Cerebral venous thrombosis and headache–a case-series. Headache. 2015;55(6):806–14. https://doi.org/10.1111/head.12599.
8. Mehta A, Danesh J, Kuruvilla D. Cerebral venous thrombosis headache. Curr Pain Headache Rep. 2019;23(7):47. https://doi.org/10.1007/s11916-019-0786-9.
9. ICHD-3. Headache attributed to cerebral venous thrombosis (CVT). In: International classification of headache disorders. 3rd ed. 2018.
10. Piazza G. Cerebral venous thrombosis. Circulation. 2012;125(13):1704–9. https://doi.org/10.1161/CIRCULATIONAHA.111.067835.
11. Olaru C, Langberg S, McCoin NS. A review of the clinical presentation, causes, and diagnostic evaluation of increased intracranial pressure in the emergency department. West J Emerg Med. 2024;25(6):1003–10. https://doi.org/10.5811/westjem.18500.
12. Saposnik G, Barinagarrementeria F, Brown RD Jr, Bushnell CD, Cucchiara B, Cushman M, deVeber G, Ferro JM, Tsai FY, American Heart Association stroke council and the council on epidemiology and prevention. Diagnosis and management of cerebral venous thrombosis: a statement for healthcare professionals from the American Heart Association/American Stroke Association. Stroke. 2011;42(4):1158–92. https://doi.org/10.1161/STR.0b013e31820a8364.
13. Russo AF. Calcitonin gene-related peptide (CGRP): a new target for migraine. Annu Rev Pharmacol Toxicol. 2015;55:533–52. https://doi.org/10.1146/annurev-pharmtox-010814-124701.

14. Hu S, Lee H, Zhao H, Ding Y, Duan J. Inflammation and severe cerebral venous thrombosis. Front Neurol. 2022;13:873802. https://doi.org/10.3389/fneur.2022.873802.
15. Li AY, Tong E, Yedavalli VS. A case-based review of cerebral venous infarcts with perfusion imaging and comparison to arterial ischemic stroke. Front Radiol. 2021;1:687045. https://doi.org/10.3389/fradi.2021.687045.
16. Bernstein C, Burstein R. Sensitization of the Trigeminovascular pathway: perspective and implications to migraine pathophysiology. J Clin Neurol. 2012;8(2):89–99. https://doi.org/10.3988/jcn.2012.8.2.89.
17. Idiculla PS, Gurala D, Palanisamy M, Vijayakumar R, Dhandapani S, Nagarajan E. Cerebral venous thrombosis: a comprehensive review. Eur Neurol. 2020;83(4):369–79. https://doi.org/10.1159/000509802.
18. Nascimento FA, Sória MG, Rizelio V, Kowacs PA. Cerebral venous thrombosis with migraine-like headache and the Trigeminovascular system. Case Rep Neurol Med. 2016;2016:2059749. https://doi.org/10.1155/2016/2059749.
19. Botta R, Donirpathi S, Yadav R, Kulkarni GB, Kumar MV, Nagaraja D. Headache patterns in cerebral venous sinus thrombosis. J Neurosci Rural Pract. 2017;8(Suppl 1):S72–7. https://doi.org/10.4103/jnrp.jnrp_339_16.
20. Duman T, Uluduz D, Midi I, Bektas H, Kablan Y, Goksel BK, Milanlioglu A, Necioglu Orken D, Aluclu U (No specific date provided). Headache as the sole presenting symptom of cerebral venous sinuses thrombosis: Subgroup analysis of data from the VENOST study.
21. Wasay M, Kojan S, Dai AI, Bobustuc G, Sheikh Z. Headache in cerebral venous thrombosis: incidence, pattern and location in 200 consecutive patients. J Headache Pain. 2010;11(2):137–9. https://doi.org/10.1007/s10194-010-0186-3. Epub 2010 Jan 29. PMID: 20112042; PMCID: PMC3452295.
22. Singh RJ, Saini J, Varadharajan S, Kulkarni GB, Veerendrakumar M. Headache in cerebral venous sinus thrombosis revisited: exploring the role of vascular congestion and cortical vein thrombosis. Cephalalgia. 2018;38(3):503–10. https://doi.org/10.1177/0333102417698707.
23. Bousser MG, Ferro JM. Cerebral venous thrombosis: an update. Lancet Neurol. 2007;6(2):162–70. https://doi.org/10.1016/S1474-4422(07)70029-7.
24. Timóteo Â, Inácio N, Machado S, Pinto AA, Parreira E. Headache as the sole presentation of cerebral venous thrombosis: a prospective study. J Headache Pain. 2012;13:487.
25. Ferro JM, Aguiar de Sousa D. Cerebral venous thrombosis: an update. Curr Neurol Neurosci Rep. 2019;19(10):74. https://doi.org/10.1007/s11910-019-0988-x.
26. Ferro JM, Bousser MG, Canhão P, Coutinho JM, Crassard I, Dentali F, di Minno M, Maino A, Martinelli I, Masuhr F, Aguiar de Sousa D, Stam J, European Stroke Organization. European stroke organization guideline for the diagnosis and treatment of cerebral venous thrombosis – endorsed by the European academy of neurology. Eur J Neurol. 2017;24(10):1203–13. https://doi.org/10.1111/ene.13381.
27. Ranjan R, Ken-Dror G, Sharma P. Pathophysiology, diagnosis and management of cerebral venous thrombosis: a comprehensive review. Medicine (Baltimore). 2023;102(48):e36366. https://doi.org/10.1097/MD.0000000000036366.
28. Coutinho JM, Ferro JM, Canhão P, Barinagarrementeria F, Bousser MG, Stam J, ISCVT Investigators. Unfractionated or low-molecular weight heparin for the treatment of cerebral venous thrombosis. Stroke. 2010;41(11):2575–80. https://doi.org/10.1161/STROKEAHA.110.588822.
29. Weimar C, Beyer-Westendorf J, Bohmann FO, Hahn G, Halimeh S, Holzhauer S, Kalka C, Knoflach M, Koennecke HC, Masuhr F, Mono ML, Nowak-Göttl U, Scherret E, Schlamann M, Linnemann B. New recommendations on cerebral venous and dural sinus thrombosis from the German consensus-based (S2k) guideline. Neurol Res Pract. 2024;6(1):23. https://doi.org/10.1186/s42466-024-00320-9.
30. Siddiqui FM, Dandapat S, Banerjee C, Zuurbier SM, Johnson M, Stam J, Coutinho JM. Mechanical thrombectomy in cerebral venous thrombosis: systematic review of 185 cases. Stroke. 2015;46(5):1263–8. https://doi.org/10.1161/STROKEAHA.114.007465.

31. Sundar K, Paulraj S, Choudhury SR, Hassan H, Sengupta J, Pattari SK. Successful endovascular treatment of cerebral venous thrombosis with a novel, larger aspiration catheter (REACT): a case report. Neurointervention. 2021;16(1):83–7. https://doi.org/10.5469/neuroint.2020.00304. Epub 2020 Dec 28. Erratum in: Neurointervention. 2021 Jul;16(2):200. https://doi.org/10.5469/neuroint.2020.00304.e1.
32. Zhongrong M, Feng L, Shengmao L, Fengshui Z. Venous sinus stent-assisted angioplasty for refractory benign intracranial hypertension. Interv Neuroradiol. 2003;9(1):79–82. https://doi.org/10.1177/159101990300900114. Epub 2004 Oct 22
33. ten Hove MW, Friedman DI, Patel AD, Irrcher I, Wall M, McDermott MP. NORDIC idiopathic intracranial hypertension study group. Safety and tolerability of acetazolamide in the idiopathic intracranial hypertension treatment trial. J Neuroophthalmol. 2016;36(1):13–9. https://doi.org/10.1097/WNO.0000000000000322.
34. NORDIC Idiopathic Intracranial Hypertension Study Group Writing Committee, Wall M, McDermott MP, Kieburtz KD, Corbett JJ, Feldon SE, Friedman DI, Katz DM, Keltner JL, Schron EB, Kupersmith MJ. Effect of acetazolamide on visual function in patients with idiopathic intracranial hypertension and mild visual loss: the idiopathic intracranial hypertension treatment trial. JAMA. 2014;311(16):1641–51. https://doi.org/10.1001/jama.2014.3312.
35. Kareemi H, Pratte M, English S, Hendin A. Initial diagnosis and management of acutely elevated intracranial pressure. J Intensive Care Med. 2023;38(7):643–50. https://doi.org/10.1177/08850666231156589.
36. Lim JX, Liu SJ, Cheong TM, Saffari SE, Han JX, Chen MW. Intracranial pressure as an objective biomarker of decompression adequacy in large territory infarction: a multicenter observational study. Front Surg. 2022;9:823899. https://doi.org/10.3389/fsurg.2022.823899.
37. Gadgil N, Aldave G, Whitehead WE, Dmytriw AA, Chen K, Orbach D, Maier I, Behme D, Fargen KM, Elijovich L, Dornbos D 3rd, Spiotta A, Kan P. Endovascular intervention for refractory pediatric cerebral venous sinus thrombosis. Pediatr Neurol. 2021;121:45–50. https://doi.org/10.1016/j.pediatrneurol.2021.05.004.

Chapter 25
Headache Attributed to Reversible Cerebral Vasoconstriction Syndrome

Marcelo Valença and Luciana Patrízia Alves de Andrade-Valença

25.1 Introduction

Reversible cerebral vasoconstriction syndrome (RCVS) is a condition characterized by recurrent episodes of thunderclap headache associated with reversible multifocal vasoconstriction of cerebral arteries [1–3]. The syndrome can occur spontaneously or be triggered by various factors, including sexual activity, antidepressants such as selective serotonin reuptake inhibitors [4, 5], immunosuppressant pharmacotherapy [6–8], vasoactive drugs [9], cocaine abuse [10], fibromuscular dysplasia [11], snakebite victims [12], Guillain–Barré syndrome [13], coronavirus 2 vaccination [14], intracranial hypotension [15], among other causes [16]. The female sex appears to be more susceptible to RCVS [17]. Cases of RCVS have been diagnosed as a rare and understudied transfusion reaction, most commonly observed in adult females after the correction of chronic, severe anemia [18, 19]. While initially underrecognized, RCVS has gained increasing attention due to its potential to cause severe neurological complications.

The first time we encountered a patient with RCVS was in 1999. She was a woman who experienced two episodes of explosive thunderclap headache occurring during separate orgasms, one during sexual intercourse and another during masturbation. Her case was published in 2004 alongside a literature review of similar cases associated with sexual activity [20]. In our article, we mentioned that we found several cases in the literature of thunderclap headache with concurrent intracranial arterial vasoconstriction unrelated to eclampsia, suggesting a distinct clinical entity. We first introduced this concept at the Brazilian Headache Congress in 2002 [21], where we proposed it as a new headache syndrome, initially named “Abrupt Severe Headache Associated with Segmental Artery Narrowing (ASHCAN).” At that time, we drafted an article outlining diagnostic criteria, clinical features, and prognostic

M. Valença (✉) · L. P. A. de Andrade-Valença
Federal University of Pernambuco, Recife, Brazil

D. Uludüz et al. (eds.), *Rare Causes of Headache Disorders*, Headache,
https://doi.org/10.1007/978-3-032-10242-3_25

factors. However, the article was not accepted for publication, with no justification provided. Years later, we eventually published our findings, contributing to the growing recognition of RCVS as a distinct neurological disorder [16].

25.2 Case Presentation

A 42-year-old woman with a history of chronic migraine-like headache and overuse of analgesics, particularly Neosaldina® (a combination of isometheptene, dipyrone sodium, and caffeine), was scheduled for elective gallbladder surgery. One week before the procedure, she took Allegra D (fexofenadine) for 7 days to manage her allergy symptoms.

During the surgery, she developed anaphylactic shock, requiring resuscitation. Following this event, she became torpid and exhibited right-sided hemiparesis. Magnetic resonance imaging (MRI) with angiography revealed multiple ischemic lesions affecting different arterial territories (Fig. 25.1), and MR angiography showed diffuse arterial narrowing in several cerebral arteries (Fig. 25.2), consistent with RCVS.

The patient deteriorated further, developing intracranial hypertension, primarily due to cerebellar edema with brainstem compression. MRI scans revealed the absence of subarachnoid cisterns, indicating a significant mass effect in the posterior fossa (Fig. 25.1b, c). An emergency posterior fossa decompressive craniectomy with duroplasty was performed to relieve pressure (Fig. 25.3).

Over the next 2 months, the patient showed gradual improvement in consciousness, initially presenting with akinetic mutism, where she failed to open her eyes but occasionally obeyed simple verbal commands. At 6 months, she regained the ability to walk and communicate verbally, though she remained somewhat apathetic with mild right-arm motor weakness. She was even able to drive under her husband's supervision.

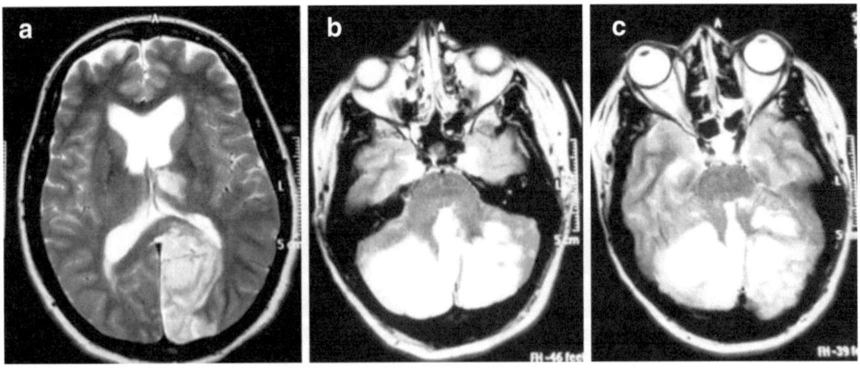

Fig. 25.1 Axial brain MRI showing ischemic areas in the left posterior cerebral artery territory, including the left thalamus (**a**), and a large cerebellar ischemic area involving both hemispheres with significant brainstem compression (**b** and **c**). Note the near-complete disappearance of the posterior fossa cisterns, suggesting severe compartmental hypertension

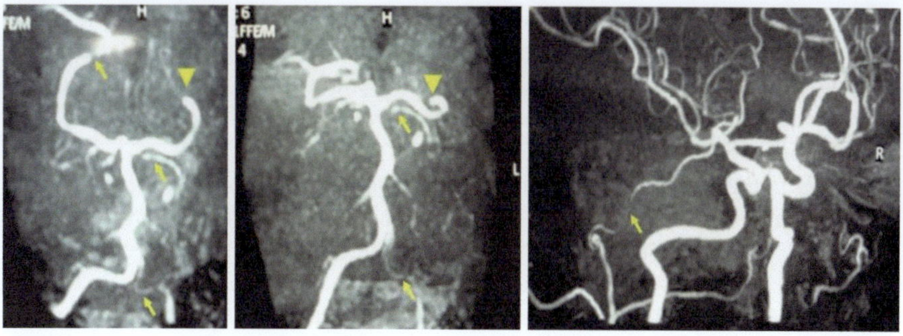

Fig. 25.2 MR angiography of the intracranial arteries and branches of the external carotid artery showing multiple constrictions or vascular lumen narrowing (arrows), predominantly affecting the posterior cerebral, middle cerebral, anterior cerebral, and left vertebral arteries. Note the significant occlusion of the left posterior cerebral artery (arrowhead), corresponding to the infarct observed in the left cerebral hemisphere within the posterior cerebral artery territory (see Fig. 25.1)

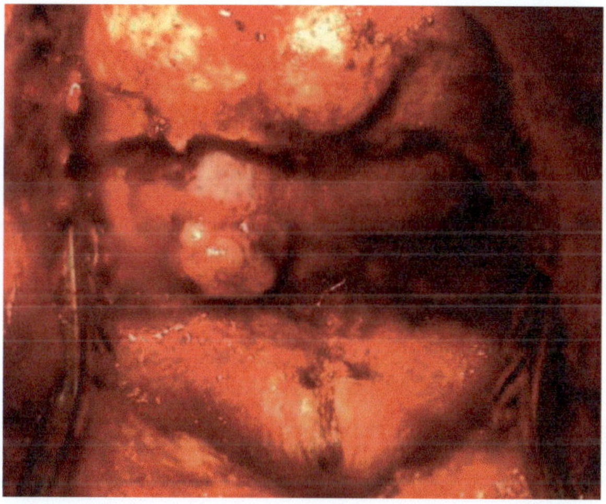

Fig. 25.3 Intraoperative image of posterior fossa craniectomy at the moment of dura mater opening, showing the spontaneous extrusion of softened ischemic cerebellar tissue due to severe intracranial hypertension

Years later, she continues to experience right homonymous hemianopia and behavioral disturbances, including irritability and reduced spontaneity.

25.3 Case Discussion

This case illustrates several important aspects of RCVS: (1) Triggering Factors: The patient had a history of medication overuse and recent exposure to fexofenadine, a medication with sympathomimetic properties. Additionally, the surgical procedure itself may have contributed to endothelial dysfunction and subsequent vasoconstriction. (2) Neurological Complications: While RCVS is often self-limiting, severe cases can lead to extensive ischemic damage, intracranial hypertension, and brainstem compression requiring surgical intervention. (3) Recovery and Sequelae: Despite significant initial deficits, the patient demonstrated substantial recovery, albeit with persistent visual and behavioral impairments. This highlights the variability in RCVS prognosis.

RCVS is thought to result from transient dysfunction of cerebrovascular tone, possibly triggered by endothelial injury, autonomic dysregulation, or vasoactive substances. The hallmark feature is the reversible nature of arterial constrictions, which typically resolve within 3 months.

RCVS shares overlapping features with other conditions, necessitating careful differentiation:

- Primary Thunderclap Headache: Unlike RCVS, these headaches do not involve arterial vasoconstriction.
- Subarachnoid Hemorrhage (SAH): RCVS can mimic SAH, but neuroimaging typically lacks hemorrhagic features.
- Posterior Reversible Encephalopathy Syndrome (PRES): Both conditions can present with similar imaging findings, but PRES is more commonly associated with hypertension and edema without arterial narrowing.
- Eclampsia: RCVS in pregnant women must be distinguished from eclampsia, which typically presents with proteinuria and hypertension.

RCVS diagnosis relies on clinical and radiological findings:

- Sudden-onset thunderclap headache, often recurrent.
- Multifocal segmental arterial narrowing on MR angiography or conventional angiography.
- Absence of aneurysmal SAH or other clear vascular pathology.
- Resolution of vasoconstriction within 3 months.

There is no specific treatment for RCVS, but supportive care includes:

- Pain management: Nonsteroidal anti-inflammatory drugs (NSAIDs) and calcium channel blockers (e.g., nimodipine) may help reduce headache frequency.
- Blood pressure control: Avoidance of excessive hypotension or hypertension.
- Withdrawal of vasoactive substances: Discontinuing triggers such as sympathomimetics, triptans, or serotonergic agents.
- Close monitoring: In severe cases, intensive care may be required to manage complications like ischemia or brain edema.

25.4 Conclusion

RCVS remains an underrecognized yet clinically significant cause of thunderclap headache. This case underscores the importance of identifying potential triggers, recognizing severe neurological complications, and providing timely intervention.

References

1. Ducros A, Boukobza M, Porcher R, Sarov M, Valade D, Bousser MG. The clinical and radiological spectrum of reversible cerebral vasoconstriction syndrome. A prospective series of 67 patients. Brain. 2007;2007(130):3091–101.
2. Singhal AB. Thunderclap headache, reversible cerebral arterial vasoconstriction, and unruptured aneurysms. J Neurol Neurosurg Psychiatry. 2002;2002(73):96; author reply –7.
3. Dodick DW. Thunderclap headache. J Neurol Neurosurg Psychiatry. 2002;2002(72):6–11.
4. Postolowski M, Shakil O, Ramachandran L, Rao CV. Reversible cerebral vasoconstriction syndrome secondary to escitalopram. Clin Med Res. 2024;22(2024):222–6.
5. Wang C, Iftekharuddin A, Fipps DC. Management of psychiatric diagnoses in reversible cerebral vasoconstriction syndrome: the dangers of worsening pathology with serotonergic medications: a case report and literature review. J Psychiatr Pract. 2024;30(2024):379–84.
6. Montarello NL, Irvine I, Warner V, Hare J, Kaye D, Cloud GC. Reversible cerebral vasoconstriction syndrome post-cardiac transplantation: a therapeutic dilemma: case report. BMC Neurol. 2024;2024(24):277.
7. Soh RJH, Lim GZ, Vijayan J, Tan K. Reversible cerebral vasoconstriction syndrome after intravenous immunoglobulin: a rare cause of headache and sudden onset weakness in a patient with Guillain-Barre syndrome. BMJ Case Rep. 2024;17(2024)
8. Wei C, Zhai F, Jia C, Zhang W, Zhou D, Zhang Y. Immunochemotherapy triggered reversible cerebral vasoconstriction syndrome in a patient with intravascular large B-cell lymphoma. Leuk Lymphoma. 2024;2024(65):848–51.
9. Osmont MN, Malrain C, Ruellan AL, Benchikh A, Herlem E, Polard E, Scailteux LM. Reversible cerebral vasoconstriction syndrome in a methylphenidate-treated patient: a case report. BMC Neurol. 2024;24(2024):494.
10. Roa CII, Rodriguez LC, Bastidas N, Vergara S, Borda S, Osorio G, et al. Reversible cerebral vasoconstriction syndrome secondary to chronic cocaine abuse: case report. Radiol Case Rep. 2025;20(2025):597–601.
11. Santos Neto EPD, Sousa IA, Ricarte IF, Pontes-Neto OM. Reversible cerebral vasoconstriction syndrome and fibromuscular dysplasia: an epiphenomenon or a causal relationship? Acta Neurol Taiwan. 2024;33(3):122–6.
12. Senthilkumaran S, Williams J, Almeida JR, Williams HF, Patel K, Thirumalaikolundusubramanian P, Vaiyapuri S. Snakebite-induced reversible cerebral vasoconstriction syndrome: Report of three cases. Toxicon. 2024;251(2024):108161.
13. Seok HY, Eun MY, Kim S, Lee JJ, Oh GR, Kim GY, Sohn SI. Reversible cerebral vasoconstriction syndrome in Guillain-Barre syndrome: a case report and literature review. Neurol Sci. 2024;45(2024):101–7.
14. Shimura M, Fujikawa H, Yazawa M, Matsumoto Y, Yamada M. An autopsy case of reversible cerebral vasoconstriction syndrome after a severe acute respiratory syndrome coronavirus 2 vaccination. Cureus. 2024;2024(16):e59311.
15. Li S, Yang Y, Zuo J, Du N, Kou G. Reversible cerebral vasoconstriction syndrome following intracranial hypotension in a postpartum patient: a case report and literature review. Front Neurol. 2023;2023(14):1281074.
16. Valenca MM, Andrade-Valenca LP, Bordini CA, Speciali JG. Thunderclap headache attributed to reversible cerebral vasoconstriction: view and review. J Headache Pain. 2008;2008(9):277–88.
17. Nelson SE. Reversible cerebral vasoconstriction syndrome and female sex: a narrative review. Stroke. 2024;2024(55):1113–7.
18. Pelham-Webb B, Guo Y, Ramirez A, Waldron E, Emmanuele V, Vargas W, Kahn J, Stone EF. When transfusion causes a splitting headache: a case report and rapid review of transfusion-associated reversible cerebral vasoconstriction syndrome. Transfusion. 2024;64(11):2038–42. https://doi.org/10.1111/trf.17984.
19. Verma A, Sharma G, Singh A, Gupta H, Singh DP, Gaidhane AM, Khatib MN, Bushi G, Sah S, Ndabashinze R. Reversible cerebral vasoconstriction syndrome following blood transfusion

in a patient with chronic anemia: a case report. Clin Case Rep. 2024;12(12):e9618. https://doi.org/10.1002/ccr3.9618.
20. Valenca MM, Valenca LP, Bordini CA, da Silva WF, Leite JP, Antunes-Rodrigues J, Speciali JG. Cerebral vasospasm and headache during sexual intercourse and masturbatory orgasms. Headache. 2004;44(2004):244–8.
21. Valença MM, Costa J, Silva WF, Andrade-Valença LPA, Wichert-Ana L, Leite JP. Cerebral arterial narrowing: differential diagnosis, pathophysiology and correlation with headache syndromes. Neurobiologia. 2002;65(2002):3–12.

Chapter 26
Cerebral Autosomal Dominant Arteriopathy and Subcortical Infarcts Leukoencephalopathy (CADASIL) Attributed Headache

Utku Topbaş, Nevra Öksüz, and Aynur Özge

26.1 Introduction

Cerebral Autosomal Dominant Arteriopathy with Subcortical Infarcts and Leukoencephalopathy (CADASIL) is a hereditary condition characterized by progressive degeneration of smooth muscle cells in the walls of small arteries. This leads to recurring strokes, cognitive decline, and characteristic white matter changes in the brain. One of the primary symptoms experienced by CADASIL patients is migraine, often with aura, which can precede other neurological manifestations by many years [1, 2]. By exploring the nuances of headaches attributed to CADASIL, this chapter aims to elucidate the implications of these findings for clinical practice and future investigations, providing a comprehensive overview of the challenges and potential strategies for managing this complex condition.

26.2 Pathophysiology

CADASIL is caused by mutations in the NOTCH3 gene, leading to abnormal protein accumulation in blood vessels. The resultant arteriopathy is characterized by thickening of vessel walls, luminal narrowing, and ultimately, reduced cerebral blood flow. This vascular pathology underlies the occurrence of migraines, which are prevalent in up to 40% of CADASIL patients. Migraines in CADASIL are often

U. Topbaş · N. Öksüz
School of Medicine, Mersin University, Mersin, Turkey

A. Özge (✉)
Mersin State Hospital, Mersin, Turkey

D. Uludüz et al. (eds.), *Rare Causes of Headache Disorders*, Headache,
https://doi.org/10.1007/978-3-032-10242-3_26

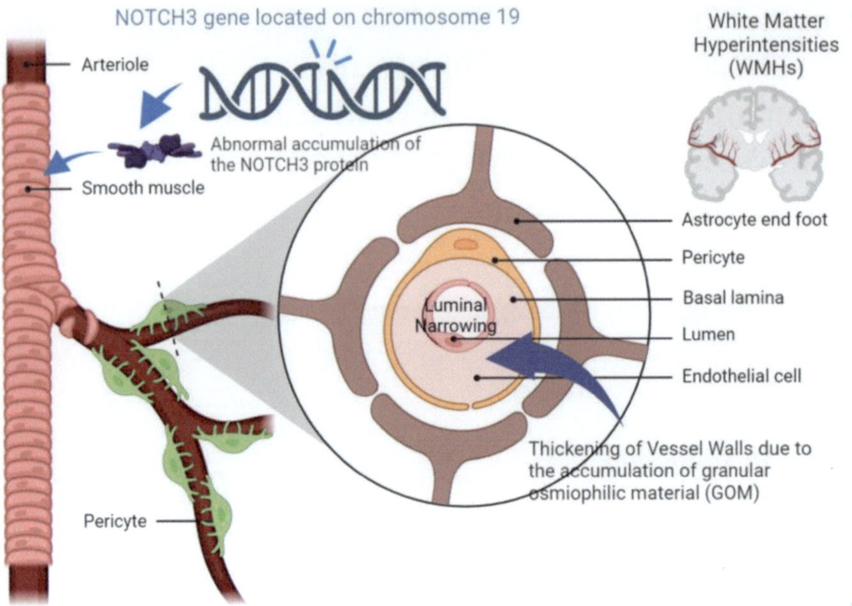

Fig. 26.1 Mechanism of CADASIL white matter intensities (WMI) causes clinical presentation

accompanied by aura and may evolve into chronic daily headaches. The headaches are typically severe and can significantly impact the quality of life of affected individuals. The presence of white matter hyperintensities (WMHs) on magnetic resonance imaging (MRI) is a hallmark of CADASIL and correlates with the frequency and intensity of migraine attacks [3–5].

Figure 26.1 visually summarizes the complex pathophysiology of CADASIL to understand the direct link between the genetic mutation and the clinical manifestations, particularly headaches.

26.3 Case Presentation

Ayşe, a 44-year-old woman, presented with a history of chronic migraines that had progressively worsened over the years. Her headaches were primarily characterized by migraine with aura, manifesting as severe, throbbing pain accompanied by visual disturbances such as flashing lights and blind spots, along with sensory changes, including tingling sensations in her limbs. These episodes often lasted several hours and were resistant to conventional migraine therapies. Over time, her migraines evolved into more persistent headaches, eventually occurring on a near-daily basis.

In addition to the headaches, Ayşe experienced cognitive decline, gait disturbances, and episodic speech difficulties, further complicating her clinical picture.

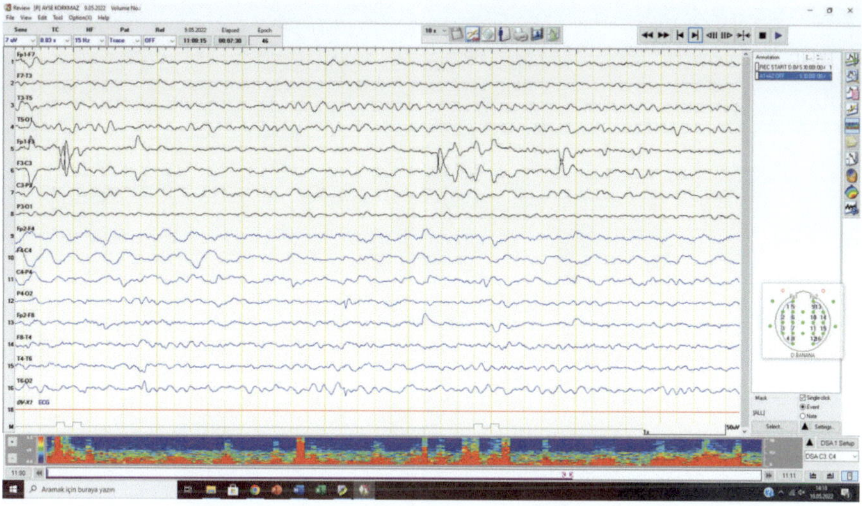

Fig. 26.2 EEG revealed diffuse slowing, consistent with an underlying encephalopathy, and intermittent temporal epileptiform discharges, particularly in the left temporal lobe

The persistence and progression of her headaches, combined with the presence of other neurological symptoms and a significant family history of dementia, strongly suggested an underlying genetic disorder. A routine electroencephalography (EEG) was performed, revealing diffuse slowing, consistent with an underlying encephalopathy, and intermittent temporal epileptiform discharges, particularly in the left temporal lobe (Fig. 26.2). These findings suggested an increased cortical irritability, which could explain some of her complex partial seizures and further supported the suspicion of a neurodegenerative or vascular etiology. The persistence and progression of her headaches, combined with the presence of other neurological symptoms, a significant family history of dementia, and these EEG findings, strongly suggested an underlying genetic disorder.

Brain MRI revealed characteristic white matter hyperintensities, particularly in the periventricular regions and corpus callosum, which, along with the identification of a pathogenic mutation in the NOTCH3 gene, confirmed the diagnosis of CADASIL (Fig. 26.3). Ayşe's headache characteristics, especially the chronic migraines with aura that were unresponsive to treatment and associated with cognitive and motor symptoms, were pivotal in prompting the consideration of CADASIL as a diagnosis.

Over time, her condition progressed to include secondary parkinsonism, polyneuropathy, complex partial epilepsy, and increasing disability. Despite medical interventions, her condition deteriorated, with recurrent falls, bradykinesia, and severe motor impairments leading to a reliance on a wheelchair.

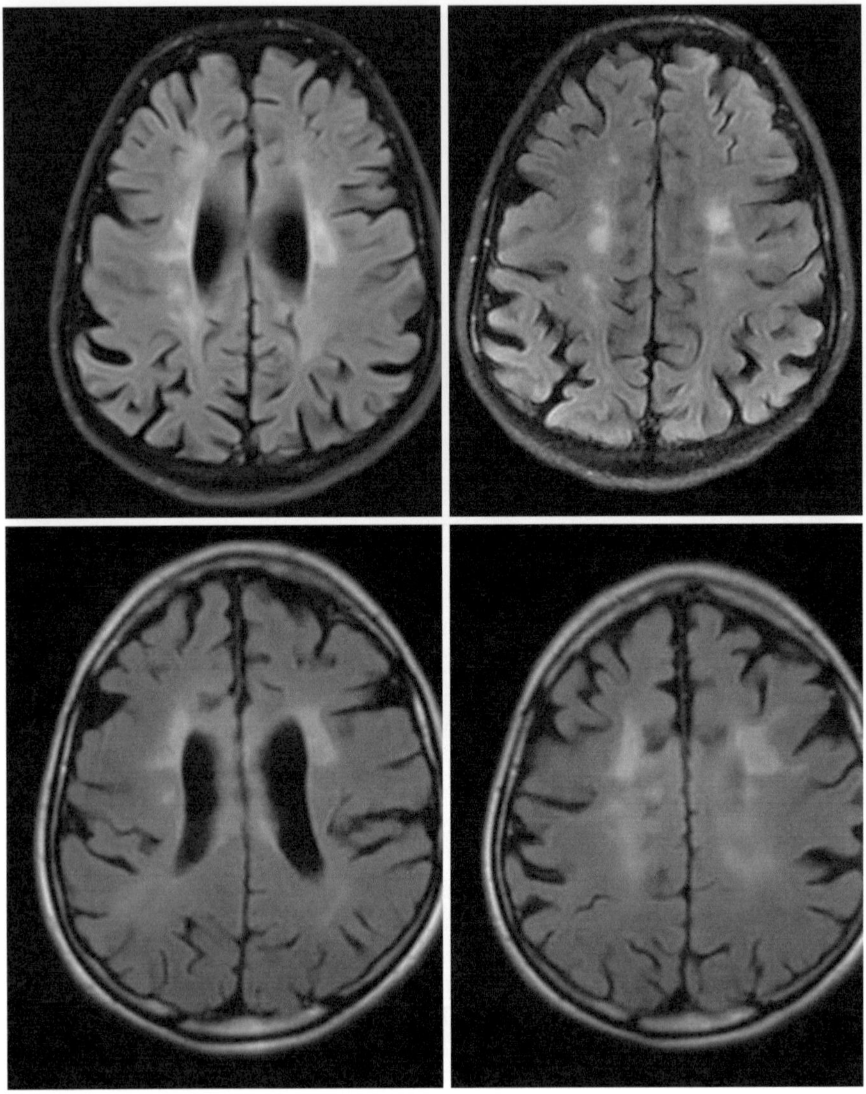

Fig. 26.3 MRI findings of our case show white matter hyperintensities, especially in the corpus callosum, and mild atrophy in the frontoparietal regions

26.4 Case Discussion

Ayşe's case illustrates the progressive nature of CADASIL, with initial manifestations of migraine evolving into more severe neurological deficits. Her clinical course highlights the importance of early diagnosis and comprehensive management in CADASIL patients, emphasizing the need for genetic testing in individuals with a family history of stroke or dementia and atypical migraine [5].

26.5 Clinical Characteristics

Headaches in CADASIL are predominantly characterized by migraine with aura, often presenting before other neurological symptoms. These migraines are typically severe, featuring visual disturbances, sensory changes, and sometimes motor symptoms, and they may be resistant to conventional therapies [1]. As CADASIL progresses, migraines can evolve into chronic daily headaches, with tension-type headaches also emerging in later stages due to cerebral microangiopathy [5]. Migraine disorders occur in 20–40% of CADASIL patients, with some cases involving status migrainous and persistent aura, highlighting the complex relationship between CADASIL and migraine [6]. The high prevalence of right-to-left shunt in CADASIL patients with migraines underscores the hereditary nature of the condition and its pathophysiological links to headaches [5, 6]. Genetic mutations, particularly in the NOTCH3 gene, are closely tied to the manifestation of chronic headaches in CADASIL, emphasizing the importance of genetic screening [7]. Understanding these genetic factors is crucial for advancing diagnostic and therapeutic strategies, as CADASIL's headache phenotype shares similarities with but diverges from typical migraine with aura [7, 8]. Additionally, acute confusional migraine (ACM) may serve as an early indicator of CADASIL, often preceding diagnosis by several years [1, 2]. Current research underscores the need to reevaluate how CADASIL-related headaches are classified, advocating for a more nuanced approach considering the genetic mechanisms underlying these headaches [1].

26.6 Diagnostic Algorithm

Step 1: Clinical Suspicion

- *Identify Key Symptoms*:
  - Migraine with aura
  - Family history of stroke or dementia

Step 2: Initial Diagnostic Workup

- *Perform Brain MRI*:
  - *Assess for White Matter Hyperintensities (WMHs)*:
    - Anterior temporal lobes
    - External capsules
    - Periventricular regions

Step 3: Genetic Testing

- *Conduct Genetic Testing*:
  - *Test* for NOTCH3 gene mutations

Step 4: Additional Diagnostic Evaluations

- *Perform* EEG:
  - *Look* for signs of encephalopathy and temporal epileptiform discharges
- *Neuropsychological* Testing:
  - *Assess* cognitive function to identify possible cognitive decline
- *Cerebrospinal* Fluid Analysis:
  - *Exclude* other differential diagnoses

Step 5: Apply ICHD-3 Diagnostic Criteria [9]

A. Typical, hemiplegic, or recurrent migraine attacks with prolonged aura
B. Presence of subcortical infarcts and leukoencephalopathy (confirmed by MRI)
C. Fulfill at least two of the following:

   First detection of migraine with aura.
   Migraine attacks with aura combined with other CADASIL manifestations (e.g., ischemic stroke, mood disorders, cognitive dysfunction).

D. Exclude more suitable diagnoses according to ICHD-3 criteria.

Step 6: Confirm Diagnosis

- Confirm CADASIL diagnosis:
  - NOTCH3 antibody testing (via immunohistochemical staining or biopsy)*

Step 7: Classification Re-evaluation

- Reassess headache classification:
  - Consider genetic mechanisms in the classification within the context of vascular disorders

**The diagnosis of this disorder is based on NOTCH3 antibodies by immunohistochemical staining or extracellular granular osmiophilic in arterial media electron for material evaluation a simple deep microscopy of the skin NOTCH3 mutations using biopsy is detected by scanning* [9].

Other investigations: EEG, neuropsychological testing, and cerebrospinal fluid analysis may aid in excluding other differential diagnoses [4, 7].

The classification of headaches associated with genetic disorders, particularly CADASIL, requires a critical re-evaluation, as highlighted by Sacco et al. [1]. Their examination of the International Classification of Headache Disorders suggests that the current categorization of CADASIL-related headaches within the framework of vascular disorders may inadequately capture the genetic mechanisms contributing to these headaches. Sacco et al. advocate for a more nuanced understanding of the etiology of these headaches, emphasizing the intersection of genetic factors and headache pathology. This perspective lays the groundwork for a comprehensive exploration of headache manifestations in CADASIL, which this chapter will further elaborate on [1, 9].

26.7 Management

Management of CADASIL-related headaches focuses on symptomatic relief and preventing stroke. The treatment regimen may include:

- Migraine Prophylaxis: Migraine prophylaxis in CADASIL patients typically includes medications such as beta-blockers, calcium channel blockers, and anti-epileptics, which may help reduce migraine frequency. Recent studies, including detailed case studies, highlight the debilitating nature of migraines in CADASIL, primarily due to vascular dysfunction linked to NOTCH3 mutations. This research underscores the refractory nature of traditional migraine treatments in these patients. It introduces calcitonin gene-related peptide (CGRP) receptor antagonists as a promising novel therapeutic approach, supported by emerging literature, for potentially improving headache management in CADASIL [10, 11].
- Antiplatelet Therapy: Aspirin is commonly used to prevent ischemic events.
- Supportive Care: Physiotherapy, speech therapy, and occupational therapy are essential in managing progressive neurological deficits.
- Genetic Counselling: Given the hereditary nature of CADASIL, counselling for family members is crucial [10, 12, 13].

26.8 Conclusion

Headaches in CADASIL represent a significant early symptom of the disease and may precede other neurological manifestations by many years. Early recognition and management are key to improving outcomes and preventing further complications. This chapter has provided an overview of the pathophysiology, case presentation, diagnostic approach, and management strategies for headaches associated with CADASIL, emphasizing the importance of a multidisciplinary approach in caring for these patients. The insights from recent literature underscore the complexity of managing CADASIL-related headaches and highlight the need for tailored therapeutic approaches that consider both the neurological and vascular challenges inherent to this condition.

References

1. Sacco S, Degan D, Carolei A. Diagnostic criteria for CADASIL in the international classification of headache disorders (ICHD-II): are they appropriate? J Headache Pain. 2010;11(3):181–6. https://doi.org/10.1007/s10194-010-0203-6. Epub 2010 Mar 12. PMID: 20224942; PMCID: PMC3451909
2. Gosalia H, Karsan N, Goadsby P. Genetic mechanisms of migraine: insights from monogenic migraine mutations. Int J Mol Sci. 2023;24(16):12697. https://doi.org/10.3390/ijms241612697.
3. Su Y, Tay VQ, Singh S, Leary MC, Koss V, Kincaid HM, Yacoub HA, Castaldo J. A retrospective review of sex differences of white matter hyperintensities in brain MRI of patients with migraine. Headache. 2024;64(6):612–23. https://doi.org/10.1111/head.14714. Epub 2024 May 24. PMID: 38785411.
4. Liem MK, Oberstein SA, van der Grond J, Ferrari MD, Haan J. CADASIL and migraine: a narrative review. Cephalalgia. 2010;30(11):1284–9. https://doi.org/10.1177/0333102410370870. PMID: 21038489.
5. Guey S, Mawet J, Hervé D, Duering M, Godin O, Jouvent E, Opherk C, Alili N, Dichgans M, Chabriat H. Prevalence and characteristics of migraine in CADASIL. Cephalalgia. 2016;36(11):1038–47. https://doi.org/10.1177/0333102415620909. Epub 2016 Jul 11. PMID: 26646784.
6. Sacco S, Rasura M, Cao M, Bozzao A, Carolei A. CADASIL presenting as status migraineurs and persisting aura without infarction. J Headache Pain. 2009;10(1):51–3. https://doi.org/10.1007/s10194-008-0079-x. Epub 2008 Oct 25. PMID: 18953486; PMCID: PMC3451763.
7. Gosalia H, Karsan N, Goadsby PJ. Genetic mechanisms of migraine: insights from monogenic migraine mutations. Int J Mol Sci. 2023;24(16):12697. https://doi.org/10.3390/ijms241612697. PMID: 37628876; PMCID: PMC10454024.
8. Ferrante E, Trimboli M, Erminio C, Martino I, Tiraboschi P. Acute confusional migraine in CADASIL: a case report and literature review. Clin Neurol Neurosurg. 2022;216:107239. https://doi.org/10.1016/j.clineuro.2022.107239. Epub 2022 Apr 6. PMID: 35413636.
9. The International Classification of Headache Disorders, 3rd edition. Cephalalgia. 2018;38(1):1–211. Jes Olesen ISSN: 0333-1024.
10. Donnini I, Nannucci S, Valenti R, Pescini F, Bianchi S, Inzitari D, Pantoni L. Acetazolamide for the prophylaxis of migraine in CADASIL: a preliminary experience. J Headache Pain. 2012;13(4):299–302. https://doi.org/10.1007/s10194-012-0426-9. Epub 2012 Feb 25. PMID: 22367627; PMCID: PMC3356473.
11. Goldstein ED, Badi MK, Meschia JF. Treating chronic migraine in CADASIL with calcitonin gene-related peptide receptor antagonism. Neurol Clin Pract. 2019;9(3):277–8. https://doi.org/10.1212/CPJ.0000000000000651. PMID: 31341718; PMCID: PMC6615658.
12. Gravesteijn G, Dauwerse JG, Overzier M, Brouwer G, Hegeman I, Mulder AA, Baas F, Kruit MC, Terwindt GM, van Duinen SG, Jost CR, Aartsma-Rus A, Lesnik Oberstein SAJ, Rutten JW. Naturally occurring NOTCH3 exon skipping attenuates NOTCH3 protein aggregation and disease severity in CADASIL patients. Hum Mol Genet. 2020;29(11):1853–63. https://doi.org/10.1093/hmg/ddz285. PMID: 31960911; PMCID: PMC7372551.
13. Yamamoto Y, Liao YC, Lee YC, Ihara M, Choi JC. Update on the epidemiology, pathogenesis, and biomarkers of cerebral autosomal dominant Arteriopathy with subcortical infarcts and leukoencephalopathy. J Clin Neurol. 2023;19(1):12–27. https://doi.org/10.3988/jcn.2023.19.1.12. PMID: 36606642; PMCID: PMC9833879.

Chapter 27
Headache Attributed to Mitochondrial Encephalopathy, Lactic Acidosis, and Stroke-Like Episodes (MELAS)

Nana Nino Tatishvili, Teona Shatirishvili, and Sofia Tatishvili

27.1 Introduction

Mitochondria are dynamic subcellular organelles with innumerable functions, including energy generation via oxidative phosphorylation (OXPHOS), calcium homeostasis, and regulation of apoptotic cell death, placing them at the center of cellular metabolism and signalling [1].

Mitochondrial diseases are caused by either a mutation in the nuclear DNA (nDNA) or mitochondrial DNA (mtDNA).

Among the systems most affected by this group of diseases, the nervous system stands out, primarily due to its high dependence on aerobic metabolism. Due to this, sleep disorders, headache, and epilepsy are common in mitochondrial disorders (MDs). These symptoms can be one of the cardinal symptoms that define some of the subtypes of these diseases, such as headache in mitochondrial encephalomyopathy with lactic acidosis and stroke-like episodes (MELAS) [2].

MDs occur in a large section of the lifespan (from the neonatal period to late adulthood), with an incidence of about 1.6/5000. In the pediatric population, the incidence ranges from 0.5 to 1.5 per 100,000. In the majority of cases, onset occurs in infancy or early childhood and is associated with high morbidity and mortality [3, 4].

The most common neurological symptoms present in the majority of children with mitochondrial disorder (MD) are muscle weakness, peripheral neuropathy, ophthalmoplegia, movement disorder, epilepsy, and headache, so the neuropediatrician must be one of the key physicians involved in the diagnosis and management of childhood-onset MDs [5].

N. N. Tatishvili (✉) · T. Shatirishvili · S. Tatishvili
David Tvildiani Medical University, Tbilisi, Georgia

D. Uludüz et al. (eds.), *Rare Causes of Headache Disorders*, Headache,
https://doi.org/10.1007/978-3-032-10242-3_27

27.2 Case Presentations

We had two patients with MD and headaches. Headache was not the dominant feature of an MD, but only an ancillary feature of the phenotype in both. The headache was not very severe, but was admitted by both, mostly between acute progressing episodes, during the stable period.

Case 27.1 Male, 5 years old, early development was normal.

At the age 5, he lost consciousness and presented with right-sided hemiparesis. At that point, a cranial magnetic resonance imaging (MRI) showed normal findings. A second episode occurred at 7 years of age: during a respiratory infection complicated with pneumonia, he transiently lost consciousness and vision. It was evaluated as an epileptic seizure, he was treated with carbamazepine, and his electroencephalography (EEG) was normal. An MRI showed non-specific changes of the bilateral occipital white matter. After this, he had periods of headache without any other signs; he could not describe the type of headache, it was of moderate severity, and sometimes nonsteroidal anti-inflammatory drugs (NSAIDs) were needed. His third episode occurred at the age of 10 years. Again, after an unspecific illness, focal convulsive status epilepticus (epilepsia partialis continua) occurred with deviation of head and eyes to the right and twitching of the right side of the face, accompanied by left-sided focal spike and slow-wave activity. All blood tests, including liver enzymes, were normal. The MRI was unchanged.

The patient was treated with i/v antiseizure medication (ASM) in the pediatric intensive care unit (PICU). Status epilepticus was not controlled. Then thiopentone anaesthesia was used. He was alert and responsive for 3 days. However, acute severe deterioration occurred, and the boy died within 10 h due to recurrent status epilepticus, acidosis, anuria, and respiratory failure.

Genetic analysis revealed that our patient and sibling had MD Alpers- and mitochondrial neurogastointestinal encephalomyopathy (MNGIE)-like disease with disturbed cerebrospinal fluid (CSF) folate transport and an unusual mode of genetic transmission of POLG mutations. In the blood DNA of our patient and his sibling, two heterozygous variants were detected, while multiplex ligation-dependent probe amplification (MLPA) analysis was normal. One of these NM_002693.2: c.680G > A p.(Arg227Gln) is a missense variant that has recently been described in three infants with mitochondrial depletion syndrome (MDS) and Alpers-Huttenlocher syndrome (AHS) [6–8] This variant was also present in blood DNA of the deceased brother but not in the parents and the healthy brother. A buccal swab, saliva, and hair bulbs of the father were also negative for this mutation. Paternal blood DNA was additionally tested by deep targeted next-generation sequencing (coverage >2500) for this POLG variant and was negative [6].

Case 27.2 A 9-year-old male patient developed bilateral sensorineural hearing loss followed by a generalized tonic–clonic seizure. From this period, he had monthly headaches without other signs, usually of moderate severity, and rare NSAIDs were

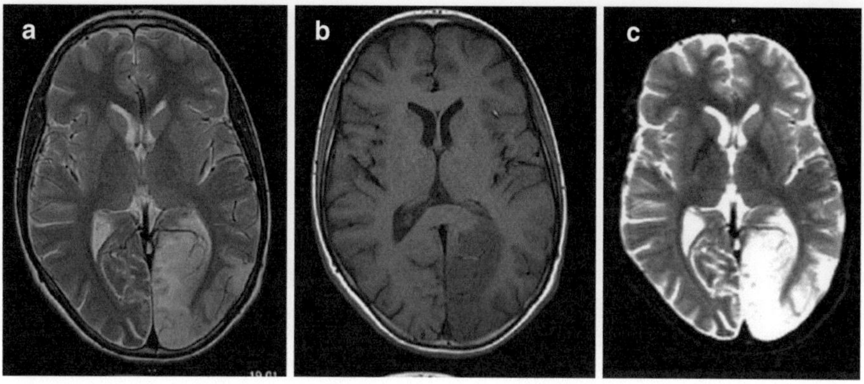

Fig. 27.1 Brain MRI: Stroke-like episode (SLE) (A-C) demonstrating hyperintensities in the left occipital and parietal lobes, extending into white matter—a suspected area of cortical and subcortical ischemia not respecting the borders of large and medium-sized arterial territories. (T. Shatirishvili et al. [6])

used. From age 15, he exhibited progressive fatigue, muscle weakness, and stroke-like episodes.

MRI revealed stroke-like lesions in the brain (Fig. 27.1). Over 2 years, he experienced multiple hospital admissions for severe symptoms including right-sided hemiparesis, hemianopia, seizures, and encephalopathy, periodically with non-migraineous headaches. Despite treatment, his condition deteriorated, leading to multi-organ failure and death at the age 16 years. Molecular genetic analysis identified a heteroplasmic m.3764C > G variant in MT-ND1.

The case was evaluated as MELAS with a new mutation [9].

27.3 Clinical Characteristics

Headache is a common feature of MD and can manifest as a migraine-like headache, cluster headache, non-classified headache, or tension headache. Headache may be the dominant feature of a MD or only an ancillary feature of the phenotype [10].

Due to the absence of a structured diagnostic headache tool, specific questionnaires, interviews, and objective clinical examination, the prevalence of headache/migraine in MDs patients fluctuates noticeably in the scientific literature [2].

Migraine may also be part of the clinical presentation of a stroke-like episode (SLE). Regarding headache, it is still unclear whether headache is a primary disorder associated with MDs or a secondary migraine-like headache caused by mitochondrial disease. In the study population, 71% (43/61) indicated headache, and 29% (18/61) reported not suffering any headache [11].

The pathophysiology of migraine-like headache is poorly understood. Still, there are indications that it is a vascular pathology, resulting in initial hyperperfusion, which results from activation of the calcitonin-related protein or enhanced influx of calcium into mitochondria, resulting in increased oxidative stress [10].

A SLE, which can have an acute or subacute neurological manifestation, typically affects young individuals and is caused by focal brain dysfunction of an epileptic nature.

MD-associated migraine tends to be chronic and more disabling than in the general population. Non-classified headache has been reported in patients carrying POLG1 mutations [10]. A higher frequency of headache, other than migraine, has also been observed in patients with MELAS syndrome, suggesting the presence of a characteristic headache subtype in these patients. In this way, mitochondrial dysfunction could be one of the pathophysiological mechanisms of headache migrainous or non-migrainous and constitute a factor of chronification and severity in this entity [2].

27.4 Discussion

Mitochondria play a central role in a variety of cellular functions, including energy generation, production of reactive oxygen species (ROS), control of Ca2+ homeostasis, and regulation of apoptosis [7].

Mitochondrial diseases are caused by either mutation in the nuclear DNA(nDNA) or mitochondrial DNA(mtDNA). The mtDNA encodes only for approximately 1% of all estimated 1500 (nuclear and mtDN encoded) proteins needed for normal structure and function of mitochondria [7, 8]. Pathogenic variants in mtDNA include single-nucleotide variants as well as single large-scale deletions/rearrangements. The integrity of mtDNA can also be affected by multiple deletions arising in the context of primary defects in one of over 30 nuclear genes that control mtDNA maintenance. This can also result in reduced mtDNA content (mtDNA depletion). According to O. Heath, R.G. Feichtinger et al. (2025), pathogenic variants in the nuclear gene POLG account for the most prevalent mtDNA maintenance defect in childhood [12].

Mitochondrial diseases presenting in childhood are characterized by clinical, biochemical, and genetic complexity. Some children are affected by well-described syndromes, and many have nonclassical multisystemic disease presentations involving any organ in the body. Each child has a unique combination of clinical features and disease trajectory, leading to enormous challenges in the diagnosis and management of these heterogeneous disorders [2].

Fifty-five percent of all participants reported a headache. Forty-eight percent of women and 31% of all men in the population reported headache as one of the five most essential complaints due to their mitochondrial disease [10].

Despite many publications about the high frequency of headache in MD, it is still unclear whether headache is a primary disorder associated with or coincidental to

MDs, mainly manifested as migraine, or a secondary migraine-like headache caused by mitochondrial disease.

The current edition of the International Classification of Headache Disorders (ICHD-3 beta) only includes headache in MELAS among headache attributed to genetic vasculopathy, without other references to headache in the context of MDs [13].

About 80% of the MD cases are associated with the pathogenic m.3243A > G mutation in the MT-TL1 gene, the first genetic defect linked to MELAS syndrome. However, other rare mtDNA mutations and recessive POLG1 mutations are well-recognized causes of SLEs [5].

POLG1 patients have an explosive onset and a rapid progression, with a higher risk of death due to status epilepticus [14], as was the case in our case 27.1. The patient developed suprarefractory status epilepticus, which led to the patient's death. Patients with the 3243A > G mutation usually show a protracted disease course with an insidious onset and mainly die from complications not related to central nervous system (CNS). Moreover, around half of POLG1 patients have no other symptoms outside of CNS features before the first SLE. The patient in case 27.1 also had purely CNS signs.

A. H. San Martin, C. D. Gonzalez et al. (2023) performed a cross-sectional cohort study. Of the 203 patients interviewed, 92 (45.3%) reported suffering regularly from headache of any type (at least one headache day per month), the prevalence being more frequent in women than in men (53.2 vs. 32.9%, respectively). Within the group of 92 patients with headaches, migraine prevalence was 35%, which is higher compared to the general population. Sixteen (69.6%) of these patients met the criteria of migraine, while the remaining seven had non-migraine-type headaches. Patients with migraine had a median of 10 headache days per month, while patients with non-migraine headaches, like our case 27.2 patient, had a median of 3 headache days per month. Both our patients had non-migrainous headaches, frequency was not high, and severity was moderate [2].

Patients with the pathogenic variant m.8344 A > G in the MTTK gene were those with the highest prevalence of headache. A total of 39 patients with the m.3243 A > G mutation in the MTTL1 gene (58.2%) presented headache, with 69% of cases fulfilling migraine criteria [2]. This prevalence was reported to be independent of sex, phenotype, or genotype, which, together with dysfunction of mitochondrial metabolism in migraine observed in several studies, supports the hypothesis that mitochondrial dysfunction could play an important role in the pathophysiology of migraine. Moreover, there is emerging evidence that monoclonal antibodies acting on calcitonin gene-related peptide (CGRP) (CGRP-mAbs), widely used in the treatment of patients with migraine, are also safe and effective in the treatment of refractory headaches associated with mitochondrial diseases. This data also supports the theory about common pathophysiological pathways between MDs and migraine.

Based on the phenotype of the patients with MD, a statistically significant relationship was found between the MELAS syndrome and the presence of headache, in contrast with other phenotypes, with a p-value of less than 0.01 [2].

The exciting fact is that in MD patients with epilepsy, myoclonus, and SLEs are more frequent in patients with headache/migraine compared to patients without it. In both of our cases, there was a combination of epilepsy (in one, myoclonus) and headache. The finding of a higher prevalence of epilepsy in the population of mitochondrial migraineurs (33.33%; 11/33) compared with non-migraineurs (11.66%; 7/60) presumably means that the association between migraine and epilepsy is not fortuitous in these patients, but could underlie common pathophysiological mechanisms [15].

It is essential to mention that the pharmacological management of MDs patients with headache/migraine could be particularly challenging, probably due to poor tolerance to drugs commonly used for headaches.

We can admit that mitochondrial dysfunction could be one of the pathophysiological mechanisms of headache/migraine, mainly through the production of ROS, apoptosis, Ca2þ homeostasis, and global increased neuronal excitability, and it can also constitute one of the mechanisms of chronification and severity of migraine.

27.5 Conclusion

Headache/migraine has a higher prevalence in MDs compared with general population-based data, independently of genotype or phenotype. Headache is not merely a phenotypic aspect of specific MDs. Still, it is rather the expression of vulnerability of the central nervous system, probably directly related to defects of the respiratory chain.

A headache can be a cardinal sign of clinical presentation, as well as an ancillary feature. It can be migrainous as well as non-migrainous or unclassified, as in our cases. New data is needed for a better understanding of pathophysiologic mechanisms and the relationship between MD and headache in mitochondrial disorders, especially in MELAS and SLE.

References

1. Rahman S. Mitochondrial disease in children. J Intern Med. 2020;287:609–33. https://doi.org/10.1111/joim.13054.
2. San Martin AH, Gonzalez CD, Conejo MM, Hernandez Salas ME, Gallego JH. Headache and sleep quality in mitochondrial diseases. Cephalalgia Rep. 2023;6:1–7.
3. Tolomeo D, Orsucci D, Nesti C, Baldacci J, Battini R, Bruno C, Bruno G, Cassandrini D, Doccini S, Donati MA, Ferrari A, Fiori S, Fiorillo C, Guerrini R, Mari F, Montomoli M, Pochiero F, Procopio E, Ruggiero L, Sampaolo S, Sicca F, Ticci C, Rubegni A, Santorelli FM. The diagnostic approach to mitochondrial disorders in children in the era of next-generation sequencing: a 4-year cohort study. J Clin Med. 2021;10(15):3222. https://doi.org/10.3390/jcm10153222.

4. Tan J, Wagner M, Stenton SL, Strom TM, Wortmann SB, Prokisch H, Meitinger T, Oexle K, Klopstock T. Lifetime risk of autosomal recessive mitochondrial disorders calculated from genetic databases. EBioMedicine. 2020;54:102730.
5. Conti F, Di Martino S, Drago F, Bucolo C, Micale V, Montano V, Siciliano G, Mancuso M, Lopriore P. Red flags in primary mitochondrial diseases: what should we recognize? Int J Mol Sci. 2023;24:16746.
6. Shatirishvili T, Katsitadze Z, Yi Shiau Ng, Achuthaprasad A, Alston CL, Blakey E, Turnbull DM, Bregvadze K, Tkemaladze T, Tatishvili NN. Novel m.3764C>G variant in MT-ND1 linked to severe MELAS syndrome: a case report. Brain Dev Case Rep. 2025;3:100059.
7. Tiehuis LH, Koene S, Saris CGJ, Janssen MCH. Mitochondrial migraine; a prevalence, impact and treatment efficacy cohort study. Mitochondrion. 2020;53:128–32.
8. El-Hattab AW, Craigen WJ, Scaglia F. Mitochondrial DNA maintenance defects. Biochim Biophys Acta (BBA) – Mol Basis Dis. 2017;1863(6):1539–55.
9. Korinthenberg R, Kirschner J, Eckenweiler M, Steinfeld R, Tatishvili NN, Horvath R, Kleinle S, Abicht A. Alpers- and MNGIE-like disease with disturbed CSF folate transport and an unusual mode of genetic transmission of POLG mutations: a case report. J Int Child Neurol Assoc. 2020;20(216)
10. Finsterer J, Torres de Carvalho EH. Cerebral manifestations of mitochondrial disorders. Can J Neurol Sci. 2017;44:654–63. https://doi.org/10.1017/cjn.2017.211.
11. Burow P, Meyer A, Naegel S, Watzke S, Zierz S, Kraya T. Headache and migraine in mitochondrial disease and its impact on life—results from a cross-sectional, questionnaire-based study. Acta Neurol Belg. 2021;121:1151–6.
12. Heath O, Feichtinger Ren'e G, Achleitner MT, Hofbauer P, Doris M, Merkevicius K, Spenger J, Steinbrücker K, Steindl C, Tiefenthaler E, Mayr JA, Wortmann SB. Mitochondrial disorder diagnosis and management– what the pediatric neurologist wants to know. Eur J Paediatr Neurol. 2025;54:75–88.
13. Headache Classification Committee of the International Headache Society (IHS). The international classification of headache disorders, 3rd edition 2018.
14. Hikmat O, Naess K, Engvall M, Klingenberg C, Rasmussen M, Tallaksen CM, Brodtkorb E, Ostergaard E, de Coo IFM, Pias-Peleteiro L, Isohanni P, Uusimaa J, Darin N, Rahman S, Bindoff LA. Simplifying the clinical classification of polymerase gamma (POLG) disease based on age of onset; studies using a cohort of 155 cases. J Inherit Metab Dis. 2020;43(4):726–36. https://doi.org/10.1002/jimd.12211.
15. Catello V, Guido P, Giacomo DM, Losurdo A, Servidei S. Migraine in mitochondrial disorders: prevalence and characteristics. Cephalalgia. 2018;38(6):1093–106.

Chapter 28
Headache Attributed to Moyamoya Angiopathy

Esra Kochan Kizilkilic and Derya Uluduz

28.1 Introduction

Moyamoya disease (MMD) is a chronic, progressive cerebrovascular disorder characterized by bilateral stenosis or occlusion of the terminal portion of the internal carotid arteries (ICA) and the development of compensatory basal collateral vessels. These vessels appear as a "puff of smoke" on cerebral angiography—hence the name "Moyamoya," which means "hazy" or "smoky" in Japanese [1, 2].

While MMD is traditionally recognized for its ischemic and hemorrhagic stroke presentations, headache is an increasingly acknowledged, yet underdiagnosed, manifestation of the disease, particularly in adults [3]. Clinical series and case reports suggest that headache can be the initial and sometimes the only presenting symptom of Moyamoya disease, preceding more serious cerebrovascular events by months or even years [4, 5].

Headaches in MMD can mimic primary headache disorders, particularly migraine without aura, and are often misclassified due to overlapping clinical features such as throbbing pain, photophobia, nausea, and unilateral localization [6, 7]. In some cases, patients may be labelled as having refractory migraine or chronic tension-type headache, delaying the correct diagnosis and appropriate management [8, 9]. In a recent case series from Indonesia, Moyamoya-related headache was among the most challenging initial presentations to identify, often requiring advanced neurovascular imaging for diagnosis [10]. Headaches associated with MMD can occur both in the ischemic phase, due to cerebral hypoperfusion, and in the hemorrhagic phase, due to the rupture of fragile collateral vessels [6]. Moreover,

E. Kochan Kizilkilic · D. Uluduz (✉)
Department of Neurology, University of Health Sciences,
Prof. Dr. Cemil Tascioglu City Hospital, Istanbul, Turkey

Medical Faculty, Neurology Department, Istanbul University Cerrahpasa, Samatya, Türkiye

D. Uludüz et al. (eds.), *Rare Causes of Headache Disorders*, Headache,
https://doi.org/10.1007/978-3-032-10242-3_28

variations in headache frequency and intensity may correlate with cerebral blood flow dynamics and compensatory collateral load [8]. In pediatric populations, headache is also a common symptom of MMD, though more overt neurological deficits frequently overshadow it. An extensive review of 204 pediatric patients showed that headache was a primary complaint in nearly one-third of cases [11], emphasizing the need for age-specific diagnostic consideration.

Given the often-subtle and misleading nature of headache presentations in Moyamoya disease, clinicians must maintain a high index of suspicion, especially in cases of late-onset, changing headache patterns or those refractory to typical migraine therapies. Advanced neuroimaging remains the cornerstone of diagnosis, and timely identification may prevent progression to more debilitating vascular events [3, 7].

This chapter explores Moyamoya-related headaches through the lens of a detailed case vignette, discussing clinical features, diagnostic challenges, and the current understanding of pathophysiology and management. By shedding light on this rare but crucial cause of secondary headaches, we aim to bridge the gap between clinical suspicion and definitive diagnosis, thereby improving patient outcomes through timely intervention.

28.2 Case Presentation

A 51-year-old right-handed female patient presented to the neurology outpatient clinic with a complaint of gradually increasing frequency and intensity of headaches over the past 2–3 months. She reported that she had been experiencing headaches intermittently for the past 30 years. Initially, the headaches had a pattern consistent with episodic migraine without aura—unilateral, throbbing in character, accompanied by nausea, vomiting, and photophobia. Attacks occurred approximately one to two times per month in earlier years, lasted for about 24 h if untreated, and were typically moderate in intensity, often responsive to over-the-counter analgesics.

Interestingly, over the last 5 years, the frequency of her attacks had significantly declined, almost to the point of remission. However, during the past few months, the headache frequency abruptly increased, now occurring once or twice a week, with some attacks reaching high intensity and lasting nearly a full day, sometimes requiring her to rest in a dark room due to severe photophobia. The headache pattern remained predominantly unilateral and pulsatile, localized to the frontotemporal region. No aura, focal neurological deficits, or syncope episodes were described. There were no triggers she could identify. Despite the increased burden, she had never undergone a formal neurological evaluation or neuroimaging prior to this visit.

Her past medical history was unremarkable. She had never been diagnosed with hypertension, diabetes, or hyperlipidemia and was not on any regular medication. She denied alcohol or illicit drug use but reported smoking one pack of cigarettes per day for over 20 years. Her family history was notable for similar headaches in her mother, which had never been investigated or formally diagnosed.

Neurological examination at the time of admission was entirely normal. Routine blood work revealed no abnormalities, including thyroid function, C-reactive protein (CRP), autoimmune panels, coagulation studies, and vasculitis screening.

Initial non-contrast cranial computed tomography (CT) was normal. However, a contrast-enhanced cranial magnetic resonance imaging (MRI) was performed due to the patient's atypical headache evolution, particularly the recurrence after a prolonged quiescent phase and the increased burden. MRI revealed contrast enhancement of basal collateral vessels, along with increased fluid-attenuated inversion recovery (FLAIR) signal intensities at the level of the cerebral convexities, suggestive of slow-flow collateral channels (Figs. 28.1 and 28.2). These findings prompted further vascular imaging.

Cranial MR angiography (MRA) demonstrated bilateral occlusion of the supraclinoid segments of the internal carotid arteries (ICA), along with prominent basal collaterals, producing the characteristic "puff of smoke" appearance. Subsequent digital subtraction angiography (DSA) (Figs. 28.3 and 28.4) confirmed the diagnosis, revealing:

- Bilateral occlusion of ICA supraclinoid segments.
- Proliferation of basal collaterals adjacent to the occlusion.
- Convexity collaterals arising from the external carotid arteries.
- Posterior circulation compensation via vertebrobasilar collaterals.

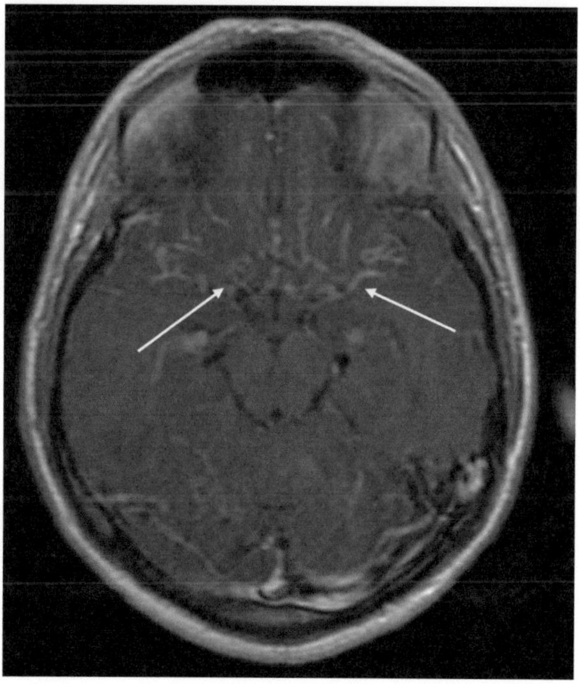

Fig. 28.1 Contast enhancement brain MRI

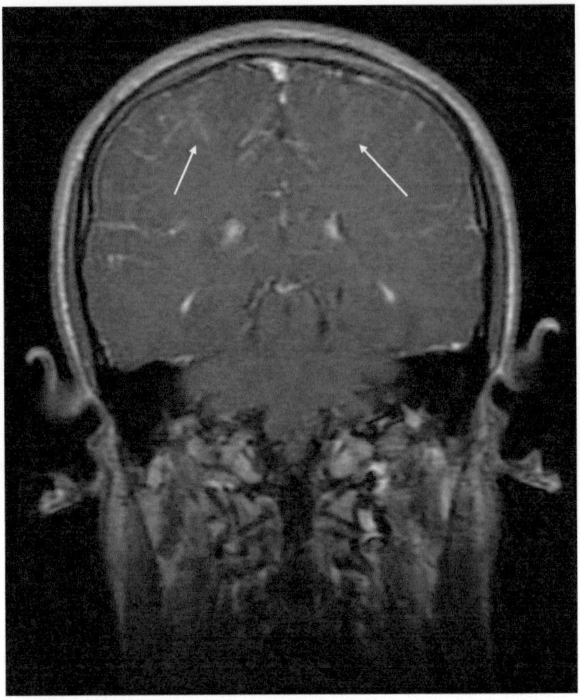

Fig. 28.2 Coronal image of contast enhancement Brain MRI

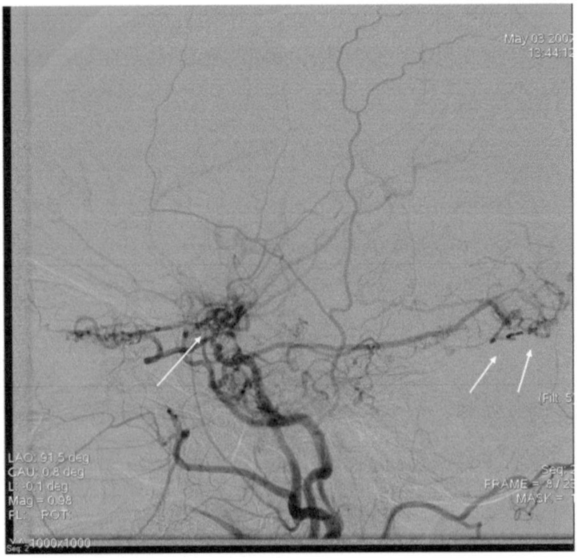

Fig. 28.3 Network of blood vessels in cerebral angiography

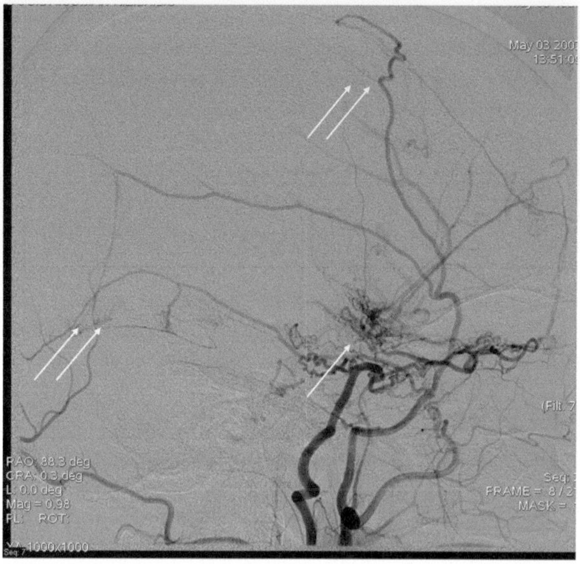

Fig. 28.4 Cerebral angiographic image of the patients

No evidence of atherosclerosis, dissection, or secondary causes such as craniopharyngioma or sickle cell disease was found. The imaging and clinical findings met the diagnostic criteria for Moyamoya disease.

Given the absence of transient ischemic attacks, strokes, or hemorrhagic events and the currently stable neurological status, no immediate surgical intervention was planned. A conservative management strategy focusing on headache control was adopted. The patient was counseled regarding the nature of Moyamoya disease and the need for regular follow-up and vascular monitoring. Symptomatic treatment with triptan alternatives and migraine prophylaxis was initiated cautiously, considering potential vasoconstrictive effects.

28.3 Case Discussion

This case highlights the often under-recognized presentation of Moyamoya disease with migraine-like headaches as the primary or even sole manifestation, particularly in adults. The long history of stable, non-disabling headaches followed by a recent, unexplained escalation in attack frequency and severity should alert the clinician to reconsider the initial diagnosis and evaluate for underlying structural or vascular abnormalities.

The absence of focal deficits or classic ischemic episodes may delay diagnosis, especially in patients with a long-standing migraine history. However, certain red flags—such as a late-onset increase in headache burden, resistance to usual medications, and headaches associated with signs of impaired cerebrovascular reserve—warrant advanced neuroimaging. In this case, progressive bilateral ICA occlusion and basal collateral formation were consistent with Moyamoya disease and dramatically changed the clinical trajectory.

While surgical revascularization is typically considered for ischemic or hemorrhagic complications, headache itself is increasingly recognized as a symptom worthy of monitoring in Moyamoya patients due to its possible association with cerebral hypoperfusion or compensatory collateral circulation overload.

28.4 Clinical Characteristics

Headache is a frequently under-recognized symptom in Moyamoya disease (MMD), often overshadowed by its more dramatic ischemic or hemorrhagic presentations. Yet, growing evidence underscores that headache may be the disease's first—and in some cases the only—manifestation, especially in adults [4–6]. As such, it carries significant diagnostic value and should prompt careful consideration in the appropriate clinical context.

The pathophysiology of Moyamoya-associated headaches is complex and multifactorial. One prominent theory involves chronic cerebral hypoperfusion, which can result in ischemia-induced activation of nociceptors in pain-sensitive intracranial structures [6]. Another mechanism includes the mechanical distension or tortuosity of collateral vessels, which may irritate the dura or surrounding tissues, triggering pain via the trigeminovascular pathway [1]. Additionally, altered cerebrovascular autoregulation and fluctuating perfusion pressures may sensitize central pain-processing networks and contribute to migrainous features [8].

In the case presented, the patient had a long history of migraine-like headaches, but a recent shift in frequency and severity suggested a secondary etiology. Such evolution in headache phenotype should be a red flag, especially in patients without prior neuroimaging or a history of progressive disease [5, 7]. Importantly, this shift represents a diagnostic opportunity: headache may act as a clinical "early warning sign" preceding irreversible ischemic events, mainly when supported by subtle imaging findings [3].

28.5 Diagnosis

The differential diagnosis for a unilateral, throbbing headache with associated nausea, vomiting, and photophobia is broad. The primary consideration is migraine without aura, given the symptomatic overlap. However, several distinguishing features can guide clinicians toward alternative diagnoses:

- Reversible Cerebral Vasoconstriction Syndrome (RCVS): Presents with recurrent thunderclap headaches, often bilateral and severe, and may include focal deficits or seizures. Unlike Moyamoya, RCVS typically has a reversible angiographic pattern over weeks [6].

- Cerebral Arterial Dissection: Especially in younger patients, carotid or vertebral dissections may cause hemicranial headaches with Horner's syndrome or focal neurological signs. MRI/MRA and vessel wall imaging help differentiate this from Moyamoya.
- Giant Cell Arthritis (GCA) is an essential consideration in patients > over 50. It presents with a new-onset headache, scalp tenderness, jaw claudication, and elevated inflammatory markers. Temporal artery biopsy and imaging are diagnostic.
- Cerebral Venous Sinus Thrombosis (CVST): Typically presents with diffuse or frontal headache, possibly with papilledema, seizures, or altered mental status. MR venography is the gold standard for diagnosis.
- Idiopathic Intracranial Hypertension (IIH): It presents with diffuse headache, visual symptoms, and papilledema, more common in obese women of childbearing age. Routine imaging with elevated opening pressure on lumbar puncture is diagnostic.
- Brain Tumors or Mass Lesions: A headache due to a mass effect is often worse in the morning or with Valsalva and may be associated with vomiting or neurological deficits.
- Primary Angiitis of the CNS (PACNS): This is rare but important. It causes subacute headaches, cognitive decline, and multifocal infarcts. Vessel imaging and, in some cases, a brain biopsy are needed to diagnose it.

When Moyamoya disease is the underlying pathology, standard migraine treatments are often inadequate or even contraindicated, particularly vasoconstrictive agents like triptans or ergot derivatives, which may exacerbate cerebral hypoperfusion [4, 5]. Thus, accurate diagnosis is not only crucial for disease monitoring and stroke prevention but also essential to tailor appropriate symptomatic treatments and avoid iatrogenic harm.

In contrast to classic migraine, Moyamoya-related headaches may lack aura and often evolve in frequency or severity over time. Moreover, they are sometimes exacerbated by physical exertion or hyperventilation, likely due to impaired vascular reactivity and decreased reserve capacity in affected territories [6]. These distinguishing features, when recognized, can guide clinicians toward timely neurovascular imaging.

Radiological imaging is pivotal in identifying Moyamoya disease and excluding other entities in this complex differential. Non-contrast CT is often normal in early stages, but MRI with FLAIR sequences may reveal slow-flow signal abnormalities and subtle ischemic changes. Magnetic resonance angiography (MRA) typically reveals stenosis or occlusion of the terminal internal carotid arteries (ICAs) and the proliferation of fine basal collateral vessels, which is often more visible with contrast-enhanced techniques [10]. Digital subtraction angiography (DSA) remains the gold standard for diagnosis, characteristically demonstrating bilateral or unilateral ICA occlusion at the supraclinoid segment; basal collateral vessels with a "puff of smoke" appearance, resulting from compensatory lenticulostriate and thalamoperforator networks; collaterals arising from the external carotid system and the vertebrobasilar circulation as disease progresses [1]. In some cases, perfusion MRI or single photon emission computed tomography (SPECT) can reveal regions of delayed cerebral blood flow and impaired vascular reactivity, offering insights into headache mechanisms and guiding surgical planning.

28.6 Conclusion

In conclusion, headache should be regarded as a potential sentinel symptom of Moyamoya disease, especially in patients with atypical features, progression of previously stable headache patterns, or resistance to standard treatments. Early neurovascular imaging and heightened clinical awareness can facilitate earlier diagnosis, allowing for timely intervention and stroke prevention [6, 8]. In this context, the neurology clinic becomes not only a place of symptom management but also of life-changing early detection.

28.7 Key Messages

- Headache can be the first and sometimes only symptom of Moyamoya disease, particularly in adult patients. Clinicians should maintain a high index of suspicion when evaluating patients with new-onset, changing, or refractory headaches.
- Migraine-like features (unilateral, throbbing pain, photophobia, nausea) are standard in Moyamoya-related headaches, which may lead to misdiagnosis and delayed imaging.
- Red flag signs, such as an abrupt increase in attack frequency, resistance to typical treatments, or changes in headache pattern after years of stability, should prompt evaluation for secondary causes, including Moyamoya disease.
- Differential diagnosis includes primary headache disorders and secondary causes such as RCVS, cerebral vasculitis, arterial dissection, CVST, and tumors. Neurovascular imaging is essential to differentiate Moyamoya from these mimics.
- Conventional migraine therapies, especially vasoconstrictors, may be inappropriate or harmful in Moyamoya disease due to compromised cerebral perfusion.
- MRI, MRA, and DSA remain the gold standards for diagnosis, with the "puff of smoke" angiographic appearance being a hallmark finding.

References

1. Kuroda S, Houkin K. Moyamoya disease: current concepts and future perspectives. Lancet Neurol. 2008;7(11):1056–66. https://doi.org/10.1016/S1474-4422(08)70240-0.
2. Research Committee on the Pathology and Treatment of Spontaneous Occlusion of the Circle of Willis; Health Labour Sciences Research Grant for Research on Measures for Infractable Diseases. Guidelines for diagnosis and treatment of moyamoya disease (spontaneous occlusion of the circle of Willis). Neurol Med Chir (Tokyo). 2012;52(5):245–66. https://doi.org/10.2176/nmc.52.245.
3. Smith ER, Scott RM. Moyamoya: epidemiology, presentation, and diagnosis. Neurosurg Clin N Am. 2010;21(3):543–51. https://doi.org/10.1016/j.nec.2010.03.007.
4. Prabhu N, et al. Unraveling the mystery: headache as a presenting symptom of moyamoya disease. J Neurol Sci. 2024;455:121659. https://doi.org/10.1016/j.jns.2023.121659.
5. Zach V, Bezov D, Lipton RB, Ashina S. Headache associated with moyamoya disease: a case story and literature review. J Headache Pain. 2010;11(1):79–82. https://doi.org/10.1007/s10194-009-0181-8.
6. Chiang CC, Shahid AH, Harriott AM, Tietjen GE, Savastano LE, Klaas JP, et al. Evaluation and treatment of headache associated with moyamoya disease – a narrative review. Cephalalgia. 2022;42(6):542–52. https://doi.org/10.1177/03331024211056250.
7. Malone M, Ritchie D. The mystery of a unilateral headache ultimately diagnosed as Moyamoya disease. Cureus. 2022;14(7):e26816. https://doi.org/10.7759/cureus.26816.
8. Gao B, Kang K, Zhang J, Zhang D, Zhao X. Clinical characteristics and long-term outcome of headaches associated with Moyamoya disease in the Chinese population – a cohort study. Front Neurol. 2020;11:605636. https://doi.org/10.3389/fneur.2020.605636.
9. Kraemer M, Lee SI, Ayzenberg I, Schwitalla JC, Diehl RR, Berlit P, et al. Headache in Caucasian patients with Moyamoya angiopathy – a systematic cohort study. Cephalalgia. 2017;37(5):496–500. https://doi.org/10.1177/0333102416643516.
10. Muljadi R, Koesbandono, Pratama TA, Octavius GS. Moyamoya disease and moyamoya syndrome: a case series from multicentre private hospitals in Indonesia. Neurocirugia (Astur : Engl Ed). Forthcoming 2024. https://doi.org/10.1016/j.neucie.2024.11.001. (DOI assumed for completion—please update when available).
11. Seol HJ, Wang KC, Kim SK, Hwang YS, Kim KJ, Cho BK. Headache in pediatric moyamoya disease: review of 204 consecutive cases. J Neurosurg Pediatr. 2005;103(5 Suppl):439–42. https://doi.org/10.3171/ped.2005.103.5.0439.

Chapter 29
Migraine-Like Aura Attributed to Cerebral Amyloid Angiopathy (CAA)

Maria Eduarda Nobre

29.1 Introduction

Cerebral amyloid angiopathy (CAA), also known as cerebral congophilic angiopathy due to the presence of abnormal amyloid aggregations demonstrated by microscopic examination of brain tissue after staining with Congo red, is a condition characterized by the deposition of amyloid-beta peptides in the walls of cerebral blood vessels. This deposition can lead to various neurological symptoms and complications, including an increased risk of hemorrhagic stroke, particularly in normotensive and elderly patients [1].

CAA has been recognized since the early twentieth century, with early observations suggesting that CAA was a likely cause of nontraumatic primary cerebral hemorrhage, producing stroke in a significant proportion of affected individuals. While CAA is more commonly associated with cognitive decline and intracerebral hemorrhages, some patients may experience migraine-like aura as a symptom [1].

29.2 Pathophysiology

Migraine aura refers to a range of neurological symptoms that typically occur before a migraine headache, including visual disturbances, sensory changes, or motor weakness. The exact mechanism by which CAA may produce migraine-like aura is not entirely understood, but it is believed to be related to the effects of amyloid deposition on vascular function and cerebral blood flow [1, 2].

Amyloids are fibrillary protein assemblies composed of monomers that form beta-sheet structures and aggregate into long fibers. In September 2020, the

M. E. Nobre (✉)
Fluminense Federal University, Rio de Janeiro, Brazil

D. Uludüz et al. (eds.), *Rare Causes of Headache Disorders*, Headache,
https://doi.org/10.1007/978-3-032-10242-3_29

International Amyloidosis Society identified 36 amyloid proteins that can cause disease in humans, six of which are associated with brain disease, either exclusively or as part of systemic involvement. CAA primarily affects small arteries and arterioles, especially in the cortex and leptomeninges. The deposition of beta-amyloid causes age-related sporadic CAA, while early-onset CAA occurs before age 50 and may include rare monogenic forms [2].

Amyloid deposition damages vessel walls, leading to thickening, hyalinization, and smooth muscle cell loss. This ultimately causes parenchymal brain injury due to both bleeding and ischemia. Sporadic beta-amyloid CAA is the most common form of cerebrovascular amyloidosis, primarily associated with brain hemorrhage and cognitive impairment, either occurring independently or alongside Alzheimer's disease. The distribution of sporadic amyloid-β CAA is predominantly posterior, with the occipital lobe most affected [2, 3].

CAA is a significant cause of intracerebral hemorrhage (ICH) in the elderly and can also lead to transient focal neurological episodes (TFNE). TFNE presents as recurrent, stereotyped attacks linked to cortical superficial siderosis (cSS). The definitions of TFNE and migraine aura—described as positive, reversible neurological symptoms following a sequential pattern according to the third edition of International Classification of Headache Disorders (ICHD-3)—overlap. The relationship between migraine and cerebrovascular disease has long been recognized, but the underlying pathophysiological basis remains unclear [4].

29.3 Case Presentation

J.S. is a 72-year-old male engineer with a history of hypertension, hyperlipidemia, and mild cognitive impairment who presented to the emergency department with complaints of visual disturbances and transient episodes of right-sided weakness occurring over the past few weeks. He described episodes lasting approximately 20–30 min, beginning with flickering lights in his left visual field that gradually progressed to blurry vision. These visual symptoms were sometimes followed by numbness and tingling in his right hand, which resolved once the visual disturbances subsided. He also reported mild frontotemporal pulsatile headache and photophobia, without accompanying nausea, which responded well to paracetamol. These episodes had occurred four times over the past month, with increasing frequency.

Neurological examination revealed that he was alert and fully oriented, with no focal neurological deficits identified. Brain magnetic resonance imaging (MRI) showed cortical and subcortical microbleeds predominantly in the occipital and parietal lobes, along with evidence of superficial siderosis. No signs of acute infarction or hemorrhage were detected. Routine blood work, including coagulation profile and metabolic panel, returned within normal limits.

Given the imaging findings, the patient's age, and cognitive history, a diagnosis of cerebral amyloid angiopathy (CAA) was considered. The nature of his transient visual and sensory symptoms—occurring in the absence of significant headache—was consistent with migraine-like aura attributed to CAA, a known but underrecognized manifestation of the disease.

29.4 Clinical Presentation

A retrospective study conducted between 2012 and 2018 investigated migraine prevalence and symptomatology in patients with familial CAA (D-CAA), correlating migraine history with ICH onset, ICH location, and cSS presence on MRI. Among 86 carriers, 48 (56%) had a positive migraine history, mostly among women (60%). According to ICHD-3 criteria, 39 (45%) had definite migraine, with all migraine sufferers experiencing aura. Specifically:

- 42% had only visual auras.
- 12% experienced additional sensory aura symptoms.
- 5% had additional aphasia.
- 24% had typical aura without headache, with 14% reporting this as their only migraine attack type.

The age of onset for migraine with aura showed two peaks: one before the third decade and another after the fourth decade. The prevalence of migraine in D-CAA was significantly higher for both men (51%) and women (59%) compared to the general Dutch population (lifetime prevalence: 13% in men and 33% in women). Notably, all D-CAA patients with migraine experienced visual aura. Single aura symptoms lasting more than 60 min were observed in 23% of patients. While prolonged aura is common in the general population, it is concerning in D-CAA carriers, as it indicates acute ICH in 55% of cases [4].

Migraine-like aura has been reported in rare monogenic cerebrovascular syndromes and may serve as an early hallmark or isolated symptom. Examples include cerebral autosomal dominant arteriopathy with subcortical infarcts and leukoencephalopathy, as well as retinal vasculopathy with cerebral leukoencephalopathy and systemic manifestations. These findings suggest a link between migraine and microvascular changes during the early stages of angiopathies [5].

Numerous monogenic disorders may manifest with aura, occasionally presenting as "true" migraine with aura, fulfilling ICHD-3 criteria. These disorders affect various biological pathways, including ion channels, vascular proteins, and mitochondrial metabolism, contributing to increased susceptibility to spreading depolarization—an underlying mechanism of aura. Therefore, a distinct clinical classification from typical migraine is warranted for patients with hereditary conditions, necessitating tailored management strategies [4, 5].

29.5 Diagnosis

Neurological symptoms, such as cerebral hemorrhagic manifestations, transient focal neurological episodes, memory clinic indicators, headache, or migraine-like aura, must be considered [2, 4].

Imaging tests, including magnetic resonance imaging (MRI) and computed tomography (CT) scans, are essential. Predominantly involving the small cortical and leptomeningeal vessels, amyloid-β CAA can be identified in life by characteristic hemorrhagic structural imaging markers on blood-sensitive MRI sequences, namely cortical superficial siderosis and lobar cerebral microbleeds. These hemorrhagic imaging markers, along with symptomatic bleeding events, such as parenchymal ICH and acute convexity subarachnoid hemorrhage, form the basis of the diagnostic Boston criteria [2–4].

Other nonhemorrhagic imaging features, such as cerebral atrophy, white matter hyperintensities, and MRI-visible perivascular spaces in the centrum semi-ovale (CSO-PVS), are also commonly observed in sporadic CAA. Although these are not necessarily specific to CAA, white matter hyperintensities in a "multispot" pattern and CSO-PVS have been included in the most recent Boston criteria (Version 2.0). There are also CT-based diagnostic criteria for CAA (the Edinburgh criteria); however, these require knowledge of the epsilon 4 allele (APOE ε4) genotype for complete application. Validation of using the imaging components alone is ongoing, but early suggestions indicate that they do possess diagnostic accuracy [2–4].

As MRI is more widely used for the clinical assessment of various neurological conditions, an increasing number of individuals are identified as having imaging features of CAA, which can be incidental or unexpected findings. Although clinical context is essential for determining their significance, in younger patients presenting with ICH, cognitive symptoms, or transient focal neurological episodes, the presence of these markers may indicate certain rare but essential causes of CAA that warrant specific and focused investigation, with implications for patients and their families [2–4].

Amyloid-PET imaging can also be helpful. However, it is essential to recognize that tracers can bind to other amyloids and are therefore not specific for amyloid-β [2].

Cerebrospinal fluid (CSF) measurement of amyloid-β markers can be valuable, although validated thresholds for the clinical diagnosis of CAA have not yet been established. The presence of CSF amyloid-β1–42 levels or a CSF amyloid-β1–42/1–40 ratio consistent with Alzheimer's disease would support a diagnosis of cerebral beta-amyloidosis [2–4].

Genetic testing may also be necessary in the context of CAA. Hereditary forms associated with mutations in genes like APP (amyloid precursor protein) or PSEN1/PSEN2 (presenilin 1/2) could be identified through genetic testing, especially if there is a family history suggesting genetic predisposition to CAA or early-onset Alzheimer's disease. Thus, genetic testing can help inform diagnosis and management for affected individuals [3–5].

Primary migraines can often present with aura symptoms (visual, sensory, or speech-related) and may occur independently of CAA. A review of the differential diagnosis of late-onset aura (LOA) indicates that TIAs, seizures, subarachnoid hemorrhage, arteriovenous malformation, dural arteriovenous fistula, patent foramen ovale, posterior circulation embolism, internal carotid artery dissection, vertebral artery dissection, carotid artery stenosis, moyamoya disease, brain tumors, and other rare disorders can also mimic migraine aura, in addition to CAA. Therefore, the diagnosis of late-life migraine accompaniments should be made by exclusion through appropriate investigations [3, 4, 6].

29.6 Treatment

The treatment of migraine-like aura associated with cerebral amyloid angiopathy (CAA) primarily aims to manage symptoms and reduce the risk of complications, as there is no specific therapy targeting the aura itself. Symptomatic treatment may include standard migraine medications if the headache follows the aura, although the aura itself typically does not respond to these treatments. Preventive strategies focus on lifestyle modifications such as maintaining proper hydration, ensuring regular sleep patterns, and avoiding known migraine triggers like stress or certain foods. It is also essential to control vascular risk factors—particularly hypertension, hyperlipidemia, and diabetes—as these can exacerbate the underlying pathology and increase the risk of cerebral hemorrhage or ischemic events.

In patients with CAA, the use of anticoagulants is generally avoided due to the heightened risk of intracerebral bleeding, unless there is a compelling indication. Education of the patient and family is a key part of the management strategy, emphasizing awareness of potential neurologic symptoms and the importance of promptly reporting any new changes. Ongoing monitoring through regular neurologic follow-up is crucial to evaluate disease progression and to adjust the treatment plan as needed.

Ultimately, management should be individualized based on the frequency and severity of aura episodes, the presence of associated headaches, and the patient's overall health status. A collaborative, multidisciplinary approach allows for a personalized care plan that addresses both the symptoms of migraine-like aura and the complexities of cerebral amyloid angiopathy.

29.7 Conclusion

Migraine with aura is an important, often inaugural symptom of CAA. Aura attacks lasting ≥60 min may signal acute ICH in CAA. Migraine with aura may be regarded as an early marker of disease in hereditary CAA, potentially preceding the occurrence of symptomatic ICH by several years [4]. Although mostly benign, late-onset aura (LOA) must be differentiated from secondary causes [6]. Blood-sensitive magnetic resonance imaging sequences are the best tools for the early detection of underlying pathology; therefore, treatment with antiplatelet or anticoagulant drugs should be avoided, as these may increase the risk of hemorrhage [6].

Management of patients with CAA and migraine-like symptoms focuses on treating underlying risk factors, monitoring for complications, and sometimes employing standard migraine treatments if warranted. However, caution is advised, as specific migraine treatments may increase the risk of hemorrhage in patients with CAA [6, 7].

References

1. Vinters HV. Cerebral amyloid angiopathy: a critical review. Stroke. 1987;18(2):311–24. https://doi.org/10.1161/01.str.18.2.311. PMID: 3551211.
2. Banerjee G, Collinge J, Fox NC, Lashley T, Mead S, Schott JM, Werring DJ, Ryan NS. Clinical considerations in early-onset cerebral amyloid angiopathy. Brain. 2023;146(10):3991–4014. https://doi.org/10.1093/brain/awad193.
3. Smith EE, Charidimou A, Ayata C, Werring DJ, Greenberg SM. Cerebral amyloid angiopathy-related transient focal neurologic episodes. Neurology. 2021;97(5):231–8. https://doi.org/10.1212/WNL.0000000000012234. Epub 2021 May 20. PMID: 34016709; PMCID: PMC8356377.
4. Koemans EA, Voigt S, Rasing I, Van Etten ES, Van Zwet EW, Van Walderveen MAA, Wermer MJH, Terwindt GM. Migraine with aura as early disease marker in hereditary Dutch-type cerebral amyloid angiopathy. Stroke. 2020;51(4):1094–9. https://doi.org/10.1161/STROKEAHA.119.028170.
5. Pensato U, Demchuk AM, Dreier JP, Brennan KC, Sacco S, Romoli M. Aura phenomenon: a proposal for an etiology-based clinical classification. J Headache Pain. 2025;26(9):1–9. https://doi.org/10.1186/s10194-024-01943-8.
6. Samanci B, Coban O, Baykan B. Late onset aura may herald cerebral amyloid angiopathy: a case report. Cephalalgia. 2016;36(10):998–1001. https://doi.org/10.1177/0333102415620253. Epub 2015 Nov 26. PMID: 26611682.
7. Paterson RW, Uchino K, Emsley HC, Pullicino P. Recurrent stereotyped episodes in cerebral amyloid angiopathy: response to migraine prophylaxis in two patients. Cerebrovasc Dis Extra. 2013;3(1):81–4. https://doi.org/10.1159/000347114. PMID: 23741226; PMCID: PMC3670647.

Chapter 30
Headache Attributed to Pituitary Apoplexy

Carolina Martins, Jesuíno Albino, Juliana Andrade, and Marcelo Valença

30.1 Introduction

Apoplexy derives from a Greek root and means "a sudden blow." In medicine, it is used to characterize the sudden onset of a set of signals and symptoms (hence, a syndrome), usually related to the infarction of hemorrhage of an organ or structure. When no anatomical findings accompany such a syndrome, the term functional apoplexy is applied.

Pituitary apoplexy, therefore, is a term used to describe a sudden constellation of signs and symptoms related to endocrinological, visual, oculomotor, or meningeal symptoms resulting from vascular changes (infarction, hemorrhage or both) within the sellar content. Apoplexy happens in the context of adenomas, Rathke cysts and several other pituitary lesions, including normal pituitary glands in especial conditions (pregnancy, puerperal period) [1]. Nevertheless, it is commonly seen in the setting of an undiagnosed pituitary adenoma [2].

The incidence of apoplexy in pituitary adenomas when considering clinical and surgical or histopathological evidence is 2–7% [3]. This combination of factors must be differentiated from the findings of hemorrhagic infarction in lesions harbored by asymptomatic patients which reach up to 25% [3]. This differentiation is paramount because the latter does not conform with a diagnosis of pituitary

C. Martins (✉) · J. Andrade · M. Valença
Department of Neuropsychiatry, Federal University of Pernambuco (UFPE), Recife, Brazil
e-mail: maria.cmlima@ufpe.br

J. Albino
Neurocirurgia Assistência e Ensino (NAE), Recife, Brazil

D. Uludüz et al. (eds.), *Rare Causes of Headache Disorders*, Headache,
https://doi.org/10.1007/978-3-032-10242-3_30

apoplexy. Pituitary apoplexy was first described as a syndrome by Pearce Bailey, in 1898 [3], it received this denomination in 1950, by Brougham et al. [4].

Lesions of the sellar and parasellar regions are a common finding in the general population and their incidental findings on cadaveric and health volunteer imaging studies vary from 1.7% to 27% [5]. On the other hand, headache as a presenting complaint among patients with pituitary lesions range from 33% to 73%, consistently higher than the prevalence of headaches in the general population, meaning that sellar lesions do cause headache—and in fact this is often the primary reason leading to the diagnosis [5]. Because scant data exist on the specific improvement of headache after surgical treatment of sellar/parasellar lesions, it remains challenging to indicate surgical resection in patients harboring these lesions—and no other sign or symptom.

Among sellar lesions, adenomas are the most frequent, occurring in 20% of the general population [6], from childhood to the elderly, and most of them being incidental and asymptomatic (at the most 5% of adenomas are symptomatic) [5]. Adenomas can be classified by (a) size—as microadenomas (less 10 mm), macroadenomas (more than 10 mm), and giant macroadenomas (more than 40 mm in greatest dimension), (b) hormonal production—as functional and non-functional, (c) histology, or (d) biologic behavior [6]. Among functional adenomas, prolactinomas are the most frequent. Prolactinomas comprise 30% of all adenomas, while nonfunctional adenomas correspond to another 25–30% [6].

This being said, apoplexy, therefore, occurs when a sellar structure—usually a pituitary adenoma—undergoes hemorrhage, infarction, or both. Most cases affect males (twice as likely to present with apoplexy) [7], during fifth or sixth decade of life, often on previously unidentified non-functional adenomas or prolactinomas.

Because apoplexy differs significantly from the incidental finding of a sellar/parasellar lesion during the investigation of a headache patient, the surgical considerations made above do not apply. It is fundamental to understand that apoplexy results in a life-threatening situation with pressing goals that take precedence over (but fortunately overlapping) with the relief of the headache.

30.2 Clinical Case

A 37-year-old male was transferred to a tertiary, neurovascular unit hours after having presented himself at his district health unit, with a sudden and severe headache, vomiting, and decrease in visual acuity. Although his admission occurred two months into the official coronavirus disease 2019 (COVID-19) pandemic period in our region—and at a time when no specific diagnostic tests were available—suspected patients were in small numbers, community spread low, and it was still possible to keep infected patients segregated within a part of our health network. The headache woke him out of sleep, and he experienced sudden vomiting at the installation of the complaints. Neurological examination at the emergency department showed Glasgow Coma Scale of 12 out of 15. He was restless and anxious, complaining of a throbbing headache. He was not cushingoid, acromegalic, or eunuchoid and no gynecomastia or galactorrhea was present. Unable to help with the bedside visual acuity test, the patient kept repeating that he could not see well, especially with his left eye. There was a sluggish light reflex bilaterally and a questionable nuchal rigidity. A subarachnoid hemorrhage was the initial diagnostic assumption, as no previous medical history of a sellar lesion existed. A computed tomography (CT) scan (Fig. 30.1A–D), however, showed an enlarged sella and an intrasellar lesion that extended to the suprasellar space and protruded towards the cavernous sinuses, particularly on the left. A bright, thin halo on the top of the lesion suggested focal subarachnoid intracranial hemorrhage. The patient was admitted to the intensive care unit (ICU) with the diagnosis of apoplectic, previously undiagnosed sellar lesion and routine preoperative exams as well as hormonal serum profile were collected. An endovenous (EV) bolus of hydrocortisone 500 mg was administered before surgery, while awaiting the results of the hormonal profile. Five hours after admission he was taken to the operating room (OR) and a microsurgical transsphenoidal surgery with endoscopic assistance performed. During surgery, the bony sellar floor was found thinned and eroded, with a tense sellar dura prolapsing towards the sphenoidal sinus. Dural opening initially relieved a liquified, reddish bloody content and further material was collected under the surgical microscope with transsphenoidal microsurgical curettes. The endoscope was introduced to explore the cavity at the end of the procedure and further laterally displaced material removed, except on the right side, where the pituitary gland seemed to have been displaced. The sella floor was closed using a bony fragment reserved from the sphenoidal rostrum during the approach, supported by Gelfoam cubes. The surgical procedure was undertaken under 150 minutes. At the immediate postop period, the patient indicated relief both of his headache and visual disturbances. The same-day postop CT scan (Fig. 30.1E–H), 17 hours after the admission CT, showed adequate sellar decompression. Preop serum profile disclosed only mild elevation of serum prolactin, compatible with infundibular compression by a non-secreting pituitary adenoma, later confirmed by histopathology. The postop period was uneventful, during which first line, EV, analgesic drugs, were administered, when needed, and were enough to control his headache. Oral hydrocortisone was swiftly tapered off while monitoring the urinary density and output. The patient was able to perform a campimetry on the third postop day. He was discharged on the fourth postop day, after repetition of the hormonal profile and having the first endocrinologic outpatient consultation scheduled within a fortnight. The first neurosurgical outpatient follow-up, scheduled in four weeks' time included evaluation of postop magnetic resonance imaging (MRI) and comparative campimetry.

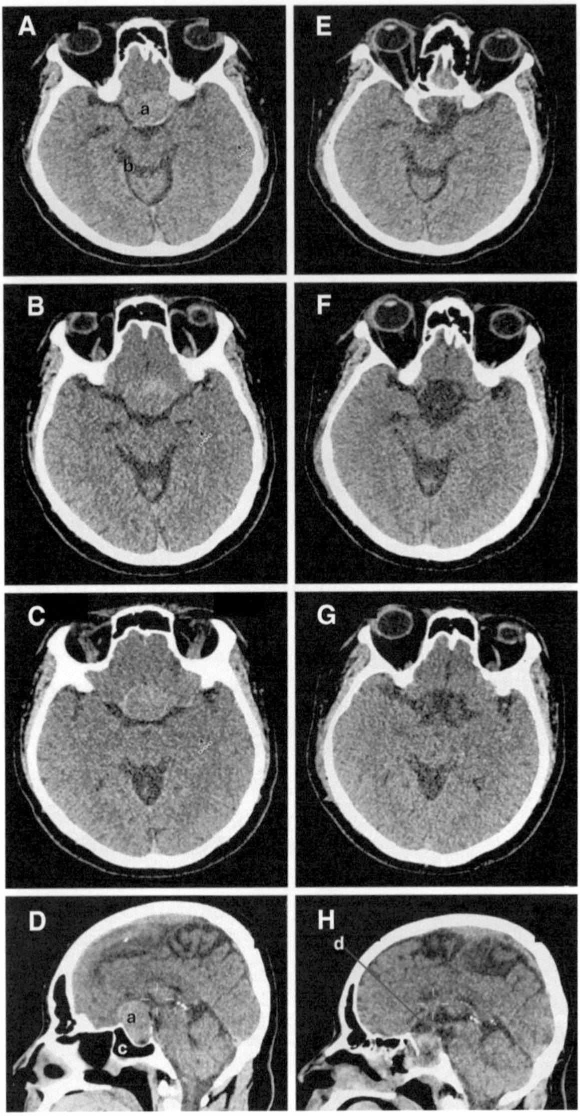

Fig. 30.1 (**A**–**D**) Emergency room (ER) admission, non-contrast CT scans on axial (**A**–**C**) and sagittal (D) planes. A predominantly hyperdense sellar lesion extended to the suprasellar area (**a**). A hyperdense halo is seen around the edges of the lesion. The floor of the III ventricle and infundibulum cannot be seen on the sagittal view, but the subarachnoid cisterns are opened (**b**), and the sulci and gyri can be delineated, suggesting an absence of significant elevation of global intracranial pressure. The floor of the sella did not—at first—seem thinned, but it was found during surgery to be eroded and breached, with a tense, bulging sellar dura protruding into the sphenoid sinus (**c**) suggesting increase intrasellar pressure. (**E**–**H**). Postoperative, non-enhanced CT scan obtained 17 hours after admission. Adequate debulking of the lesion has been achieved, but for a small remnant on the right of the sella that seemed particularly stuck during surgery. With decompression of the sella, the floor of the III ventricle and infundibulum (**d**) could then be seen (H).

30.3 Clinical Presentation

Typically, signs and symptoms of pituitary apoplexy start abruptly with (a) headache, (b) vomiting and (c) disturbance in consciousness, (d) visual disturbance (visual loss, field defects or ophthalmoplegia), and (e) acute hypopituitarism [6]. Signs and symptoms associated with pituitary apoplexy may have different proposed pathogenesis (Box 30.1).

The resulting syndrome may be mild but often presents as a catastrophic event and may be initially attributed to stroke or subarachnoid hemorrhage [2], resulting that these patients will often be seen in neurovascular reference centers—as happened in the index-case, presented above.

Pituitary apoplexy was the clinical manifestation that led to the diagnosis of a pituitary lesion in more than 80% of cases [3] and in up to 97.4% of patients [4].

Box 30.1 Signs and symptoms associated with pituitary apoplexy and their proposed pathogenesis

Headache	Intrasellar contents rapidly increase in size leading to dural stretching Pain is transmitted through meningeal nerves supplying the central skull base dura	Sellar wall enlargement causes displacement of the superior division of the trigeminal nerve (CNV1) within the cavernous sinus	With vomiting and altered consciousness, the headache can be part of intracranial hypertensive syndrome that can be due to enlargement of sellar contents only, to subarachnoid hemorrhage or obstructive hydrocephalus
Nausea and vomiting	With headache and altered consciousness, nausea and vomiting can be part of intracranial hypertensive syndrome	Can signal adrenal insufficiency	Can signal hypothalamic dysfunction
Visual field defects	Optic nerve, chiasm, or tract impingement by upward displacement of intrasellar contents		
Reduced visual acuity	As a part of CNII deficit syndrome can be cause by optical apparatus Displacement		
Reduced level of consciousness	With headache, nausea, and vomiting can be part of intracranial hypertensive syndrome	Due to hypothalamic involvement	Due to adrenal insufficiency

Although headache is described as the earliest symptom [3], present in most (84–89.8%) [5, 8] or all patients [9] with apoplexy—while visual loss and ophthalmoparesis are only described in 52–57% of the patients at presentation [9, 10]—the type, localization, and severity of the headache are seldom detailed.

The literature available mentions sudden and severe headache that can be retro-orbital, bifrontal, or diffuse [3] and combined with nausea and vomiting. Apoplexy patients usually describe a significant short duration of the headache (1–10 days) than the non-apoplexy patients harboring sellar lesions (4 days–30 years) [5].

Cranial nerve palsy may involve III, IV, and VI, and usually signal the extension of apoplectic tumor to a specific cavernous sinus compartment [11–13]. In the case of early III nerve involvement, superolateral expansion may displace the nerve, which is located horizontally in the same plane as the pituitary gland [10] and against its entry dural point (the oculomotor porus) at the cavernous sinus oculomotor trigone [14]. An ischemic cranial nerve syndrome can also result from compression of dural arteries supplying the transdural, cavernous segments of these nerves. Because these vessels arise at the cavernous segment of the internal carotid artery and also supply the meningeal layers in the central skull base [15] a similar pathophysiology can explain the headache and ophthalmoparesis in apoplectic patients.

Hypopituitarism is usually considered when there is proof of biochemical deficiency of at least one endocrine axis. When prolactin is elevated, a differentiation should be made between the elevation related to infundibular compression of the pituitary stalk which decreases dopamine inhibition to the pituitary gland (levels of less than 250 ng/mL) and an elevation that signals a prolactin-secreting tumor (higher than 1000 ng/mL) [16].

Patients with pituitary apoplexy and low serum prolactin at presentation are deemed to have the highest intrasellar pressure and be prone to poor recovery [3] after decompressive surgery, making their management even more time pressing, explaining the expedite treatment offered to our case-example.

Secondary electrolyte abnormalities and acid–base imbalance are usually responsible for other life-risking findings as arrhythmia [17], but bradycardia may result from distortion of III ventricular walls and resulting hypothalamic dysfunction.

Acute secondary adrenal insufficiency is seen in approximately two-third of apoplectic patients and can be a major source of mortality [3]. Hypocortisolemia renders vasculature less responsive to pressor effects of catecholamines, which results in hemodynamic instability. It also augments vasopressin release from the posterior pituitary lobe inhibiting water excretion and resulting in dilution hyponatremia. Particularly in patients undergoing surgery and additional metabolic requirements, prompt empirical corticosteroid replacement should be undertaken, with hydrocortisone intravenously at first, but orally as soon as viable and possible. If the oral route remains closed, the intramuscular route should be elected instead, because of the saturation kinetics of cortisol binding globulin [3]. Once recovered from acute stress, the hydrocortisone should be quickly tapered. For biochemically-proven insufficient-patients, a standard maintenance dose is 20–30 mg per day, orally, usually divided into three doses, and reevaluation of adrenocorticotropic hormone (ACTH) reserve reassessed at three months follow-up [3].

The headache pathogenesis in an apoplexy can be multifactorial: (a) with the vascular changes taking place in the sella, a sudden surge in the sellar pressure, distending its meningeal walls is a possible mechanism—this hypothesis is reinforced by the fact that sellar decompression is usually able to improve this symptom, and (b) the hemorrhagic changes happening within the sella may reach the subarachnoidal space. Both hypotheses uphold in the case presented: intraoperative findings consistent with elevated intrasellar pressure were seen in our patient, as well as meningeal signs at admission and a certain amount of blood in the basal cisterns was deemed present in the initial CT. Although transop intrasellar pressure recordings have been reported, this method still awaits further validation [5] to become routinely used.

30.4 Differential Diagnosis

Because pituitary apoplexy syndrome may share a commonality of symptoms and signs with other common neurological emergencies such as subarachnoid hemorrhage, bacterial meningitis or stroke [3], this diagnosis may be delayed or missed.

Most apoplexies seem spontaneous, but causal roles have been identified in up to 40% of cases [3]. These range from the most frequent—hypertension—through a wide array of contributing factors, including dopamine agonist therapy (bromocriptine and cabergoline) [1], estrogen treatment, radiation therapy of pituitary tumors [1], head trauma, thrombocytopenia, lymphocytic leukemia, sickle cell anemia [4], pregnancy, arteriography, lumbar puncture, myelography, pneumoencephalography, recent surgery, use of anticoagulants, increased intracranial pressure, and pituitary function tests [1, 18], to the least common—major surgery [3]; causal factors abound.

Factors implied on the pathogenesis of apoplexy include (a) the close relationship between the portal vessels and the diaphragm sellae, (b) the critical size of a tumor inside a semi-rigid sella and (c) the tumor metabolic activity versus its vascularization. Some other factors seem to be implied in specific cases. Vascular endothelial growth factor messenger RNA may be increased, particularly in nonfunctioning pituitary adenomas [4].

All these factors for pituitary apoplexy can be arranged into four groups: (a) vascular flux reduction (as in surgical procedures, radiotherapy and after spinal anesthesia), (b) acute increase in blood flow (physical activity and systemic hypertension), (c) pituitary stimulation (as in pituitary function tests), and (d) coagulation disturbances (thrombocytopenia and anticoagulation) [4].

Considering the association of apoplexy and pituitary function tests [18], one should remember that the thyrotropin-releasing hormone (TRH) effect in elevating serum norepinephrine may trigger vasospasm. It can also act directly activating the tumor cells, resulting in higher metabolic demand. Both effects being therefore implicated in apoplectic events.

In apoplexy related to dopamine agonists therapy (bromocriptine and cabergoline) [1], the resulting apoptosis of lactotroph cells reduces metabolic demands and angiogenesis is inhibited, but it is the imbalance between the two that leads to infarctions with hemorrhage or hemorrhage only [1]. In bromocriptine long-term usage, it is the rapid shrinkage of tumor cells and perivascular accumulation of fluid the implicated factors. The disruption of tissue textures seems to be the factor causing hemorrhage within the lesion, but the hypotension induced effect caused by this drug has also been suggested as causal factor in the circulatory disturbances within the capillaries of the region [18]. Cystic degeneration within the prolactinoma which is being treated with a dopamine antagonist, particularly cabergoline, signals previous intratumoral hemorrhage and is considered a predisposition to the development clinical pituitary apoplexy [1].

30.5 Diagnosis

Unenhanced tomogram (CT) is often the first study performed. Although it is fairly sensitive to demonstrate the sellar lesion, usually disclosing a variably hyperdense mass in the sella [6] and suprasellar regions, it is not infrequent that it fails in presenting a small hemorrhage or infarction [18]; therefore, it is the combination of an acute syndrome and a sellar tumor on CT that underscores the diagnosis of pituitary apoplexy and treatment decisions can be made with CT in centers where MRI is not readily available.

MRI is considered the exam of choice and can identify intrinsic hemorrhage, necrosis and provide data on adjacent structures [6]. The findings will depend on the size of tumor, extent of hemorrhage/necrosis, and timing of examination, because—like hemorrhage elsewhere in the brain—the MRI appearance depends on the stage of hemoglobin degradation. Gadolinium IV administration discloses areas of necrosis or infarct that—differently from normal pituitary tissue—stays hypointense.

Endocrinologic assessment involves establishing a hormonal serum profile (serum prolactin, testosterone/estrogen, luteinizing hormone, follicle-stimulating hormone, free thyroxine, thyroid stimulating hormone, growth hormone, insulin-like growth factor-1 and cortisol).

Preop evaluation includes blood count, kidney and liver function, electrolytes, glucose, and coagulation profile.

Early register of the visual fields should be obtained whenever possible but should not postpone treatment. This rationale is based on the observation that significant improvement has been observed in patients rendered blind by the apoplexy if early decompression is undertaken [3]. Campimetry studies performed on the days following surgery can be used as set-point for visual field follow-up, because although improvement is seen in the immediate postoperative period, it often continues for several weeks afterwards [3].

30.6 Treatment

Although alleviating the headache is undoubtedly a focus in the management of these patients, it is not the main priority:

Pituitary apoplexy is a life-threatening complication in which reaching clinical stability, relief of the elevated intracranial pressure, and decompression of the optical apparatus takes clear precedence and should not be delayed longer than the time to stabilize the patient. It is also true that because of the pathogenesis involved in this type of headache (Table 30.1), prioritizing the goal just presented also relieves the headache.

It has been a rule of thumb in the field that if the apoplectic patient has no visual deficits or is making neurological improvements, a conservative treatment may be established. Surgical intervention, by an experienced surgical team, is required whenever the patient presents with visual deficits or deteriorates within the frame of a previously established conservative treatment. Visual field defects and ocular palsy seem to benefit the most from surgical treatment, but there is also a tendency for a protective effect of surgery on visual acuity and pituitary function [19]. Intractable headaches were also listed as indications for surgery in 7.7% of pituitary apoplexy patients [4], but are usually seconded by other indications for surgery.

A lot has been debated about the timing of surgery in apoplectic patients [3, 20]. Urgent decompressive transsphenoidal surgery [4] is the denomination given for the surgical treatment performed within hours (in a semi-elective regimen, as reported in our patient), on the same day or a maximum of 24 hours after the ictus. It is our experience, as well as others [4] that timing of surgery and extent of preop deficits are important factors influencing the final outcome of these patients, and considering headache, early surgery results in prompt control or shortening of the analgesic requirements. A semi-elective regimen takes advantage of a harmonic structure existing within a neurosurgical department in which—while the patient is being stabilized and initially evaluated by the on-call neurosurgical and ICU teams—the group with experience in sellar surgery and handling of the specific equipment is being deployed, in a sequential fashion, to benefit the patient and provide prompt and qualified care as have happened in our case-example.

Surgery (transcranial, transsphenoidal microscopic or endoscopic) resulted in improvement of visual function in 73–80% of cases [18, 21], but the best results are to be expected the sooner visual decompression is performed, particularly in patients presenting with blindness [21]. The goals of the procedure should be debulking of the lesion and decompression of intracranial structures, while avoiding complications that may keep the patient in the ICU, as postoperative fistula (and the following meningitis) or diabetes insipidus.

Transient diabetes insipidus is noted in the postoperative period in up to 16% of patients with pituitary apoplexy [3]. In our department, besides the usual monitoring of serum indicators, urinary output and density have been carefully followed, sometimes only to witness an interval of insufficiency that is but a few hours-long and swiftly recovered in the cases in which the pituitary gland and its stalk are anatomically preserved, suggesting that in fact transient diabetes insipidus can be much more frequent than reported in literature. However, diabetes insipidus is a dreaded complication to be dealt with when it is permanent, taking a considerable tool on the life of the patient, family, and on the health system.

30.7 Conclusion

Patients with pituitary apoplexy should have endocrine, biochemical assessment of pituitary function, formal assessment of visual acuity and fields four to eight weeks after the event. MRIs are recommended three to six months after apoplexy and annually for five years, then two-yearly.

Residual tumor should be followed. Tumor regression after apoplexy is a well-known phenomenon with a clear pathophysiology but is definitely not a done deal. The fate of such a tumor after apoplexy lies on its molecular signature, size of residue, and extent of hemorrhage or infarction [8] and recurrences are also recognized. In such cases, redo surgery or radiotherapy might be indicated [3], depending on the type of lesion.

References

1. Chng E, Dalan R. Pituitary apoplexy associated with cabergoline therapy. J Clin Neurosci. 2013;20:1637–43. https://doi.org/10.1016/j.jocn.2013.02.027.
2. Laws E. Surgical management of pituitary apoplexy. In: Primer on cerebrovascular diseases. Academic; 1997.
3. Rajasekaran S, Vanderpump M, Baldeweg S, Drake W, Reddy N, Lanyon M, et al. UK guidelines for the management of pituitary apoplexy pituitary apoplexy guidelines development group: may 2010. Clin Endocrinol. 2011;74:9–20. https://doi.org/10.1111/j.1365-2265.2010.03913.x.
4. Gondim JA, de Albuquerque LAF, Almeida JP, Bulcao T, Gomes E, Schops M, et al. Endoscopic Endonasal surgery for treatment of pituitary apoplexy: 16 years of experience in a specialized pituitary Center. World Neurosurg. 2017;108:137–42. https://doi.org/10.1016/j.wneu.2017.08.131.
5. Jahangiri A, Wagner JR, Chin AT, Han SW, Tran MT, Miller LM, et al. Incidence of headache as a presenting complaint in over 1000 patients with sellar lesions and factors predicting postoperative improvement. Clin Neurol Neurosurg. 2015;132:16–20. https://doi.org/10.1016/j.clineuro.2015.02.006.
6. Chapman PR, Singhal A, Gaddamanugu S, Prattipati V. Neuroimaging of the pituitary gland: practical anatomy and pathology. Radiol Clin North Am. 2020;58:1115–33. https://doi.org/10.1016/j.rcl.2020.07.009.
7. Martinez-Perez R, Kortz MW, Carroll BW, Duran D, Neill JS, Luzardo GD, et al. Coronavirus disease 2019 and pituitary apoplexy: a single-Center case series and review of the literature. World Neurosurg. 2021;152:e678–87. https://doi.org/10.1016/j.wneu.2021.06.004.
8. Almeida JP, Sanchez MM, Karekezi C, Warsi N, Fernández-Gajardo R, Panwar J, et al. Pituitary apoplexy: results of surgical and conservative management clinical series and review of the literature. World Neurosurg. 2019;130:e988–99. https://doi.org/10.1016/j.wneu.2019.07.055.

9. Oyesiku NM, Tindall GT. Pituitary apoplexy: syndromes and surgical management. Clin Neurol Neurosurg. 1997;99:S243–4. https://doi.org/10.1016/s0303-8467(97)82413-4.
10. Rosso M, Ramaswamy S, Sucharew H, Vagal A, Anziska Y, Levine SR. Isolated third cranial nerve palsy in pituitary apoplexy: case report and systematic review. J Stroke Cerebrovasc Dis. 2021:30. https://doi.org/10.1016/j.jstrokecerebrovasdis.2021.105969.
11. Campero A, Martins C, Yasuda A, Rhoton AL Jr. Microsurgical anatomy of the diaphragma sellae and its role in directing the pattern of growth of pituitary adenomas. Neurosurgery. 2008;62 https://doi.org/10.1227/01.neu.0000317321.79106.37.
12. Campero A, Campero AA, Martins C, Yasuda A, Rhoton AL Jr. Surgical anatomy of the dural walls of the cavernous sinus. J Clin Neurosci. 2010;17 https://doi.org/10.1016/j.jocn.2009.10.015.
13. Yasuda A, Campero A, Martins C, Rhoton AL Jr, Ribas GC. The medial wall of the cavernous sinus: microsurgical anatomy. Neurosurgery. 2004;55:179.
14. Martins C, Yasuda A, Campero A, Rhoton AL Jr. Microsurgical anatomy of the oculomotor cistern. Neurosurgery. 2006;58 https://doi.org/10.1227/01.NEU.0000204673.55834.BE.
15. Martins C, Yasuda A, Campero A, Ulm AJ, Tanriover N, Rhoton A. Microsurgical anatomy of the dural arteries. Neurosurgery. 2005;56 https://doi.org/10.1227/01.NEU.0000144823.94402.3D.
16. Zaidi HA, Cote DJ, Castlen JP, Burke WT, Liu YH, Smith TR, et al. Time course of resolution of hyperprolactinemia after Transsphenoidal surgery among patients presenting with pituitary stalk compression. World Neurosurg. 2017;97:2–7. https://doi.org/10.1016/j.wneu.2016.09.066.
17. Mlawa G, Rehman F. Pituitary tumours and bradycardia/complete heart block-an association or incidental findings? Endocr Abstr. 2017; https://doi.org/10.1530/endoabs.50.p301.
18. Masago A, Ueda Y, Umemura S. Pituitary apoplexy after pituitary function test: a report oftwo cases and review of literature. Surg Neurol. 1995:158–65.
19. Tu M, Lu Q, Zhu P, Zheng W. Surgical versus non-surgical treatment for pituitary apoplexy: a systematic review and meta-analysis. J Neurol Sci. 2016;370:258–62. https://doi.org/10.1016/j.jns.2016.09.047.
20. Sahyouni R, Goshtasbi K, Choi E, Mahboubi H, Le R, Khahera AS, et al. Vision outcomes in early versus late surgical intervention of pituitary apoplexy: meta- analysis. World Neurosurg. 2019;127:52–7. https://doi.org/10.1016/j.wneu.2019.03.133.
21. Lubbe DE, Mankahla N, Carrara H, Semple P. Surgical intervention for binocular blindness in pituitary apoplexy. Interdiscip Neurosurg. 2019:18. https://doi.org/10.1016/j.inat.2019.100490.

Part V
Headache Attributed to Non-vascular Intracranial Disorder

Chapter 31
Headache Attributed to Low Cerebrospinal Fluid (CSF) Pressure

Marcio Nattan Portes Souza and Diogo Guilherme Leão Edelmuth

31.1 Introduction

Spontaneous intracranial hypotension (SIH) is an underdiagnosed secondary headache condition caused by spontaneous cerebrospinal fluid (CSF) leakage, resulting in a spectrum of diverse symptoms and radiological findings. The most common clinical manifestation is orthostatic headache, and the first step of investigation is the brain magnetic resonance imaging (MRI). Advances in imaging and understanding of the underlying mechanisms, including cerebrospinal fluid (CSF)–venous fistulas (CVF), have improved diagnostic accuracy; however, management remains challenging, particularly in patients with complex presentations or comorbidities. This chapter explores the pathophysiology, clinical presentation, diagnostic approaches, and treatment strategies for SIH, grounded in a real-world case that highlights the importance of specialized care, multidisciplinary evaluation, and targeted imaging techniques. Through this lens, we aim to provide clinicians with practical insights and an evidence-based framework to recognize and manage this condition effectively across a range of clinical settings.

31.2 Pathophysiology

Currently, three different etiologies of SIH are recognized: (1) CSF leak due to a nerve root sleeve diverticulum, (2) CSF leak due to an osteophyte spur, and (3) CSF–venous fistula (CVF)(1). In all types, there is a CSF leak from the subarachnoid space to either the epidural space or the intravenous compartment. Despite the CSF volume loss, intracranial pressure measured by lumbar puncture is usually

M. N. P. Souza (✉) · D. G. L. Edelmuth
Hospital Israelita Albert Einstein, Hospital das Clinicas FMUSP, São Paulo, Brazil

D. Uludüz et al. (eds.), *Rare Causes of Headache Disorders*, Headache,
https://doi.org/10.1007/978-3-032-10242-3_31

normal, due to compensatory mechanisms including an increase in intracranial venous volume, which can be identified in some cases by prominent intracranial venous engorgement [1–3]. One important concept is that skull-base CSF leaks typically do not present with the typical symptoms of SIH or neuroimaging signs. Therefore, in cases of SIH presentation, the target of investigation and treatment should be at the spinal levels [4].

31.3 Case Presentation

A 72-year-old man with a history of chronic kidney disease following unilateral nephrectomy, splenomegaly, and prior malignancies (including bladder, renal, intestinal, and prostate cancer) presented with a sudden onset of daily headache, predominantly orthostatic, worsening in the upright position and alleviating with recumbency. He had no previous history of headaches. Brain MRI at the time revealed bilateral subdural hematomas and diffuse pachymeningeal thickening, findings suggestive of spontaneous intracranial hypotension (SIH) (Fig. 31.1).

Spine MRI did not present any longitudinal epidural collection (Fig. 31.2).

After the first week, there was spontaneous improvement in symptoms. A few days later, following a minor motor vehicle accident, the patient experienced clinical deterioration characterized by exacerbation of headaches, postural instability, gait disturbances, and altered level of consciousness. Brain computed tomography (CT) showed enlargement of the subdural hematomas, requiring urgent neurosurgical drainage (Fig. 31.3).

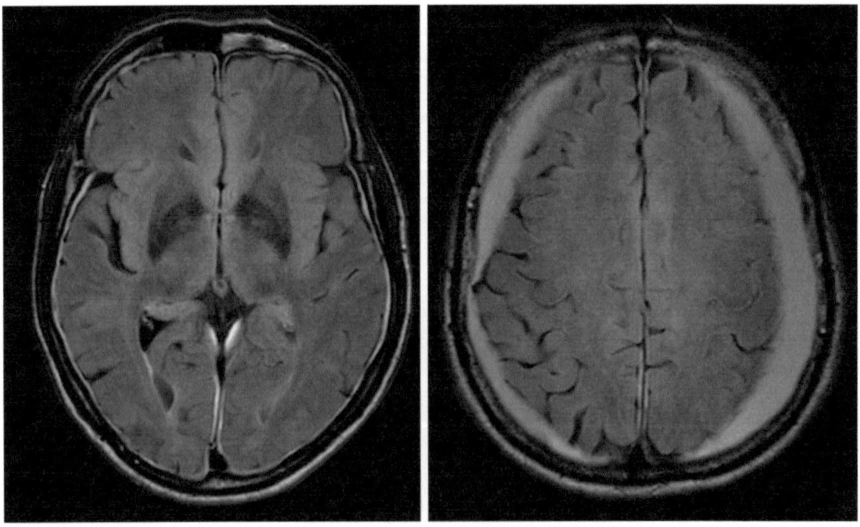

Fig. 31.1 Axial fluid-attenuated inversion recovery (FLAIR) image shows diffuse pachymeningeal thickening and bilateral subdural effusions/hematomas

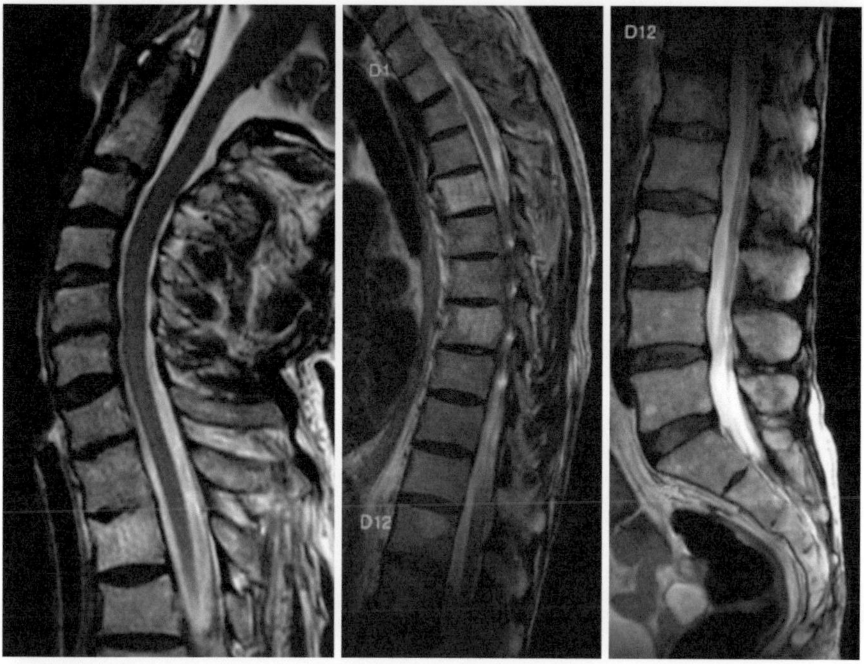

Fig. 31.2 Spine MRI sagittal T1 showing absence of longitudinal epidural collection

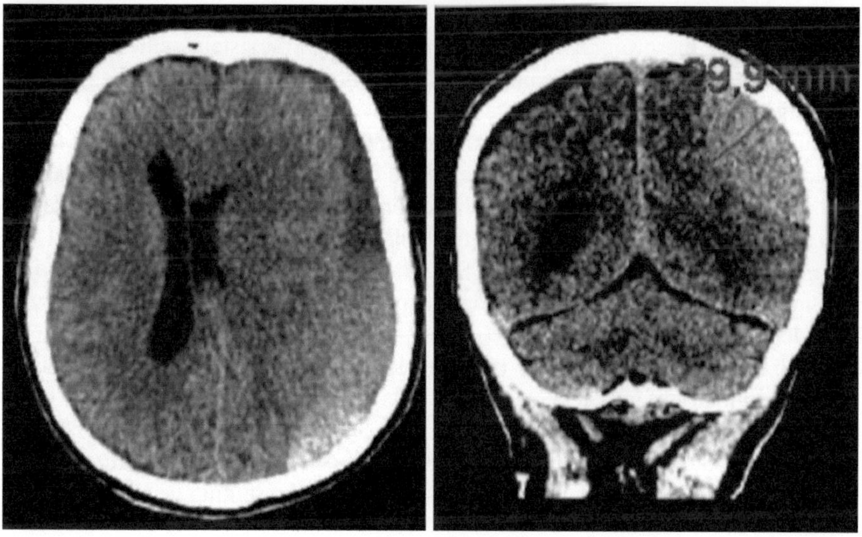

Fig. 31.3 Brain CT showing left hematoma with shift of the midline suggestive of hypertensive hematoma

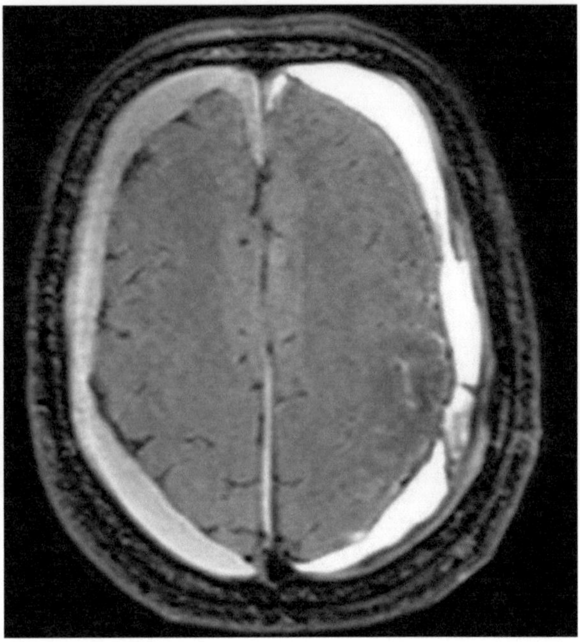

Fig. 31.4 Axial FLAIR showing bilateral subdural hematoma

The postoperative course was complicated by delayed surgical site infection and subsequent bacterial meningitis, necessitating further surgical interventions, including craniectomy and drainage repositioning. Although the headaches initially improved after these procedures, the patient reported persistent asthenia and discrete proximal weakness in the upper limbs, and brain MRI continued to show findings suggestive of SIH (Fig. 31.4).

An epidural blood patch (EBP) was considered at that time. Still, due to the comorbidities and the absence of an epidural collection at the first spine image, a second opinion was sought in a specialized center. Considering the typical presentation at the beginning of the evolution, the typical findings of the first Brain MRI, the absence of an identifiable epidural CSF collection and the persistence of signs of SIH in the last Brain MRI after surgery, the possibility of a CSF–venous fistula was considered.

A first computed tomography (CT) myelography was performed with contrast injection in the right lateral decubitus position and did not reveal any definite cerebrospinal fluid–venous fistula (Fig. 31.5). However, subtle linear contrast enhancement was observed near the left T10–T11 neural foramen (at the emergence of the left T10 nerve root), with delayed washout, possibly representing veins of the intervertebral venous plexus.

After two days, a second CT myelography was performed in the left lateral decubitus position, and it revealed a CSF–venous fistula at the level of T10–T11 (Fig. 31.6).

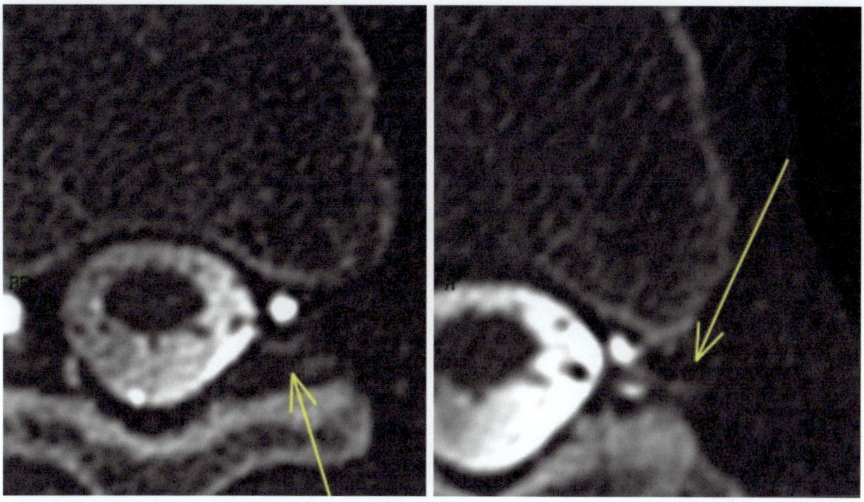

Fig. 31.5 Dynamic CT myelography showing delayed washout contrast in the left intervertebral venous plexus

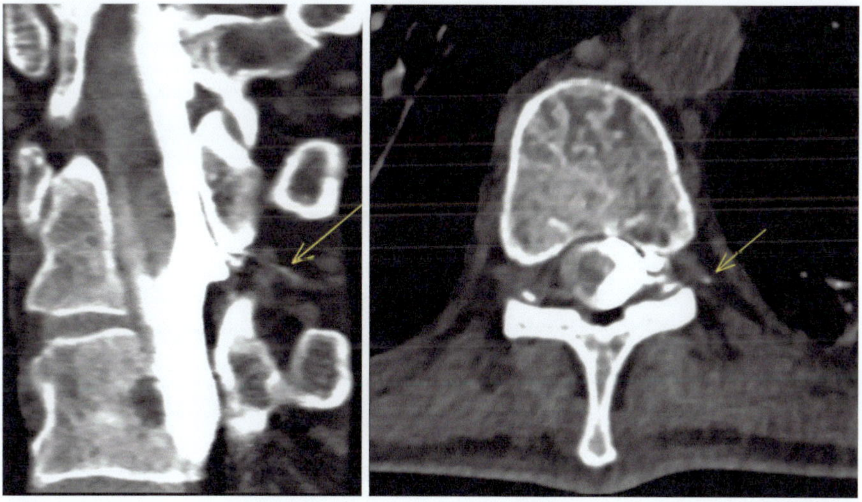

Fig. 31.6 Dynamic CT myelography showing contrast showing CVF at the level of T10-T11

Once the diagnosis of CSF–venous fistula was confirmed, the patient underwent transvenous embolization (Fig. 31.7).

He showed progressive improvement, with complete clinical recovery after two weeks. A control brain MRI demonstrated improvement in SIH signs and complete resolution of the subdural hematomas (Fig. 31.8).

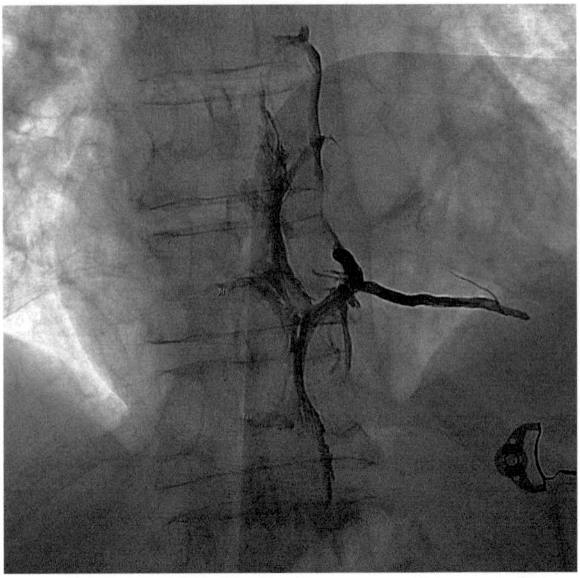

Fig. 31.7 CVF embolization with Onyx

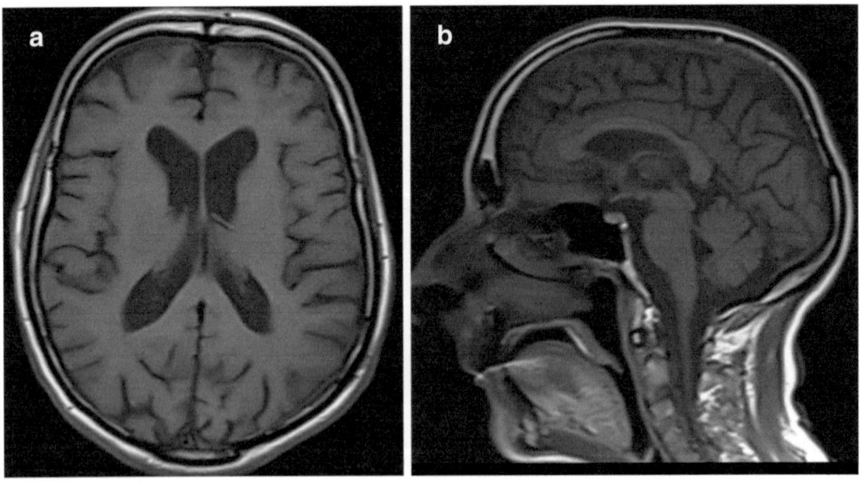

Fig. 31.8 Post-treatment brain MRI. (**a**) Axial T1-weighted image showing resolution of the subdural collection. (**b**) Sagittal T1-weighted image showing resolution of brain sagging

31.4 Case Discussion

This case demonstrated a typical presentation of SIH, with new-onset daily orthostatic headache. The patient's advanced age and comorbidities increased the complexity of management, and the worsening of the subdural hematoma represented a life-threatening complication that was successfully treated. An important insight from this case is that not all SIH patients present with spinal longitudinal epidural collection (SLEC), which is particularly true for virtually all cases of CSF–venous fistula. Adding further complexity, the first dynamic lateral decubitus CT myelography did not show the fistula. However, considering the specificity of the clinical and radiological presentation, the care team decided to repeat the exam, switching the decubitus side. This decision proved crucial to identifying the CSF–venous fistula. After successful embolization, the patient showed complete clinical and radiological improvement. The case highlights the importance of managing complex cases of SIH in specialized centers, where patients may have access to well-trained, multidisciplinary teams that can improve diagnostic accuracy and prognosis.

31.5 Clinical Presentation

Orthostatic headache is the most common symptom of SIH, being present in 75–97% of patients [5, 6]. However, the duration of symptoms may change the typical orthostatic presentation. In one study, over 93% of patients evaluated with <10 weeks since the beginning of symptoms presented with orthostatic headache, whereas it was present in only 62.5% of those who were evaluated with >10 weeks [7]. Other common signs and symptoms are nausea, neck pain or stiffness, hearing disturbances, dizziness, and tinnitus [5]. Other rare presentations include movement disorders, nonorthostatic headache, and cognitive symptoms mimicking frontotemporal dementia [5].

Patients with SIH may also present acute and chronic complications. The most frequent acute complication is subdural hematoma, which is present in up to 40% of patients, and usually is laminar, but occasionally may have high volume and require urgent intervention [5]. More rarely, patients with SIH may be complicated by cerebral venous thrombosis [6]. Chronic complications include superficial siderosis and brachial amyotrophy [8].

31.6 Diagnosis and Treatment

The diagnosis of SIH may be simple in cases with typical presentation, but it often presents challenges that may be related to atypical presentations, most commonly the absence of a clear orthostatic headache, and to difficulties in accessing adequate investigation. Therefore, it has appropriately been proposed that the diagnostic rationale must consider the context of healthcare delivery. In this context, we propose a diagnostic algorithm that considers both non-specialized and specialized centers [9].

For all patients presenting with clinical suspicion, brain MRI with contrast should be considered. The diagnosis is confirmed by signs of SIH in the brain MRI or by documented low CSF pressure (< 60 mm CSF) [10, 11]. The most common signs of SIH on brain MRI are diffuse pachymeningeal enhancement, intracranial venous engorgement, enlarged pituitary gland, subdural collection, and brain sagging [5]. Other findings may include effacement of the suprasellar cistern, reduction in the prepontine cistern, and decreased mamillopontine distance [12].

Conservative treatment consists of bed rest, hydration (2–2.5 L/day), and avoidance of Valsalva maneuvers. Although ineffective in over 75% of patients with SIH, it is considered the first-line option for those within two weeks of symptom onset [5, 9].

Epidural blood patch (EBP) consists of the injection of autologous blood in the epidural space. It is widely considered the first choice of treatment in patients who have a diagnosis of SIH and have an unavailable spine MRI. A non-targeted blood patch consists of any EBP that is performed without an invasive myelography to confirm the precise leak site. Several studies have shown that a non-targeted blood patch may be successful for up to 67% of patients [5]. In non-specialized centers, for patients who have no or sub-optimal improvement, a second EBP should be considered [9]. High-volume EBP (≥ 20 mL) has higher rates of success [5].

Spine MRI is increasingly considered necessary as an initial step in the investigation of SIH, when available [3]. The presence of a spinal longitudinal epidural collection (SLEC) suggests that the etiology is either a CSF leak from a nerve root sleeve diverticulum or an osteophyte spur. In such cases, epidural blood patching (targeted or non-targeted) and surgery should be considered, depending on the clinical context and local availability. When spine MRI shows no signs of SLEC, a CVF should be suspected, and patients should be referred to specialized centers for further evaluation with either dynamic lateral decubitus CT myelography (DL-CTM) or digital subtraction myelography (DSM) [9]. Once the CVF is documented, treatment options include surgery and intravascular embolization.

Algorithm

Non-specialized Center

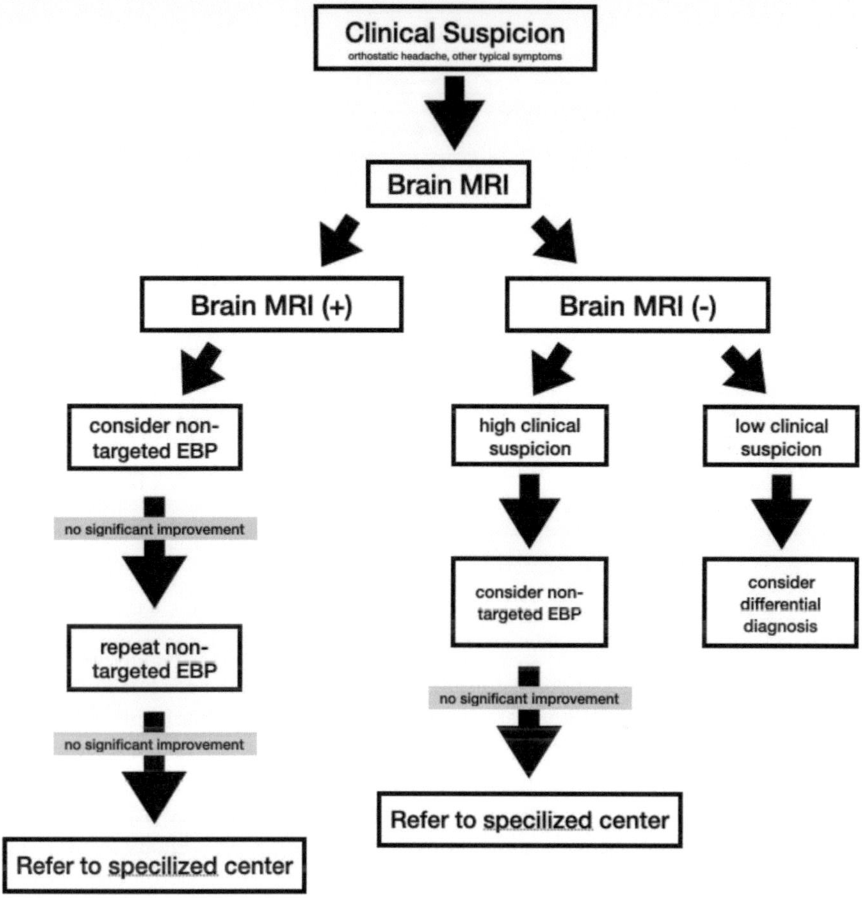

Specialized Center

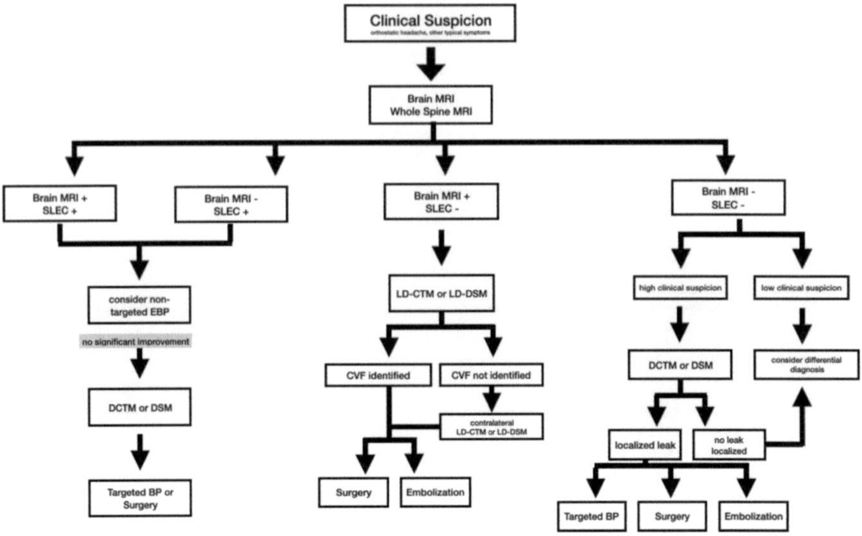

31.7 Conclusion

Spontaneous intracranial hypotension (SIH) is an increasingly recognized cause of secondary headache, with orthostatic headache being its most characteristic feature. Early recognition is crucial to prevent potentially severe complications, such as subdural hematomas, and to guide appropriate investigation. This chapter has outlined the pathophysiology, clinical presentation, diagnostic approach, and treatment strategies for SIH, illustrated by a complex case involving a CSF–venous fistula. The case reinforces the importance of specialized centers and advanced imaging techniques in achieving an accurate diagnosis, particularly in atypical or refractory presentations. Insights from recent advances in the understanding of SIH highlight the evolving landscape of management, underscoring the need for individualized and multidisciplinary care approaches to improve patient outcomes.

References

1. Amrhein TJ, Kranz PG. Spontaneous intracranial hypotension: imaging in diagnosis and treatment. Radiol Clin North Am. 2019;57:439–51. Elsevier Inc. https://doi.org/10.1016/j.rcl.2018.10.004.
2. Kranz PG, Tanpitukpongse TP, Choudhury KR, Amrhein TJ, Gray L. How common is normal cerebrospinal fluid pressure in spontaneous intracranial hypotension? Cephalalgia. 2016;36(13):1209–17.

3. Farnsworth PJ, Madhavan AA, Verdoorn JT, Shlapak DP, Johnson DR, Cutsforth-Gregory JK, Brinjikji W, Lehman VT. Spontaneous intracranial hypotension: updates from diagnosis to treatment. Neuroradiology. 2023;65(2):233–43. https://doi.org/10.1007/s00234-022-03079-5.
4. Schievink WI, Schwartz MS, Maya MM, Moser FG, Rozen TD. Lack of causal association between spontaneous intracranial hypotension and cranial cerebrospinal fluid leaks. J Neurosurg. 2012;116(4):749–54. Available from: http://www.ncbi.nlm.nih.gov/pubmed/22264184.
5. D'Antona L, Jaime Merchan MA, Vassiliou A, Watkins LD, Davagnanam I, Toma AK, Matharu MS. Clinical presentation, investigation findings, and treatment outcomes of spontaneous intracranial hypotension syndrome: a systematic review and meta-analysis. JAMA Neurol. 2021;78(3):329–37. https://doi.org/10.1001/jamaneurol.2020.4799.
6. Mehta D, Cheema S, Glover S, Qureshi AM, Davagnanam I, Kamourieh S, Sayal P, Toma A, Lagrata S, Joy C, Duncan C, Anderson J, Davies B, Dorman PJ, Angus-Leppan H, Walkden J, Rohrer J, Matharu MS. Defining the typical characteristics of orthostatic headache in patients with spontaneous intracranial hypotension. Cephalalgia. 2025;45(1):3331024241308154. https://doi.org/10.1177/03331024241308154.
7. Häni L, Fung C, Jesse CM, Ulrich CT, Miesbach T, Cipriani DR, Dobrocky T, Z'Graggen WJ, Raabe A, Piechowiak EI, Beck J. Insights into the natural history of spontaneous intracranial hypotension from infusion testing. Neurology. 2020;95(3):e247–55. https://doi.org/10.1212/WNL.0000000000009812.
8. Schievink WI, Maya M, Moser F, Nuño M. Long-term risks of persistent ventral spinal CSF leaks in SIH: superficial Siderosis and Bibrachial Amyotrophy. Neurology. 2021;97(19):E1964–70.
9. Cheema S, Anderson J, Angus-Leppan H, Armstrong P, Butteriss D, Carlton Jones L, Choi D, Chotai A, D'Antona L, Davagnanam I, Davies B, Dorman PJ, Duncan C, Ellis S, Iodice V, Joy C, Lagrata S, Mead S, Morland D, Nissen J, Pople J, Redfern N, Sayal PP, Scoffings D, Secker R, Toma AK, Trevarthen T, Walkden J, Beck J, Kranz PG, Schievink W, Wang SJ, Matharu MS. Multidisciplinary consensus guideline for the diagnosis and management of spontaneous intracranial hypotension. J Neurol Neurosurg Psychiatry. 2023;94(10):835–43. https://doi.org/10.1136/jnnp-2023-331166.
10. Schievink WI, Ropper AH, editors. Spontaneous Intracranial Hypotension. N Engl J Med. 2021;385(23):2173–8. Available from: http://www.nejm.org/doi/10.1056/NEJMra2101561.
11. Olesen J, Headache Classification Committee of the International Headache Society (IHS). The international classification of headache disorders, 3rd edition. Cephalalgia. 2018;38(1):1–211. Available from: http://journals.sagepub.com/doi/10.1177/0333102417738202.
12. Dobrocky T, Grunder L, Breiding PS, Branca M, Limacher A, Mosimann PJ, Mordasini P, Zibold F, Haeni L, Jesse CM, Fung C, Raabe A, Ulrich CT, Gralla J, Beck J, Piechowiak EI. Assessing spinal cerebrospinal fluid leaks in spontaneous intracranial hypotension with a scoring system based on brain magnetic resonance imaging findings. JAMA Neurol. 2019;76(5):580–7. https://doi.org/10.1001/jamaneurol.2018.4921.

Chapter 32
Headache Attributed to Neurosarcoidosis

Mohamad Ali Hussein, Marco Antonio Nihi, and Camila Carneiro Ferreira

32.1 Introduction

Sarcoidosis is an immune-mediated disorder characterized by granulomatous inflammation of affected organs [1]. Neurological involvement of sarcoidosis (neurosarcoidosis) can involve the central nervous system or peripheral nervous system. Meningitis accounts for 10–20% of cases of neurosarcoidosis [2], which may or may not be associated with other types of involvement, such as cranial neuropathy (50–75%), myelopathy (5–26%), and peripheral neuropathy (2–86%) [3]. In leptomeningeal presentation, patients typically present with subacute to chronic onset of headache, constitutional symptoms, and signs of meningeal irritation [4]. By exploring the nuances of headaches attributed to neurosarcoidosis, this chapter aims to elucidate the implications of these findings for clinical practice and future investigations, providing a comprehensive overview of the challenges and potential strategies for managing this complex condition.

32.2 Pathophysiology

The International Classification of Headache Disorders, third edition (ICHD-3) classifies the headache related to neurosarcoidosis as headache attributed to noninfectious inflammatory Diseases and it may result from several pathophysiological mechanisms, depending on the neurological structures involved by granulomatous severity, such as granulomatous meningitis, intracranial hypertension, hydrocephalus, central neuropathic pain, and headache secondary to use of corticosteroids.

M. A. Hussein (✉) · M. A. Nihi · C. C. Ferreira
Neurological Institute of Neurology of Curitiba, Curitiba, Brazil

D. Uludüz et al. (eds.), *Rare Causes of Headache Disorders*, Headache,
https://doi.org/10.1007/978-3-032-10242-3_32

Neurosarcoidosis is an essential cause of noninfectious meningitis, especially drug-induced aseptic meningitis [5]. The major causative agents are nonsteroidal anti-inflammatory drugs (NSAIDs), antimicrobials, intravenous immunoglobulin, intrathecal agents, vaccines, and several other less frequently reported agents. One of the pathophysiological hypotheses is related to immunological mechanisms with hypersensitivity reaction, since the symptoms begin quickly after the medication ingestion. This can be explained through the hapten theory, in which a drug could act as a hapten that binds to intravascular proteins, prompting the immune system to subsequently recognize those proteins as foreign antigens [6].

In cases of intracranial hypertension, headache may be explained by parenchymal edema, increased cerebral blood volume, excessive cerebrospinal fluid (CSF) production, compromised cerebrospinal fluid reabsorption, and venous outflow obstruction [6]. There are also several other hypotheses to explain the pathophysiological mechanisms of headaches in patients diagnosed with neurosarcoidosis, such as those attributed to lymphocytic hypophysitis, intracranial neoplasm, epileptic seizures, and Chiari malformations type I. However, there is still a lack of studies that can explain the real mechanism of this condition.

32.3 Case Presentation

Ucb, a 38-year-old woman, presented with a history of a subacute onset of migraine-pattern headache, characterized by pulsating pain of high intensity, associated with nausea and photophobia, without aura symptoms. Initially, the pain lasted from hours to days, but it progressed to chronicity, with daily headaches. In addition to the headache, the patient reported worsening vertigo and gait ataxia that had been progressively deteriorating. During the first few months, she attended several emergency departments, being treated for a diagnosis of migraine. When the episodes began to exhibit signs and symptoms of cerebellar origin vertigo, such as multidirectional and non-fatigable nystagmus, axial ataxia, and accentuated limb ataxia, the patient underwent further investigation with a magnetic resonance imaging (MRI) of the brain, which revealed leptomeningeal enhancement in the brainstem and cerebellum (see Fig. 32.1). Extending the investigation with MRI of the spinal column also showed altered contrast enhancement at the cervical spinal cord level (see Fig. 32.1). A lumbar puncture was performed, revealing pleocytosis (93 cells) with a predominance of lymphomonocytic cells, as well as an increase in protein content in the sample (223 g/L). Following a hypothesis of granulomatous disease, screening for other systemic inflammatory foci was conducted, which returned negative. This led to a meningeal biopsy, which, in addition to the clinical findings, confirmed the diagnosis of neurosarcoidosis, as it found non-necrotizing granulomas, with no other foci of systemic disease identified.

After treatment with pulsotherapy, with methylprednisolone, the patient exhibited symptomatic improvement, maintaining the same imaging pattern for several months, until a reduction in contrast uptake in the leptomeninges was observed. She

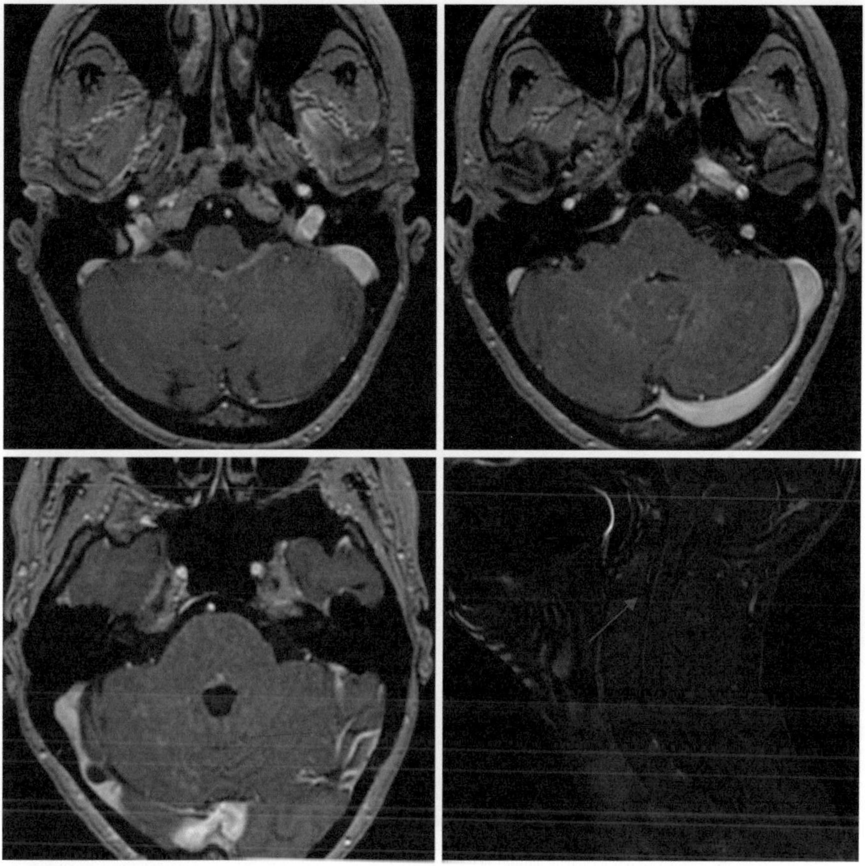

Fig. 32.1 MRI findings of our case show cerebellar leptomeningeal enhancement, in the brainstem and in the cervical spinal cord

initiated treatment with methotrexate, achieving satisfactory disease control, with only one relapse during follow-up so far, also treated with pulsotherapy, with no significant sequelae remaining.

32.4 Case Discussion

The presented case illustrates a phenotypic manifestation of leptomeningitis in a case of neurosarcoidosis without systemic involvement. The inflammatory nature of the disease leads to a clinical presentation characterized by relapses, which typically respond well to corticosteroid treatment. Neurosarcoidosis is a rare disease with a broad phenotypic spectrum; for this reason and others, there is still no consensus on the best approach to monitor and treat these patients. The case presented exemplifies a phenotype with a lower potential for generating sequelae, as it may occur in patients who exhibit lesions of structures such as the optic nerve and intramedullary lesions. In this case, we emphasize that leptomeningeal involvement may present with symptoms that closely resemble those of a first migraine attack.

32.5 Headache Characteristics of Neurosarcoidosis

Headache is a common neurological symptom of neurosarcoidosis, and it can present as a new-onset headache, worsening headache, or a chronic type of headache. Several headache patterns can be observed, and their characteristics will depend on the brain lesion location: leptomeningeal involvement, supratentorial tumor-like lesions, and involvement of cranial nerves. Furthermore, pain patterns that resemble migraine and tension type headache have been reported [7].

In that regard, more important than evaluating the quality of headaches is to correlate the evidence of causality of the development/worsening of headache with the onset of neurosarcoidosis symptoms, and to evaluate the improvement of headache with the start of neurosarcoidosis treatment.

32.6 Diagnosis

Neurosarcoidosis is a diagnosis of exclusion, especially in individuals with a personal or family history of systemic sarcoidosis. Clinical presentation is variable, with neurological manifestations that may include persistent and refractory headache, cranial nerve palsies (particularly facial and optic neuropathies), myelopathy, seizures, cognitive dysfunction, and autonomic disturbances. Associated symptoms can include persistent fatigue, affective disturbances, and cognitive alterations. Meningeal involvement can lead to secondary intracranial hypertension, while hypothalamic–pituitary dysfunction may cause endocrine disorders such as diabetes insipidus or adrenal insufficiency [3, 8].

Laboratory findings may include anemia, lymphopenia, and elevated inflammatory markers such as CRP, ESR, NS, IGRA, PCR, HTLV, SLE, IgG, CGRP, and protein electrophoresis (EFPTN), though these are nonspecific. Elevated concentrations of angiotensin-converting enzyme (ACE) and serum lysozyme have been associated with active systemic sarcoidosis, serving as potential biomarkers to support the diagnostic evaluation. Examination of cerebrospinal fluid (CSF) may demonstrate lymphocytic pleocytosis, hypoglycorrhachia, and increased protein concentration, findings that can support the diagnosis of NS. Other highly specific tests for ruling out differential diagnoses include CSF protein electrophoresis, IgG index, oligoclonal bands (with corresponding serum), tuberculosis screening via IGRA and PCR, and serologies for HIV, HTLV, SLE, Lyme, and syphilis [10, 11, 17].

Although not part of standard diagnostic criteria, certain genetic variants, such as HLA-DRB103 and HLA-DRB115, may confer disease predisposition. Genetic testing may be helpful in cases with strong suspicion but no systemic evidence of sarcoidosis [3].

32.7 Additional Diagnostic Evaluations

Gadolinium-enhanced MRI of the brain, columns, and orbit is a key imaging modality for evaluating neurological involvement in NS, frequently revealing diffuse leptomeningeal enhancement and, in some cases, pachymeningeal thickening. Additional findings may include inflammatory periventricular lesions and cranial nerve involvement, particularly affecting the optic nerve. FDG-PET may also assist in detecting systemic inflammatory activity [12, 13].

High-resolution computed tomography (CT) of the thorax can provide additional diagnostic insights, particularly in assessing pulmonary involvement, which may reinforce systemic disease characterization. This technique has demonstrated high sensitivity for detecting mediastinal and hilar adenopathy, aiding in differential diagnosis. In combination with bronchoalveolar lavage and immunocytochemistry, CD4:CD8 ratio assessments have been proposed as supportive diagnostic markers [14].

32.8 Apply ICHD-3 Diagnostic Criteria [9]

- Any headache fulfilling criterion C
- NS has been diagnosed
- Evidence of causation demonstrated by at least two of the following:
  - A headache has developed in temporal relation to the onset of NS
  - Either or both of the following: (a) Headache has significantly worsened in parallel with worsening of NS, (b) Headache has significantly improved in parallel with improvement in NS
  - One or more cranial nerve palsies accompany headache
- Not better accounted for by another ICHD-3 diagnosis.

A definitive diagnosis of NS relies on a combination of clinical, laboratory, and imaging findings. When diagnostic uncertainty remains, performing a meningeal biopsy can be considered to confirm the presence of non-caseating granulomas, which is considered the gold standard method. When a direct CNS biopsy is unfeasible, obtaining tissue samples from peripheral lymph nodes, pulmonary structures, or other extracranial sites exhibiting systemic involvement may contribute to the diagnostic assessment of NS [15].

32.9 Classification Re-evaluation

- *Histopathological investigation*: Confirmation of non-caseating granulomas as a complementary criterion.
- *Clinical and neuroimaging correlation*: Leptomeningeal and pachymeningeal involvement may modify headache presentation.
- *Complementary laboratory tests*: ACE levels and CSF analysis as non-mandatory criteria for differentiating other inflammatory diseases.

Reevaluation should include continuous monitoring of therapeutic response. Changes in headache frequency and intensity may indicate the need for treatment adjustments or suggest the coexistence of other secondary headaches. Thus, the diagnostic and classificatory approach to headaches in NS should not only consider current ICHD-3 criteria but also the underlying pathophysiological mechanisms of granulomatous inflammation and its impact on cerebral hemodynamics. Clinical evolution and treatment response should be monitored, with periodic reassessment of therapeutic adjustments, particularly in refractory cases.

32.10 Management

The management of NS is based on controlling inflammatory responses and addressing symptomatic manifestations to improve patient outcomes. Corticosteroids remain the first-line therapy, typically initiated with prednisone at 0.25–1 mg/kg/day, followed by a gradual tapering based on clinical response. In severe cases, high-dose intravenous methylprednisolone (1 g/day for 3–5 days) may be required. For patients with refractory disease, immunosuppressants such as methotrexate, azathioprine, mycophenolate mofetil, or biologic agents like infliximab and adalimumab are therapeutic alternatives [3, 11, 16].

Headache management should begin with the exclusion of secondary intracranial hypertension. Mild-to-moderate headaches may respond to nonsteroidal anti-inflammatory drugs (NSAIDs), while triptans may be considered for severe migraine-like headaches. In patients requiring preventive therapy, anticonvulsants such as topiramate and valproic acid, tricyclic antidepressants, and CGRP antagonists represent viable options for reducing headache frequency and severity. Considering the overlap with primary headache disorders, treatment strategies should be customized based on individual patient profiles and associated comorbidities.

32.11 Conclusion

NS is a granulomatous inflammatory disorder affecting the central nervous system, often presenting with complex and refractory headache syndromes that pose diagnostic and therapeutic challenges. Diagnosis can be complex and requires a thorough assessment that integrates clinical history, specialized laboratory testing, cerebrospinal fluid analysis, and advanced neuroimaging modalities. Therapeutic approach should prioritize sustained immunosuppression alongside targeted headache management, ensuring continuous monitoring to reduce relapse risk and prevent neurological deterioration.

References

1. Valeyre D, Prasse A, Nunes H, Uzunhan Y, Brillet PY, Müller-Quernheim J. Sarcoidosis. Lancet. 2014;383(9923):1155–67. https://doi.org/10.1016/S0140-6736(13)60680-7.
2. Joseph FG, Scolding NJ. Neurosarcoidosis: a study of 30 new cases. J Neurol Neurosurg Psychiatry. 2009;80(3):297–304. https://doi.org/10.1136/jnnp.2008.151977.
3. Bradshaw MJ, Pawate S, Koth LL, Cho TA, Gelfand JM. Neurosarcoidosis: pathophysiology, diagnosis, and treatment. Neurol Neuroimmunol Neuroinflamm. 2021;8(6):e1084. https://doi.org/10.1212/NXI.0000000000001084.
4. Stern BJ, Aksamit A, Clifford D, Scott TF, Neurosarcoidosis Study Group. Neurologic presentations of sarcoidosis. Neurol Clin. 2010;28(1):185–98. https://doi.org/10.1016/j.ncl.2009.09.012.
5. Fritz D, Voortman M, van de Beek D, Drent M, Brouwer MC. Many faces of neurosarcoidosis: from chronic meningitis to myelopathy. Curr Opin Pulm Med. 2017;23(5):439–46. https://doi.org/10.1097/MCP.0000000000000401.
6. Obermann M, Holle D, Naegel S, Diener HC. Headache attributable to nonvascular intracranial disorders. Curr Pain Headache Rep. 2011;15(4):314–23. https://doi.org/10.1007/s11916-011-0193-3.
7. Curone M, Tullo V, Peccarisi C, Bussone G, D'Amico D. Headache as presenting symptom of neurosarcoidosis. Neurol Sci. 2013;34(Suppl 1):S183–5. https://doi.org/10.1007/s10072-013-1423-8.
8. Voortman M, Stern BJ, Saketkoo LA, Drent M. The burden of neurosarcoidosis: essential approaches to early diagnosis and treatment. Semin Respir Crit Care Med. 2020;41(5):641–51. https://doi.org/10.1055/s-0040-1710576.
9. Pawate S, Moses H, Sriram S. Presentations and outcomes of neurosarcoidosis: a study of 54 cases. QJM. 2009;102(7):449–60. https://doi.org/10.1093/qjmed/hcp042.
10. Nowak DA, Widenka DC. Neurosarcoidosis: a review of its intracranial manifestation. J Neurol. 2001;248(5):363–72. https://doi.org/10.1007/s004150170184.
11. Joseph FG, Scolding NJ. Sarcoidosis of the nervous system. Pract Neurol. 2007;7(4):234–44. https://doi.org/10.1136/jnnp.2007.124263.
12. Bathla G, Singh AK, Policeni B, Agarwal A, Asrani AV, Khandelwal A. Imaging of neurosarcoidosis: common, uncommon, and rare. Clin Radiol. 2016;71(1):96–106. https://doi.org/10.1016/j.crad.2015.09.007.
13. Fritz D, van de Beek D, Brouwer MC. Clinical features, treatment and outcome in neurosarcoidosis: systematic review and meta-analysis. BMC Neurol. 2016;16:220. https://doi.org/10.1186/s12883-016-0741-x.

14. Headache Classification Committee of the International Headache Society (IHS). The international classification of headache disorders, 3rd edition. Cephalalgia. 2018;38(1):1–211. https://doi.org/10.1177/0333102417738202.
15. Kidd DP. Neurosarcoidosis: clinical manifestations, investigation and treatment. Pract Neurol. 2020;20(3):199–212. https://doi.org/10.1136/practneurol-2019-002349.
16. Baughman RP, Wells AU. Advanced sarcoidosis. Curr Opin Pulm Med. 2019;25(5):497–504. https://doi.org/10.1097/MCP.0000000000000612.
17. Stern BJ, Royal W 3rd, Gelfand JM, Clifford DB, Tavee J, Pawate S, Berger JR, Aksamit AJ, Krumholz A, Pardo CA, Moller DR, Judson MA, Drent M, Baughman RP. Definition and consensus diagnostic criteria for neurosarcoidosis: from the Neurosarcoidosis Consortium Consensus Group. JAMA Neurol. 2018;75(12):1546–53. https://doi.org/10.1001/jamaneurol.2018.2295.

Chapter 33
Headache with Neurological Deficits and CSF Lymphocytosis (HaNDL Syndrome)

Amr Hassan, Rehab Magdy, and Mona Hussein

33.1 Introduction

Headache with neurological deficits and cerebrospinal fluid (CSF) lymphocytosis (HaNDL syndrome) is a rare disorder first described in the early 1980s and also known as pseudomigraine with temporary neurological symptoms and lymphocytic pleocytosis (PMP) [1, 2]. In 1995, it was given its current name [3]. Mounting evidence confirms that its incidence is higher between the third and fourth decades, with an age range of 5–52 years. No significant sex predominance has been reported [2, 3]. Up to 25% of the published cases were pediatric cases [4].

This benign syndrome is usually characterized by recurrent migraine-like headaches, transient neurological deficits, for example, hemiparesis, hemihypothesia, aphasia, visual impairment, or dysphagia, along with CSF lymphocytic pleocytosis. HaNDL syndrome is currently classified among secondary headaches attributed to "non-infectious, inflammatory intracranial disease." Despite its classification as a secondary headache, the current definition of HaNDL does not specify a definite causal agent [5]. This chapter aims to shed light on this underdiagnosed disorder and to emphasize its practice essentials, potential diagnostic challenges, and management strategies.

A. Hassan (✉) · R. Magdy
Cairo University, Giza, Egypt
e-mail: amrhasanneuro@kasralainy.edu.eg

M. Hussein
Beni-Suef University, Beni Suef, Egypt

D. Uludüz et al. (eds.), *Rare Causes of Headache Disorders*, Headache,
https://doi.org/10.1007/978-3-032-10242-3_33

33.2 Pathophysiology

The exact cause of HaNDL syndrome still remains unclear, but various theories exist about the etiology. Initially, it was assumed to be secondary to an infectious agent (probably viral) due to frequent viral prodrome in up to 25–40% of cases, self-limiting monophasic course, and CSF lymphocytic pleocytosis. Some recent studies have found calcium channel autoantibodies, CACNA1H, in some patients with HaNDL. Furthermore, some other findings using protein microarray screening revealed the identification of autoantibodies to three DNA repair proteins (mitogen-activated protein kinase-4, DNA-dependent protein kinase catalytic subunit, DNA excision repair protein ERCC6). DNA repair protein antibodies can signify DNA damage and inflammatory causes of HaNDL [6]. Therefore, it is postulated that viral infection is implicated in the production of autoantibodies against vascular and neuronal antigens, which subsequently induce aseptic leptomeningeal vasculitis via a spreading depression-like mechanism (Fig. 33.1) [7, 8].

On the one hand, previous studies mentioned the association between vasomotor changes and HaNDL pathophysiology. Global hemispheric hypoperfusion pattern supporting secondary oligemia induced by a hemispheric wave of cortical spreading depression (CSD) had been speculated in a study that showed direct spread of CSD-induced vasomotor changes across the anomalous vasculature [9, 10].

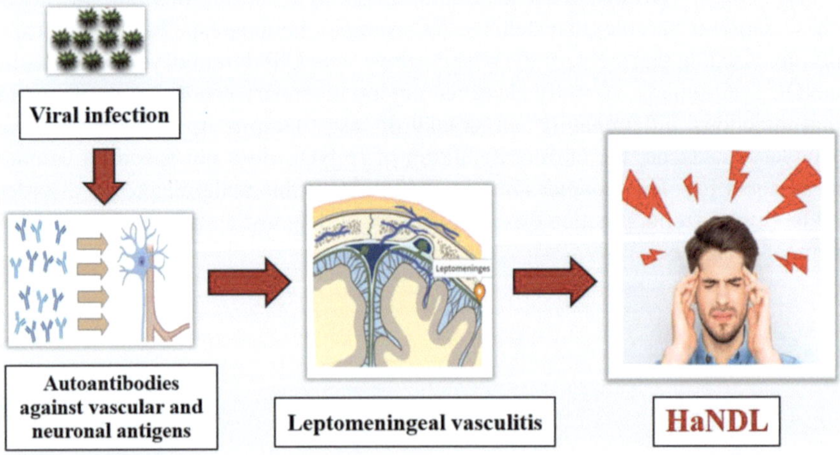

Fig. 33.1 Pathophysiology of HaNDL syndrome

33.3 Case Presentation

Sara, a 33-year-old female, presented to the emergency room with a severe unilateral throbbing headache associated with photophobia, nausea, vomiting, and mild neck meningism accompanied by new-onset expressive dysphasia and right-sided weakness of four hours duration. She had an irrelevant medical history except for being diagnosed previously by her family doctor as having migraine with aura. Such a diagnosis was made based on a history of three episodes of headache with the same phenotype described above, but with a milder intensity occurring over a month earlier. Each episode was preceded by several hours of numbness in the right arm. In all three episodes, she recovered fully in 5–12 hours.

On clinical examination, she was alert, fully oriented and attentive. Her vital signs were completely normal. Neurological examination revealed right-sided mild weakness, graded 4/5 using the Medical Research Council (MRC) grading system and expressive dysphasia. There was no papilledema nor signs of meningeal irritation.

Laboratory workup was within normal ranges, including complete blood count, liver and kidney function tests, serum electrolytes, glucose, coagulation profile, erythrocyte sedimentation rate, and C-reactive protein. The urine toxicology screen was also negative.

Brain computed tomography (CT) and magnetic resonance imaging (MRI) were unremarkable. The possibility of vascular insult, such as subarachnoid hemorrhage (SAH), reversible cerebral vasoconstriction syndrome (RCVS), or cerebral venous sinus thrombosis (CVST) versus central nervous system (CNS) infection, was raised. Accordingly, MRI-SWI, CT angiography, venography, and a lumbar puncture (LP) were performed.

All vascular imaging workup was also unremarkable. However, a few minutes after angiography, the patient had ongoing right hemiparesis graded 2/5 using the MRC grading system, and eventually, she became agitated. Therefore, MRI brain and CT angiography were repeated under general anesthesia to exclude vasospasm or iatrogenic arterial dissection. Both were also normal.

CSF analysis revealed pleocytosis of 96 cells per microliter with predominated lymphocytes (97%). Protein levels were mildly elevated at 48 mg/dL, with glucose levels normal to contemporary plasma values. Xanthochromia testing was negative. CSF gram stain and polymerase chain reaction (PCR) testing for Herpes Simplex Virus (HSV) and Varicella Zoster Virus (VZV) were negative.

However, after six hours, the patient improved gradually till complete recovery in twelve hours, and even the headache subsided. CSF was repeated at this point, and all CSF parameters returned to normal levels. Accordingly, a diagnosis of HaNDL was established.

33.4 Clinical Characteristics

As its name implies, the characteristic presentation of HaNDL includes recurrent attacks of severe headache, transient neurological symptoms, and CSF lymphocytic (>15 white cells/mL) [11]. The most reported neurological symptoms in HaNDL are hemiparesis, hemi-paraesthesia, and dysphasia [12]. Other manifestations, such as diminution of vision, homonymous hemianopsia, sixth nerve palsy, and central retinal vein occlusion, have also been described [2, 3]. HaNDL may be occasionally associated with papilledema and manifestations of increased intracranial pressure (ICP) [13]. Some rare manifestations such as acute confusional state and behavioral abnormalities have been also reported [14]. The neurological symptoms usually last from 15 to 120 minutes, with a range between five minutes and three days [3]. Former reports declared that HaNDL usually has a monophasic course; however, some patients may experience recurrent episodes. The neurological deficits may vary from one episode to another [3].

The headache of HaNDL is mostly migraine-like. It may be unilateral or bilateral, characterized by throbbing, and moderate-to-severe in intensity [3]. Thunderclap onset is rare [15]. It is often associated with nausea/vomiting and photophobia. It typically lasts from one hour to one week. Typically, the headache follows the neurological symptoms by 15–60 minutes; however, occasionally, the headache may precede the neurological symptoms [1, 2]. In addition to cerebrospinal fluid (CSF) lymphocytosis (up to 760 cells/μL), there are elevations of CSF total protein (up to 250 mg/dL) in more than 90% of cases and of CSF pressure (up to 400 mm CSF) in more than 50% of cases. Routine CT and MRI scans (with or without intravenous contrast) and angiography are invariably normal when performed interictally; however, brain imaging during an episode may reveal delayed brain perfusion, without increased diffusion-weighted imaging changes, and narrowing of cerebral arteries. However, gray matter edema and sulcal enhancement have been described in some patients. Microbiological studies have been uniformly normal. Electroencephalography (EEG) and single-photon emission computed tomography (SPECT) scans may reveal focal areas of abnormality consistent with the focal neurological deficits [6, 11].

33.5 Diagnostic Algorithm

Step 1: Clinical Suspicion

- *Identify Key Symptoms*:
- Episodes of transient neurological deficits, including motor, sensory, aphasia, and, less frequently, visual, lasting several hours, accompanied or followed by moderate-to-severe headache.

Step 2: Initial Diagnostic Workup

- *Perform Brain CT and MRI*:
  - *Exclude*:
    - Subarachnoid hemorrhage (SAH)
    - Reversible cerebral vasoconstriction syndrome (RCVS)
    - Cerebral venous sinus thrombosis (CVST)
    - CNS infection.

Step 3: CSF Examination

- *Conduct CSF Analysis*:
  - Measure the opening pressure
  - Assess protein, glucose, red and white cell count.
  - Exclude xanthochromia
  - Microscopy and culture (to exclude viral, fungal, treponemal and mycobacterial infection)
  - PCR testing for viruses (e.g., HSV, VZV, and enterovirus)
  - Anti-N-methyl-D-aspartate (NMDA) receptor antibodies: Anti-NMDA receptor encephalitis may present as a severe multistage neuropsychiatric syndrome that could be similar to HaNDL

Step 4: Additional Diagnostic Evaluations

- Perform CT Angiography:
  - Look for aneurysms or other vascular malformations
- EEG and SPECT scans may show focally abnormal areas consistent with the focal neurological deficits.

Step 5: Apply the International Classification of Headache Disorders, third edition (ICHD-3) Diagnostic Criteria [11]

A. Episodes of migraine-like headache fulfilling criteria B and C
B. Both of the following:
   1. Accompanied or shortly preceded by onset of at least one of the following transient neurological deficits lasting >4 hours
      (a) Hemiparaesthesia
      (b) Dysphasia
      (c) Hemiparesis
   2. Associated with cerebrospinal fluid (CSF) lymphocytic pleocytosis (>15 white cells per μL), with negative etiological studies

C. Evidence of causation demonstrated by either or both of the following:
    1. Headache and transient neurological deficits have developed or significantly worsened in temporal relation to onset or worsening of the CSF lymphocytic pleocytosis, or led to its discovery
    2. Headache and transient neurological deficits have significantly improved in parallel with improvement in the CSF lymphocytic pleocytosis

D. Not better accounted for by another ICHD-3 diagnosis.

33.6 Treatment

HaNDL syndrome is a self-limited disorder with a favorable outcome. Therefore, pharmacological therapy is typically limited to the symptomatic treatment of headaches. Once the diagnosis of HaNDL has been established, reassurance of the patients should be done as they may experience further attacks that can occur weeks or months following the first attack. The rare occurrence of risks and complications of HaNDL syndrome should also be explained to the patient and their family. Apart from the dramatic and sudden onset, the condition is self-limited and rarely causes lifelong complications.

Antiepileptic and migraine prevention can help prevent acute attacks because of their close association with migraine-like headaches. However, the response of these drugs is difficult to compare with the natural progression of the disease itself due to their self-limiting property [2].

Urgent re-evaluation for elevated intracranial pressure is recommended for recurring headaches or developing visual symptoms after recovery from HaNDL. Short- to medium-term management with CSF drainage and acetazolamide is needed to prevent visual loss [16].

In a case report, a patient was treated with ibuprofen (400 mg, 3 times per day) with excellent response and remained asymptomatic and free of any relapse for 6 months [12].

33.7 Conclusion

HaNDL syndrome usually presents as headache episodes with neurological symptoms and considerable cerebrospinal fluid lymphocytosis but no signs of central nervous system infection. At the same time, MRIs of the brain are normal. Although the etiology is still uncertain, viral infection is one of the factors for consideration. Due to similarities of symptoms with other neurological disorders, it is essential to rule out more serious diseases. Patients with HaNDL syndrome should be educated about the nature of the disease and must be well informed about the benign and self-limiting nature of the disease. The prognosis is excellent, and symptoms typically resolve within 1–3 weeks. Apart from the dramatic and sudden onset, the condition is self-limited and rarely causes lifelong complications.

References

1. Bartleson JD, Swanson JW, Whisnant JP. A migrainous syndrome with cerebrospinal fluid pleocytosis. Neurology. 1981;31(10):1257–62.
2. Berg MJ, Williams LS. The transient syndrome of headache with neurologic deficits and CSF lymphocytosis. Neurology. 1995;45(9):1648–54.
3. Gómez-Aranda F, Cañadillas F, Martí-Massó JF, Díez-Tejedor E, Serrano PJ, Leira R, Gracia M, Pascual J. Pseudomigraine with temporary neurological symptoms and lymphocytic pleocytosis. A report of 50 cases. Brain. 1997;120(Pt 7):1105–13. https://doi.org/10.1093/brain/120.7.1105.
4. Al-Chalabi M, Hegde P, Asghar F, Aladamat N, Delcimmuto N, Gharaibeh K, Samara M, Esengul Y, Mahfooz N, Sheikh A. Transient headache and neurological deficits with cerebrospinal fluid lymphocytosis syndrome: a comprehensive systematic review of 93 patients from 57 studies. Cephalalgia. 2023;43(4):3331024231157694. https://doi.org/10.1177/03331024231157694.
5. Al Hadidi M, Meng WD, Jumean K, Hawatmeh A. Syndrome of transient headache and neurologic deficits with cerebrospinal fluid lymphocytosis masquerading as meningitis in HIV patient. Ann Transl Med. 2017;5(6):138.
6. Erdağ E, Çelebisoy N, Yüceyar AN, Kürtüncü M, Vural B, Tüzün E. Antibodies to DNA repair proteins in headache with neurological deficits and cerebrospinal fluid lymphocytosis (HaNDL) patients. Acta Neurol Belg. 2015;115(2):137–40.
7. Kappler J, Mohr S, Steinmetz H. Cerebral vasomotor changes in the transient syndrome of headache with neurologic deficits and CSF lymphocytosis (HaNDL). Headache. 1997;37(8):516–8.
8. Pascual J, Valle N. Pseudomigraine with lymphocytic pleocytosis. Curr Pain Headache Rep. 2003;7(3):224–8.
9. Burke MJ, Lamb MJ, Hohol M, Lay C. Unique CT perfusion imaging in a case of HaNDL: new insight into HaNDL pathophysiology and vasomotor principles of cortical spreading depression. Headache. 2017;57(1):129–34.
10. Smail RC, Baird-Gunning J, Drummond J, Ng K. A case report of a transient splenial lesion related to HaNDL syndrome. Cephalalgia. 2020;40(10):1119–22.
11. Headache Classification Committee of the International Headache Society (IHS). The international classification of headache disorders, 3rd edition. Cephalalgia. 2018;38(1):1–211.
12. Salazar-Orellana JLI, Prado-Miranda G, Maldonado-Ortiz A. Agraphia: presenting feature of syndrome of transient headache and neurological deficits with cerebrospinal fluid lymphocytosis (HaNDL). Cureus. 2021;13(2):e13178.
13. Morrison DG, Phuah HK, Reddy AT, Dure LS, Kline LB. Ophthalmologic involvement in the syndrome of headache, neurologic deficits, and cerebrospinal fluid lymphocytosis. Ophthalmology. 2003;110(1):115–8. https://doi.org/10.1016/s0161-6420(02)01444-6.
14. Mateo I, Pinedo A, Gómez-Beldarrain M, García-Moncó JC. Estado confusional agudo secundario a síndrome de cefalea y déficit neurológicos transitorios con linfocitosis en líquido cefalorraquídeo [Acute confusional state secondary to transient headache and neurological deficits with cerebrospinal fluid lymphocytosis]. Neurologia. 2004;19(10):763–5.
15. Parasram M, Malhotra A, Yoo AS, Mir SA. HaNDL syndrome presenting with thunderclap headache. Case Rep Neurol Med. 2021;2021:9925004. https://doi.org/10.1155/2021/9925004.
16. Mulroy E, Yap J, Danesh-Meyer H, Anderson N. Symptomatic intracranial hypertension during recovery from the syndrome of headache with neurologic deficits and cerebrospinal fluid lymphocytosis (HANDL). Pract Neurol. 2017;17(2):145–8.

Chapter 34
Headache Attributed to Chiari Malformation Type I (CM1)

Claudia Baptista Tavares

34.1 Introduction

Chiari malformation, also known as Arnold-Chiari malformation, is a congenital or acquired anomaly of the hindbrain, described in autopsies in 1891 by the Austrian pathologist Hans Chiari [1]. He identified four distinct anatomical variations characterized by displacement of the cerebellar tonsils beyond the foramen magnum [2, 3].

This chapter discusses the most common form, *Chiari malformation type 1 (CM1)*, in which only the cerebellar tonsils extend below the level of the foramen magnum. CM1 may occur in isolation or be associated with syringomyelia—a disorder characterized by the development of a fluid-filled cavity (syrinx) within the spinal cord, usually resulting from disrupted cerebrospinal fluid (CSF) flow at the craniocervical junction. This condition may arise from a congenitally small posterior fossa or be acquired due to changes in intracranial pressure that lead to displacement of the cerebellar tonsils [1, 4].

Cerebellar tonsillar herniation may obstruct the foramina of Luschka and Magendie and impair the circulation of the cerebrospinal fluid (CSF) between the fourth ventricle and the spinal subarachnoid space (Fig. 34.1). This disruption may lead to the formation of syringomyelia, usually at the cervical region of the spinal cord or, in rare cases, the brainstem [4].

CM1 is more prevalent in women than men, and the peak age of presentation is 41 years in adults and 8 years in children [5].

CM1 is radiologically defined when the cerebellar tonsils project five millimeters or more below the level of the foramen magnum (Fig. 34.2). Although often an incidental finding on neuroimaging, it may cause significant symptoms, with headache being the most common complaint [6].

C. B. Tavares (✉)
Fluminense Federal University, School of Medicine, Niteroi, Rio de Janeiro, Brazil

D. Uludüz et al. (eds.), *Rare Causes of Headache Disorders*, Headache,
https://doi.org/10.1007/978-3-032-10242-3_34

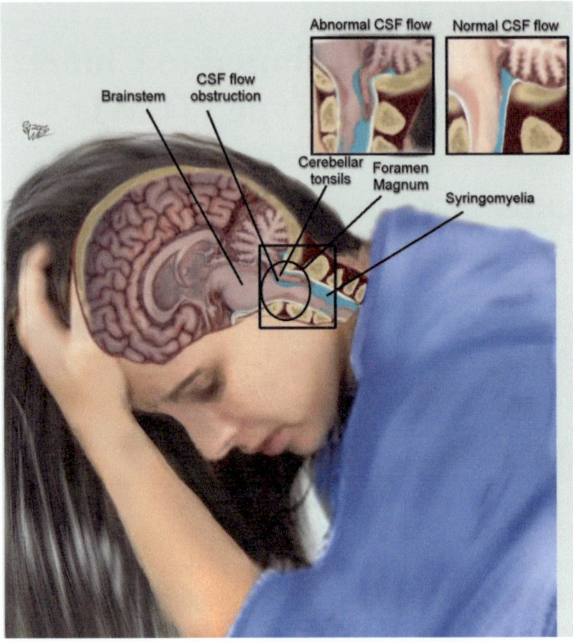

Fig. 34.1 Mechanisms proposed in CM1: Key pathophysiological aspects observed in CM1, including cerebellar tonsil herniation and CSF flow obstruction. The image also depicts syringomyelia, a condition that may occur in some cases of CM1. The two highlighted panels at the top compare altered CSF flow patterns typically observed in CM1 with normal flow dynamics, emphasizing the impact of tonsillar descent on craniospinal fluid circulation

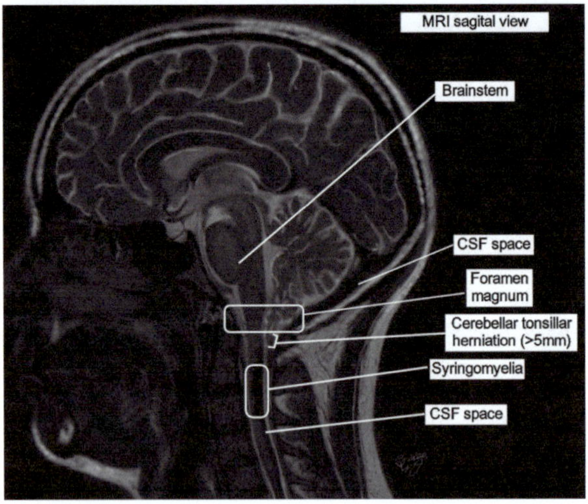

Fig. 34.2 MRI of a patient with CM1: T2-weighted midsagittal MRI demonstrating tonsillar descent and CSF space reduction at the foramen magnum

Given the variability of symptoms and the possibility of overlapping with primary headaches, a proper understanding of the underlying mechanisms of CM1 is essential. This chapter aims to discuss the mechanisms to prevent misdiagnoses and help distinguish headaches related to Chiari malformation from other types of headaches, thus contributing to a more accurate and practical approach to patient management.

34.2 Pathophysiology

In CM1, headaches are usually located in the occipital region and tend to be triggered or intensified by Valsalva maneuvers, such as coughing, sneezing, or physical exertion, leading to increased intracranial pressure [7]. The following main mechanisms are involved in this pain (Fig. 34.1):

1. Disruption of CSF flow: Cerebellar tonsillar herniation can obstruct CFS circulation at the craniocervical junction and lead to increased intracranial pressure and worsened headaches, especially during Valsalva maneuvers. This obstruction disrupts the normal CSF flow between the posterior fossa and spinal cord, creating an abnormal pressure gradient [8]. Studies employing cine magnetic resonance imaging (cine MRI) have demonstrated altered CSF flow in CM1 patients, characterized by turbulent jets and increased velocity in the foramen magnum. These disturbances may result in repetitive microtrauma to the upper cervical spinal cord and brainstem, contributing to the pathophysiology of the disease [9, 10].
2. Brainstem and spinal cord compression: Direct mechanical compression affects pain pathways, contributing to chronic headache and associated neurological symptoms.
3. Dural stretching and irritation: The caudal descent of the cerebellar tonsils and restricted CSF flow may lead to compensatory reductions in intracranial pressure in the posterior fossa and cause mechanical traction on pain-sensitive structures, such as the dura mater and cranial base vessels. This mechanism may explain orthostatic headaches in CM1 cases without syringomyelia [4].
4. Venous congestion and increased intracranial pressure: Impaired CSF flow may contribute to venous hypertension, further exacerbating headaches [4].
5. Altered central sensitization: Evidence suggests that CM1 may lead to hyperexcitability of the trigeminovascular system, similar to mechanisms observed in chronic migraine. Functional neuroimaging studies also indicated increased connectivity between the trigeminal nucleus and structures involved in chronic pain processing (e.g., thalamus and insular cortex) in CM1 patients [11, 12]. This finding may explain the presence of migraine-like headaches in some cases.

34.3 Case Presentation

A 42-year-old woman with no prior comorbidities presented with a history of moderate and intermittent occipital headache since the age of 37, which had become more frequent over the past six months, dizziness, and postural instability. The patient reported intense bilateral pain in the occipital region, pulsatile at times and constrictive at others, that worsened with Valsalva maneuvers (coughing, sneezing, and physical exertion) and was partially relieved by rest. She also reported intermittent upper limb (UL) paresthesia and episodes of hand numbness upon waking.

Despite having no family history of Chiari malformation, her mother had a diagnosis of chronic migraine.

A neurological exam revealed preserved strength and sensation throughout the body, a negative Romberg sign, subjective complaints of postural instability, increased deep tendon reflexes in the UL (bilateral biceps reflex), and reduced tactile discrimination.

MRI of the posterior fossa and cervical spine showed cerebellar tonsils descent of seven millimeters below the level of the foramen magnum. Additionally, there was a syrinx cavity extending from the C2 to C6 vertebrae and partial obstruction of cerebrospinal fluid (CSF) flow at the craniocervical junction. Cine MRI also showed increased flow velocity in turbulent jets. The diagnosis was a headache attributed to CM1. Gabapentin was initiated to modulate pain and paresthesia, and acetazolamide to reduce CSF flow obstruction and relieve the headache.

After six months of conservative treatment, the patient presented a 50% reduction in headache episodes but remained highly symptomatic during exertion, with episodes of incapacitating headaches impacting quality of life, along with hyperreflexia and paresthesia in UL.

A possible neurosurgical intervention was discussed with the patient, and a posterior fossa decompression with suboccipital craniectomy and duraplasty was planned (Fig. 34.2). The decision to perform a dural opening in association was based on studies suggesting a higher rate of headache relief and lower risk of recurrence compared with bone-only decompression.

Six months post-surgery, the patient reported complete resolution of headaches and significant improvement in sensory symptoms. The follow-up MRI showed a normalization of the CSF flow at the craniocervical junction.

34.4 Case Discussion

Based on clinical and imaging findings, the central diagnostic hypothesis was *headache attributed to CM1*, according to the International Classification of Headache Disorders [13]. The presence of occipital pain triggered by Valsalva, neurological symptoms, and the impact on CSF flow confirmed the dysfunction at the craniocervical junction. MRI is an advanced diagnostic tool that allows for detailed evaluation of the posterior fossa anatomy, craniocervical junction integrity, and CSF pulsatile flow. In this case, it was crucial to distinguish CM1 with CSF flow restriction from cases without relevant hemodynamic impact. Changes in CSF dynamics correlate more strongly with symptoms than the extent of cerebellar tonsil descent [10].

The management of headaches in CM1 must consider the severity of symptoms, the presence of neurological signs, and the impact on quality of life. For patients without severe neurological deficits, conservative pharmacological treatment with central pain modulators and/or CSF flow regulators is recommended first.

34.5 Characteristics of Headache Related to CM1

CM1-related headaches have distinct characteristics [13]:

- Location: Occipital or suboccipital, often radiating to the vertex or frontal regions.
- Onset and duration: Typically chronic, with episodic exacerbations.
- Triggering factors: Valsalva maneuvers (coughing, sneezing, and straining) or neck movements.
- Associated symptoms: Neck pain, dizziness, nystagmus, sleep disturbances, and autonomic dysfunction.

34.6 Diagnostic Algorithm

Step 1: Clinical suspicion.
Identify key symptoms:

- Suboccipital headache aggravated by Valsalva maneuvers.
- Neck pain and stiffness.
- Occasional vertigo or balance issues.
- Neurological signs, such as nystagmus, gait instability, hyperreflexia, and paresthesia.

Step 2: Initial diagnostic workup.

- Perform brain MRI to assess tonsillar descent: more than five millimeters is considered significant.
- Cine MRI to evaluate CSF flow dynamics.

Step 3: Genetic testing.

- Considered in cases with syndromic characteristics or family history. Use next-generation sequencing to investigate mutations in the OLFML2A, SLC4A9, and COL4A1 genes [14].

Step 4: Additional diagnostic evaluations.

- Ophthalmologic assessment if papilledema is suspected [15].

Step 5: Apply third edition of International Classification of Headache Disorders (ICHD-3) diagnostic criteria (ICHD, 2018).
According to the ICHD-3, CM1-related headache should:

1. Be associated with CM1 findings on MRI.
2. Improve after decompression surgery.
3. Have a characteristic location and trigger profile.

CM1-related headache should be excluded if:

1. Another headache disorder better explains the symptoms.
2. MRI shows secondary tonsillar descent due to altered CSF pressure.
3. The headache lacks CM1-specific characteristics, such as Valsalva triggers or improvement after decompression.

Step 6: Confirm the diagnosis.

- Integrate clinical and imaging findings.

Step 7: Classification re-evaluation.

- Differentiate between symptomatic and incidental CM1.

Headaches associated with CM1 may be confused with primary headache, migraine, tension-type headache, or occipital neuralgia. However, some characteristics may help to perform a differential diagnosis of migraine, which is more prevalent [13]:

- Triggering: CM1 headache is typically triggered by Valsalva maneuvers, which are different from migraine.
- Pain location: Although migraine may present with associated occipital pain, CM1-related headache frequently extends to the neck and shoulders.
- Response to treatment: Patients with CM1 are usually resistant to triptans and occipital blockages, but they may have significant relief after surgical decompression of the posterior fossa.

A recent machine learning-based neuroimaging study identified structural brain changes as potential biomarkers for differentiating between primary and secondary headaches in CM1 [16].

34.7 Treatment

1. Pharmacological treatment

   Among the available drugs, the following can be highlighted:

- *Gabapentin* (300–900 mg/day) acts on the hyperexcitability of the upper cervical spine and can reduce associated paresthesia [17].
- *Topiramate* (50–100 mg/day) is a modulator of glutamate that reduces central sensitization. It may also reduce segmental pressure of the CSF and alleviate headaches [18].
- *Acetazolamide* (250–500 mg/day) may help alleviate headache symptoms, particularly in patients with signs of intracranial hypertension. Its mechanism involves direct inhibition of cerebrospinal fluid secretion at the choroid plexus, leading to sustained intracranial pressure reduction for up to 10 hours and an approximate 40% decrease in CSF flow [19].
- *P2X7 receptor antagonists*, such as JNJ-47965567, lead to cytokine release (interleuin-1β (IL-1 β), tumor necrosis factor-α [TNF-α], and IL-6) associated

with neuropathic pain and hypersensitization of the trigeminovascular pathway. A review suggested that P2X7 receptor antagonists may reduce microglial inflammatory responses and have shown significant analgesic potential in experimental models of neuropathic pain and chronic headache [20].

- *Anti-Calcitonin Gene-Related Peptide (CGRP) monoclonal antibodies* (erenumab, fremanezumab, and galcanezumab) are used for refractory migraines and provide sustained improvement in pain frequency and intensity [21]. While studies for CM1 are still limited, the use of anti-CGRP may be a viable alternative for patients with persistent post-surgical headaches or headaches unresponsive to conventional therapy.

2. *Other therapeutic approaches*

   Physical therapy and lifestyle modifications: Although high-quality evidence is lacking, physical therapy focused on postural correction and cervical stabilization is often considered in clinical practice. Lifestyle adjustments such as avoiding activities that increase intrathoracic and intracranial pressure are also recommended based on pathophysiological rationale.
3. *Surgical treatment*

   Posterior fossa decompression (Fig. 34.3): The standard approach to relieve tonsillar herniation in severe or progressive cases. Posterior fossa decompression with or without duraplasty are indicated in patients with (1) disabling headache, particularly when triggered by Valsalva maneuvers (e.g., coughing, sneezing,

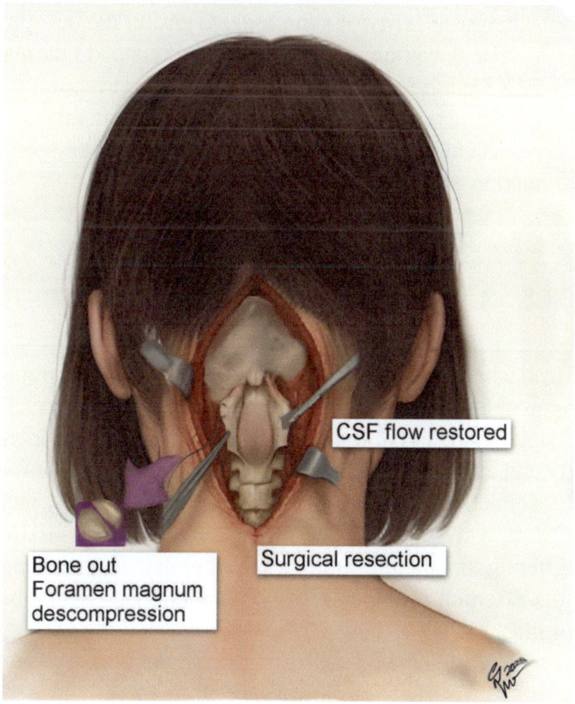

Fig. 34.3 Decompression surgery for CM1: Representation of the posterior fossa decompression procedure with duraplasty, highlighting anatomical landmarks and expected CSF restoration

and exertion); (2) significant CSF flow restriction at the foramen magnum on cine-MRI; (3) progressive syringomyelia; and (4) progressive neurological deficits, including cervicomedullary myelopathy, brainstem dysfunction (hyperreflexia, paresthesias, and motor deficits), cerebellar symptoms (ataxia, dysmetria, and nystagmus), autonomic dysfunction (blood pressure instability and neurogenic syncope), central sleep apnea, neurogenic dysphagia with no other identified cause, and craniovertebral deformity impacting CSF dynamics.

Studies indicated that up to 80% of patients subjected to posterior fossa decompression presented sustained headache improvement, especially those with significant CSF flow obstruction before the surgery [22, 23].

Duraplasty: Expansion of the dura mater to improve CSF flow.

Despite a higher risk of complications, posterior fossa decompression with duraplasty has been associated with better clinical outcomes in patients with syringomyelia [24].

Cervical fusion: In cases of atlantoaxial instability, cervical fusion may be considered a treatment option. Vertebral fusions, such as atlas assimilation and C2–3 fusion, may represent adaptive responses to chronic craniovertebral junction instability. From this perspective, isolated atlantoaxial fixation could stabilize the region and reverse associated neural and musculoskeletal changes, including those observed in patients with CM1 [25].

CM1 can be managed conservatively or through surgical decompression, with the latter being more effective in symptomatic patients with cough-induced headaches and progressive syringomyelia [26]. Treatment selection must consider the severity of symptoms to ensure the best prognosis.

The development of new biomarkers and pharmacological therapies, such as P2X7 inhibitors and anti-CGRP, may represent a promising avenue for managing refractory headaches, particularly in patients unresponsive to surgery or with persistent pain after decompression. However, specific studies in Chiari malformation are still lacking [20, 21].

34.8 Conclusion

Headache in CM1 represents a diagnostic and therapeutic challenge that requires approaches beyond conventional imaging findings. The clinical case presented, despite being hypothetical, was created based on evidence to illustrate the complexity and emphasize the need for an individualized approach.

This chapter explored the key aspects of CM1, including central sensitization, CSF flow dysfunction, the role of cine MRI in assessing CSF flow obstruction, and different therapeutic strategies. Rather than categorizing patients in clinical profiles, it is essential to understand how the disease affects their functionality and quality of life.

Treatment must be adjusted for each case. For patients with mild-to-moderate symptoms, conservative strategies might effectively control headaches, reduce neuroinflammation, minimize central sensitization, and optimize CSF dynamics. For severe cases with significant functional impairment, surgical decompression remains the best option. Nevertheless, decision-making should go beyond rigid protocols and consider the patient holistically (i.e., history, symptoms, and impact of headaches on daily life).

With advances in the understanding of CM1 and its neurological implications, emerging neuroimaging tools and biomarkers may enhance diagnostic accuracy and optimize therapeutic strategies. The main challenge remains balancing scientific evidence with a patient-centered approach. This chapter highlights the importance of a multidisciplinary perspective that integrates technical expertise with personalized treatment to improve clinical outcomes for these patients.

References

1. Chiari H. Ueber Veränderungen des Kleinhirns infolge von Hydrocephalie des Grosshirns. Dtsch Med Wochenschr. 1891;17:1172–5.
2. McClugage SG, Oakes WJ. The Chiari I malformation. J Neurosurg Pediatr. 2019;24(3):217–26. https://doi.org/10.3171/2019.5.PEDS18382.
3. Moro ERP, Teive HAG, Souza SMP, Lambrecht F, Werneck LC. Malformação de Chiari tipo I: relato de dois casos com apresentações clínicas pouco usuais. Arq Neuropsiquiatr. 1999;57(3A):666–71. https://doi.org/10.1590/S0004-282X1999000400021
4. Friedlander RM. Congenital and acquired Chiari syndrome. N Engl J Med. 2024;390(23):2191–8. https://doi.org/10.1056/NEJMra2308055.
5. Arnautovic A, Splavski B, Boop FA, Arnautovic KI. Pediatric and adult Chiari malformation Type I surgical series 1965–2013: a review of demographics, operative treatment, and outcomes. J Neurosurg Pediatr. 2015;15(2):161–77. https://doi.org/10.3171/2014.10.PEDS14295.
6. Stovner LJ. Headache associated with the Chiari type I malformation. Headache. 1993;33(4):175–81. https://doi.org/10.1111/j.1526-4610.1993.hed33040175.x.
7. Martins HAL, Ribas VR, Lima MDC, Oliveira DA, Viana MT, Ribas KHS. Cefaleia precipitada por manobras de Valsalva em pacientes com malformação congênita de Chiari tipo I. Arq Neuropsiquiatr. 2010;68(3):406–9. https://doi.org/10.1590/S0004-282X2010000300015.
8. McGirt MJ, Nimjee SM, Floyd J, Bulsara KR, George TM. Correlation of cerebrospinal fluid flow dynamics and headache in Chiari I malformation. Neurosurgery. 2005;56(4):716–21.
9. Oldfield EH, Muraszko K, DeMonte F, Menezes A. Pathophysiology of Chiari I malformation-related headache: an MRI study. N Engl J Med. 1994;331(17):1081–6. https://doi.org/10.1056/NEJM199410273311701.
10. Quigley MF, Iskandar B, Quigley MA, Nicosia M, Haughton V. Cerebrospinal fluid flow in foramen magnum: temporal and spatial patterns at MR imaging in volunteers and in patients with Chiari I malformation. Radiology. 2004;232(1):229–36.
11. Yuan Z, Wang W, Zhang X, Bai X, Tang H, Mei Y, Zhang P, Qiu D, Zhang X, Zhang Y, Yu X, Sui B, Wang Y. Altered functional connectivity of the right caudate nucleus in chronic migraine: a resting-state fMRI study. J Headache Pain. 2022;23(1):154. https://doi.org/10.1186/s10194-022-01506-9.
12. Islam J, Rahman MT, Elina KC, Park YS. Deciphering the functional role of insular cortex stratification in trigeminal neuropathic pain. J Headache Pain. 2024;25:76. https://doi.org/10.1186/s10194-024-01784-5.

13. Headache classification Committee of the International Headache Society (IHS). The international classification of headache disorders, 3rd edition. Cephalalgia. 2018;38(1):1–211. https://doi.org/10.1177/0333102417738202.
14. Yan RE, Chae JK, Dahmane N, Ciaramitaro P, Greenfield JP. The genetics of Chiari 1 malformation. J Clin Med. 2024;13(20):6157. https://doi.org/10.3390/jcm13206157.
15. Shaikh AG, Ghasia FF. Neuro-ophthalmology of type 1 Chiari malformation. Expert Rev Ophthalmol. 2015;10(4):351–7. https://doi.org/10.1586/17469899.2015.1057505.
16. Rahman Siddiquee MM, Shah J, Chong C, Nikolova S, Dumkrieger G, Li B, Wu T, Schwedt TJ. Headache classification and automatic biomarker extraction from structural MRIs using deep learning. Brain Commun. 2022;5(1):fcac311. https://doi.org/10.1093/braincomms/fcac311.
17. Kraychete DC, Sakata RK, Lannes LOC, Bandeira ID, Sadatsune EJ. Dor crônica persistente pós-operatória: o que sabemos sobre prevenção, fatores de risco e tratamento? Rev Bras Anestesiol. 2016;66(5):505–12. https://doi.org/10.1016/j.bjan.2014.12.002.
18. Scotton WJ, Botfield HF, Westgate CS, Mitchell JL, Yiangou A, Uldall MS, Jensen RH, Sinclair AJ. Topiramate is more effective than acetazolamide at lowering intracranial pressure. Cephalalgia. 2019;39(2):209–18. https://doi.org/10.1177/0333102418776455.
19. Barbuskaite D, Oernbo EK, Wardman JH, Jenkins VG, Damkier HH, Malte H, MacAulay N. Acetazolamide modulates intracranial pressure directly by its action on the cerebrospinal fluid secretion apparatus. Fluids Barriers CNS. 2022;19(1):53. https://doi.org/10.1186/s12987-022-00348-6.
20. Hu SQ, Hu JL, Zou FL, Liu JP, Luo HL, Hu DX, Wu LD, Zhang WJ. P2X7 receptor in inflammation and pain. Brain Res Bull. 2022;187:199–209. https://doi.org/10.1016/j.brainresbull.2022.07.006.
21. Aditya S, Rattan A. Advances in CGRP monoclonal antibodies as migraine therapy: a narrative review. Saudi J Med Med Sci. 2023;11(1):11–8. https://doi.org/10.4103/sjmms.sjmms_95_22.
22. Moniruzzaman S, Kaipainen A, Tervonen J, Huttunen J, Jyrkkänen HK, Huuskonen TJ, Rantala S. Long-term outcome of operated Chiari I patients between 2005 and 2020 in eastern Finland. Acta Neurochir. 2024;166(1):115. https://doi.org/10.1007/s00701-024-05999-y.
23. Raza-Knight S, Mankad K, Prabhakar P, Thompson D. Headache outcomes in children undergoing foramen magnum decompression for Chiari I malformation. Arch Dis Child. 2017;102(3):238–43. https://doi.org/10.1136/archdischild-2016-310662.
24. Lin W, Duan G, Xie J, Shao J, Wang Z, Jiao B. Comparison of results between posterior fossa decompression with and without duraplasty for the surgical treatment of Chiari malformation type I: a systematic review and meta-analysis. World Neurosurg. 2017;108:943–950.e1. https://doi.org/10.1016/j.wneu.2017.10.161.
25. Goel A. Cervical fusion as a protective response to craniovertebral junction instability: a novel concept. Neurospine. 2018;15(4):323–8. https://doi.org/10.14245/ns.1836236.118.
26. Chavez A, Roguski M, Killeen A, Heilman C, Hwang S. Comparison of operative and non-operative outcomes based on surgical selection criteria for patients with Chiari I malformations. J Clin Neurosci. 2014;21(12):2125–31. https://doi.org/10.1016/j.jocn.2014.06.009.

Part VI
Headache Attributed to a Substance or Its Withdrawal

Chapter 35
Headache Attributed to a Substance or Its Withdrawal: Carbon Monoxide (CO)-Induced Headache

Esra Aciman Demirel

35.1 Introduction

Carbon monoxide (CO) is a gaseous signaling molecule that is endogenously produced in the human body by the enzyme heme oxygenase [1]. CO functions as a gas carrier, playing a role in nociception, neurotransmission, and cerebral hemodynamics [2]. Additionally, CO has been identified as a pain-modulating neurotransmitter [3]. Exposure to CO can result in various neurological effects. A well-documented effect of CO exposure is the manifestation of headaches [4]. Typically, CO levels between 10% and 20% have been shown to induce mild headaches devoid of accompanying gastrointestinal and neurological symptoms. Levels between 20% and 30% have been associated with moderate-to-throbbing headaches and irritability. Levels of 30–40% have been associated with severe headaches, nausea, vomiting, and blurred vision. Levels exceeding 40% often result in a lack of reported headaches due to altered consciousness [5]. Levels between 50% and 60% frequently lead to myocardial ischemia, ventricular arrhythmias, pulmonary edema, lactic acidosis, hypotension, coma, seizures, and death [6].

Carbon monoxide-induced headache is a type of headache that is caused by exposure to carbon monoxide. This headache typically resolves on its own within 72 hours after the exposure is eliminated from the body [5]. Headache is frequently the initial and most prevalent symptom of CO poisoning, which can lead to neurological and systemic complications if left untreated.

E. A. Demirel (✉)
Zonguldak Bulent Ecevit University, School of Medicine, Zonguldak, Turkey

D. Uludüz et al. (eds.), *Rare Causes of Headache Disorders*, Headache,
https://doi.org/10.1007/978-3-032-10242-3_35

35.2 Pathophysiology of Carbon Monoxide-Induced Headaches (Fig. 35.1)

The pathophysiology of CO-induced headaches involves several mechanisms:

1. *CO Binding to Hemoglobin*
   - CO binds to hemoglobin 200–250 times more strongly than oxygen, forming carboxyhemoglobin (COHb) [7].
   - This reduces the blood's ability to carry and deliver oxygen to tissues, leading to cellular hypoxia [3, 4].
2. *Hypoxia in the Brain*
   - Decreased oxygen delivery results in *cerebral hypoxia*, leading to neuronal stress and metabolic dysfunction.
   - The occurrence and severity of CO-induced headache depend on both the COHb level (the severity of hypoxia) and the amount of free CO reaching the nervous system [3, 4].

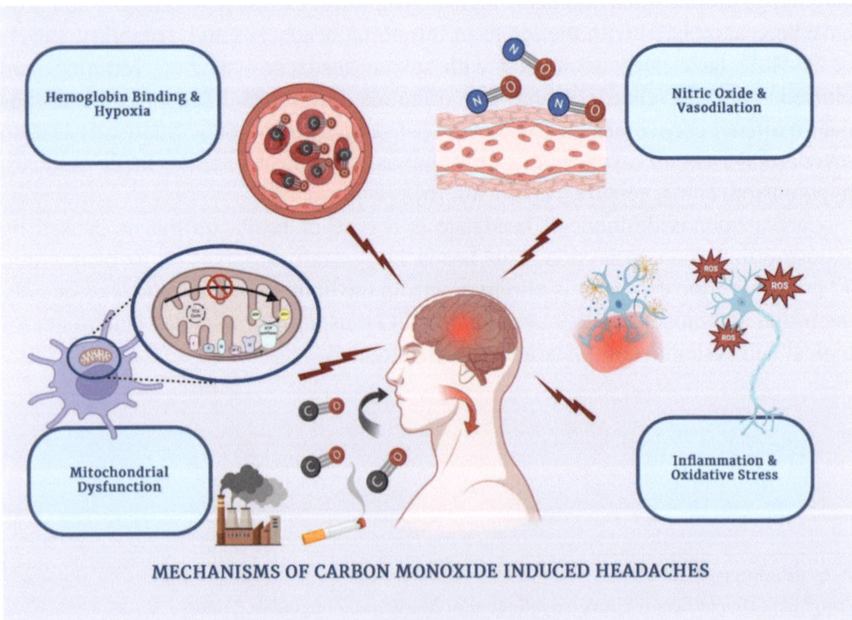

Fig. 35.1 Mechanism of carbon monoxide-induced headaches

3. *Vasodilation and Increased Blood Flow*

   - Hypoxia caused by CO exposure leads to compensatory cerebral vasodilation, increasing cerebral blood flow (CBF) in an attempt to deliver more oxygen.
   - This vasodilation, mediated by nitric oxide (NO) and other pathways, increases intracranial pressure (ICP), leading to headaches [3, 4, 8].

4. *Mitochondrial Dysfunction*

   - CO also binds to *cytochrome c oxidase*, an enzyme in the mitochondrial electron transport chain. CO inhibits cytochrome c oxidase.
   - This disrupts ATP production, causing energy failure in neurons and leading to headache and neurological symptoms and worsening headache symptoms.
   - Hypoxia and the CO toxicity directly on mitochondria cause glutamate release, which activates N-methyl-d-aspartate (NMDA) receptors, further leading to neurologic injury [9].

5. *Inflammation*

   - CO exposure triggers oxidative stress, damaging brain cells and increasing inflammatory mediators.
   - This can irritate pain-sensitive structures in the brain, contributing to headache and neuroinflammation [9].

6. *Neurotransmitter Imbalance*

   - CO has been identified as a neurotransmitter that modulates pain [9].
   - It is endogenously produced and affects pain transmission via cyclic guanosine monophosphate. It shows a strong affinity for the heme in soluble guanylate cyclase. This affinity activates soluble guanylate cyclase, leading to increased production of cyclic guanosine monophosphate and glutamate release [9].
   - CO interacts with nitric oxide, which plays an important role in the mechanisms underlying migraine formation [8]. This interaction causes dilation of cerebral vessels and the formation of free radicals, leading to headaches [4, 8].

Figure visually summarizes the complex pathophysiology of carbon monoxide-induced headaches.

35.3 Case Presentation

A 46-year-old female patient presented to the emergency department due to smoke inhalation. The incident occurred during the night while she was asleep, following a fire that broke out due to an explosion from a mobile phone battery. The patient did not notice the fire while sleeping and was awakened by her husband, who had just returned home from work and saw the house filled with smoke. Upon waking, she became aware that the entire house was engulfed in smoke. Emergency services were called, and she was promptly brought to the hospital. Upon evaluation, the patient complained of a persistent, throbbing headache accompanied by dizziness and nausea. She denied any significant past medical history and was a non-smoker. Her vital signs on admission were blood pressure, 130/85 mm Hg; heart rate 95 beats per minute; respiratory rate, 20 breaths per minute; and oxygen saturation, 97% on room air. Neurological examination revealed no abnormalities.

- Arterial blood gas (ABG) analysis revealed a carboxyhemoglobin (COHb) level of 14% (normal <2% in non-smokers).
- Electrocardiogram (ECG) was normal.
- Chest X-ray showed no abnormalities.
- Complete blood count and metabolic panel were within normal limits.
- Brain magnetic resonance imaging (MRI) was normal.

She was immediately placed on 100% high-flow oxygen via a non-rebreather mask, which helps expedite CO elimination. Symptomatic treatment for headache and nausea was provided. She was admitted for follow-up in the hospital by anesthesia. After six hours of oxygen therapy, the patient's symptoms improved significantly, and his COHb levels decreased to 5%. Following the administration of treatment, the patient's headaches were alleviated, and they were fully resolved within 24 hours. The patient was discharged from the hospital. One week later, she underwent a neurological evaluation at the outpatient neurology clinic. During this evaluation, no headaches or additional neurological symptoms were observed.

35.4 Case Discussion

This case highlights the importance of promptly recognizing and treating carbon monoxide poisoning, even in the absence of severe symptoms. A high index of suspicion, the appropriate use of carboxyhemoglobin measurements, timely administration of oxygen therapy, and meticulous follow-up are imperative to ensure optimal patient outcomes.

35.5 Headache Characteristics of CO-Induced Headache

A carbon monoxide (CO)-induced headache typically presents with distinctive features that help in its recognition and differentiation from other headache types. It is often described as a dull, continuous pain affecting both sides of the head, with moderate-to-severe intensity. The headache tends to worsen with physical activity, and it is commonly accompanied by nausea and vomiting [4, 8]. The frontal region (forehead) is the most frequently reported site of pain, although it can be diffuse and involve multiple areas of the head [4, 10]. Studies show that 66% of patients report frontal pain, while 41% describe the pain as throbbing.

Associated symptoms often include a range of neurological and systemic signs, such as dizziness, weakness, confusion, blurred vision, and shortness of breath, which may accompany or even precede the headache [4, 10]. The onset of symptoms usually occurs within 12 hours of CO exposure, and resolution is expected within 72 hours after the exposure ends.

One of the key diagnostic clues is the rapid improvement of symptoms following the administration of 100% oxygen, which helps distinguish CO-induced headaches from other types. Interestingly, recent studies indicate that symptom severity correlates more strongly with the duration of CO exposure than with the level of carboxyhemoglobin (COHb) in the blood [4].

35.6 Third Edition of International Classification of Headache Disorders (ICHD-3) Diagnostic Criteria [5]

8.1.3 Carbon Monoxide (CO)-ınduced Headache

Diagnostic Criteria:

A. Bilateral headache fulfilling criterion C
B. Exposure to carbon monoxide (CO) has occurred
C. Evidence of causation demonstrated by all of the following:
    1. Headache has developed within 12 hours of exposure to CO
    2. Headache intensity varies with the severity of CO intoxication
    3. Headache has resolved within 72 hours of elimination of CO
D. Not better accounted for by another ICHD-3 diagnosis.

Acute CO poisoning is diagnosed by anamnesis and clinical suspicion. There are no standard criteria or laboratory tests for diagnosing acute CO poisoning. COHb levels measured in blood gas are partially related to the degree of intoxication. Oxygen pressure measurements tend to be normal because PO_2 reflects O_2 dissolved in the blood and CO does not affect this measurement [6].

Carbon monoxide hemoglobin (COHb) levels are of critical importance in the diagnosis of CO poisoning. Non-smokers typically exhibit levels of less than 2%, while smokers generally display levels of 5–10%. Levels exceeding 10–15% suggest the presence of poisoning, and levels above 25% are considered severe and potentially fatal. The severity of poisoning can be gauged by the COHb levels, which in turn inform treatment methods. Carboxyhemoglobin levels above 25% are considered potentially fatal and require treatment with hyperbaric oxygen treatment [11, 12].

Lesions seen on neuroimaging are as varied as the spectrum of clinical signs and symptoms observed after CO poisoning. There are no pathognomonic radiographic changes seen on computed tomography. Magnetic resonance imaging (MRI) is a sensitive imaging method that identifies cerebral lesions in the acute period of CO poisoning. It was determined that acute CO poisoning may lead to acute brain damage, and 40.6% would be detected in brain MRIs taken in patients during the acute phase [10, 13].

35.7 Treatment

35.7.1 Oxygen Therapy (100% Oxygen)

The primary therapeutic intervention for cases of CO poisoning is the administration of 100% oxygen. The administration of high-concentration oxygen has been demonstrated to facilitate the rapid displacement of CO from hemoglobin, thereby enabling the restoration of normal oxygen-carrying capacity in the blood. The administration of oxygen is a primary treatment for CO poisoning. The rapid displacement of CO from the hemoglobin in the blood facilitates the restoration of normal oxygen-carrying capacity. Oxygen therapy accelerates the elimination of CO from the body, as CO is excreted through the lungs [11, 14].

In a study by Okan et al., it was demonstrated that the use of "oxygen only" was as adequate as the combination of "oxygen plus metoclopramide" or "oxygen plus metamizole sodium" in treating headaches induced by CO poisoning [14].

Carboxyhemoglobin levels above 25% are considered potentially fatal and require treatment with hyperbaric oxygen treatment [11, 12].

35.8 Conclusion

Carbon monoxide-induced headache is a common and early symptom of CO poisoning that requires prompt recognition and intervention. The pathophysiology involves multiple mechanisms, including hypoxia, cerebral vasodilation, mitochondrial dysfunction, oxidative stress, and neurotransmitter imbalances. Although COHb levels are helpful for diagnosis, they do not always correlate with symptom severity, making clinical judgment essential.

Oxygen therapy remains the primary and most effective treatment, facilitating rapid CO elimination and symptom resolution. This case underscores the importance of timely diagnosis and management in preventing potential neurological sequelae. Clinicians should maintain a high index of suspicion for CO poisoning in patients presenting with unexplained headaches, particularly those with a relevant exposure history. Increased awareness and education about CO toxicity are crucial for both healthcare professionals and the general public to ensure early detection and prevention of CO-related morbidity and mortality.

References

1. Arngrim N, Schytz HW, Britze J, Vestergaard MB, Sander M, Olsen KS, Olesen J, Ashina M. Carbon monoxide inhalation induces headache in a human headache model. Cephalalgia. 2018;38(4):697–706. https://doi.org/10.1177/0333102417708768.
2. Ghanizada H, Arngrim N, Schytz HW, Olesen J, Ashina M. Carbon monoxide inhalation induces headache but no migraine in patients with migraine without aura. Cephalalgia. 2018;38(13):1940–9.
3. Arngrim N, Schytz HW, Hauge MK, Ashina M, Olesen J. Carbon monoxide may be an important molecule in migraine and other headaches. Cephalalgia. 2014;34:1169–80. https://doi.org/10.1177/0333102414534085.
4. Hwang H, Lee S, Heo YW, Ha WS, Kim KM, Cha YS. Carbon monoxide poisoning is associated with increased risk of migraine in the long term: a nationwide population-based cohort study. Front Toxicol. 2025;7:1532584. https://doi.org/10.3389/ftox.2025.1532584.
5. ICHD-3 beta. The International Classification of Headache Disorders 3rd edition (beta version). Cephalalgia. 2013;33:629–808.
6. Quinn DK, McGahee SM, Politte LC, Duncan GN, Cusin C, Hopwood CJ, Stern TA. Complications of carbon monoxide poisoning: a case discussion and review of the literature. Prim Care Companion J Clin Psychiatry. 2009;11(2):74–9. https://doi.org/10.4088/pcc.08r00651.
7. Coburn RF. Karbon monoksit toksisitesinin mekanizmaları. Prev Med Baltim. 1979;8:310–22.
8. Mustafa AK, Gadalla MM, Snyder SH. Signaling by gasotransmitters. Sci Signal. 2009;2(68):re2. https://doi.org/10.1126/scisignal.268re2.
9. Rose JJ, Wang L, Xu Q, McTiernan CF, Shiva S, Tejero J, Gladwin MT. Carbon monoxide poisoning: pathogenesis, management, and future directions of therapy. Am J Respir Crit Care Med. 2017;195(5):596–606. https://doi.org/10.1164/rccm.201606-1275CI. Erratum in: Am J Respir Crit Care Med. 2017;196(3):398-399. 10.1164/rccm.
10. Hampson NB, Hampson LA. Characteristics of headache associated with acute carbon monoxide poisoning. Headache. 2002;42(3):220–3.
11. Nguyen DD, Nguyen PS, Anh Lam NH. Carbon monoxide poisoning with neurological, ocular, and myocardial damage: a case report. Asia Pacific journal of Med Toxicol. 2024;13(4):167.
12. Afzal M, Agarwal S, Elshaikh RH, Babker AMA, Choudhary RK, Prabhakar PK, Zahir F, Sah AK. Carbon monoxide poisoning: diagnosis, prognostic factors, treatment strategies, and future perspectives. Diagnostics. 2025;15(5):581. https://doi.org/10.3390/diagnostics15050581.
13. Kavak N, Doğan B, Sultanoğlu H, Kavak RP, Özdemir M. Clinical and magnetic resonance imaging findings of patients with acute carbon monoxide poisoning. Konuralp Med J. 2020;12(3):443–50. https://doi.org/10.18521/ktd.735274.
14. Ocak T, Tekin E, Basturk M, Duran A, Serinken M, Emet M. Treatment in carbon monoxide poisoning patients with headache: a prospective, multicenter, double-blind, controlled clinical trial. Am J Emerg Med. 2016;34(11):2140–5. https://doi.org/10.1016/j.ajem.2016.08.002.

Chapter 36
Cocaine-Induced Headache

Utku Topbaş and Aynur Özge

36.1 Introduction

Headache attributed to a substance or its withdrawal is a distinct diagnostic category in the International Classification of Headache Disorders, third edition (ICHD-3), encompassing headaches triggered by the use or cessation of various pharmacological and non-pharmacological agents [1]. Among these, cocaine-induced headache represents a relatively rare but clinically relevant condition, mainly due to the growing global use of cocaine and its neurovascular complications [2].

Cocaine acts as a powerful sympathomimetic agent by inhibiting the reuptake of dopamine, norepinephrine, and serotonin, leading to heightened adrenergic activity and resultant vasoconstriction, blood pressure elevation, and neuronal excitability, all of which are implicated in the pathogenesis of acute headache [2, 3]. While some users report cocaine as a headache reliever—particularly in the context of cluster headache management via intranasal administration—others develop new-onset or worsening headaches shortly after use [4]. These headaches are typically bilateral, throbbing in nature, and of moderate severity, developing within an hour of cocaine use and resolving within 72 h, as defined by the ICHD-3 criteria [1].

Chronic cocaine use has also been associated with more serious complications, such as reversible cerebral vasoconstriction syndrome (RCVS), intracerebral hemorrhage, arterial dissection, and structural white matter changes observable via neuroimaging [5–8]. These findings underscore the complexity and potential severity of

U. Topbaş
Toros State Hospital, Mersin, Turkey

A. Özge (✉)
Mersin State Hospital, Mersin, Turkey

D. Uludüz et al. (eds.), *Rare Causes of Headache Disorders*, Headache,
https://doi.org/10.1007/978-3-032-10242-3_36

cocaine's impact on the central nervous system. Cocaine's role in triggering seizures and psychiatric agitation further complicates its clinical presentation [2, 9].

Despite its inclusion in formal headache classifications, cocaine-induced headache remains underrecognized in clinical settings due to factors such as patient reluctance to disclose substance use and overlapping symptoms with other neurological or psychiatric conditions [10]. Moreover, regional variations in cocaine purity and use patterns may influence its clinical effects and reporting [11]. Considering these challenges, a high index of suspicion and careful history-taking are essential when evaluating patients presenting with acute headache in emergency or critical care settings.

This chapter presents a detailed case illustrating the complex interplay between acute headache, seizure activity, and underlying vascular pathology in the context of recent crack cocaine use, offering an opportunity to review diagnostic and therapeutic approaches for this uncommon but essential headache subtype.

36.2 Pathophysiology

Cocaine, chemically known as benzoylmethylecgonine, is an ester alkaloid derived from the leaves of the coca plant. Due to its ester structure and high bioavailability, cocaine can easily cross cell membranes and quickly produce systemic and neurological effects. It can be administered to the body through various routes: intranasal (snorting), inhalation (crack), oral consumption, and intravenous (IV) injection [12].

Cocaine causes significant vasoconstriction in the central nervous system and inhibits the reuptake of the neurotransmitters dopamine and noradrenaline in presynaptic neurons. This leads to an excessive accumulation of dopamine and noradrenaline in the synaptic cleft, which further intensifies the vasoconstriction. Additionally, cocaine stimulates the release of noradrenaline and adrenaline from the adrenal medulla, which enhances systemic vasoconstriction. The increased levels of dopamine in the mesolimbic pathway and the nucleus accumbens are responsible for pleasurable and addictive effects. The metabolites of cocaine, namely benzoylecgonine and ecgonine, also lead to vasoconstriction. Since these metabolites have longer half-lives, the secondary effects of vasoconstriction continue even after the initial effects of cocaine have faded [2].

So far, three different types of headache associated with cocaine use have been described. Type 1 usually occurs after intravenous or inhaler use. Immediately after ingestion, a bilateral throbbing headache of moderate intensity occurs which may last up to three days. This pain may be accompanied by focal neurologic findings. Severe vasoconstriction occurs immediately after cocaine ingestion. This leads to transient ischemia caused by the increase in noradrenaline in the presynaptic cleft, which results in pain. Additionally, cocaine enhances calcium-mediated contractility in vascular smooth muscle cells, thereby deactivating the compensatory vasomotor mechanisms. As a result of prolonged vasoconstriction, complications such as stroke, subarachnoid hemorrhage, and RCVS can be seen after this type of headache [2, 13].

Type 2 headache usually occurs in individuals who engage in binge intranasal usage of cocaine. The headache disappears temporarily after intranasal intake and intensifies after 45–90 minutes. After each intranasal intake, the headache is alleviated and becomes more severe with the next intranasal intake. Intranasal use of cocaine in patients with cluster-type headache may be due to the acute anesthetic effect of cocaine in the sphenopalatine ganglion. The reduction in headache is explained by an increase in presynaptic serotonin in the acute use of cocaine. Increased levels of serotonin can improve pain by activating the 5-HT1B and 5-HT1D receptors in the trigeminal ganglia, similar to the action of triptans. However, with prolonged cocaine use, there is a secondary depletion of presynaptic serotonin, which can lead to an exacerbation of pain [2, 13, 14].

Type 3 headache is a type of headache related to cocaine withdrawal rather than cocaine use. Chronic use of cocaine causes upregulation of postsynaptic dopaminergic, serotoninergic, and noradrenergic receptors. Therefore, these neurotransmitters are depleted in the presynaptic cleft faster than usual. Headaches begin 2–4 weeks after cocaine withdrawal and can persist for up to 9 months. This type of headache is included in the ICHD-3 headache attributed to withdrawal from chronic use of other substance [1, 2, 13].

36.3 Case Presentation

A 29-year-old male named Mehmet was brought to the emergency unit by his wife. She reported that her husband had been behaving strangely, yelling at her for no apparent reason and continuously pacing around the house. He was experiencing a bilateral throbbing headache on his temporoparietal region rated as 6 out of 10 in severity, accompanied by nausea. However, he did not have photophobia, phonophobia, or osmophobia. Mehmet appeared agitated, mildly confused, and disoriented regarding time. His pupils were mid-dilated bilaterally, and his skin was dry. Both the Brudzinski and Kernig signs were negative, and he exhibited no neck stiffness. The fundoscopic examination showed no signs of papilledema. At the time of admission, his blood pressure was recorded as 150/87 mm Hg, and his body temperature was 37 °C. Blood tests indicated that his creatinine kinase levels were moderately elevated, three times higher than the standard upper limit. Both he and his wife denied using any substances. However, his medical records indicated that he was currently on probation for illicit drug use. Twelve months ago, he had a seizure after using drugs and was discharged with levetiracetam. He refused to take any medications as advised by the doctors. After one hour, his headache worsened without changing in characteristics. We administered 1000 mg of intravenous paracetamol for his headache and performed a computed tomography (CT) scan. The CT revealed a space-occupying mass lesion in the left temporal lobe, with no hemorrhages detected. Upon returning to the CT room and then to the emergency room, the patient experienced generalized tonic–clonic seizures that lasted for one minute. We administered IV diazepam to treat the seizures, but he did not respond to verbal stimuli for one hour following the first seizure. He then had a second seizure episode, leading us to confirm status epilepticus. We treated him with 15 mg/kg of IV phenytoin over 45 minutes and subsequently transferred him to the intensive care unit (ICU). We collected a urine sample to send to a toxicology laboratory for substance use screening. A lumbar puncture could not be performed due to the presence of a temporal mass lesion. Instead, we conducted an urgent magnetic resonance imaging (MRI) with contrast and MRA to rule out the possibility of subarachnoid hemorrhage. The MRI revealed a lesion in the left temporal lobe that resembled a vascular abnormality (see Fig. 36.1). The MRA showed no signs of an aneurysm or arterial rupture; it only revealed vascular and microvascular tangles in the left temporal lobe, with no extravascular contrast enhancement, consistent with arteriovenous malformation (AVM; see Fig. 36.2).

In the ICU, his mental status returned to baseline after 12 hours. He was awake but extremely agitated, attacking everyone around him and yelling. He even began to harm himself by hitting the medical staff. We consulted the psychiatry department, and they advised starting treatment with 5 mg of haloperidol and 5 mg of biperiden administered intramuscularly. We initiated the treatment, and he soon fell asleep again.

After another 10 hours, he woke up and complained of a headache and nausea. He finally admitted that he had smoked two crack cocaine cigarettes two hours before arriving at the emergency unit. His headache remained the same as it had been at the beginning: a bilateral, throbbing pain in the temporal regions. The pain was moderately severe, so we treated him with IV dexketoprofen. By the next day, his headache had entirely resolved. A urine sample revealed the presence of cocaine metabolites. He refused further treatment and wanted to go home. We informed him

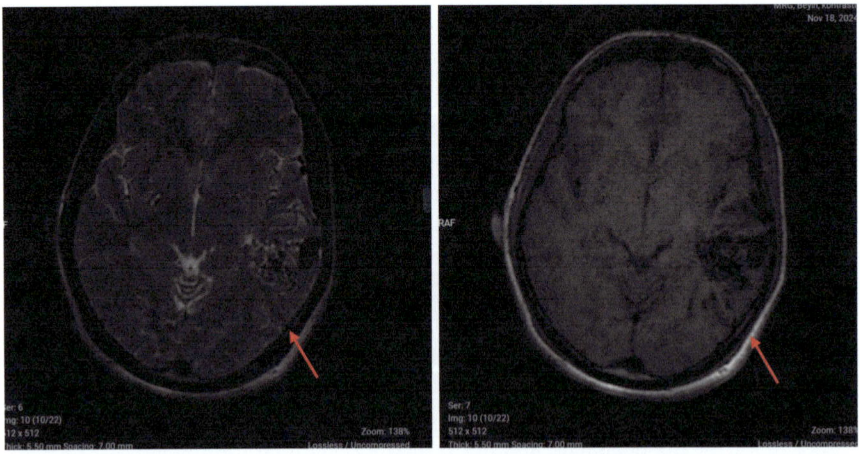

Fig. 36.1 MRI with non-contrast revealed left temporal T1 and T2 hypointensities (red arrows) resembling berry-like vascular structures. MRI Magnetic resonance imaging

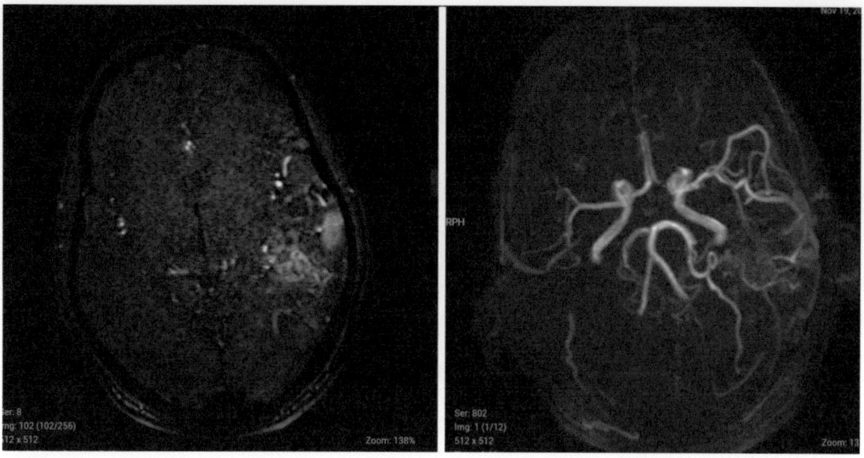

Fig. 36.2 MRA shows intravascular contrast enhancements and microvascular tangles on the left MCA. Findings consistent with left temporal lobe arteriovenous malformation. MCA Middle cerebral artery, MRA Magnetic resonance angiography

of the risks associated with refusing tests and treatment. After he had signed the necessary forms, we discharged him with a prescription for valproic acid, 500 mg to be taken twice daily.

36.4 Clinical Presentation (Table 36.1)

Cocaine-induced headache remains a diagnostically challenging entity due to its variable clinical manifestations and frequent overlap with other neurological or psychiatric conditions. According to the ICHD-3 criteria, such headaches typically present within one hour of cocaine administration and resolve spontaneously within 72 hours [1]. However, real-life clinical presentations, such as the case described here, often deviate from textbook definitions, involving more complex symptomatology and overlapping syndromes.

Cocaine exerts its effects primarily through the inhibition of monoamine reuptake, resulting in intense sympathomimetic stimulation. This neurochemical surge may contribute to vasoconstriction, hypertension, and increased excitatory neurotransmission, mechanisms implicated in the pathogenesis of cocaine-related headache [2]. Furthermore, cocaine use has been associated with serious cerebrovascular complications, including reversible cerebral vasoconstriction syndrome (RCVS), arterial dissections, and intracranial hemorrhages, particularly in chronic or high-dose users [3–5].

Table 36.1 Diagnostic criteria of cocaine-induced headache according to the ICHD-3

8.1.5 Cocaine-induced headache
Description:
Headache developing within 1 hour of, and caused by, administration of cocaine by any route. It resolves spontaneously within 72 hours
Diagnostic criteria:
A. Any headache fulfilling criterion C
B. Any route has administered cocaine
C. Evidence of causation demonstrated by all of the following:
1. Headache has developed within 1 hour of cocaine administration
2. Headache has resolved within 72 hours after cocaine administration
3. Headache has at least one of the following four characteristics:
(a) Bilateral
(b) Mild-to-moderate intensity
(c) Pulsating quality
(d) Aggravated by physical activity
D. Not better accounted for by another ICHD-3 diagnosis
Comment: *The principal routes of cocaine administration are oral ("chewing"), intranasal ("snorting"), intravenous ("mainlining"), and inhalation (smoking)*

36.5 Diagnostic Algorithm

Neuroimaging findings in patients presenting with headaches and cocaine use vary widely. In some cases, cocaine can unmask or exacerbate pre-existing vascular malformations, such as arteriovenous malformations (AVMs) or berry aneurysms, by triggering acute hypertensive episodes [2]. Cocaine-induced cerebral vasculopathy may be reversible, but the risk of permanent structural damage, particularly in the white matter, has been demonstrated using diffusion tensor imaging techniques [6].

36.6 Treatment

Interestingly, cocaine is paradoxically used in some clinical contexts as an abortive agent for cluster headaches due to its local vasoconstrictive and anesthetic effects when applied intranasally [7]. However, such off-label applications are not without risk and may lead to cranial nerve complications or dependency [7, 8].

Seizure activity, often observed in patients with acute cocaine toxicity, may be the result of direct cortical excitability or secondary to vascular insults [2]. The presence of psychiatric agitation or psychosis, as seen in the described patient, also aligns with the known neurobehavioral sequelae of cocaine use, further complicating the diagnostic picture [2, 9].

From a public health perspective, rising trends in cocaine purity and regional variability in its street formulations must be considered as they can influence both the potency and the pattern of adverse effects [10]. Despite the clinical relevance, cocaine-induced headache is likely underdiagnosed, partly due to patient hesitancy to report substance use and the lack of awareness among healthcare providers [2]. Psychosocial interventions and pharmacologic strategies remain central to addressing cocaine addiction, yet effective management of headache in this population remains an area requiring further study [11, 15].

36.7 Conclusion

- Cocaine-induced headache is a recognized secondary headache disorder under ICHD-3, yet remains underdiagnosed due to patient non-disclosure and clinical overlap with other neuropsychiatric conditions.
- Cocaine's neurovascular effects, including vasoconstriction, excitotoxicity, and hypertension, are central to headache pathophysiology and may precipitate life-threatening complications such as RCVS, intracerebral hemorrhage, or arterial dissections.
- Neuroimaging plays a crucial role in excluding structural lesions and vascular abnormalities in patients presenting with headaches and a history of cocaine use.
- Cocaine use may unmask latent cerebrovascular pathologies, such as arteriovenous malformations, which can exacerbate clinical presentation and complicate management.
- While intranasal cocaine has historically been used in procedures and cluster headache management, this practice carries risks, including cranial nerve involvement and dependency.
- Seizure activity and psychiatric agitation are common comorbidities, underscoring the need for a multidisciplinary approach involving neurology, emergency medicine, and psychiatry.
- Epidemiological studies are needed to determine the true prevalence and patterns of cocaine-induced headaches in different populations, especially in emergency settings.
- Further research into biomarkers and neuroimaging correlates may help differentiate cocaine-induced headaches from other secondary headaches and identify high-risk patients early.
- The development of specific clinical protocols for headache evaluation in individuals with known or suspected substance use could improve detection and reduce complications.
- There is a need for prospective studies evaluating the effectiveness of different acute and preventive headache treatments in the context of active or past cocaine use.
- As substance abuse trends evolve, longitudinal studies assessing the impact of changing cocaine purity and formulations on neurological outcomes, including headache, are warranted.

- Finally, integration of addiction services with headache and emergency care may offer a more holistic treatment model, improving long-term outcomes for patients with substance-induced neurological symptoms.

References

1. Headache Classification Committee of the International Headache Society (IHS). The international classification of headache disorders, 3rd edition. Cephalalgia. 2018;38(1):1–211. https://doi.org/10.1177/0333102417738202. PMID: 29368949.
2. Farooque U, Okorie N, Kataria S, Shah SF, Bollampally VC. Cocaine-induced headache: a review of pathogenesis, presentation, diagnosis, and management. Cureus. 2020;12(8):e10128. https://doi.org/10.7759/cureus.10128. PMID: 33005542; PMCID: PMC7524019.
3. Roa CH, Rodríguez LC, Bastidas N, Vergara S, Borda S, Osorio G, Gómez MF, González V, Aldana JC. Reversible cerebral vasoconstriction syndrome secondary to chronic cocaine abuse: case report. Radiol Case Rep. 2024;20(1):597–601. https://doi.org/10.1016/j.radcr.2024.10.095. PMID: 39583229; PMCID: PMC11583687.
4. Alenzi F, D'Cruz DP. Reversible cerebral vasoconstriction syndrome and Raynaud's phenomenon: is there a link between the pathogeneses of their underlying complex etiology? A case report and literature review. Diagnostics (Basel). 2023;13(18):2951. https://doi.org/10.3390/diagnostics13182951. PMID: 37761318; PMCID: PMC10528332.
5. Abdulnabi KF, Alalawi WF, Ahmed SMS, Abdulla KM, Abdultawab AA. Cocaine-induced bilateral internal carotid artery dissection: a case report. Cureus. 2023;15(11):e48548. https://doi.org/10.7759/cureus.48548. PMID: 38084188; PMCID: PMC10710747.
6. Hodges CB, Steinberg JL, Zuniga EA, Ma L, Bjork JM, Moeller GF. Chronic cocaine use and white matter coherence: a diffusion tensor imaging study. J Stud Alcohol Drugs. 2023;84(4):585–97. https://doi.org/10.15288/jsad.21-00410. Epub 2023 Feb 22. PMID: 36971714; PMCID: PMC10488304
7. Davis PM, Riddle ML. Pupil-sparing cranial nerve III palsy after intranasal cocaine treatment for cluster headache. J Am Coll Emerg Phys Open. 2020;1(5):935–7. https://doi.org/10.1002/emp2.12074. PMID: 33145543; PMCID: PMC7593431.
8. McGrath J, McGrath A, Burdett J, Shokri T, Cohn JE. Investigation of topical intranasal cocaine for sinonasal procedures: a randomized, phase III clinical trial. Int Forum Allergy Rhinol. 2020;10(8):981–90. https://doi.org/10.1002/alr.22561. Epub 2020 May 8. PMID: 32384578.
9. Buchholz J, Saxon AJ. Medications to treat cocaine use disorders: current options. Curr Opin Psychiatry. 2019;32(4):275–81. https://doi.org/10.1097/YCO.0000000000000518. PMID: 31008728.
10. Verri P, Rustichelli C, Ferrari A, Marchesi F, Baraldi C, Licata M, Vandelli D, Palazzoli F, Potì F, Silingardi E. Seizures of illicit substances for personal use in two Italian provinces: analysis of trends by type and purity from 2008 to 2017. Subst Abuse Treat Prev Policy. 2019;14(1):41. https://doi.org/10.1186/s13011-019-0229-y. PMID: 31533834; PMCID: PMC6751801.
11. De Crescenzo F, Ciabattini M, D'Alò GL, De Giorgi R, Del Giovane C, Cassar C, Janiri L, Clark N, Ostacher MJ, Cipriani A. Comparative efficacy and acceptability of psychosocial interventions for individuals with cocaine and amphetamine addiction: a systematic review and network meta-analysis. PLoS Med. 2018;15(12):e1002715. https://doi.org/10.1371/journal.pmed.1002715. PMID: 30586362; PMCID: PMC6306153.
12. Zimmerman JL. Cocaine intoxication. Crit Care Clin. 2012;28(4):517–26. https://doi.org/10.1016/j.ccc.2012.07.003. Epub 2012 Aug 30. PMID: 22998988.

13. Dhuna A, Pascual-Leone A, Belgrade M. Cocaine-related vascular headaches. J Neurol Neurosurg Psychiatry. 1991;54(9):803–6. https://doi.org/10.1136/jnnp.54.9.803. PMID: 1955899; PMCID: PMC1014520.
14. Cameron C, Kelly S, Hsieh SC, Murphy M, Chen L, Kotb A, Peterson J, Coyle D, Skidmore B, Gomes T, Clifford T, Wells G. Triptans in the acute treatment of migraine: a systematic review and network meta-analysis. Headache. 2015;55(Suppl 4):221–35. https://doi.org/10.1111/head.12601. Epub 2015 Jul 14. PMID: 26178694.
15. Chaudhary SC, Sawlani KK, Malhotra HS, Apurva NS, Rao PK. Cocaine abuse: an unusual association. J Assoc Physicians India. 2016;64(11):77–9. PMID: 27805341.

Part VII
Headache Attributed to Disorder of Homoeostasis

Chapter 37
Headache Attributed to Airplane Travel

Hilton Mariano da Silva Júnior and Leticia Bragalia Passarella

37.1 Introduction

Aeroplane headache (AH), or headache attributed to aeroplane travel, is a distinct and fascinating type of head pain that occurs exclusively during air travel. First described in 2004 by Atkinson and Lee [1], AH has since gained recognition as a specific clinical condition, characterized by sudden, severe headaches triggered by changes in cabin pressure. Although air travel is now one of the safest and most widely used forms of transportation, moving millions of people worldwide daily, these debilitating headaches during certain flight phases remain underrecognized and often misunderstood. Initially, AH caught the medical community's attention through isolated case reports and small-scale clinical studies [2], providing a limited understanding of its causes, symptoms, and potential treatments. Only after larger studies were conducted was AH officially acknowledged as a distinct medical condition. This milestone led to its inclusion in the International Classification of Headache Disorders, third edition (ICHD-3) [3], providing standardized diagnostic criteria that have guided further research and clinical identification. Before this classification, the absence of clear diagnostic guidelines made it difficult to distinguish AH from other types of headaches, like migraines, tension headaches, or sinus-related pain, which can present with comparable symptoms. Growing awareness of AH has opened up new investigation paths into its epidemiology, underlying mechanisms, and management strategies, underscoring its importance in clinical practice and public health. Research shows that AH most often occurs during aircraft descent, strongly linked to rapid shifts in cabin and atmospheric pressure. The pain is characteristically described as sharp, pulsating, or stabbing, often affecting just one side of the head, especially around the forehead and eye.

H. M. da Silva Júnior (✉) · L. B. Passarella
Pontifical Catholic University of Campinas, School of Medicine, Sao Paulo, Brazil

D. Uludüz et al. (eds.), *Rare Causes of Headache Disorders*, Headache,
https://doi.org/10.1007/978-3-032-10242-3_37

Yet, despite these advances, much remains unknown about the precise mechanisms behind AH. Possible factors include sinus barotrauma, cerebral blood vessel dilation, and individual anatomical differences. Managing AH is still a challenge, with treatments based mainly on case reports and clinical observations rather than solid randomized controlled trials (RCTs). Some medications, like non-steroidal anti-inflammatory drugs (NSAIDs), triptans, and nasal decongestants, have shown promise, particularly when taken before a flight, but standardized treatment protocols are still lacking. There is a strong need for further research to better understand and manage this condition.

This chapter aims to present a comprehensive and updated review of AH, encompassing its epidemiology, pathophysiological theories, diagnostic criteria, and current therapeutic strategies. The goal is to provide healthcare professionals with practical tools to identify, diagnose, and manage AH effectively, ultimately improving the quality of life and travel experience for affected patients. The potential impact of this research on patient care is significant and should not be underestimated.

37.2 Pathophysiology

The exact pathophysiology of aeroplane headache (AH) remains incompletely understood. However, several mechanisms have been proposed to explain its origin, with most hypotheses emphasizing the interaction between cabin pressure changes and individual anatomical or physiological predisposition.

1. *Sinus Barotrauma Due to Cabin Pressure Changes*

One of the most broadly accepted mechanisms is sinus barotrauma resulting from rapid cabin pressure fluctuations during takeoff and landing. These pressure shifts may provoke an imbalance between the atmospheric pressure and the pressure within the paranasal sinuses, leading to nasal mucosal damage, local inflammation, and activation of pain pathways [9, 14]. Berligen and Mungen [5] proposed that AH commonly results from the temporary local inflammation caused by hypoxia or dryness in the sinus mucosa or sinus barotrauma. They advocate that their treatment findings in patients support this hypothesis. According to them, AH did not occur in 95% of the patients in their subsequent flights when they received naproxen sodium (550 mg) one hour before takeoff. In a person who suffers from AH, it was proposed that there are possible anatomical variations, particularly in the ethmoidal sinuses, causing reduced patency of the nasal pathways and making it difficult to equalize pressure during ascent or descent. The ethmoidal air cells and arteries, innervated by the ethmoidal nerve (a branch of the ophthalmic division of the trigeminal nerve), may become sensitized due to barotrauma, triggering inflammatory responses and activating both the trigeminovascular system and trigeminocervical complex, leading to the typical fronto-orbital pain seen in AH. Additionally, negative pressure within the sinuses may contribute to tissue inflammation and a "vacuum effect," thereby further intensifying pain. Although many AH patients consistently show normal findings on ENT (ear, nose, and throat) workup, this may reflect mild (first-degree) barotrauma not detectable through routine diagnostics [8, 12].

2. *Cerebral Vasodilation and Prostaglandin E2 (PGE2) Release*

Cerebral vasodilation is at the core of an additional proposed mechanism for AH. Fluctuations in atmospheric pressure may induce vasodilation of cerebral arteries, possibly mediated by prostaglandin E2 (PGE2), a powerful vasodilator produced by mast cells and cerebral endothelial cells. In the experimental study by Bui et al. [15], 14 participants were evaluated using a pressure chamber to simulate (AH) conditions. The study included seven individuals with a history of AH and seven healthy controls, with a mean age of 24 years (±1.6), comprising four males and 10 females. All participants in the AH group developed headache attacks during the simulated flight, while none of the control group experienced symptoms. The AH attacks were mostly fronto-orbital, unilateral, and described as stabbing or pulsating, with severe or moderate intensity. Biomarker analysis showed that cortisol and prostaglandin E2 (PGE2) levels were significantly elevated in AH patients compared to controls, and oxygen saturation (SPO) was markedly lower in the AH group during the simulated flight. These findings suggest that AH predominantly affects young adults and is associated with physiological changes during pressure alterations, supporting the use of pressure chamber models to study AH mechanisms and potential therapeutic targets. PGE2 may induce vasodilation and activate perivascular sensory afferents, contributing to headache generation. Furthermore, local sinus inflammation during AH episodes could stimulate PGE2 release, supporting its potential role as a biomarker and mediator in AH pathophysiology [14].

3. *Cerebral Vasoconstriction (Controversial Hypothesis)*

Although less supported, some evidence suggests cerebral vasoconstriction may contribute to AH. Hiraga et al. [16] reported the case of a 74-year-old woman who presented with thunderclap headache during aeroplane descent. A magnetic resonance angiography showed segmental vasoconstriction of cerebral vessels that improved 9 days after onset. Nevertheless, this hypothesis remains controversial, as AH clinical features differ from those of reversible cerebral vasoconstriction syndrome (RCVS), particularly concerning shorter attack duration (typically <30 minutes) and absence of postictal headache [17].

4. *Psychological Factors (Anxiety and Stress)*

Anxiety and mental stress have been found at higher rates in patients with AH attacks, hence making these potential influencing factors to the development of AH. Psychological stress and anxiety are also recognized as possible contributing factors. Anticipatory anxiety, notably in individuals with prior painful episodes, may exacerbate AH symptoms or even act as a trigger. The fear of flying and associated somatic responses may amplify pain perception in susceptible individuals [18]. Besides, Bui et al. [15] demonstrated that cortisol a primary stress hormone released by the hypothalamic–pituitary–adrenal (HPA) axis was significantly elevated in AH patients when subjected to barometric pressure changes mimicking aeroplane ascent and descent.

5. *Hypoxia*

Although hypoxia is not prominently featured in recent AH pathophysiological models, cabin pressure changes may indirectly reduce oxygen availability, potentially affecting individuals who are sensitive to hypoxia. While not a primary mechanism, hypoxia may act synergistically with other factors in some cases [2, 5].

6. *Anatomical and Environmental Factors*

Structural abnormalities, such as nasal septum deviation, frontal sinus polyps, or mucosal edema, may impede normal sinus ventilation and pressure equalization, predisposing to AH. Furthermore, environmental factors including aircraft type, speed, angle of ascent/descent, and cabin pressurization systems may influence the occurrence and severity of AH episodes [5].

7. *Differential Diagnosis and Secondary Causes*

According to ICHD-3, AH is classified as a primary headache. However, it is crucial to exclude secondary causes, particularly acute and chronic sinusitis, nasal or sinus masses, and RCVS. Serial imaging studies (e.g., magnetic resonance imaging [MRI], MRA) may be required when clinical suspicion persists [8].

8. *Inflammatory Processes*

An inflammatory component is also suspected in AH pathogenesis, supported by the observed benefit of NSAIDs (e.g., ibuprofen, naproxen) in some cases [8]. The role of local inflammation, whether initiated by barotrauma, vascular changes, or both, remains a subject of ongoing investigation.

In summary, the pathophysiology of AH appears to be multifactorial, possibly involving sinus barotrauma triggered by rapid changes in cabin pressure. This leads to local inflammation, trigeminal nerve activation, and potential vasodilation of cerebral arteries. The imbalance between intrasinus and external cabin pressure is believed to be a key factor. Nevertheless, further research is needed to elucidate the underlying mechanisms of this condition fully.

37.3 Case Presentation

A 45-year-old woman presented to our private clinic with a history of headache attacks that occur during aeroplane flights. Such attacks started six months previously and never came outside of plane flights. The patient regularly flies from Brazil to the USA for family reasons every two weeks. The attacks began during takeoff and before landing. The headache was left-sided, orbitofrontal, sometimes also placed in the vertex, was pulsatile in quality, had moderate-to-severe intensity, and was associated with nausea, photophobia, and phonophobia. The attacks usually last

45 minutes. Headache spontaneously improved within 30 minutes after the ascent or descent of the aeroplane. The patient tried over-the-counter medications, such as paracetamol, dipyrone, ibuprofen, and acetylsalicylic acid (isolated or in combination), to take before and during the flight, with a slight response. She has a previous history of systemic arterial hypertension. The neurological examination showed no abnormalities. An extensive neurological and otolaryngological workup was unremarkable. The patient's clinical picture fulfills the International Classification of Headache Disorders-3 criteria for AH. Naratriptan 2.5 mg was prescribed 30 minutes before the flight and landing. The patient reported no more headaches during takeoff and landing. She had tried this therapeutic approach at least 10 times until our last communication.

Some studies have investigated the epidemiology of AH, although clear epidemiological data are still limited. It is critical to consider that much of the initial epidemiological data on aeroplane headache was derived from case series and small cohort studies. Chronologically, the epidemiologic landmarks of headache attributed to aeroplane travel are as follows:

- 2004: A 28-year-old man experienced severe jabbing headaches over the forehead and between the eyes during aeroplane ascent and descent, resolving at cruising altitude. It was the first description of "headache associated with aeroplane travel" in the literature [1].
- 2006: Six cases of AH were reported [2]. All patients were male, with a mean age of 37.3 years (ranging from 33 to 42 years), and the mean age of headache onset was 35.4 years. The average disease duration was 2.1 years, varying from 7 months to 4 years.
- 2008: A cohort study by Potasman et al. [4] found that approximately 5.7% of 906 air travelers attending a travel clinic for a wide range of other complaints were affected by AH. The mean age was 33.3 ± 14.2 years (range 18–91 years). It is a noteworthy clinical condition among individuals who frequently travel by air. A significant female predominance was observed, and 19.2% of individuals with AH also had a formal diagnosis of migraine.
- 2011: Berilgen and Müngen [5] studied 33 patients with AH, of whom 28 were men (85%) and 5 were women (15%). The mean age of the patients was 33.1 ± 8.2 years, and headaches typically began suddenly during the descent phase of flights, although some occurred during the ascent phase. The authors proposed preliminary diagnostic criteria and possible mechanisms of etiopathogenesis for headaches associated with aeroplane travel.
- 2011: İpekdal et al. [6] reported five patients (three women and two men) suffering from AH, the mean age was approximately 30 years (from 27 to 32). All patients experienced headaches exclusively during aeroplane ascent or descent.
- 2012: Mainardi et al. [7] evaluated 75 patients with AH, with a male predominance (61.3%) and a mean age of 36.5 years. Most patients (88%) developed headaches after their first flight, and over half (54.6%) had coexisting primary headaches, mainly tension-type and migraine without aura.

- 2013: The third edition of the International Classification of Headache Disorders (ICHD-3) recognized headache attributed to aeroplane travel as a distinct type of secondary headache [2].
- 2016: Bui et al.'s Danish survey [8] included 21 patients (9 males, 12 females) with a mean age of 39 ± 14 years among 254 Scandinavian air travelers. The 21 participants (8.3%) fulfilled the aeroplane headache (AH) diagnostic criteria defined by ICHD-3.
- 2017: Bui et al. [9] analyzed 39 scientific papers representing 275 patients. This review highlights the initially reported male predominance; however, as more case reports emerged, no significant gender predominance was observed. The median age at diagnosis was 28.7 ± 4.8 years.
- 2018: The third edition of the International Classification of Headache Disorders (ICHD-3) was published [10].
- 2018: In the first multicentric survey on aeroplane headache (AH) in a pediatric population, De Carlo et al. [11] evaluated 320 children with primary headaches who had travelled by aeroplane, identifying 15 cases (4.7%) of AH. The mean age at headache onset was 7.2 years, and the mean age at recruitment was 12.4 years, with a marked female predominance (80%).
- 2020: Lima et al. [12] conducted a prospective, cross-sectional study involving Brazilian medical students who had traveled by aeroplane at least three times. The study included 155 participants, among whom 14.2% (22/155) reported experiencing headache attributed to aeroplane travel (AH), corresponding to 7.5% of all flights (80/1070 trips). Among those affected, 63.6% (14/22) were men and 36.4% (8/22) were women, indicating a slight male predominance, although this difference did not reach statistical significance. The mean age of individuals with AH was 22.4 years for those experiencing headaches during takeoff or landing, and 23 years for those reporting headaches during the cruise phase, consistent with the overall young demographic of the medical student population. Notably, most headaches (77.3%) occurred during takeoff and landing, highlighting these flight phases as primary triggers for AH.
- 2022: In an extensive cross-sectional study, Konrad et al. [13] assessed 50,000 airline passengers and found a 0.2% prevalence of aeroplane headache (AH), much lower than previous reports. The mean age of affected individuals was 41.8 years, with no significant difference in gender. Most headaches began during periods of pressure change (79.2%) and were short-lived (lasting ≤30 minutes in 82.2%).

The prevalence of headache attributed to aeroplane travel varies between studies, possibly due to the different populations studied and data acquisition methodologies. While initially thought to affect adult males more, more recent data suggest there might not be a significant gender predominance in adults. In children with primary headaches, it is more prevalent in females and presents distinct characteristics. More population-based studies are needed to determine the exact prevalence in the general population and to better understand the risk factors and clinical features of this condition.

37.4 Headache Characteristics

The typical clinical picture of AH is a sudden, severe, and strictly unilateral pain, typically located in the frontal, orbital, or fronto-orbital regions, and closely linked to aeroplane travel, particularly during takeoff and landing [4, 5, 7–9]. It lasts a few to 30 minutes, sometimes accompanied by ipsilateral nasal congestion or lacrimation. The pain is frequently described as sharp, stabbing, jabbing, or pulsating, with moderate-to-severe intensity, and usually resolves spontaneously within 5–30 minutes after pressure stabilization. Seldom are migraine-like symptoms like nausea, photophobia, and phonophobia present. AH primarily affects young to middle-aged adults, with some studies suggesting a slight male predominance, though more recent data indicate no significant gender difference. Its hallmark is the exclusive occurrence during flights, without headache episodes outside air travel. Aeroplane headache is a primary headache under the International Classification of Headache Disorders (ICHD-3):

10.1.2 Headache Attributed to Aeroplane Travel
Description:

Headache, often severe, usually unilateral and periocular and without autonomic symptoms, occurring during and caused by aeroplane travel. It remits after landing.

Diagnostic criteria:

A. At least two episodes of headache fulfilling criterion C
B. The patient is traveling by aeroplane
C. Evidence of causation demonstrated by at least two of the following:
    1. Headache has developed during the aeroplane flight
    2. Either or both of the following:
        (a) Headache has worsened in temporal relation to ascent following takeoff and/or descent before landing of the aeroplane
        (b) Headache has spontaneously improved within 30 minutes after the ascent or descent of the aeroplane is completed
    3. Headache is severe, with at least two of the following three characteristics:
        (a) Unilateral location[1]
        (b) Orbitofrontal location[2]
        (c) Jabbing or stabbing quality[3]
D. Not better accounted for by another ICHD-3 diagnosis[4].

Notes:

1. Side-shift between different flights occurs in around 10% of cases.
2. Parietal spread may occur.
3. Pulsation (throbbing) may also be noted.
4. In particular, sinus disorder should be excluded.

37.5 Case Discussion

Our case demonstrates various distinctive features supporting the diagnosis of aeroplane headache (AH), by the International Classification of Headache Disorders, third edition (ICHD-3, code 10.1.2). The headache presents an exclusive temporal relationship with aeroplane travel, specifically during takeoff and landing, directly correlating with cabin pressure changes. The pain is strictly unilateral, localized to the orbitofrontal and vertex regions, which aligns with the typical distribution described in AH. The headache is characterized by a pulsatile quality, with moderate-to-severe intensity, and demonstrates spontaneous resolution shortly after cabin pressure stabilizes. The absence of headache attacks outside of flights reinforces the situational and mechanically triggered nature of this condition. Although associated migrainous symptoms, including nausea, photophobia, and phonophobia, are not universally reported in AH, their presence in this case may reflect individual variation in pain processing. Additionally, neurological, otolaryngological, and imaging evaluations were unremarkable, ruling out other structural or sinus-related causes.

37.6 Treatment

Many medications have been used to treat and prevent aeroplane headache (AH), with variable degrees of reported efficacy according to different sources [7, 14, 18, 19]. These pharmacological approaches include non-steroidal anti-inflammatory drugs (NSAIDs), triptans, and nasal decongestants. However, it is essential to emphasize that most of the available evidence regarding the effectiveness and use of these medications is derived from case reports, small case series, and retrospective studies. While these sources offer valuable insights into possible treatment options, they are limited by their observational nature and small sample sizes, which prevent broader generalizations. Therefore, randomized controlled trials (RCTs) are critically needed to establish more definitive and evidence-based treatment guidelines for managing aeroplane headache. Robust clinical studies would help determine the most effective medications, appropriate dosing regimens, and preventive strategies, ultimately improving the care and quality of life for individuals affected by this condition. Until such data are available, therapeutic approaches to AH will remain based on empirical evidence and individual patient responses as observed in clinical practice. The pharmacological and non-pharmacological approaches to treat AH are shown in Tables 37.1, 37.2 and 37.3:

Table 37.1 Preventive treatment

Class	Examples	How to use	Evidence/Comments
Triptans	Naratriptan 2.5 mg, sumatriptan 50–100 mg, zolmitriptan 2.5 mg	Take 30–60 minutes before takeoff and/or landing	According to case reports, the most effective prophylaxis is long-acting triptans, which are preferred
NSAIDs	Ibuprofen 400–600 mg, naproxen 500 mg	Take 1 hour before flight	Variable efficacy; may help in milder cases
Combination (triptan + NSAID)	Naratriptan + ibuprofen, etc.	Take before flight	Anecdotal reports suggest possible additive effect
Nasal decongestants	Pseudoephedrine 60–120 mg, oxymetazoline nasal spray	Use 30–60 minutes before flight	It may help if sinus barotrauma is suspected; there is limited evidence

Table 37.2 Acute treatment

Class	Examples	Evidence/Comments
Analgesics	Paracetamol 1 g, dipyrone (Metamizole)	Often insufficient alone but may help in mild cases
NSAIDs	Ibuprofen, naproxen	It may offer partial relief but is less effective than prophylactic triptans
Triptans	Sumatriptan 50 mg oral or 6 mg subcutaneous	If not used preventively, may be attempted as rescue

Table 37.3 Non-pharmacological approaches

Approach	Description
Pressure equalization techniques	Yawning, swallowing, chewing gum, and using the Valsalva maneuver
Nasal saline sprays	To improve sinus drainage before/during flight
Behavioral strategies	Stress/anxiety management for psychological components
Avoidance of known triggers	Choosing seats near the wing, avoiding flights during respiratory infections

37.7 Conclusion

Aeroplane headache (AH) is a unique, under-recognized condition that can cause significant distress during air travel. Recognizing AH as a distinct headache entity has advanced understanding, classification, and therapeutic approaches. Prophylactic measures with NSAIDs and triptans, possibly combined with nasal decongestants, are currently the most effective strategies. More controlled studies are needed to confirm optimal treatments and elucidate the underlying mechanisms of AH, to improve patient outcomes and comfort during flights.

References

1. Atkinson V, Lee L. An unusual case of an airplane headache. Headache. 2004;44(5):438–9. https://doi.org/10.1111/j.1526-4610.2004.04087.x.
2. Berilgen MS, Müngen B. Headache associated with airplane travel: report of six cases. Cephalalgia. 2006;26(6):707–11. https://doi.org/10.1111/j.1468-2982.2006.01096.x.
3. Headache classification Committee of the International Headache Society (IHS). The international classification of headache disorders, 3rd edition (beta version). Cephalalgia. 2013;33(9):629–808. https://doi.org/10.1177/0333102413485658.
4. Potasman I, Rofe O, Weller B. Flight-associated headaches-prevalence and characteristics. Cephalalgia. 2008;28(8):863–7. https://doi.org/10.1111/j.1468-2982.2008.01638.x.
5. Berilgen MS, Mungen B. A new type of headache associated with airplane travel: preliminary diagnostic criteria and possible mechanisms of aetiopathogenesis. Cephalalgia. 2011;31(12):1266–73. https://doi.org/10.1177/0333102411418804. Epub 2011 Aug 9
6. Ipekdal HI, Karadaş Ö, Öz O, Ulaş ÜH. Can triptans safely be used for airplane headache? Neurol Sci. 2011;32(6):1165–9. https://doi.org/10.1007/s10072-011-0603-7. Epub 2011 May 10. PMID: 21556868.
7. Mainardi F, Lisotto C, Maggioni F, Zanchin G. Headache attributed to airplane travel ('airplane headache'): clinical profile based on a large case series. Cephalalgia. 2012;32(8):592–9. https://doi.org/10.1177/0333102412441720. Epub 2012 Apr 5. PMID: 22492425.
8. Bui SBD, Petersen T, Norgaard Poulsen J, Gazerani P. Headaches attributed to airplane travel: a Danish survey. J Headache Pain. 2016;17(1):33. https://doi.org/10.1186/s10194-016-0628-7. PMID: 27165237; PMCID: PMC4864431.
9. Bui SBD, Gazerani P. Headache attributed to airplane travel: diagnosis, pathophysiology, and treatment: a systematic review. J Headache Pain. 2017;18(1):84. https://doi.org/10.1186/s10194-017-0788-0. PMID: 28801043; PMCID: PMC5556684.
10. Headache Classification Committee of the International Headache Society (IHS). The international classification of headache disorders, 3rd edition. Cephalalgia. 2018;38(1):1–211. https://doi.org/10.1177/0333102417738202.
11. De Carlo D, Toldo I, Tamborino AM, Bolzonella B, Ledda MG, Margari L, Raieli V, Santucci M, Sciruicchio V, Vecchio A, Zanini S, Sartori S, Gatta M, Verrotti A, Battistella PA. Headache attributed to aeroplane travel: the first multicentric survey in a paediatric population affected by primary headaches. J Headache Pain. 2018;19(1):108. https://doi.org/10.1186/s10194-018-0939-y.
12. Lima GAM, Vasconcelos Júnior FCF, Morais IMA, Cruz VT, Krymchantowski AG, Jevoux C, Krymchantowski A, Silva-Néto RP. Prevalence of headache attributed to airplane travel among medical students in Brazil. Headache. 2020;60(10):2406–12. https://doi.org/10.1111/head.13983.
13. Konrad F, Moritz A, Moritz M, Keunecke JG, Tischler F, Prottengeier J. The epidemiology of airplane headache: a cross-sectional study on point prevalence and characteristics in 50,000 travelers. Cephalalgia. 2022;42(10):1050–7. https://doi.org/10.1177/03331024221092408.
14. Mainardi F, Maggioni F, Lisotto C, Zanchin G. Diagnosis and management of headache attributed to airplane travel. Curr Neurol Neurosci Rep. 2013;13(3):335. https://doi.org/10.1007/s11910-012-0335-y.
15. Bui SBD, Petersen T, Poulsen JN, Gazerani P. Simulated airplane headache: a proxy for identifying underlying mechanisms. J Headache Pain. 2017;18(1):9. https://doi.org/10.1186/s10194-017-0724-3. PMID: 28148172; PMCID: PMC5286638.
16. Hiraga A, Aotsuka Y, Koide K, Kuwabara S. Reversible cerebral vasoconstriction syndrome precipitated by airplane descent: case report. Cephalalgia. 2017;37(11):1102–5. https://doi.org/10.1177/0333102416665226. Epub 2016 Sep 7
17. Mainardi F, Maggioni F, Zanchin G. Reversible cerebral vasoconstriction syndrome (RCVS) and headache attributed to aeroplane travel (AH): does a link exist? Cephalalgia. 2017;37(13):1311–2. https://doi.org/10.1177/0333102416677967. Epub 2016 Nov 12

18. Nierenburg H, Jackfert K. Headache attributed to airplane travel: a review of literature. Curr Pain Headache Rep. 2018;22(7):48. https://doi.org/10.1007/s11916-018-0701-9.
19. Koçer A. Airplane headache and its management with oxymetazoline nasal spray: a case report. J Headache Pain. 2020;21(1):151. https://doi.org/10.1186/s10194-020-01211-8. PMID: 33302898; PMCID: PMC7731784.

Chapter 38
Diving Headache

Juliana Ramos de Andrade, Marcos Antônio Inácio de Oliveira Filho, and Marcelo Valença

38.1 Introduction

Headache attributed to disorders of homeostasis, as classified by the International Classification of Headache Disorders, 3rd edition (ICHD-3), encompasses a group of secondary headaches triggered by physiological imbalances such as hypoxia, hypercapnia, and pressure changes [1]. Within this category, diving headache (DH) represents a rare but clinically relevant phenomenon associated with the specific environmental and metabolic challenges encountered during scuba diving.

Although often considered benign, diving headaches (DH) may reflect a range of underlying mechanisms, including carbon dioxide retention (hypercapnia) due to inadequate ventilation of compressed gases, barotrauma involving the sinuses or middle ear, decompression illness, arterial gas embolism, or the exacerbation of pre-existing primary headache disorders such as migraine [2–4].

Among these, hypercapnia is the most consistently implicated etiology, typically presenting as a bilateral, pulsatile headache during or shortly after a dive. Rapid symptom resolution with the administration of 100% oxygen has been documented, reinforcing its metabolic origin [3]. In other cases, headache may result from mask compression, cervical muscle strain, or psychological tension, especially in novice divers with anxiety or fear of marine life [5].

A retrospective review of incident reports published by Divers Alert Network (DAN) International between 2001 and 2009 revealed that the absolute number and

J. R. de Andrade · M. A. I. de Oliveira Filho
Federal University of Pernambuco, Recife, Pernambuco, Brazil

M. Valença (✉)
Federal University of Pernambuco, Recife, Pernambuco, Brazil

Center of Excellence in the Treatment of Migraine and Other Headache Disorders, Hospital Esperança, Recife, Pernambuco, Brazil

D. Uludüz et al. (eds.), *Rare Causes of Headache Disorders*, Headache,
https://doi.org/10.1007/978-3-032-10242-3_38

relative percentage of headaches reported as the primary complaint in diving-related incidents were consistently low. In 2001, 64 out of 1480 incidents (4.3%) involved headache. This proportion peaked in 2002, with 57 cases among 573 incidents (10%), and gradually declined over subsequent years. By 2008 and 2009, the number of headache-related incidents dropped significantly, with only 12 and 17 cases reported, respectively, representing 0.1 and 0.15% of the total incidents [2–7]. These findings suggest a downward trend in reported diving-related headaches, reinforcing the impression that DH is a relatively rare occurrence.

Accurate diagnosis requires a detailed clinical history and neurological examination, particularly in the presence of focal neurological signs, which may indicate serious conditions that require urgent hyperbaric treatment [3]. Although DH is rare, its clinical relevance lies in the need to differentiate benign headache from life-threatening complications.

38.2 Pathophysiology

The pathophysiology of diving headache is multifactorial, involving a combination of physiological and environmental stressors specific to the underwater setting. These headaches can occur at various phases of the dive and are influenced by changes in ambient pressure, altered gas composition, cold exposure, physical exertion, and individual predispositions such as primary headache disorders. A solid understanding of the underlying mechanisms is essential for accurate diagnosis, effective management, and the development of preventive strategies, especially for recreational or occupational divers at higher risk.

Hypercapnia, or elevated carbon dioxide levels, is one of the most well-established causes of diving headache. It results from inadequate ventilation of compressed gases, often due to shallow breathing or poorly adjusted equipment, leading to CO_2 accumulation. The consequent cerebral vasodilation increases intracranial pressure, triggering headache symptoms that are usually diffuse, throbbing, and accompanied by confusion or malaise. Oxygen administration is the treatment of choice in such cases, as it helps lower carbon dioxide levels and rapidly alleviates symptoms [2, 4].

Barotrauma is another frequent cause, particularly involving the middle ear or paranasal sinuses. Failure to properly equalize pressure during descent can create a vacuum effect, resulting in mucosal stretching, localized pain, and headache, often in the frontal or temporal regions. In more severe cases, such as barotrauma affecting the sphenoid sinus, vital adjacent neurovascular structures may be involved, leading to vertigo, nausea, or even neurological deficits [3, 8, 9]. On ascent, expanding gas trapped in these cavities may exert mechanical pressure, further intensifying the headache.

Additional contributors to diving headache include external compression from tight-fitting equipment, cold-water exposure, and physical exertion. Cold-stimulus headaches and exertional headaches are typically benign and self-limiting but can be distressing for divers [2, 10]. Furthermore, individuals with a history of primary headache disorders such as migraine or tension-type headache may experience exacerbations triggered by the diving environment [11]. While most diving headaches are benign, serious conditions like decompression sickness or arterial gas embolism must always be ruled out, particularly in the presence of neurological symptoms [3, 4, 8]. A comprehensive understanding of these mechanisms is crucial for clinicians to distinguish between benign and potentially life-threatening causes and to ensure safe diving practices.

Diving headache does not follow a single, well-defined clinical phenotype. Reported cases typically involve pain that begins during or shortly after diving, with locations ranging from frontal and occipital to diffuse. The quality of the pain varies—pulsatile or pressing in nature—and its intensity ranges from mild to severe, often lasting from a few minutes to several hours. In some cases, the headache is aggravated by equipment use, pre-dive anxiety, or equalization maneuvers.

The multifactorial origin of DH includes potential triggers such as:

- CO_2 retention due to hypoventilation
- Sinus or middle ear barotrauma
- Cervical muscle tension
- Psychological stress
- Environmental conditions (cold water, depth, physical exertion)

Cases attributed to hypercapnia often respond quickly to 100% oxygen therapy, reinforcing the metabolic nature of some DH subtypes.

Most frequently, DH is observed in individuals with a history of primary headache disorders—particularly migraine—suggesting that diving may act as a trigger rather than an independent cause.

38.3 Case Presentation

A representative case report is not presented in this chapter due to the absence of a typical clinical pattern and the heterogeneous nature of DH. Instead, we present a clinical observation based on prospective field data.

In 2013, a cohort of 50 recreational divers without a prior history of migraine was prospectively assessed for headache occurrence within 24 hours post-dive. The sample consisted predominantly of males (90%), with a mean age of approximately 33 years. Pre-dive anxiety was commonly reported, and 52% of participants used medications to prevent motion sickness (e.g., meclizine). All participants provided informed consent.

None of the divers reported headache during or after the dive. This finding supports the hypothesis, also observed in retrospective DAN data, that scuba diving under safe, controlled conditions does not induce headache in healthy, non-migraine individuals.

Unfortunately, we were not able to include a case of a patient with this type of headache. Instead, we chose to present a study involving several individuals who had undergone professional diving. However, none of them reported experiencing headache. There may be a selection bias, as individuals who have previously experienced this type of headache may avoid diving exposure.

38.4 Clinical Presentation

Diving headache remains a rare secondary headache disorder, more often associated with individual susceptibility and situational stressors than with the diving activity itself. Retrospective data from DAN International (2001–2009) demonstrate low absolute and relative frequencies of headache reported as a primary complaint. These values are notably lower than the general population prevalence of headache in Brazil (15.2%), suggesting a low burden of DH.

This discrepancy may be due to underreporting, preemptive exclusion of chronic headache sufferers from diving, and adherence to medical advice discouraging dives deeper than 18 meters for individuals with migraine. The absence of headache in the 2013 prospective cohort further supports the conclusion that scuba diving is not an independent trigger of headache in individuals without primary headache disorders.

Nonetheless, headache occurring during or after diving should always be evaluated carefully, especially when accompanied by focal neurological symptoms, as these may indicate serious complications such as arterial gas embolism or decompression illness. In such cases, immediate referral to a hyperbaric facility is warranted.

38.5 Diagnostic Algorithm

The diagnosis DH is straightforward, as it refers to any headache precipitated by the act of diving. Since it is a multifactorial condition, the associated signs and symptoms will vary depending on the underlying cause. For example, it may result from a tight-fitting mask, barotrauma-related otitis, or be triggered in individuals with a predisposition to migraine.

A. Any headache fulfilling criterion C
B. Both of the following:

    1. The patient is diving at a depth > 10 meters
    2. No evidence of decompression illness

C. Evidence of causation demonstrated by at least one of the following:

1. Headache has developed during the dive
2. Either or both of the following:
3. (a) Headache has worsened as the dive is continued
4. (b) Either of the following:
5. Headache has spontaneously resolved within three days of completion of the dive
6. Headache has remitted within one hour after treatment with 100% oxygen
7. At least one of the following symptoms of CO_2 intoxication:
   (a) Mental confusion
   (b) Light-headedness
   (c) Motor incoordination
   (d) Dyspnoea
   (e) Facial flushing

D. Not better accounted for by another ICHD-3 diagnosis.

38.6 Treatment

Treatment begins with immediate removal of the individual from the act of diving, always observing the necessary protocols for a slow ascent from deeper waters to avoid complications such as gas embolism. Depending on the underlying cause, specific treatment will be required.

38.7 Conclusion

Diving headache is a rare and multifactorial entity, more commonly affecting individuals with pre-existing primary headache disorders such as migraine. Evidence from both retrospective DAN reports and a prospective cohort study indicates that, when conducted under standard safety protocols, scuba diving does not independently cause headache in healthy individuals.

The absence of a typical clinical presentation justifies the decision to forgo a standard case report in this chapter. Instead, we emphasize the need for individualized assessment and awareness of risk factors. Preventive strategies—such as proper screening, adherence to dive safety standards, and counseling for migraineurs—remain effective measures to minimize the occurrence of DH.

References

1. Headache Classification Committee of the International Headache Society (IHS). The International Classification of Headache Disorders, 3rd edition (beta version). Cephalalgia. 2013;33(9):629–808.
2. Cheshire WP, Ott MC. Headache in divers. Headache. 2001;41(3):235–47.
3. Cheshire WP. Headache and facial pain in scuba divers. Curr Pain Headache Rep. 2004;8(4):315–20.
4. Burkett JG, Nahas-Geiger SJ. Diving headache. Curr Pain Headache Rep. 2019;23(7):46.
5. Di Fabio R, Vanacore N, Davassi C, Serrao M, Pierelli F. Scuba diving is not associated with high prevalence of headache: a cross-sectional study in men. Headache. 2012;52(3):385–92.
6. Durham PL, Cady R. Insights into the mechanism of OnabotulinumtoxinA in chronic Migraine. Headache. 2011;51(10):1573–7.
7. Lantéri-Minet M. The role of general practitioners in Migraine management. Cephalalgia. 2008;28(2_suppl):1–8.
8. Newton HB. Neurologic complications of scuba diving. Am Fam Physician. 2001;63(11):2211–8.
9. Schipke JD, Cleveland S, Drees M. Sphenoid sinus barotrauma in diving: case series and review of the literature. Res Sports Med. 2018;26(1):124–37.
10. Indo T, Takahashi A. Swimmer's migraine. Headache. 1990;30(8):485–7.
11. Beduhn B, Roe G, Furst W, Lewno A. Head pain in the competitive aquatic athlete—an approach to a differential diagnosis and management. Curr Sports Med Rep. 2022;21(11):398–404.

Chapter 39
Dialysis Headache

Ana Luisa de Lima Antoniazzi and Andre Cleriston Jose dos Santos

39.1 Introduction

Chronic kidney disease (CKD) is a significant public health concern, with a high global prevalence (850 million people in 2022, 7–12%) [1, 2]. A considerable proportion of these patients progress to end-stage renal disease (ESRD), requiring renal replacement therapy (hemodialysis, peritoneal dialysis, or kidney transplantation). Among these, hemodialysis remains the most widely available and commonly used treatment, having saved millions of lives since its implementation in the 1940s [3].

Patients undergoing hemodialysis often experience a range of systemic and neurological symptoms, with headache being the most frequently reported [4]. Studies dating back to the 1970s have characterized a distinct type of headache associated with hemodialysis [5]. This chapter provides a concise review of hemodialysis-related headache, discussing its clinical implications and future research directions.

39.2 Pathophysiology of Dialysis Headache

The pathophysiology of hemodialysis-related headache is multifactorial, with several mechanisms proposed to explain its occurrence [6]. Patients with CKD are predisposed to neurological symptoms due to endothelial dysfunction, neurotoxin accumulation, and electrolyte imbalances [7, 8]. Additionally, those undergoing

A. L. de Lima Antoniazzi (✉)
Member of Brazilian Headache Society, Ribeirão Preto, Brazil

A. C. J. dos Santos
Department of Neurology at the Hospital das Clínicas, Ribeirão Preto Medical School – University of São Paulo, Ribeirão Preto, Brazil

D. Uludüz et al. (eds.), *Rare Causes of Headache Disorders*, Headache,
https://doi.org/10.1007/978-3-032-10242-3_39

hemodialysis experience acute homeostatic alterations, which may contribute to headache development.

In a seminal 1972 study, Bana et al. suggested that hemodialysis-related headaches might be linked to "dialysis disequilibrium syndrome" [5]. This syndrome is characterized by mental confusion, nausea, and headache occurring during or after dialysis. The rapid removal of urea and the production of idiogenic osmoles in the brain create a gradient between the blood and brain, resulting in water influx into brain tissue, leading to edema and increased intracranial pressure [9]. However, Bana also hypothesized that additional mechanisms were involved, as headache frequently occurred in isolation and often resembled other primary headache disorders, such as migraine and tension-type headache. Subsequent research has confirmed his hypothesis, revealing multiple contributing factors.

Several elements have been implicated in dialysis headache, including dialysate composition, electrolyte imbalances, vasoactive substances, cerebrovascular regulation, hemodynamic changes, and variations in fluid balance [10].

One study reported that patients undergoing bicarbonate dialysis experienced fewer headaches compared to those receiving acetate dialysis [11]. However, a more recent study found no significant difference related to dialysate composition [4]. Regarding the hemodialysis technique, evidence suggests that online hemodiafiltration offers substantial protection against headache development when compared to conventional methods [12].

Electrolyte disturbances, such as low pre-dialysis sodium levels, magnesium fluctuations, and urea and renin concentrations, have been identified as risk factors for dialysis headache [6, 13–15]. The ultrafiltration rate also appears to be a contributing factor, with slower rates tending to cause fewer headaches [10, 16]. Blood pressure (BP) variability, both pre-dialysis hypertension and intradialytic hypotension, has also been linked to headache occurrence [4, 6, 17].

Vasoactive substances, such as nitric oxide and bradykinin, exhibit elevated levels during hemodialysis and have been implicated in other primary headaches [18]. These substances alter cerebrovascular regulation, as demonstrated by a transcranial Doppler ultrasound study by Sousa Melo et al., which revealed reduced middle cerebral artery pulsatility in patients experiencing dialysis headache compared to those without headache [19]. Additionally, increased levels of substance P and calcitonin gene-related peptide (CGRP) have been associated with headache onset before or after dialysis [20]. The role of CGRP was confirmed in a recent study that evaluated patients with hemodialysis-induced headaches without a history of primary headaches, also demonstrating higher levels in those experiencing headaches [21].

39.3 Case Presentation

A 51-year-old female teacher with a history of hypertension, type 2 diabetes mellitus, and generalized anxiety disorder, had no prior history of headaches. She also had no family history of migraine or other primary headaches. Due to end-stage renal disease, she initiated hemodialysis three times per week, with each session lasting 4 hours.

She reported a unilateral frontal headache (without a preferential side), pulsating in nature, and of severe intensity (8/10 on the Visual Analog Scale—VAS), typically beginning 2–3 hours after the start of the dialysis session. The headache was not associated with photophobia or phonophobia and tended to persist for 6–8 hours after the session in the absence of treatment. It significantly impacted her quality of life to the extent that she described it as the most bothersome symptom during hemodialysis sessions.

No significant changes in blood pressure were observed before, during, or after hemodialysis. Additionally, sodium, potassium, magnesium, urea, calcium, and other electrolyte levels remained within normal limits. Neurological examination was unremarkable. However, given the recent onset of headache and her concern about secondary causes, a brain magnetic resonance imaging (MRI) was performed, revealing only mild microangiopathy (Fazekas 2).

During dialysis sessions, the pain improved, though usually incompletely, with intravenous dipyrone (2 g). The patient also noted that when the headache persisted for several hours after dialysis, she occasionally used an over-the-counter analgesic (Dorflex®: dipyrone 300 mg, caffeine 50 mg, and orphenadrine 35 mg), which provided relief in some instances.

39.4 Case Discussion

This case illustrates a common presentation of hemodialysis headache. A clear temporal relationship was observed, with the pain beginning during dialysis sessions and typically resolving within a few hours after their completion. The headache intensity ranged from moderate to severe, significantly affecting the patient's quality of life.

Although the headache was unilateral and pulsatile, it lacked additional features characteristic of migraine or tension-type headache. Notably, the pain pattern did not follow a specific characteristic and could even mimic other primary headache disorders.

Blood pressure remained controlled and did not show significant fluctuations during dialysis sessions, ruling out hypertensive crisis as a potential cause. The patient reported symptom relief with a common analgesic and a caffeine-containing medication but did not exhibit excessive caffeine consumption, limiting her intake to a maximum of two cups per day. This level of intake also did not meet the criteria for caffeine withdrawal headache.

Despite partial relief with these medications, the improvement was often incomplete. This, combined with the significant impact of the headache on her quality of life, making it the most distressing symptom during hemodialysis, highlights the importance of further research and the development of more effective prophylactic and abortive treatment strategies.

39.5 Characteristics of Dialysis Headache

The prevalence of hemodialysis-related headache ranges from 6.6% to 70% among patients undergoing maintenance hemodialysis [5, 6, 13, 17–19, 22–25]. Older studies reported higher prevalence rates, while recent research suggests a decline, potentially due to advancements in dialysis technology and changes in diagnostic criteria under the third edition of the International Classification of Headache Disorders (ICHD-3). Over the past 5 years, prevalence rates have ranged from 8.7% to 49% [6, 19, 26]. There does not appear to be a preferential involvement based on sex, although some studies suggest a slightly higher prevalence in men [10]. Hemodialysis headache can also occur in children. In a 2017 study, Davidovits et al. examined 60 children with CKD and found a prevalence of 43.3% [24].

Hemodialysis-related headache is typically of moderate-to-severe intensity, significantly impacting quality of life. It begins during the dialysis session, most commonly occurring some hours after its initiation, usually after the third hour [19]. The pain has no specific characteristics but is commonly located in the frontal and temporal regions bilaterally. It may also affect the occipital area or present unilaterally. The headache may be pulsatile, pressure-like, or tightening in nature, resembling tension-type or migraine-like headaches. In severe cases, nausea and vomiting may accompany the headache [18, 19]. The duration of symptoms varies, lasting an average of 3–7 hours post-dialysis but sometimes persisting up to 72 hours.

Interestingly, approximately 20–23% of affected patients have no prior history of primary headache disorders [18, 27]. However, patients with pre-existing headache disorders may experience exacerbations or alterations in their headache patterns after starting hemodialysis. The causal link between hemodialysis and headache is reinforced by observations that headaches often resolve or revert to pre-dialysis characteristics following successful kidney transplantation [7].

39.6 ICHD-3 Diagnostic Criteria [28]

Headache with no specific characteristics, occurring during and caused by hemodialysis. It resolves spontaneously within 72 hours after the hemodialysis session has ended.

39.6.1 Diagnostic Criteria

A. At least three episodes of acute headache fulfilling criterion C
B. The patient is on hemodialysis
C. Evidence of causation demonstrated by at least two of the following:
    1. Each headache has developed during a session of hemodialysis
    2. Either or both of the following:
        (a) Each headache has worsened during the dialysis session
        (b) Each headache has resolved within 72 hours after the end of the dialysis session
    3. Headache episodes cease altogether after successful kidney transplantation and termination of hemodialysis
D. Not better accounted for by another ICHD-3 diagnosis.

Note: Caffeine is rapidly removed by dialysis: 8.3.1 *Caffeine-withdrawal headache* should be considered in patients who consume large quantities of caffeine.

39.7 Diagnostic Algorithm

Step 1: Identification of Headache in Hemodialysis Patients

- Presence of recurrent headache episodes during hemodialysis sessions.

Step 2: Identification of Differential Diagnoses

- Monitor blood pressure before, during, and after hemodialysis.
- Differentiate from hypertensive crisis headache without hypertensive encephalopathy (acute systolic BP ≥180 mm Hg and/or diastolic BP ≥120 mm Hg), per ICHD-3 criteria 10.3.2.
- Ensure the patient does not consume excessive caffeine (defined as ≥6 cups of coffee/day) [19, 29].
- If the patient presents with severe symptoms of dialysis disequilibrium syndrome, such as altered consciousness or seizures unexplained by electrolyte disturbances, brain imaging is warranted.

Step 3: Confirmation of ICHD-3 Diagnostic Criteria
Step 4: Identification of Predisposing Factors

- Assess for significant electrolyte imbalances (sodium, magnesium, urea, calcium) before and during hemodialysis.
- Monitor weight and hydration status pre- and post-hemodialysis, as large fluctuations predispose to headache.

- Observe blood pressure variability, as both pre-dialysis hypertension and intradialytic hypotension are contributing factors.

39.8 Management of Dialysis Headache

The management of dialysis headache primarily focuses on identifying and mitigating predisposing factors. Current recommendations include limiting excessive caffeine intake, maintaining appropriate fluid balance, and optimizing blood pressure and electrolyte levels. However, research on specific pharmacological treatments remains limited [10].

Anecdotal reports suggest that caffeine may be beneficial for alleviating acute symptoms. However, a recent randomized controlled trial failed to demonstrate a higher incidence of headache among caffeine consumers [30]. Additionally, there are reports of symptomatic relief with dipyrone, a non-narcotic analgesic with antipyretic and antispasmodic properties. While dipyrone is widely used in Brazil, its availability is restricted in several countries [17, 31].

The role of triptans in dialysis headache remains unexplored, as does the use of nonsteroidal anti-inflammatory drugs (NSAIDs), which are generally avoided in patients with chronic kidney disease due to potential nephrotoxicity and cardiovascular risks. Although a case report described headache relief with dihydroergotamine [32], ergot alkaloids are contraindicated in this patient population due to the risk of arteriovenous fistula thrombosis.

Evidence regarding prophylactic treatment is similarly scarce. One report suggested potential benefits from chlorpromazine and angiotensin-converting enzyme inhibitors [33]. Additionally, anecdotal accounts describe the use of topiramate, nortriptyline, and amitriptyline [31], though robust clinical data are lacking.

To date, CGRP-blocking monoclonal antibodies have not been investigated as a prophylactic treatment for dialysis headache. Given their pathophysiological rationale, they represent a promising therapeutic option. Studies by Alessandri et al. [20] and Gursoy et al. [21] have strongly implicated CGRP in dialysis-related headache, providing a solid foundation for future clinical trials exploring anti-CGRP therapies as a potential prophylactic strategy.

39.9 Conclusion

Dialysis headache remains a prevalent yet underrecognized complication of hemodialysis, with multifactorial pathophysiology and significant implications for patient quality of life. Although progress has been made in understanding its mechanisms, further research is needed to optimize preventive and therapeutic strategies. Enhanced recognition and targeted interventions can potentially improve the well-being of patients undergoing hemodialysis.

References

1. Romagnani P, Remuzzi G, Glassock R, Levin A, Jager KJ, Tonelli M, Massy Z, Wanner C, Anders HJ. Chronic kidney disease. Nat Rev Dis Primers. 2017;3:17088. https://doi.org/10.1038/nrdp.2017.88.
2. Romagnani P, Agarwal R, Chan JCN, Levin A, Kalyesubula R, Karam S, Nangaku M, Rodríguez-Iturbe B, Anders HJ. Chronic kidney disease. Nat Rev Dis Primers. 2025;11(1):8. https://doi.org/10.1038/s41572-024-00589-9.
3. Kolff WJ, Berk HTJ, Welle NM, Van Der Ley AJW, Van Dijk EC, Van Noordwijk J. The artificial kidney: a dialyser with a great area. Acta Med Scand. 1944;117(2):121–34.
4. Göksan B, Karaali-Savrun F, Ertan S, Savrun M. Haemodialysis-related headache. Cephalalgia. 2004;24(4):284–7.
5. Bana DS, Yap AU, Graham JR. Headache during hemodialysis. Headache J Head Face Pain. 1972;12(1):1–14.
6. Xiong Y, You N, Liao R, Wu L, Liu Y, Ling Z, Yu Y. Association of intradialysis blood sodium level, blood pressure variability, and hydration status with hemodialysis-related headache: a prospective cohort study. J Headache Pain. 2023;24(1):166. https://doi.org/10.1186/s10194-023-01701-2.
7. Viticchi G, Falsetti L, Salvemini S, Bartolini M, Ranghino A, Buratti L, Silvestrini M. Headache changes after kidney transplant. Acta Neurol Belg. 2022;122(1):83–90. https://doi.org/10.1007/s13760-021-01637-x.
8. Maggioni F, Mantovan MC, Rigotti P, Cadrobbi R, Mainardi F, Mampreso E, Ermani M, Cortelazzo S, Zanchin G. Headache in kidney transplantation. J Headache Pain. 2009;10(6):455–60. https://doi.org/10.1007/s10194-009-0148-9. Epub 2009 Aug 27. P.
9. Lu R, Kiernan MC, Murray A, Rosner MH, Ronco C. Kidney–brain crosstalk in the acute and chronic setting. Nat Rev Nephrol. 2015;11(12):707–19.
10. Barber M. Dialysis headache: an updated literature review. Curr Pain Headache Rep. 2025;29(1):16.
11. Neyer U, Wöss E, Haller R, Kröss R. [Headache and EEG changes caused by acetate and bicarbonate dialysis]. Acta Med Austriaca. 1983;10(1):15–23.
12. Hazim A, Adarmouch L, Eloury A, Aasfara J, Asly M, Slassi I. Hemodialysis-related headache: still a challenge in 2020? Effect of conventional versus online hemodiafiltration from a study in Casablanca, Morocco. Artif Organs. 2021;45(6):602–7.
13. Yang Y, Meng F, Zhu H, Zhang L, Lu G, Xiao S, He J, Yu S, Liu R. The applicability research of the diagnostic criteria for 10.2 Heamodialysis-related headache in the international classification of headache disorders-3rd edition. J Headache Pain. 2023;24(1):19. https://doi.org/10.1186/s10194-023-01548-7.
14. Bana DS, Graham JR. Renin response during hemodialysis headache. Headache J Head Face Pain. 1976;16(4):168–72.
15. Bana DS, Graham JR. Plasma 18 Hydroxy- II - Deoxycorticosterone in dialysis patients with headache. Headache J Head Face Pain. 1978;18(1):23–5.
16. Chou JA, Kalantar-Zadeh K. Volume balance and intradialytic ultrafiltration rate in the hemodialysis patient. Curr Heart Fail Rep. 2017;14(5):421–7.
17. Antoniazzi AL, Bigal ME, Bordini CA, Speciali JG. [Headache and hemodialysis: evaluation of the possible triggering factors and of the treatment]. Arq Neuropsiquiatr. 2002;60(3-A):614–8.
18. de Lima Antoniazzi AL, Corrado AP. Dialysis headache. Curr Pain Headache Rep. 2007;11(4):297–303.
19. Sousa Melo E, Pedrosa RP, Carrilho Aguiar F, Valente LM, Sampaio Rocha-Filho PA. Dialysis headache: characteristics, impact and cerebrovascular evaluation. Arq Neuropsiquiatr. 2022;80(2):129–36.
20. Alessandri M, Massanti L, Geppetti P, Bellucci G, Cipriani M, Fanciullacci M. Plasma changes of calcitonin gene-related peptide and substance P in patients with dialysis headache. Cephalalgia. 2006;26(11):1287–93.

21. Gürsoy G, Karadağ S, Köse Ş, Şakacı T, Koçak SY, Döventaş YE, Oktar AÇ, Bayar MD. The role of calcitonin gene-related peptide and substance P in the pathogenesis of dialysis headache. Hemodial Int. 2024;28(1):85–91. https://doi.org/10.1111/hdi.13120.
22. Stojimirovic B, Milinkovic M, Zidverc-Trajkovic J, Trbojevic-Stankovic J, Maric I, Milic M, Andric B, Nikic P. Dialysis headache in patients undergoing peritoneal dialysis and hemodialysis. Ren Fail. 2015;37(2):241–4. https://doi.org/10.3109/0886022X.2014.982486.
23. Antoniazzi AL, Bigal ME, Bordini CA, Tepper SJ, Speciali JG. Headache and hemodialysis: a prospective study. Headache J Head Face Pain. 2003;43(2):99–102.
24. Davidovits M, Eidlitz MT. Headache in pediatric and adolescent patients with chronic kidney disease, with and without hemodialysis: a comparative cohort study. Cephalalgia. 2018;38(5):883–91.
25. Jesus ACFD, Oliveira HA, Paixão MOR, Fraga TP, Barreto FJN, Valença MM. Clinical description of hemodialysis headache in end-stage renal disease patients. Arq Neuropsiquiatr. 2009;67(4):978–81.
26. Chhaya KT, Mankad S, Shah MK, Patel M, Desai D, Desai SD. Headache associated with hemodialysis in patients with end-stage renal disease in India: a common yet overlooked comorbidity. Ann Indian Acad Neurol. 2022;25(1):82–7.
27. Sav MY, Sav T, Senocak E, Sav NM. Hemodialysis-related headache. Hemodial Int. 2014;18(4):725–9.
28. The International Classification of Headache Disorders, 3rd edition (beta version). Cephalalgia Int J Headache. 2013;33(9):629–808.
29. Freedman ND, Park Y, Abnet CC, Hollenbeck AR, Sinha R. Association of coffee drinking with total and cause-specific mortality. N Engl J Med. 2012;366(20):1891–904.
30. Aoun MH, Hilal N, Beaini C, Sleilaty G, Hajal J, Boueri C, Chelala D. Effects of caffeinated and decaffeinated coffee on hemodialysis-related headache (CoffeeHD): a randomized multicenter clinical trial. J Ren Nutr. 2021;31(6):648–60. https://doi.org/10.1053/j.jrn.2021.01.025.
31. Sousa Melo E, Carrilho Aguiar F, Sampaio Rocha-Filho PA. Dialysis headache: a narrative review. Headache J Head Face Pain. 2017;57(1):161–4.
32. Levin M. Resident and fellow section. Headache J Head Face Pain. 2013;53(1):181–5.
33. Leinisch-Dahlke E, Schmidt-Wilcke T, Krämer B, May A. Improvement of dialysis headache after treatment with ACE-inhibitors but not angiotensin II receptor blocker: a case report with pathophysiological considerations. Cephalalgia. 2005;25(1):71–4.

Chapter 40
Headache Attributed to Pheochromocytoma

Christina I. Deligianni and Theodoros Mavridis

40.1 Introduction

Pheochromocytomas are rare neuroendocrine tumors that secrete catecholamines and arise from the adrenal medulla, representing approximately 80–85% of such neoplasms [1]. When these tumors originate instead from extra-adrenal chromaffin cells of the sympathetic or parasympathetic ganglia in the chest, abdomen, pelvis, head, or neck, they are referred to as paragangliomas [2]. They are responsible for producing excessive amounts of catecholamines (adrenaline, noradrenaline, dopamine) and their metabolites (metanephrines, normetanephrines) These tumors, though uncommon, are of significant clinical importance due to their potential to cause life-threatening hypertension and a wide range of systemic clinical manifestations, and because they represent a potentially treatable condition. Among the various symptoms, headache is a frequently reported complaint in patients with pheochromocytoma [2]. This chapter provides an overview of the disease, exploring the mechanisms underlying headache in pheochromocytoma individuals, its variant clinical presentations, diagnosis assessment, and management strategies.

C. I. Deligianni (✉)
Neurology Department, Athens Naval Hospital, Athens, Greece

1st Department of Neurology, Eginition Hospital, National and Kapodistrian University of Athens, Athens, Greece

T. Mavridis
Neurology Department, Tallaght University Hospital, Dublin, Ireland

D. Uludüz et al. (eds.), *Rare Causes of Headache Disorders*, Headache,
https://doi.org/10.1007/978-3-032-10242-3_40

40.2 Pathophysiology of Pheochromocytoma-Related Headaches

The pathophysiology of headache induction in pheochromocytoma is not fully understood. It is primarily related to the excessive secretion of catecholamines, such as epinephrine and norepinephrine, particularly during paroxysmal episodes of hormone secretion, leading to vasoconstriction and an abrupt rise in blood pressure. High blood pressure results in endothelial damage, leading to alterations in cerebral blood flow, which in turn may induce headaches [3]. Other potent vasodilator agents secreted by the adrenal gland, such as adrenomedullin, which belongs to the calcitonin gene-related peptide (CGRP) superfamily of vasoactive peptide hormones could induce headache, via the activation of the trigeminovascular system, which is also activated by high levels of catecholamines (dopamine and norepinephrine) in the synaptic dopaminergic and noradrenergic clefts of pain matrix pathways [4, 5].

40.3 Case Presentation

A 22-year-old non-smoker male with no previous medical history presented to the emergency department with a severe, right-sided, throbbing headache lasting 76 h. The pain was rated as 10/10 in intensity and accompanied by photophobia, phonophobia, and persistent nausea. He denied prior episodes of similar headaches. There was no trauma, fever, or illicit drug use. His family history included his mother suffering from chronic migraine. He received oral sumatriptan 50 mg and naproxen 500 mg twice daily and metoclopramide 10 mg four times daily for nausea over 4 days at home without meaningful relief. In the emergency department, pain improved only slightly to 7–9/10. On examination, he was diaphoretic with a blood pressure of 220/122 mmHg, heart rate 95 bpm, oxygen saturation (SpO_2) 99%, and temperature 36.8 °C. The neurological examination revealed only a fine tremor in the upper limbs, with no focal neurological deficits. Due to the absence of a headache history and the presence of red flag symptoms (neurological signs, systemic involvement, and new headache), further evaluation was necessary. Routine blood tests and magnetic resonance imaging (MRI) of the brain were unremarkable. Despite symptomatic treatment with intravenous dexketoprofen and dexamethasone (which reduced pain to 2/10), blood pressure remained elevated at 200/110 mmHg. Given the triad of headache, sustained hypertension, and diaphoresis, workup for pheochromocytoma was initiated. A 24-hour urinary catecholamine profile revealed elevated metanephrine (600 μg/24 h) and normetanephrine (1200 μg/24 h). Urine norepinephrine, epinephrine, and dopamine were also elevated. Contrast-enhanced computed tomography (CT) of the abdomen and pelvis showed a 5 cm right adrenal mass consistent with pheochromocytoma. Fludeoxyglucose-18-positron emission tomography (FDG-PET) ruled out metastatic disease or extra-adrenal paragangliomas. Metoclopramide was promptly discontinued due to its potential to precipitate catecholaminergic crises [6]. The patient was started on an α-blocker with doxazosin, followed by a β-blocker with metoprolol. Blood pressure gradually improved.

After appropriate preoperative preparation, he underwent successful laparoscopic adrenalectomy. Histopathology confirmed pheochromocytoma. Postoperatively, the patient made a full recovery. Antihypertensive medications were tapered and discontinued. He has remained normotensive and free of headache episodes since. Despite the absence of clinical features suggestive of a hereditary syndrome, genetic testing for common mutations associated with pheochromocytoma/paraganglioma (Von Hippel–Lindau [VHL], REarranged during Transfection/multiple endocrine neoplasia [RET/MEN2], neurofibromatosis type 1 [NF1]) was conducted and returned negative [7].

40.4 Case Discussion

This case illustrates the necessity of following the criteria of the International Classification of Headache Disorders (ICHD) for diagnosing headache syndromes, particularly when a secondary cause is possible [8]. While migraine-like headaches and migraine status are typically seen in patients with established migraine, their occurrence in a patient without prior headache history should prompt evaluation for secondary causes. The presence of SNNOOP10 red flags appropriately guided further workup [9]. Pheochromocytoma should be considered in patients with episodic headache, especially when associated with hypertension and autonomic features [10–12]. Metoclopramide, commonly used for migraine-associated nausea, can provoke hypertensive crises in this context and should be avoided [6]. Early diagnosis and surgical resection of pheochromocytoma are curative in most cases [13]. Genetic testing remains essential for ruling out syndromic associations, even in apparently sporadic presentations.

40.5 Headache Characteristics of Pheochromocytoma

Headaches in patients with Pheochromocytoma can vary in presentation. Typically, these headaches are associated with other classic symptoms of catecholamine excess, including hypertension, sweating, palpitations, anxiety/ panic-like symptoms, and flushing. It is the most common symptom (39.5%) [14]. It is predominantly characterized by it is paroxysmal manifestation in 51–80% of patients suffering from pheochromocytoma [8]. Headache intensity is usually severe, the location is frontal or occipital, and has pulsating or constant features. The duration of the headache is distinctive, lasting less than 15 min in 50% of patients, while in 70% lasts less than an hour. It could be accompanied by anxiety, tremor, visual disturbances, nausea, vomiting, abdominal/chest pain, flashing/blanching face, and rarely by paresthesias [8]. These symptoms often occur in episodes, with periods of remission between attacks. Nevertheless, some patients may experience more persistent, non-paroxysmal symptoms. A headache is present in close temporal relation to a blood pressure rise and improves with normalization of the blood pressure.

However, there are cases reported with atypical clinical manifestations of headache type, mimicking other types of headaches, especially when other systemic symptoms do not accompany them.

40.5.1 Diagnostic Algorithm

Step 1: Clinical Suspicion

- Apply a detailed clinical evaluation including patient's history, general physical examination, neurological examination, fundoscopy [15]
- *Identify Key Symptoms:*
  - Arterial hypertension, palpitation, anxiety, sweating, flashing/blanching face during the attack
  - Family history of hereditary syndromes: multiple endocrine neoplasia (MEN) type 2, Von Hippel–Lindau (VHL) syndrome, and neurofibromatosis type 1 (NF1)

Step 2: Initial Diagnostic Workup

- *Perform brain computed tomography (CT)*
  - Exclude other causes of thunderclap headache, for example, subarachnoid hemorrhage (SAH), other intracranial hemorrhages, cerebral venous thrombosis (CVT), brain tumor, central nervous system (CNS) infections, posterior reversible encephalopathy syndrome (PRES)
- *Perform lumbar puncture (LP)*
  - If brain CT is not diagnostic
  - Measure opening pressure, cell count, protein, glucose, inspect visually xanthochromia, test for CNS infections
- *Perform contrast-enhanced brain magnetic resonance imaging (MRI) and noninvasive vascular imaging of the head and neck (e.g., magnetic resonance angiography [MRA], CT angiography [CTA]).*
  - If brain CT and LP are not diagnostic
  - Exclude other diagnoses

Step 3: Biochemical Testing

- *Measure plasma or 24-hour urine metanephrine levels* [16]
  - It is the gold standard for the diagnosis of pheochromocytoma

Step 4: Additional Diagnostic Evaluations

- *Perform either contrast enhanced CT or MRI for the initial anatomical localization of the tumor*

  - Abdomen and pelvis imaging is most commonly used

- *Perform functional imaging to clearly establish the diagnosis* [17]
  - If the tumor is extra-adrenal, additional imaging with 123I-metaiodobenzylguanidine (MIBG) scintigraphy may be helpful for locating tumors outside of the adrenal glands.
  - 18F-FDG PET scan is the most accessible tracer and is playing an increasingly important role in PCC/ PGL imaging [17].

Step 5: Apply ICHD-3 Diagnostic Criteria [8]

A. Recurrent discrete short-lasting headache episodes fulfilling criterion C
B. Pheochromocytoma has been demonstrated
C. Evidence of causation demonstrated by at least two of the following:

   1. Headache episodes in temporal relation to development of the pheochromocytoma, or led to its discovery
   2. Either or both of the following:

      (a) Individual headache episodes develop in temporal relation to abrupt rises in blood pressure
      (b) Individual headache episodes remit in temporal relation to normalization of blood pressure

   3. Headache is accompanied by at least one of the following:

      (a) Sweating
      (b) Palpitations
      (c) Anxiety
      (d) Pallor

   4. Headache episodes remit entirely after removal of the pheochromocytoma

D. Exclude more suitable diagnoses according to ICHD-3 criteria

Step 6: Confirm Diagnosis

- Combination of clinical suspicion, application of ICHD-3 criteria, biochemical testing, and imaging studies.

Other investigations: *Genetic testing* may be indicated in certain cases, particularly in patients with familial syndromes, such as multiple endocrine neoplasia (MEN) type 2. Pheochromocytomas are also associated with mutations in genes locations: SDHB (succinate dehydrogenase subunit B or complex II of the mitochondrial respiratory chain), SDHC (subunit C), SDHD (subunit D), VHL (Von Hippel-Lindau), RET (REarranged during Transfection), and NF1 (neurofibromatosis type 1), and the very recently reported susceptibility genes SDHAF2 (succinate dehydrogenase complex assembly factor 2, also called SDH5), TMEM127 (transmembrane protein 127), SDHA (subunit A), and MAX (MYC associated factor X).

40.6 Treatment

The treatment of headache in pheochromocytoma is focused on controlling the underlying cause—excess catecholamine secretion—and managing the associated hypertension. Several therapeutic strategies are employed:

1. Antihypertensive therapy: α-blockers, such as phenoxybenzamine, are used to control hypertension and prevent the vasoconstrictive effects of excessive catecholamines. These medications also help alleviate headaches by reducing blood pressure fluctuations.
2. Heart rate: β-blockers (e.g., propranolol) can be added to control tachycardia and reduce the adrenergic stimulation that contributes to the headache. Nevertheless, β-blockers should never be started before α-blockers, as unopposed alpha-adrenergic stimulation may worsen the hypertensive crisis.
3. Surgical resection: The definitive treatment for pheochromocytoma is surgical resection of the tumor, which leads to normalization of catecholamine levels and, therefore, most patients experience resolution of symptoms, including headaches.
4. Management of hypertensive crises: Intravenous medications such as nitroprusside or labetalol may be used to control acute blood pressure elevations, which can also lead to headache relief if present.

40.7 Conclusion

Headache is a common but often overlooked symptom in patients with pheochromocytoma, and it is essential to consider this diagnosis in patients presenting with unexplained headache, primarily when associated with other systemic symptoms such as hypertension, palpitations, and sweating. Clinical suspicion leads to early diagnosis and treatment, which are crucial for preventing complications and improving outcomes. Physicians must be vigilant when evaluating prolonged headaches in the emergency setting. Medical management, including alpha and beta blockade, followed by surgical resection of the tumor, remains the cornerstone of treatment. Prompt recognition and appropriate intervention can provide significant relief from the debilitating symptoms associated with this rare but significant condition.

References

1. Anyfanti P, Mastrogiannis K, Lazaridis A, Tasios K, Vasilakou D, Kyriazidou A, Aroutsidis F, Pavlidou O, Papoutsopoulou E, Tiritidou A, Kotsis V, Triantafyllou A, Zarifis I, Douma S, Gkaliagkousi E. Clinical presentation and diagnostic evaluation of pheochromocytoma: case series and literature review. Clin Exp Hypertens. 2023;45(1):2132012. https://doi.org/10.1080/10641963.2022.2132012.

2. Farrugia FA, Martikos G, Tzanetis P, Charalampopoulos A, Misiakos E, Zavras N, Sotiropoulos D. Pheochromocytoma, diagnosis and treatment: review of the literature. Endocr Regul. 2017;51(3):168–81. https://doi.org/10.1515/enr-2017-0018.
3. Gupta PK, Marwaha B. Pheochromocytoma. [Updated 2024 Nov 7]. In: StatPearls [Internet]. Treasure Island (FL): StatPearls Publishing; 2025 Jan-. Available from: https://www.ncbi.nlm.nih.gov/books/NBK589700/.
4. Ghanizada H, Al-Karagholi MA, Arngrim N, Mørch-Rasmussen M, Walker CS, Hay DL, Ashina M. Effect of adrenomedullin on migraine-like attacks in patients with migraine: a randomized crossover study. Neurology. 2021;96(20):e2488–99. https://doi.org/10.1212/WNL.0000000000011930. Epub 2021 Apr 7. PMID: 33827963.
5. D'Andrea G, D'Arrigo A, Dalle Carbonare M, Leon A. Pathogenesis of migraine: role of neuromodulators. Headache. 2012;52(7):1155–63. https://doi.org/10.1111/j.1526-4610.2012.02168.x. Epub 2012 Jun 1. PMID: 22671857.
6. Leonard JB, Munir KM, Kim HK. Metoclopramide induced pheochromocytoma crisis. Am J Emerg Med. 2018;36(6):1124.e1–2.
7. Neumann HPH, Young WF Jr, Eng C. Pheochromocytoma and Paraganglioma. N Engl J Med. 2019;381(6):552–65.
8. The International Classification of Headache Disorders, 3rd edition. Cephalalgia. 2018;38(1):1–211. Jes Olesen ISSN: 0333-1024.
9. Do TP, Remmers A, Schytz HW, Schankin C, Nelson SE, Obermann M, Hansen JM, Sinclair AJ, Gantenbein AR, Schoonman GG. Red and orange flags for secondary headaches in clinical practice: SNNOOP10 list. Neurology. 2019;92(3):134–44. https://doi.org/10.1212/WNL.0000000000006697.
10. Bravo EL, Gifford RW Jr. Pheochromocytoma. Endocrinol Metab Clin N Am. 1993;22(2):329–41.
11. Manger WM, Gifford RW. Pheochromocytoma. J Clin Hypertens (Greenwich). 2002;4(1):62–72.
12. Bravo EL. Pheochromocytoma: new concepts and future trends. Kidney Int. 1991;40(3):544–56.
13. Nehs MA, Ruan DT. Minimally invasive adrenal surgery: an update. Curr Opin Endocrinol Diabetes Obes. 2011;18(3):193–7.
14. Ando Y, Ono Y, Sano A, Fujita N, Ono S, Tanaka Y. Clinical characteristics and outcomes of pheochromocytoma crisis: a literature review of 200 cases. J Endocrinol Investig. 2022;45(12):2313–28. https://doi.org/10.1007/s40618-022-01868-6. Epub 2022 Jul 20. PMID: 35857218.
15. Schwedt TJ. Thunderclap Headache. Continuum (Minneap Minn). 2015;21(4 Headache):1058–71. https://doi.org/10.1212/CON.0000000000000201. PMID: 26252591.
16. Patel D, Phay JE, Yen TWF, Dickson PV, Wang TS, Garcia R, Yang AD, Solórzano CC, Kim LT. Update on pheochromocytoma and paraganglioma from the SSO endocrine/head and neck disease-site work group. Part 1 of 2: advances in pathogenesis and diagnosis of pheochromocytoma and paraganglioma. Ann Surg Oncol. 2020;27(5):1329–37. https://doi.org/10.1245/s10434-020-08220-3. Epub 2020 Feb 28. PMID: 32112212; PMCID: PMC8655649.
17. Taïeb D, Timmers HJ, Hindié E, Guillet BA, Neumann HP, Walz MK, Opocher G, de Herder WW, Boedeker CC, de Krijger RR, Chiti A, Al-Nahhas A, Pacak K, Rubello D, European Association of Nuclear Medicine. EANM 2012 guidelines for radionuclide imaging of phaeochromocytoma and paraganglioma. Eur J Nucl Med Mol Imaging. 2012;39(12):1977–95. https://doi.org/10.1007/s00259-012-2215-8. Epub 2012 Aug 28. PMID: 22926712; PMCID: PMC4714772.

Chapter 41
Headache Attributed to Hypertensive Encephalopathy

Mario Fernando Prieto Peres

41.1 Introduction

Headaches are one of the most common symptoms seen in emergency departments. However, when associated with an acute rise in blood pressure and neurological changes, it can signal a life-threatening condition called hypertensive encephalopathy. This syndrome is characterised by a breakdown in cerebral autoregulation leading to vasogenic oedema and, if not recognised promptly, can lead to seizures, coma or death [1, 2].

Within the spectrum of hypertensive crises, hypertensive encephalopathy stands out because of its complex clinical-radiological overlap with other neurological emergencies. It can present with acute or subacute onset of headache, visual disturbances, altered mental status and even focal neurological deficits—features that often mimic stroke, pre eclampsia/eclampsia or cerebral venous thrombosis [3, 4]. The most recognised radiological correlate is posterior reversible encephalopathy syndrome (PRES), which is associated with reversible vasogenic oedema, predominantly in the parieto-occipital lobes [5–7]. However, PRES represents only one aspect of the spectrum of hypertensive encephalopathy and should not be considered synonymous with it [8, 9].

Clinical diagnosis is further challenged by the broad differential diagnosis, particularly in special populations such as pregnant women, where the distinction between hypertensive encephalopathy, eclampsia and migraine with aura may be blurred [10, 11]. In addition, unusual imaging patterns—including brainstem,

M. F. P. Peres (✉)
Elect International Headache Society, Institute of Psychiatry, University of Sao Paulo, Sao Paulo, Brazil

Hospital Israelita Albert Einstein, Sao Paulo, Brazil

D. Uludüz et al. (eds.), *Rare Causes of Headache Disorders*, Headache,
https://doi.org/10.1007/978-3-032-10242-3_41

cerebellar, spinal cord and frontal lobe involvement—may be seen in hypertensive encephalopathy, which may delay diagnosis [12–14].

Emerging evidence also suggests that reversible cerebral vasoconstriction syndrome (RCVS) may coexist with or mimic hypertensive encephalopathy, especially when it presents with thunderclap headache and dynamic vascular changes on magnetic resonance (MR) angiography [15–17].

This chapter focuses on headaches attributed to hypertensive encephalopathy, illustrated through a representative clinical case involving a third-trimester pregnant woman with hypertensive crisis and radiological features of PRES. Beyond the classical narrative, we will explore atypical imaging patterns, potential overlaps with RCVS and diagnostic dilemmas in differential diagnosis, particularly in pregnancy-related hypertensive states. We will also provide practical clinical guidance on neuroimaging, ophthalmological signs and management strategies to prevent irreversible neurological damage.

41.2 Pathophysiology (Fig. 41.1)

Hypertensive encephalopathy is a neurologic emergency that lies on the spectrum of hypertensive crises. Its pathophysiology is primarily attributed to the failure of cerebral autoregulation under acute, severe blood pressure elevations. This leads to a

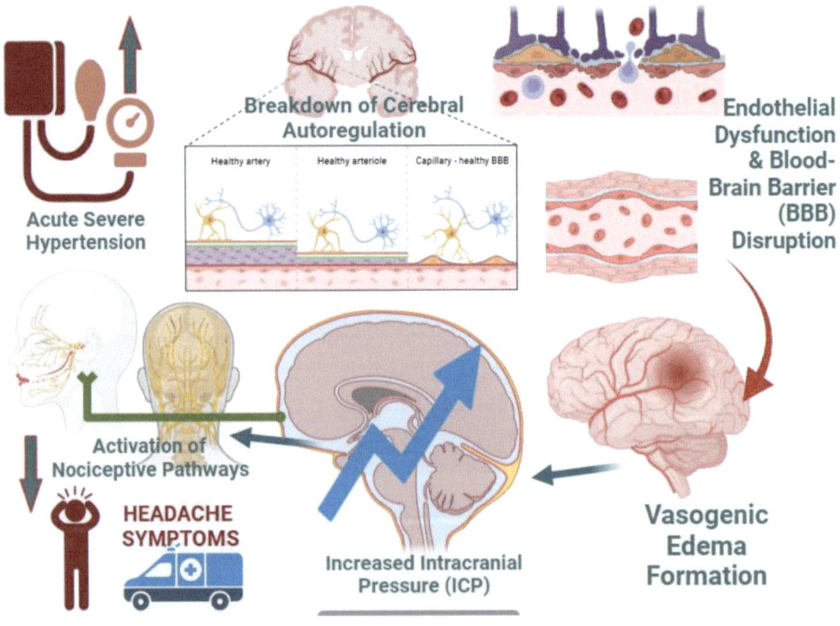

Fig. 41.1 Pathophysiological mechanism of headache in hypertensive encephalopathy. (*This figure was created on the Biorender*)

hyperperfusion state, endothelial dysfunction and leakage of plasma and proteins into the interstitial space, resulting in vasogenic oedema, most prominent in posterior brain regions due to their relatively sparse sympathetic innervation [5, 7]. While posterior reversible encephalopathy syndrome (PRES) is the most widely recognised neuroimaging pattern of this process, not all hypertensive encephalopathy cases meet the PRES criteria. Conversely, not all cases of PRES are of hypertensive origin [6, 8].

41.3 Case Presentation

Zeynep, a 42-year-old woman in her 32nd week of pregnancy with her third child, presented to the emergency department with a sudden and intensely distressing headache that had started approximately 2 hours prior. She described the onset as abrupt and explosive, 'as if something burst inside my head', with immediate full intensity. The pain was primarily located at the occipital region, radiating upward and forward toward the vertex and bilateral temples. She noted that it throbbed and pulsed with each heartbeat, but with periods where it felt like a tightening band pressing against her skull.

She rated the headache intensity as 9 out of 10, unresponsive to rest or the paracetamol she had taken at home. Unlike previous mild, tension-type headaches during her earlier pregnancies, this episode was profoundly different in both quality and severity. Associated symptoms included nausea, phonophobia and dizziness, particularly when changing positions. She also reported neck stiffness and a feeling of restlessness, frequently shifting in bed and unable to find relief. She denied fever, trauma or preceding aura symptoms. While visual blurring and flashing lights were present, she was more troubled by a heavy, internal head pressure and a sense of 'mental fog' that made it difficult to concentrate or respond promptly to questions.

She had no prior history of hypertension or migraines but had missed several prenatal follow-ups. Her two previous pregnancies were uncomplicated.

On examination, she was hypertensive with a blood pressure of 210/120 mmHg and mildly confused. Neurologically, she had brisk deep tendon reflexes and bilateral ankle clonus. An ophthalmological bedside exam revealed mild bilateral papilledema. Visual acuity was decreased but correctable, and she had difficulty with visual field testing. The fundoscopic examination showed blurred disc margins and venous engorgement, with mild flame-shaped haemorrhages suggestive of grade II hypertensive retinopathy.

A comprehensive neuroimaging workup was performed. MRI Brain (T2-FLAIR-diffusion) The MRI findings in this case are highly consistent with posterior reversible encephalopathy syndrome (PRES) secondary to hypertensive encephalopathy. On T2-weighted and fluid-attenuated inversion recovery (FLAIR) sequences, there are bilateral, symmetrical hyperintense signal changes predominantly involving the parieto-occipital lobes, affecting both the cortical and subcortical white matter. These regions demonstrate no mass effect or enhancement, and the pattern is typical for vasogenic oedema. Additionally, subtle hyperintensities in the cerebellar hemispheres—particularly on the right—further support a posterior circulation vulnerability. Diffusion-weighted imaging (DWI) shows mild hyperintensities without corresponding low signal on apparent diffusion coefficient (ADC) maps; instead, the ADC values are elevated, indicating facilitated diffusion and confirming the presence of vasogenic rather than cytotoxic oedema. The absence of true diffusion restriction effectively rules out acute infarction. These findings reflect the pathophysiology of PRES, in which severe hypertension overwhelms the cerebral autoregulatory mechanisms, especially in posterior circulation territories with relatively less sympathetic innervation, leading to transient blood–brain barrier disruption and fluid extravasation into the interstitium. Collectively, the imaging demonstrates the classic radiologic pattern of PRES, supporting a diagnosis of reversible vasogenic oedema due to hypertensive encephalopathy. Given the clinical and radiological findings, Zeynep was diagnosed with hypertensive encephalopathy in the context of severe preeclampsia, with radiological features of PRES.

Treatment was initiated with intravenous labetalol to stabilise her blood pressure and magnesium sulphate for seizure prophylaxis. Obstetrics was consulted immediately. After maternal stabilisation, she was transferred to the high-risk maternal care unit. Delivery planning was initiated in close collaboration with the perinatology team.

Over the next 72 hours, the intensity of her headache gradually lessened, and her visual symptoms began to resolve. Serial ophthalmological assessments showed improving disc clarity and resolution of venous dilation. A follow-up MRI 1 month later revealed partial regression of the T2-FLAIR abnormalities.

41.4 Clinical Presentation

Headache is often the earliest and most prominent symptom in hypertensive encephalopathy. It may precede more overt signs, such as altered mental status, visual disturbances or seizures, as a crucial diagnostic clue [1, 10]. The headache is typically bilateral, throbbing and in the occipital region, though variations exist. The presence of a new-onset severe headache, particularly in a patient with markedly elevated blood pressure and neurological complaints, should prompt urgent investigation for hypertensive encephalopathy [16].

The headache phenomenology in hypertensive encephalopathy may mimic or overlap with other secondary headache causes, especially in pregnant or peripartum individuals. This emphasises the need for structured symptom evaluation and a high index of suspicion in emergency and primary care settings.

41.5 Differential Diagnosis

- Preeclampsia/Eclampsia: Both share overlapping features with hypertensive encephalopathy, including elevated blood pressure, headache and visual disturbances. However, systemic findings such as proteinuria, elevated liver enzymes and thrombocytopenia help differentiate them [3].
- Reversible Cerebral Vasoconstriction Syndrome (RCVS): It is characterised by thunderclap headaches and reversible narrowing of cerebral arteries. MRA is critical in identifying dynamic segmental vasoconstriction [15].
- Cerebral Venous Sinus Thrombosis (CVST): It can present with subacute headache and visual symptoms, sometimes with preserved consciousness. MRV is essential for differentiation.
- Hypertensive Intracerebral Haemorrhage: It often presents with sudden, focal deficits and altered consciousness. Non-contrast computed tomography (CT) is the first-line investigation in suspected cases.
- Pituitary Apoplexy and Posterior Fossa Mass Lesions: Although less common, these should be considered in cases of headaches with visual loss, particularly in pregnant women.
- Primary Headaches Exacerbated by Blood Pressure Elevation: Migraine, tension-type and cluster headaches can all trigger transient increases in blood pressure, but in these cases, the hypertension is usually secondary, not causal.

However, the diagnostic process is complicated by the broad differential diagnosis of headaches in hypertensive and pregnant patients. In pregnant individuals like the case presented, differentials include preeclampsia/eclampsia, cerebral venous sinus thrombosis (CVST), reversible cerebral vasoconstriction syndrome (RCVS), pituitary apoplexy and even migraine with aura. Each may present with similar neurological signs and symptoms, including headache, visual changes and altered consciousness [3, 11].

Differentiating hypertensive encephalopathy from eclampsia is particularly critical in obstetric patients. Both conditions may involve elevated blood pressure, seizures and cerebral oedema, yet eclampsia often includes additional systemic features such as proteinuria, hepatic dysfunction and thrombocytopenia. Neuroimaging in both conditions may show PRES patterns, further complicating the diagnosis. Nonetheless, the presence of isolated neurological symptoms with a radiologic PRES pattern, in the absence of systemic signs, leans toward primary hypertensive encephalopathy [4].

Similarly, RCVS is a significant diagnostic consideration. Thunderclap headache is the hallmark of RCVS, and MRA often reveals segmental vasoconstriction in cerebral arteries, a finding that may also be observed in hypertensive encephalopathy [15]. Both syndromes may coexist or mimic each other, especially in postpartum or peripartum patients. The key distinction lies in the dynamic reversibility of vascular narrowing in RCVS and the dominant oedema patterns in PRES-like hypertensive encephalopathy [5, 6].

Imaging plays a pivotal role in diagnosis. MRI is superior to CT in detecting the hallmark vasogenic oedema of hypertensive encephalopathy. Typical findings include bilateral, symmetrical hyperintensities in the parieto-occipital white matter on T2- and FLAIR-weighted sequences. However, less typical presentations involve the frontal lobes, cerebellum, brainstem and spinal cord. Imaging abnormalities may persist long after symptom resolution, especially in chronic or undertreated conditions [14].

Ophthalmological examination is another essential, often underutilised, diagnostic tool. Papilledema and hypertensive retinopathy provide real-time evidence of elevated intracranial pressure and systemic vascular injury. In the case of hypertensive encephalopathy, findings such as blurred disc margins, venous engorgement, flame haemorrhages or cotton wool spots reinforce the urgency of neurological evaluation [2, 4].

41.6 Conclusion

In summary, headache is not merely a symptom in hypertensive encephalopathy—it is a diagnostic cornerstone. Its characteristics, evolution and associated findings guide the clinician toward or away from competing diagnoses. It is key to timely diagnosis and management to understand its role, alongside careful systemic evaluation, neuroimaging and fundoscopic examination. Failure to act on these early clues can lead to irreversible cerebral injury, seizures or death [13, 17].

41.7 Key Messages

- Headache can be the earliest and most critical clue in diagnosing hypertensive encephalopathy. New-onset severe headache in the presence of acute hypertension should prompt urgent neurological evaluation.
- Hypertensive encephalopathy is pathophysiologically distinct from but radiologically overlapping with posterior reversible encephalopathy syndrome (PRES). Not all PRES is hypertensive in origin, and not all cases of hypertensive encephalopathy manifest as classical PRES.
- In pregnant patients, hypertensive encephalopathy should be differentiated from preeclampsia/eclampsia, cerebral venous sinus thrombosis, RCVS and migraine with aura. Systemic findings and dynamic neuroimaging features aid in differential diagnosis.
- MRI with advanced sequences (T2-FLAIR, DWI, MRA, MRV) is essential for identifying vasogenic oedema, ruling out infarction or haemorrhage and evaluating vascular changes suggestive of RCVS or CVST.

- Ophthalmological examination, including fundoscopy, is a valuable bedside tool. Papilledema and hypertensive retinopathy findings can guide urgency and indicate elevated intracranial pressure.
- Prompt treatment, including blood pressure control and seizure prophylaxis, can lead to complete recovery and radiological reversal in most cases, especially when diagnosed early.

References

1. Potter T, Agarwal A, Schaefer TJ. Hypertensive encephalopathy. 2024 Feb 2. In: StatPearls [Internet]. Treasure Island (FL): StatPearls Publishing; 2025 Jan–. PMID: 32119386.
2. Tsou TP, Yen ZS, Fang CC, Chen SC, Chen WJ. Hypertensive encephalopathy. J Emerg Med. 2004;27(1):85–6. https://doi.org/10.1016/j.jemermed.2004.02.014. PMID: 15219310.
3. Astarita A, Covella M, Vallelonga F, Cesareo M, Totaro S, Ventre L, Aprà F, Veglio F, Milan A. Hypertensive emergencies and urgencies in emergency departments: a systematic review and meta-analysis. J Hypertens. 2020;38(7):1203–10. https://doi.org/10.1097/HJH.0000000000002372. PMID: 32510905.
4. Christopoulou F, Rizos EC, Kosta P, Argyropoulou MI, Elisaf M. Does this patient have hypertensive encephalopathy? J Am Soc Hypertens. 2016;10(5):399–403. https://doi.org/10.1016/j.jash.2016.01.020. Epub 2016 Jan 29. PMID: 26896240.
5. Triplett JD, Kutlubaev MA, Kermode AG, Hardy T. Posterior reversible encephalopathy syndrome (PRES): diagnosis and management. Pract Neurol. 2022;22(3):183–9. https://doi.org/10.1136/practneurol-2021-003194. Epub 2022 Jan 19. PMID: 35046115.
6. Ando Y, Ono Y, Sano A, Fujita N, Ono S. Posterior reversible encephalopathy syndrome: a review of the literature. Intern Med. 2022;61(2):135–41. https://doi.org/10.2169/internalmedicine.7520-21. Epub 2021 Jul 17. PMID: 34275982; PMCID: PMC8851194.
7. Fugate JE, Rabinstein AA. Posterior reversible encephalopathy syndrome: clinical and radiological manifestations, pathophysiology, and outstanding questions. Lancet Neurol. 2015;14(9):914–25. https://doi.org/10.1016/S1474-4422(15)00111-8. Epub 2015 Jul 13. Erratum in: Lancet Neurol. 2015 Sep;14(9):874. https://doi.org/10.1016/S1474-4422(15)00195-7. PMID: 26184985.
8. Mirza A. Posterior reversible encephalopathy syndrome: a variant of hypertensive encephalopathy. J Clin Neurosci. 2006;13(5):590–5. https://doi.org/10.1016/j.jocn.2005.03.042. PMID: 16769518.
9. Schwartz RB, Jones KM, Kalina P, Bajakian RL, Mantello MT, Garada B, Holman BL. Hypertensive encephalopathy: findings on CT, MR imaging, and SPECT imaging in 14 cases. AJR Am J Roentgenol. 1992;159(2):379–83. https://doi.org/10.2214/ajr.159.2.1632361. PMID: 1632361.
10. Tang-Wai DF, Phan TG, Wijdicks EF. Hypertensive encephalopathy presenting with thunderclap headache. Headache. 2001;41(2):198–200. https://doi.org/10.1046/j.1526-4610.2001.111006198.x. PMID: 11251706.
11. Minville V, N'Guyen L, Coustet B, Fourcade O, Samii K. Hypertensive encephalopathy mimicking postdural puncture headache in a parturient beyond the edge of reproductive age. Anesth Analg. 2004;99(6):1873–4. https://doi.org/10.1213/01.ANE.0000137806.09323.36. PMID: 155620.
12. Nagato M, Takahashi Y, Yoshioka M, Nambu M. A case of hypertensive encephalopathy with extensive spinal lesions on MRI. Brain Dev. 2010;32(7):598–601. https://doi.org/10.1016/j.braindev.2009.07.002. Epub 2009 Sep 5. PMID: 19733990.

13. Ille O, Woimant F, Pruna A, Corabianu O, Idatte JM, Haguenau M. Hypertensive encephalopathy after bilateral carotid endarterectomy. Stroke. 1995;26(3):488–91. https://doi.org/10.1161/01.str.26.3.488. PMID: 7886730.
14. Ito S, Ito T, Tamura N, Uchiyama T, Mori M, Hattori T. Chronic hypertensive encephalopathy showing only headache: report of a case with long-standing brain MR abnormalities suggesting extensive vasogenic edema. Eur Neurol. 2005;53(4):220–2. https://doi.org/10.1159/000086736. Epub 2005 Apr 4. PMID: 16015008.
15. Perillo T, Paolella C, Perrotta G, Serino A, Caranci F, Manto A. Reversible cerebral vasoconstriction syndrome: review of neuroimaging findings. Radiol Med. 2022;127(9):981–90. https://doi.org/10.1007/s11547-022-01532-2. Epub 2022 Aug 6. PMID: 35932443; PMCID: PMC9362037.
16. Spierings EL. Acute and chronic hypertensive headache and hypertensive encephalopathy. Cephalalgia. 2002;22(4):313–6. https://doi.org/10.1046/j.1468-2982.2002.00333.x. PMID: 12100095.
17. Grönbaek E. Acute and chronic hypertensive headache and hypertensive encephalopathy. Cephalalgia. 2003;23(3):238–9; author reply 239. https://doi.org/10.1046/j.1468-2982.2003.04851.x. PMID: 12662195.

Chapter 42
Headache Attributed to Preeclampsia or Eclampsia

Andressa Regina Galego and Eliana Meire Melhado

42.1 Introduction

This chapter aims to provide a comprehensive exploration of rare headache disorders through practical diagnostic approaches and case-based learning, offering valuable insights for clinicians and researchers.

It is well known that headaches are a condition commonly associated with pregnancy, often as an isolated and benign symptom [1]. However, headaches can also be a sign of more severe pathologies, such as preeclampsia and eclampsia, which are significant complications with substantial morbidity and mortality [1]. Preeclampsia and related hypertensive disorders of pregnancy affect up to 10% of pregnancies. Neurological complications seen in association with preeclampsia include seizures (eclampsia), arterial ischemic stroke, reversible cerebral vasoconstriction syndrome (RCVS), posterior reversible encephalopathy syndrome (PRES), cervical artery dissection, cerebral venous sinus thrombosis, subarachnoid hemorrhage (SAH), and intracerebral hemorrhage (ICH) [1]. Of these, ICH is the most devastating, directly causing up to 70% of deaths from preeclampsia [1].

Preeclampsia, which typically occurs after the 20th week of gestation, is characterized by high blood pressure and the presence of proteinuria, potentially leading to serious and significant complications for both the mother and the baby [2, 3]. Eclampsia, on the other hand, results from the progression of preeclampsia, culminating in the presence of seizures, which can lead to maternal and fetal death [2, 3]. Risk factors for the neurovascular complications of preeclampsia include older age, non-white race, heart disease, chronic hypertension, infections, prothrombotic and

A. R. Galego
Department of Neurology, Base Hospital, São José do Rio Preto, São Paulo, Brazil

E. M. Melhado (✉)
Department of Neurology, UNIFIPA (Padre Albino University Center), Catanduva, São Paulo, Brazil

D. Uludüz et al. (eds.), *Rare Causes of Headache Disorders*, Headache,
https://doi.org/10.1007/978-3-032-10242-3_42

hypercoagulable states, and a history of migraine [2, 3]. Migraine is associated with an increased risk of both hypertensive disorders of pregnancy and maternal stroke [2, 3].

When discussing headaches attributed to preeclampsia and eclampsia, it refers to one of the neurological symptoms that can result from both increased blood pressure and endothelial dysfunction [4]. This specific type of headache can vary significantly in presentation, duration, and characteristics [4]. Therefore, the presence of headaches during pregnancy should be a warning sign, especially when accompanied by other clinical and laboratory signs and symptoms [4].

Hypertensive disorders during pregnancy are reported to affect approximately 10–20% of pregnancies in the United States [5].

42.2 Pathophysiology

Preeclampsia is a progressive multisystem disorder characterized by the development of hypertension and proteinuria or organ failure after 20 weeks of gestation, during pregnancy, labor, or postpartum [6]. It is believed that a combination of maternal and fetal/placental factors is the cause [6]. Abnormalities in placental vasculature can lead to relative hypoxia, ischemia, or placental hyperperfusion, resulting in the release of antiangiogenic factors into the maternal circulation, altering the mother's systemic endothelial function and causing hypertension and other manifestations of the disease (hematological, neurological, cardiac, pulmonary, renal, and hepatic) [6].

Preeclampsia can be broadly categorized into two subtypes: early-onset preeclampsia (or placental) and late-onset preeclampsia (or maternal) [7]. Both appear to have distinct etiologies and phenotypes. In terms of early-onset type, the defective placenta is attributed to the development of preeclampsia [7]. Examination of the placenta in preeclampsia reveals numerous placental infarcts and arterial sclerosis [7]. This is accompanied by placental hypoperfusion due to altered trophoblastic invasion and, therefore, placental ischemia [7]. Maternal preeclampsia arises due to the interplay between a healthy placenta and maternal factors that ultimately lead to microvascular damage [7]. This may be due to maternal endothelial dysfunction [7]. Since maternal preeclampsia occurs later in the gestational period, it can be managed expectantly until 37 weeks of gestation [7]. Maternal preeclampsia occurs during the later stages of pregnancy, causing little or no change in arterial conversion, thus maintaining placental perfusion [7].

The underlying mechanism of the association between eclampsia and epilepsy is unclear [6]. However, hypertensive disorders during pregnancy, particularly eclampsia, are associated with impaired cerebral autoregulation, blood–brain barrier disruption, and neuroinflammation, which are possible underlying causes for the formation of cerebral edema [6]. Furthermore, preeclampsia and eclampsia can result in irreversible subclinical cerebral infarcts found in areas of cerebral edema [6]. These findings are significant and may be linked to the association with an increased risk of epilepsy in women with preeclampsia and eclampsia [6]. In other conditions associated with acute brain injury, such as sepsis, a similar association with late epilepsy has been found [6].

42.3 Case Presentation

Patient: MCG, Female, 25 years old

Gestational History: Pregnancies in 2018 and 2023

42.4 Clinical History and Progression

First Pregnancy (2018)

- 08-23-2018—Consultation (28 weeks gestation)
- History of migraine with aura since childhood, with significant worsening from the fourth month of gestation.
- Episodes of right hemicrania, sometimes on the left.
- Aura accompanied by numbness in hands and feet, and blurred vision, lasting up to 6 hours.
- During the week of consultation: migraine attacks with aura for three consecutive days, associated with nausea, vomiting, photophobia, and phonophobia.
- One episode with temporary hemiplegia and speech difficulty.
- Improvement only with hospital medication (Decadron, Dramin, Tramal, glucose).
- Diagnosis: Migraine with aura aggravated in the second half of pregnancy without hypertensive disorder.
- Management: Pyridoxine hydrochloride 250 mg, coenzyme Q10 150 mg for prevention and acute treatment: Dipyrone drops + dimenhydrinate for pain.
- 09-24-2018—Consultation (37 weeks gestation)
  - Reduced frequency of attacks (3 events in the past month: 2 with aura, 1 without aura).
  - Preventive formula maintained, physiotherapy recommended.
- 10-25-2018—Consultation
  - No attacks in recent weeks.
  - Complaints of tension headache for 1 week.
  - Foot edema and stretching difficulties.
  - Advised to discontinue preventive vitamins.
- 11-22-2018—Telephone contact (postpartum)
  - Cesarean delivery on 08/11/2018.
  - Postpartum headache, with prolonged aura.
  - Medication: Dipyrone, ibuprofen 400 mg, ondansetron 4 mg.

Second Pregnancy (2023–2024)

- 06-06-2023—Consultation (age 25)
- No preventive medication since 2018.
- Used copper intrauterine device (IUD) in 2019, removed for new pregnancy attempt.
- Increase in attack frequency last month (1x/week, some severe).
- Attacks without aura: occipital pain with persistent discomfort.
- Attacks with aura: blurred vision, pre-crisis hand paresthesia lasting 30 minutes.
- Prescription: Nortriptyline 0 mg/night, Sumax Pro + Meclin 25 mg for pain, dipyrone 1 g for mild pain.
- Significant improvement observed.
- 01-11-2024—Consultation (15 weeks gestation)
  - Pregnant at 15 weeks using vitamins.
  - Return of symptoms: prolonged visual aura (>1 hour), right-sided paresthesia.
  - Episode of migraine with aphasic aura.
  - Medications used: Ibuprofen 600 mg, dipyrone, tramadol.
  - Emotional complaint: Pain impacting conjugal relationship.
  - Conducted anesthetic blocks without corticosteroids.
- 01-24-2024—Consultation (17 weeks gestation)
  - Improvement after block on 11/01, 10 pain-free days.
  - Current diagnosis: Migraine with aura, worsening during pregnancy.
  - Management: Monitoring, anesthetic blocks as needed, guidance on hydration and proper nutrition.
  - Conducted additional blocks in 03/24 and 05/24.
- 06-30-2024—38 weeks—Normal delivery
  - In the week prior to delivery, experienced foot edema, persistent nuchal headache without aura, and was hypertensive in obstetric consultation 170/110 mmHg.
  - Obstetrician prescribed methyldopa, scheduled cesarean for 07/01, but went into labor on 06/30 with a normal delivery.
  - Postpartum, experienced persistent nuchal headache, high blood pressure, lower limb edema, and proteinuria; diagnosed with late gestational and immediate postpartum preeclampsia, treated with methyldopa and candesartan.
  - Despite significant nuchal pain, migraine was controlled with serial blocks.
  - Improvement and recovery observed within a month, followed by cardiologic monitoring to verify the need for continued antihypertensive therapy. After 90 days (October 2024), antihypertensives were discontinued, patient began physical activity amidst maternal obligations, breastfeeding, and baby care.

42.5 Case Discussion

The patient has a history of migraine with and without aura, with significant worsening during the second half of the first pregnancy and the first half of the second pregnancy. She experienced attacks with focal neurological phenomena, including transient hemiplegia and aphasia. Preventive treatment was not maintained consistently after the first delivery, leading to an increased frequency of attacks.

In the second pregnancy, late-onset preeclampsia was observed, requiring intervention. The patient requires neurological monitoring and tailored interventions. She remains under observation for the frequency of migraine attacks.

42.6 Clinical Presentation

Patients with preeclampsia often present with complaints of new-onset headaches not explained by any other diagnosis (i.e., a history of headaches or migraines) that do not respond to medication [8]. This complaint may or may not be accompanied by additional reports of visual disturbances [8]. Patients may also experience epigastric pain associated with nausea or vomiting [8]. Shortness of breath and a perceived increase in swelling, both worsening compared to baseline pregnancy-related symptoms, may also be reported [8].

In patients with preeclampsia, the most prevalent indicators in history typically include the onset of a recent headache resistant to analgesics [8]. Preeclampsia can be asymptomatic or cause edema or excessive sudden weight gain (>5 lbs per week) [9]. Non-dependent edema, such as facial and hand edema (rings may no longer fit on fingers), is more specific than dependent edema [8].

Eclampsia manifests as generalized (tonic–clonic) seizures [8].

Preeclampsia with severe features can cause organ damage; these characteristics may include severe headache, visual disturbances, confusion, hyperreflexia, pain in the epigastric or right hypochondrium region (reflecting hepatic ischemia or capsular distension), nausea and/or vomiting, dyspnea [reflecting pulmonary edema, acute respiratory distress syndrome (ARDS), or cardiac dysfunction secondary to increased afterload], oliguria (reflecting decreased plasma volume or acute ischemic tubular necrosis), and, rarely, stroke [8].

Patients presenting with any unique feature or a combination of these complaints should undergo a thorough physical examination [8]. This begins with an assessment of vital signs, specifically blood pressure [8]. Patients with systolic blood pressure (SBP) ≥140 mmHg or diastolic blood pressure (DBP) ≥90 mmHg should raise suspicion for preeclampsia [8]. In patients 20 weeks gestation or more, blood pressure readings on two occasions at least 4 hours apart should warrant further diagnostic investigation [8].

The recent reevaluation of diagnostic blood pressure readings has expanded to include sustained hypertensive readings after repeated measurements to allow timely intervention with antihypertensive therapy [8]. These blood pressure readings include SBP ≥160 mmHg or DBP ≥110 mmHg. According to the American College of Obstetricians and Gynecologists (ACOG), patients previously diagnosed with gestational hypertension presenting with these severe blood pressures should be diagnosed with preeclampsia with severe features, regardless of other diagnostic criteria [8].

When patients present with dyspnea, auscultation and percussion of the lungs should be performed to examine pulmonary disturbances [8]. An assessment of edema should also be completed, specifically evaluating areas of dependent edema (gravity-related), such as the lower extremities, or independent edema, such as in the face or hands [8].

While preeclampsia often presents with a notable history and physical signs and symptoms, there are several atypical presentations [8].

42.7 Diagnostic Algorithm [9]

The diagnostic criteria for headaches attributed to preeclampsia or eclampsia are outlined in the "International Classification of Headache Disorders" (ICHD) under the following classification:

10. Headache Attributed to Disorder of Homoeostasis

    10.3.4 Headache Attributed to Preeclampsia or Eclampsia [9]

Description:

Headache, typically bilateral and pulsating, occurring in women during pregnancy or the immediate puerperium (up to 4 weeks postpartum) with preeclampsia or eclampsia. It resolves following the resolution of preeclampsia or eclampsia [9].

Diagnostic Criteria:

A. Headache in a woman who is pregnant or in the puerperium, fulfilling criterion C [9].
B. Preeclampsia or eclampsia has been diagnosed [9].
C. Evidence of causation demonstrated by at least two of the following:

   Headache developed in temporal relation to the onset of the preeclampsia or eclampsia [9].

   1. Either or both of the following:
      (a) Headache has significantly worsened in parallel with worsening of the preeclampsia or eclampsia [9].
      (b) Headache has significantly improved or resolved in parallel with improvement in or resolution of the preeclampsia or eclampsia [9].
   2. Headache has at least two of the following three characteristics:
      (a) Bilateral location [9].
      (b) Pulsating quality [9]

(c) Aggravated by physical activity [9].

D. Not better accounted for by another ICHD-3 diagnosis [9].

Comments:

Preeclampsia and eclampsia appear to involve a strong maternal inflammatory response, with broad systemic immunological activity [9]. A placenta seems essential for their development, although case reports indicate that eclampsia can occur in the puerperium as well as during pregnancy. Preeclampsia and eclampsia are multisystem disorders with various forms [9]. Their diagnosis requires hypertension (>140/90 mmHg) documented on two blood pressure readings at least 4 hours apart, or a rise in diastolic pressure of 15 mmHg or systolic pressure of 30 mmHg, coupled with urinary protein excretion >0.3 g/24 hours [9]. Additionally, tissue edema, thrombocytopenia, and abnormalities in liver function can occur [9].

42.8 Preeclampsia

Preeclampsia is diagnosed with the new onset after 20 weeks of gestation of hypertension [blood pressure plus unexplained new-onset proteinuria (>300 mg/24 hours or urine protein/creatinine ratio ≥ 0.3) and/or signs of target organ damage] [10]. Proteinuria is defined as >300 mg/24 hours [10]. The absence of proteinuria in less precise tests (e.g., urine dipstick tests, urinalysis) does not rule out preeclampsia [10].

In the absence of proteinuria, preeclampsia can be diagnosed if pregnant women meet diagnostic criteria for new-onset hypertension and exhibit signs of new-onset target organ damage [10].

Signs or symptoms of target organ damage may include one or more of the following [10]:

- Thrombocytopenia (platelets <100 × 10^9/L)

Impaired liver function (aminotransferase >2 times normal) not explained by alternative diagnoses [10].

Severe and persistent right upper quadrant pain or epigastric pain unresponsive to medications [10].

Renal insufficiency (serum creatinine >1.1 mg/dL or doubling of serum creatinine in the absence of kidney disease) [10].

Pulmonary edema [10].

New-onset headache unresponsive to medication and unexplained by alternative diagnoses [10].

Visual disturbances [10].

Other Diagnostic Categories of Preeclampsia Include

(H = hemolysis; EL = evated liver enzymes; LP =low platelet count) (HELLP) Syndrome: Classified as a severe form of preeclampsia and diagnosed when all of the following are present [11]: lactate dehydrogenase (LDH) ≥ 600 IU/L;

aminotransferases >2 times normal; and platelets <100 × 10^9/L. HELLP syndrome may have atypical clinical presentations, with the absence of hypertension or proteinuria in up to 15% of patients [11].

Preeclampsia Superimposed on Chronic Hypertension Diagnosed when a patient known to have chronic hypertension develops one of the following after 20 weeks [12]: new unexplained proteinuria or worsening proteinuria; elevation of blood pressure above baseline; or signs of target organ damage. Women with chronic hypertension are at high risk of preeclampsia and should be closely monitored. An elevated uric acid level suggests a diagnosis of superimposed preeclampsia, rather than just chronic hypertension [12].

Patients with any type of preeclampsia are at risk of developing eclampsia [8]. Sometimes, eclampsia occurs before the diagnosis of preeclampsia [8].

42.9 Eclampsia

Eclampsia is defined as new-onset tonic–clonic, focal, or multifocal seizures without other known causes (e.g., epilepsy, cerebral ischemia or arterial infarction, intracranial hemorrhage, or drug use) [8].

42.10 Fetal Assessment

The fetus is evaluated using non-stress tests or biophysical profiles (including the assessment of amniotic fluid volume) and tests that estimate fetal weight [8].

The link between migraine and adverse pregnancy outcomes, especially hypertensive disorders such as gestational hypertension and preeclampsia, may involve factors like inflammation, endothelial dysfunction, and platelet activation [13]. Individuals with migraine often exhibit cardiovascular risk factors, such as obesity and chronic hypertension, increasing obstetric risks [13]. These adverse outcomes and migraine are associated with elevated risks of heart disease and ischemic stroke, suggesting a common etiology [13]. In a study with 30,555 pregnancies, pre-pregnancy migraine was associated with 17% higher risks of preterm birth, 28% of gestational hypertension, and 40% of preeclampsia [13]. Migraine with aura was more associated with preeclampsia than without aura, while risks of hypertension and preterm birth were similar regardless of migraine type [13]. Pre-pregnancy migraine history is a significant clinical marker of obstetric risk for vascular complications in pregnancies, independent of other established risk factors [13].

Researchers investigated the relationship between gestational hypertension, preeclampsia, and eclampsia with neurological disorders following childbirth [6]. Utilizing data from the National Patient Registry, the study included 648,385 women with no prior history of chronic hypertension or neurological disorders [6].

The findings revealed an increased risk of migraine, headache, epilepsy, sleep disorders, and mental fatigue among women with hypertensive complications during pregnancy [6]. Compared to normotensive pregnancies, the risk of developing such conditions was 27% higher for gestational hypertension, 32% for preeclampsia, and 70% for eclampsia [6]. The most pronounced association was between eclampsia and epilepsy, with a fivefold increased risk. Women with preeclampsia and preterm delivery showed a higher risk of migraine and headache than those with term delivery [6]. The researchers emphasize the need for postpartum follow-up for these women to identify neurological symptoms early [6]. Given the impact on quality of life, medical attention is crucial [6]. Future studies are necessary to understand the mechanisms involved and develop preventive strategies [6]. These findings justify additional investigations and underscore the importance of continuous monitoring of these women for post-gestational hypertension neurological complications [6].

42.11 Treatment

The treatment of preeclampsia begins with early diagnosis and intervention, focusing on adequate blood pressure control and seizure prevention [8]. The definitive treatment for preeclampsia is delivery [8]. However, the risk of premature delivery is weighed against gestational age, fetal growth restriction, fetal distress, and the severity of preeclampsia. Immediate delivery after maternal stabilization (e.g., seizure control, initiation of blood pressure management) is indicated for [8]:

- Gestation of ≥37 weeks
- Severe preeclampsia if gestation is ≥34 weeks [8]
- Deterioration of renal, pulmonary, cardiac, or hepatic functions (including HELLP syndrome) [8]
- Concerning results from fetal monitoring or testing [8]
- Eclampsia [8]

Patients with eclampsia or severe preeclampsia are typically admitted to a special maternal care unit or intensive care unit (ICU) [8]. Pregnant women between 34 and <37 weeks of gestation who do not require immediate delivery are hospitalized for assessment, at least initially [8]. If the maternal and fetal state is reassuring, outpatient treatment is possible, which includes modified activity, blood pressure measurements, laboratory monitoring, non-stress fetal tests, and medical consultations at least once per week [8]. If no criteria for severe preeclampsia develop, delivery can occur (e.g., by induction) at 37 weeks [8]. In pregnancy with <34 weeks, if delivery can be safely delayed, corticosteroids are administered for 48 hours to accelerate fetal lung maturity [8]. Corticosteroids may be given to some stable patients after 34 weeks and before 36 weeks of gestation if they have not been administered earlier [8].

42.12 Antihypertensive Management [8]

Blood pressure control includes immediate antihypertensive management in cases of severe hypertension (≥160 mmHg systolic and/or ≥110 mmHg diastolic), along with maintenance antihypertensive management in the antepartum or postpartum period, depending on the specific diagnosis of preeclampsia [8]. Antihypertensive effective medications without adverse effects on the fetus include [8]:

- Beta-blockers, such as labetalol
- Calcium channel blockers, such as nifedipine
- Alpha-2 agonists, such as clonidine
- Vasodilators, such as hydralazine [8]

Commonly used medications for treating severe hypertension include intravenous (IV) labetalol, IV hydralazine, or immediate-release oral nifedipine [8]. Although no evidence suggests a benefit of any IV medication as an initial choice for antihypertensive management, the choice is often dictated by the presence of IV access at the time of diagnosis, with oral nifedipine favored when IV access is unavailable [8]. Commonly used medications for maintaining blood pressure include oral labetalol, extended-release nifedipine, and extended-release clonidine [8].

42.13 Treatment of Eclampsia

Seizures in eclampsia are a medical emergency and require immediate treatment to prevent maternal and fetal mortality [14]. The management approach should balance immediate support measures, seizure control, prevention of recurrent seizures, ensuring safe and optimized delivery, and closely monitored postpartum care [14].

Eclampsia treatment Includes [14]:

- Initial Support Measures: Call for assistance, manage seizures, prevent injuries, ensure airway and oxygenation, and monitor vital signs and conduct laboratory studies [14].
- Magnesium Sulfate: Preferred over other anticonvulsant treatments for preventing eclampsia-related seizures [14]. Magnesium sulfate is administered primarily to prevent further convulsive activities, not to stop the current seizure [14]. The standard recommended loading dose is 6 g IV over 15–20 minutes, followed by a maintenance dose of 2 g/hour [14]. In patients without IV access, a loading dose of 10 g intramuscularly, followed by a maintenance dose of 5 g intramuscularly every 4 hours, can be used as an alternate regimen [14]. In patients with contraindications to magnesium sulfate (e.g., myasthenia gravis, hypocalcemia, renal insufficiency, cardiac ischemia, atrioventricular block, or myocarditis), alternative anticonvulsant therapies (e.g., phenytoin and diazepam) may be considered [14]. Levetiracetam may be preferable in patients with myasthenia gravis, a condition that can be exacerbated by phenytoin [14].

- Recurrent Seizures: If seizures occur, consider administering an additional 2 to 4 g of magnesium sulfate over 5 minutes [14]. If seizures persist after 20 minutes or more than two seizures occur despite magnesium therapy, recommend lorazepam 4 mg IV over 3 to 5 minutes [14].

Fetal Monitoring
During seizures, fetal heart rate decelerations, bradycardia, or tachycardia secondary to maternal hypoxia and hypercapnia may occur [14]. Uterine contractions may increase but usually resolve when maternal condition stabilizes [14].

Postpartum Management
Magnesium sulfate is recommended to prevent eclamptic seizures in postpartum patients with new-onset hypertension and neurological symptoms (e.g., headaches and blurred vision) or severe preeclampsia features [14].

42.14 Conclusion

The relationship between migraine and preeclampsia presents significant clinical concerns for the management of pregnant women. Understanding this association is critical because both conditions can have profound effects on maternal and fetal health. Preeclampsia remains a leading cause of maternal and neonatal morbidity and mortality, and migraines can exacerbate the risk of hypertensive disorders during pregnancy.

Key Insights and Lessons Learned
- Interconnected Pathophysiology: Both migraine and preeclampsia share pathophysiological traits, such as inflammation and endothelial dysfunction, which underscore the importance of vigilant monitoring and management strategies during pregnancy.
- Risk Factors: Women with a history of migraine, particularly with aura, are at increased risk of developing preeclampsia. This information can guide risk stratification and monitoring during prenatal care.
- Impact on Outcomes: Migraine during pregnancy is associated with adverse outcomes, including increased risks of preterm birth, gestational hypertension, and preeclampsia. These outcomes necessitate a proactive and preventive approach in clinical practice.

Recommendations for Clinical Practice
- Enhanced Monitoring: Healthcare professionals should consider enhanced monitoring for women with a history of migraine, especially those with aura, to detect early signs of hypertensive disorders.
- Individualized Care: Management should be tailored to individual risk profiles, with adjustments in treatment plans as necessary, including the potential use of antihypertensive medications and seizure prevention strategies where appropriate.
- Preventive Interventions: Exploring and implementing specific antenatal interventions could prove beneficial in reducing the risk of adverse outcomes for both the mother and the baby.

References

1. Hasegawa J, Ikeda T, Sekizawa A, Tanaka H, Nakata M, Murakoshi T. Maternal death due to stroke associated with pregnancy-induced hypertension. Circ J. 2015;79:1835–40.
2. Liang C-C, Chang S-D, Lai S-L, Hsieh C-C, Chueh H-Y, Lee T-H. Stroke complicating pregnancy and the puerperium. Eur J Neurol. 2006;13:1256–60.
3. Brusse IA, Kluivers ACM, Zambrano MD, Shetler K, Miller EC. Neuro-obstetrics: a multidisciplinary approach to care of women with neurologic disease. Handb Clin Neurol. 2020;171:143–60.
4. Afridi SK. Current concepts in migraine and their relevance to pregnancy. Obstet Med. 2018;11:154–9.
5. Garovic Vesna D, White William M, Vaughan L, Saiki M, Parashuram S, Garcia-Valencia O, et al. Incidence and long-term outcomes of hypertensive disorders of pregnancy. J Am Coll Cardiol. 2020;75:2323–34.
6. Tadese M, Damesa Wassihun A, Solomon Guta S, Wakie Gelmesa E, Tessema Solomon D, Endale A. Maternal deaths and preeclampsia: a retrospective study in Ethiopia. BMJ Open. 2024;14(3):e081901. https://doi.org/10.1136/bmjopen-2023-081901. PMID: 38553084; PMCID: PMC10982730.
7. Karrar Saad A, Martingano David J, Hong Philip L. Preeclampsia. In: StatPearls [Internet]. Treasure Island (FL): StatPearls Publishing; 2024 Jan–. Available from: https://www.ncbi.nlm.nih.gov/books/NBK554392/.
8. The Merck Manual of Diagnosis and Therapy. Pré-eclâmpsia e eclâmpsia: Complicações em obstetrícia. Disponível em: https://www.msdmanuals.com/pt/profissional/ginecologia-e-obstetr%C3%ADcia/complica%C3%A7%C3%B5es-pr%C3%A9-natais/pr%C3%A9-ecl%C3%A2mpsia-e-ecl%C3%A2mpsia#Tratamento_v1074563_pt.
9. Headache Classification Committee of the International Headache Society (IHS). The international classification of headache disorders, 3rd edition (ICHD-3). Cephalalgia. 2018;38(1):1–211. https://doi.org/10.1177/0333102417738202.
10. American College of Obstetrics and Gynecology (ACOG). ACOG practice bulletin, number 222: gestational hypertension and preeclampsia. Obstet Gynecol. 2020;135(6):e237–60. https://doi.org/10.1097/AOG.0000000000003891.
11. Martin JN Jr, Rinehart BK, May WL, Magann EF, Terrone DA, Norman PH. The spectrum of severe preeclampsia: comparative analysis by HELLP syndrome classification. Am J Obstet Gynecol. 1999;180:1373–84. https://doi.org/10.1016/S0002-9378(99)70022-0.
12. Lim KH, Friedman SA, Ecker JL, Ling K, Kilpatrick SJ. The clinical utility of serum uric acid measurements in hypertensive diseases of pregnancy. Am J Obstet Gynecol. 1998;178(5):1067–71. https://doi.org/10.1016/s0002-9378(98)70549-6.
13. Purdue-Smithe AC, Stuart JJ, Farland LV, Kang J-H, Harriott AM, Rich-Edwards JW, Rexrode K. Prepregnancy migraine, migraine phenotype, and risk of adverse pregnancy outcomes. Neurology. 2023;100(14):e1464–73. https://doi.org/10.1212/WNL.0000000000206831. PMID: 36657989; PMCID: PMC10104618.
14. Magley M, Hinson Melissa R. Eclampsia. In: StatPearls [Internet]. Treasure Island (FL): StatPearls Publishing; 2024. Updated. Available from: https://www.ncbi.nlm.nih.gov/books/NBK554392/.

Chapter 43
Headache Attributed to Hypothyroidism

Pablo Guarisco Ferreira, Edivan Rodrigo de Paula Ramos, and Alcântara Ramos de Assis César

43.1 Introduction

Hypothyroidism is an endocrinopathy characterized by reduced action of the thyroid hormones triiodothyronine (T3) and thyroxine (T4). In most cases, the reduced action of these hormones is associated with a reduction in their production. It can be caused by dysfunction of the thyroid (primary), pituitary (secondary), or hypothalamus (tertiary). When secondary or tertiary, it is also common to find changes in other hormones in the hypothalamic–pituitary axis. In clinical practice, the majority of cases of hypothyroidism are primary and, in these cases, an increase in serum thyroid-stimulating hormone (TSH) levels is observed. This chapter will focus on the primary form. The disease is more common in females, older individuals (≥ 65 years) and white ethnicities [1, 2]. It is a syndrome with a wide range of signs and symptoms, affecting several systems, including the nervous system.

Regarding chronic headaches, a bidirectional and comorbid relationship is observed between both conditions. The association has been reported since the twentieth century, with the publication of Fenichel in 1948 [3]. However, only in 1998, with greater laboratory technology to measure hormonal levels, based on the study by Moreau and colleagues [4], was it possible to define a headache attributed to hypothyroidism (HAH).

P. G. Ferreira
Nucleus of Studies on Headache and Cranial Pain in Western Paraná, Federal University of Paraná, Toledo, Paraná, Brazil

E. R. de Paula Ramos
Federal University of Paraná, Toledo, Paraná, Brazil

A. R. de Assis César (✉)
Coordinator of the Nucleus of Studies on Headache and Cranial Pain in Western Paraná, Neurology at the Federal University of Paraná, Toledo, Paraná, Brazil

D. Uludüz et al. (eds.), *Rare Causes of Headache Disorders*, Headache,
https://doi.org/10.1007/978-3-032-10242-3_43

Although HAH is a rare entity in the general population, headache is a common complaint in patients with hypothyroidism, and it is estimated that up to a third of patients may present HAH [4, 5], both in overt and subclinical forms. Furthermore, hypothyroidism and primary headache disorders, especially migraine, are often comorbid, so that migraine patients are at increased risk of developing clinical or subclinical hypothyroidism [5–9]. Additionally, hypothyroidism is a significant risk factor for the onset of new daily persistent headache [10].

Currently, in the International Classification of Headache Disorders 3rd edition (ICHD-3), HAH is included in the group of headaches secondary to homeostasis disorders and is defined as a headache usually bilateral and non-pulsatile, in patients with hypothyroidism and with remission after normalization of thyroid hormone levels [11]. Although common and with established diagnostic criteria, this etiology is still undervalued and under-investigated. Thus, the objective of this chapter is to specifically address this topic, from suspected diagnosis to correct management.

43.2 Pathophysiology

Although the pathophysiological basis of HAH remains unknown, alterations in peripheral craniofacial nociception (via trigeminovascular and trigeminocervical complexes) and in central pain modulation are observed.

Nociception of the face and intracranial structures occurs through afferent branches of the trigeminal nerve: ophthalmic (V1), maxillary (V2), and mandibular (V3); the remainder of the head, through the cervical nerves. The dura mater and intracranial arteries are innervated primarily by thinly myelinated (Aδ) and unmyelinated (C) fibers of the V1 division and, to a lesser extent, by the other branches. These fibers contain vasoactive substances (substance P [SP], calcitonin gene-related peptide [CGRP]) and, through vascular and neural receptors (neurokinin-1 [NK-1], CGRPr, $5\text{-HT}_{1B/D}$, P2X, P2Y, and others), modify vascular tone in an antidromic direction; among these, serotonergic receptors exert an inhibitory function, promoting antinociception through vasoconstriction (post-junctional 5-HT_{1B} receptors) and also by blocking neurogenic inflammation (pre-junctional 5-HT_{1D} receptors), in contrast to the others mentioned. In an orthodromic direction, the nociceptive nerve impulse goes towards the trigeminal ganglion, where, together with the trigeminal facial afferents, it continues in the pons towards the nucleus of the spinal trigeminal tract, mainly in the caudal subnucleus. The union of this subnucleus with the nuclei of the first cervical nerves forms the trigeminocervical complex, a continuum that receives nociception from the entire head and neck. In this region, nerve transmission occurs to second-order neurons via glutamate and its N-methyl-D-aspartate (NMDA) and metabotropic glutamate (mGluR) receptors, also modulated by inhibitory (gamma-aminobutyric acid, γ-aminobutyric acid A/B [$\text{GABA}_{A/B}$],

$5\text{-HT}_{1A/F}$) and excitatory (P2X, CGRPr) receptors, and follows to the thalamus via the trigeminothalamic tract and, subsequently, to the somatosensory cortex. This, in turn, emits direct and indirect descending projections that modulate trigeminal nociception, mediated in particular by GABA, serotonin and glutamate [13–16].

The main mechanism proposed for HAH involves the serotonergic dysfunction present in both conditions: headache and hypothyroidism. Regarding thyroid hormones, a strong correlation has been experimentally observed between serum T4 and 5-HT levels and in the central nervous system (cerebral cortex, thalamus, hypothalamus, midbrain, pons and in specific regions such as the dorsal raphe nucleus), inversely to TSH levels [17, 18], so that hypothyroid individuals present lower concentrations and action of this neurotransmitter [19–24]. This reduced serotonergic tone is reversible with hormonal treatment, both in the laboratory and clinically, in rats and humans [25–28].

At the receptor level, resulting from the decrease in serotonin levels, there may be a reduction in the action of 5-HT_{1B} and 5-HT_{1D}, with a consequent increase in the release of CGRP and SP. In contrast, a modulation in the expression and function of 5-HT_{2A} receptors was observed, with downregulation in the cerebral cortex of hypothyroid rats compared to the control groups [29, 30], which was reversible after T3 replacement [29, 31]. However, an older study showed the opposite result, although without comparison with control groups [25]. This receptor is present in the hippocampus, somatosensory and prefrontal cortex, and agonism acts on the modulation of CGRP, with pro-nociceptive stimulus; its antagonism is associated with the reduction in inflammatory and neuropathic pain [32–36]. Alterations in the expression of these receptors may pathologically modulate pain sensitivity, facilitating trigeminal pain mechanisms. Therefore, it is postulated that pain improvement after treatment with levothyroxine may result from the correction of serotonergic dysfunction, especially in conditions with characteristics similar to migraine [4, 5].

Another pathophysiological possibility of HAH is a possible dysfunction in the purinergic system. Rats with hypothyroidism present alterations in the metabolism of ATP (pro-nociceptive action via P2X receptors) and adenosine (antinociceptive action via A1 receptors), as well as in the nociceptive threshold throughout life [37, 38]. In humans, the use of A1 receptor agonist GR79236 inhibits trigeminal nociception [39]. Furthermore, another hypothesis is that it may be due to a "mass effect" secondary to possible pituitary gland hyperplasia [40, 41]. However, the compressive effect appears to be less critical than hormonal changes and genetic predispositions [41, 42].

In addition to these mechanisms, genetic studies have found a significant causal relationship between hypothyroidism (primary and secondary) and headache, and a negative relationship compared to hyperthyroidism. As for migraine, candidate genes have been found (methylenetetrahydrofolate reductase [MTHFR] and Apolipoprotein E [APOE] E2/E4), and some authors suggest polygenic factors throughout the genome [43–45]. However, studies are still incipient.

43.3 Case Presentation

A female patient, 35 years old, from southern Brazil, was referred for neurological clinical care due to the development of a chronic headache that had started 8 months ago. She reported pressure-like holocranial pain, initially mild-to-moderate in intensity, with almost daily frequency. She did not report any factors that improved or worsened her condition and denied any significant impact on her daily activities. In addition to the pain, she complained of tiredness and sadness.

For the past 6 months, the patient has reported worsening pain intensity, with daily moderate intensity (6 out of 10), with episodes of severe intensity (8 out of 10) about three times per month. He denied nausea, vomiting, photophobia, phonophobia, osmophobia, motor or visual changes before or during the attacks. He also denied worsening pain with movement. Furthermore, he reported worsening fatigue, with a more depressed mood and daytime sleepiness (Epworth 10), despite adequate sleep. In addition, he noticed that since the onset of the condition he had gained about 6 kg for no apparent reason, associated with persistent constipation, hair loss, drier skin than usual and greater sensitivity to cold, although without change in body temperature. He has been using propranolol 80 mg/day for 3 months, prescribed by the primary care doctor, without improvement in his condition. During pain crises, she used Paracetamol 750 mg about three times a week, with partial improvement of the pain. She denied using other medications during the period. Due to the persistence of the headache, there is a significant deterioration in quality of life and work performance. Regarding her medical history, she denies having had frequent or similar headaches in the past. She denied having had previous surgeries, smoking, or drinking alcohol. She works as a secretary in an accounting office and reports a sedentary lifestyle and a diet rich in carbohydrates. Her mother has hypothyroidism in her family. She denied migraine or other chronic diseases in the family.

On the physical examination, she was in good general condition, but looked tired. Her skin was dry, with no apparent lesions, and her hair was brittle. Her body mass index was 32, and her axillary temperature was 36.6 °C. The neurological examination was normal, with no motor or sensory deficits or altered reflexes. There were no trigger points or pain on palpation in the occipital nerves. Palpation of the thyroid revealed a slight, painless increase. No other changes. The patient presented laboratory tests collected a few weeks ago, with a TSH level of 12.1 mIU/L; he also brought a complete blood count, leukogram, salivary cortisol and fasting blood glucose levels requested by the primary care physician, without changes. Laboratory tests and a cranial magnetic resonance imaging (MRI) were requested for further investigation.

One week after the first consultation, the patient presented the MRI, with no changes; laboratory tests revealed hypothyroidism, with TSH 14.8 mIU/L (elevated), free T4 (fT4): 0.3 ng/dL (reduced), prolactin 20 ng/mL (normal) and positive anti-thyroid peroxidase (anti-TPO) antibodies.

Then, treatment was started with levothyroxine 50 μg/day, propranolol was maintained and paracetamol was replaced with naproxen 500 mg up to 2×/day, if pain was present. Patients were instructed to fill out a headache diary. After four weeks, the patient reported a decrease in pain intensity (4 out of 10) and frequency (3–4 times per week). Eight weeks after the initial consultation, the levothyroxine dose was adjusted to 75 µg/day, based on TSH levels, and the propranolol dose was reduced to 40 mg/day, with gradual tapering.

After 12 weeks of starting treatment, the patient reported a significant improvement in headache frequency (2–3 days per month), always of mild intensity (2 out of 10), without the need for analgesics, reduced fatigue, improved mood, sleep disturbance (Epworth 4) and willingness to perform daily tasks. She also reported a loss of 4 kg, with an improvement in constipation and the sensation of cold. As for the exams, the levels of TSH (2.3 mIU/L) and fT4 (1.1 ng/dL) were normalized.

43.4 Case Discussion

In this case, we have a 35-year-old woman with the onset of persistent daily headaches, which progressively worsened and impacted daily activities. The patient also presented nonspecific symptoms suggestive of thyroid dysfunction: fatigue, sleep disturbance, mood dysfunction, constipation, intolerance to cold, recent weight gain, dry skin and hair loss.

Based on the clinical history, causes of secondary headache should be investigated, also using complementary tests (imaging and/or laboratory tests) aimed at the suspected diagnosis. In this case, the possibility of a headache attributed to pituitary adenoma, for example, was excluded due to the absence of abnormalities in the MRI of the skull, in addition to the clinical incompatibility. Primary causes become less likely due to the chronology of symptom onset and clinical improvement with hormonal treatment. Other differential diagnoses should always be considered, as will be demonstrated below. Another relevant factor in the case presented is the use of propranolol. It is a beta-blocker medication frequently used in the treatment of chronic headaches. Still, it is also used in cases of thyrotoxicosis, as it reduces the conversion of T4 to T3, with an increase in the formation of reverse T3 (inactive form). Therefore, its use can worsen cases of hypothyroidism [12].

43.5 Clinical Manifestations

The main feature of HAH is its chronological correspondence with hypothyroidism [11]. It presents as a new headache that began together with other symptoms of the thyroid disorder, classically in the first 2 months [4], or as a clinical worsening of a primary headache already present, also with a temporal relationship to hypothyroidism [5]. Therefore, the associated symptoms are non-specific and result from the slowdown in metabolic processes (such as tiredness, cold intolerance, constipation and weight gain), the accumulation of substances in the interstitial space (edema, dry and rough skin, and hair loss) in addition to neurological conditions such as headache, carpal tunnel syndrome, encephalopathy and even myxedema coma [1, 5, 38].

In contrast, the clinical characteristics of headache are varied. The ICHD-3, according to the study by Moreau and colleagues (1998), characterizes it as a bilateral and constant headache (without paroxysms) [4]; in addition, it has classically been described as having mild-to-moderate intensity, non-pulsatile, without nausea, vomiting or photophobia. However, the study by Lima Carvalho and colleagues (2017), cited in ICHD-3, found a different clinical presentation, characterized by a predominance of a pulsating, unilateral headache lasting 4–72 hours, of moderate-to-severe intensity, accompanied by nausea and/or vomiting [5]. Therefore, given the possibility of clinical variability, the correct characterization of the symptoms of pain crises and the onset of hypothyroidism is essential.

43.6 Diagnosis

The diagnosis of HAH is made using the criteria established in ICHD-3 (Table 43.1), considering the chronology of headache onset, associated symptoms, and the laboratory diagnosis of hypothyroidism (TSH and fT4). Another relevant test in the etiological definition is the antithyroid peroxidase (anti-TPO) antibody, which denotes autoimmune etiology (Hashimoto's thyroiditis). Table 43.2 demonstrates diagnostic possibilities according TSH and fT4 serum levels.

It is important to emphasize that other conditions that may occur with headache and thyroid disorders must be evaluated, such as pituitary adenoma, vascular anatomical changes in the head and neck [46], post-infectious thyroiditis, use of

Table 43.1 Diagnostic criteria according to ICHD-3

A	Headache fulfilling criterion C
B	Hypothyroidism has been demonstrated
C	Evidence of causation demonstrated by at least two of the following:
	1. Headache has developed in temporal relation to the onset of the hypothyroidism, or led to its discovery
	2. Either or both of the following
	(a) Headache has significantly worsened in parallel with worsening of the hypothyroidism (b) Headache has significantly improved or resolved in parallel with improvement in or resolution of the hypothyroidism
	3. Headache has either or both of the following characteristics:
	(a) Bilateral location (b) Constant over time
D	Not better accounted for by another ICHD-3 diagnosis

Table 43.2 Diagnostic according to TSH and fT4 serum levels

	TSH < 0.4 mUI/L	TSH normal	TSH > 4.5 mUI/L
fT4 below normal range	Repeat exam	Repeat exam	Overt hypothyroidism
fT4 within normal range	Subclinical hyperthyroidism	Euthyroid	Subclinical hypothyroidism
fT4 above normal range	Hyperthyroidism	Consider overtreatment	Consider overtreatment

Adapted from Wilson et al [48].

medications (such as amiodarone and dopaminergic antagonists), adrenal insufficiency [47], or even other primary and secondary headaches that may be presenting as comorbidity to hormonal dysfunction.

43.7 Treatment

HAH treatment consists of resolving the underlying condition, combined with controlling comorbidities. In this case, treatment of primary hypothyroidism is through oral thyroid hormone replacement in the form of levothyroxine. The pill must be taken on an empty stomach, with water and at least 30 minutes before the next meal. The initial dose for the overt form in young adults is usually 1.6 μg/kg/day; elderly patients or those with coronary artery disease should start with a lower dose (12.5–25 μg/day) [49]. The dose of the drug must be evaluated and, if necessary, adjusted based on clinical and laboratory responses (TSH measurement until normal serum levels) every 2 months until improvement is observed [38, 49]. A reassessment to check clinical response, however, must be carried out at the end of the first month of treatment.

Regarding pain crises, most patients report significant improvement in the first 2 months after starting therapy; within 12 months, the disappearance or substantial reduction in the duration and intensity of pain is expected [4, 5]. Furthermore, treatment with levothyroxine is equally effective in both overt and subclinical forms [5].

In addition to hormone replacement therapy, analgesics such as naproxen can be used initially for support in pain crises until the condition effectively improves. Regardless, the patient should be monitored for long-term management of the disorders and ensure adequate management.

43.8 Conclusion

HAH presents as a new headache that began concomitantly with symptoms of hypothyroidism, or as the clinical worsening of a primary headache already present, also in temporal relation to the thyroid disorder. The pathophysiology of HAH is unknown, but there is evidence that it is mainly due to serotonergic dysfunction in hypothyroidism. Diagnosis is made through laboratory testing with TSH and fT4 levels. Treatment is thyroid hormone replacement therapy in the form of levothyroxine. Patients with partial improvement should be further investigated for possible comorbidities, such as sleep disorders, depressive syndromes, or primary headaches. Therefore, given the clinical variability presented, we suggest that TSH and fT4 levels be measured in all investigations of secondary headache, considering not only the diagnosis of HAH but also the bidirectional relationship between hypothyroidism and other headaches.

References

1. Chaker L, Bianco AC, Jonklaas J, Peeters RP. Hypothyroidism. Lancet. 2017;390(10101):1550–62. https://doi.org/10.1016/S0140-6736(17)30703-1. Epub 2017 Mar 20. PMID: 28336049; PMCID: PMC6619426.
2. Hollowell JG, Staehling NW, Flanders WD, Hannon WH, Gunter EW, Spencer CA, Braverman LE. Serum TSH, T(4), and thyroid antibodies in the United States population (1988 to 1994): National Health and Nutrition Examination Survey (NHANES III). J Clin Endocrinol Metab. 2002;87(2):489–99. https://doi.org/10.1210/jcem.87.2.8182.
3. Fenichel NM. Chronic headache due to masked hypothyroidism. Ann Int Med. 1948;29:456–60.
4. Moreau T, Manceau E, Giroud-Baleydier F, Dumas R, Giroud M. Headache in hypothyroidism, prevalence and outcome after thyroid hormone therapy. Cephalalgia. 1998;18:687–9.
5. de Lima Carvalho MF, de Medeiros JS, Valença MM. Headache in recent onset hypothyroidism: prevalence, characteristics and outcome after treatment with levothyroxine. Cephalalgia. 2017;37(10):938–46. https://doi.org/10.1177/0333102416658714.
6. Spanou I, Bougea A, Liakakis G, Rizonaki K, Anagnostou E, Duntas L, Kararizou E. Relationship of migraine and tension-type headache with hypothyroidism: a literature review. Headache. 2019;59(8):1174–86. https://doi.org/10.1111/head.13600.
7. Martin AT, Pinney SM, Xie C, Herrick RL, Bai Y, Buckholz J, Martin VT. Headache disorders may be a risk factor for the development of new onset hypothyroidism. Headache. 2017;57(1):21–30. https://doi.org/10.1111/head.12943. Epub 2016 Sep 27.
8. Lisotto C, Mainardi F, Maggioni F, Zanchin G. The comorbidity between migraine and hypothyroidism. J Headache Pain. 2013;14(Suppl 1):P138. https://doi.org/10.1186/1129-2377-14-S1-P138.
9. Fallah R, Mirouliaei M, Bashardoost N, Partovee M. Frequency of subclinical hypothyroidism in 5- to 15-year-old children with migraine headache. J Pediatr Endocrinol Metab. 2012;25(9–10):859–62. https://doi.org/10.1515/jpem-2012-0121.
10. Bigal ME, Sheftell FD, Rapoport AM, Tepper SJ, Lipton RB. Chronic daily headache: identification of factors associated with induction and transformation. Headache. 2002;42(7):575–81. https://doi.org/10.1046/j.1526-4610.2002.02143.x.
11. Headache Classification Committee of the International Headache Society (IHS). The international classification of headache disorders, 3rd edition. Cephalalgia. 2018;38(1):1–211.
12. Wiersinga WM. Propranolol and thyroid hormone metabolism. Thyroid. 1991;1(3):273–7.
13. Messlinger K, Dux M. Functional anatomy of trigeminovascular pain. In: Neurobiological basis of migraine. Wiley; 2017. p. 1–29.
14. Goadsby PJ, Holland PR, Martins-Oliveira M, Hoffmann J, Schankin C, Akerman S. Pathophysiology of migraine: a disorder of sensory processing. Physiol Rev. 2017;97(2):553–622. https://doi.org/10.1152/physrev.00034.2015.
15. Machado ABM, Haertel LLM. Neuroanatomia funcional. 4th ed. São Paulo: Atheneu; 2021.

16. Vincent MB. Fisiopatologia da enxaqueca. Arq Neuropsiquiatr. 1998;56:841–51.
17. Aloisi AM, Vodo S, Buonocore M. Pain and thyroid hormones. Neurol Sci. 2013;34:1501–8.
18. Bauer M, Whybrow PC. Thyroid hormone, neural tissue and mood modulation. World J Biol Psychiatry. 2001;2:59–69.
19. Hassan WA, Aly MS, Rahman TA, Shahat AS. Impact of experimental hypothyroidism on monoamines level in discrete brain regions and other peripheral tissues of young and adult male rats. Int J Dev Neurosci. 2013;31(4):225–33. https://doi.org/10.1016/j.ijdevneu.2013.02.001.
20. Stipcevic T, Kusacic-Kuna S, Dezeljin M, Dodig D, Korsic M, Pivac N, Muck-Seler D. Platelet serotonin concentration and monoamine oxidase activity in hypothyroid patients. Horm Res. 2009;71(4):207–12. https://doi.org/10.1159/000201109. Epub 2009 Mar 4.
21. Bortolotto VC, Pinheiro FC, Araujo SM, Poetini MR, Bertolazi BS, de Paula MT, Meichtry LB, de Almeida FP, de Freitas CS, Jesse CR, Prigol M. Chrysin reverses the depressive-like behavior induced by hypothyroidism in female mice by regulating hippocampal serotonin and dopamine. Eur J Pharmacol. 2018;822:78–84. https://doi.org/10.1016/j.ejphar.2018.01.017.
22. Ito JM, Valcana T, Timiras PS. Effect of hypo- and hyperthyroidism on regional monoamine metabolism in the adult rat brain. Neuroendocrinology. 1977;24(1):55–64. https://doi.org/10.1159/000122696.
23. Tousson E, Ibrahim W, Arafa N, Akela M. Monoamine concentrations changes in the PTU-induced hypothyroid rat brain and the ameliorating role of folic acid. Hum Exp Toxicol. 2011;31(3):282–9. https://doi.org/10.1177/0960327111405863.
24. Zhang Q, Feng JJ, Yang S, Liu XF, Li JC, Zhao H. Lateral habenula as a link between thyroid and serotoninergic system modiates depressive symptoms in hypothyroidism rats. Brain Res Bull. 2016;124:198–205.
25. Sandrini M, Vitale G, Vergoni AV, Ottani A, Bertolini A. Effect of acute and chronic treatment with triiodothyronine on serotonin levels and serotonergic receptor subtypes in the rat brain. Life Sci. 1996;58(18):1551–9. https://doi.org/10.1016/0024-3205(96)00129-4.
26. Hela D, Smith S. The effects of acute and repeated administration of T3 to mice on 5-HT1 and 5-HT2 function in the brain and its influence on the actions of repeated electroconvulsive shock. Neuropharmacology. 1988;27(12):1239–48. https://doi.org/10.1016/0028-3908(88)90026-3.
27. Yu D, Zhou H, Yang Y, Jiang Y, Wang T, Lv L, Zhou Q, Yang Y, Dong X, He J, Huang X, Chen J, Wu K, Xu L, Mao R. The bidirectional effects of hypothyroidism and hyperthyroidism on anxiety- and depression-like behaviors in rats. Horm Behav. 2015;69:106–15. https://doi.org/10.1016/j.yhbeh.2015.01.003.
28. Cleare AJ, McGregor A, Chambers SM, Dawling S, O'Keane V. Thyroxine replacement increases central 5-hydroxytryptamine activity and reduces depressive symptoms in hypothyroidism. Neuroendocrinology. 1996;64(1):65–9. https://doi.org/10.1159/000127099.
29. Kulikov A, Moreau X, Jeanningros R. Effects of experimental hypothyroidism on 5-HT1A, 5-HT2A receptors, 5-HT uptake sites and tryptophan hydroxylase activity in mature rat brain1. Neuroendocrinology. 1999;69(6):453–9. https://doi.org/10.1159/000054449.
30. Jin Z, Ling J, Yu J, He M, Ni P, Zhang F, Wang Y. Serotonin 2A receptor function and depression-like behavior in rats model of hypothyroidism. Exp Brain Res. 2021;239(8):2435–44. https://doi.org/10.1007/s00221-021-06129-1.
31. Kulikov AV, Jeanningro R. Vliianie gipertireoidizma na 5-HT1A-, 5-HT2A-retseptory i belok-transporter serotonina v golovnom mozgu krys [Effect of hypothyroidism on 5-HT1A-, 5-HT2A-receptors and serotonin transporter in the rat brain]. Rossiiskii fiziologicheskii zhurnal imeni IM Sechenova. 2000;86(3):312–9.
32. Huang J, Fan Y, Jia Y, Hong Y. Antagonism of 5-HT(2A) receptors inhibits the expression of pronociceptive mediator and enhances endogenous opioid mechanism in carrageenan-induced inflammation in rats. Eur J Pharmacol. 2011;654(1):33–41. https://doi.org/10.1016/j.ejphar.2010.12.007.
33. Wang D, Gao Y, Ji H, Hong Y. Topical and systemic administrations of ketanserin attenuate hypersensitivity and expression of CGRP in rats with spinal nerve ligation. Eur J Pharmacol. 2010;627(1–3):124–30. https://doi.org/10.1016/j.ejphar.2009.11.011.

34. Okamoto K, Imbe H, Morikawa Y, Itoh M, Sekimoto M, Nemoto K, Senba E. 5-HT2A receptor subtype in the peripheral branch of sensory fibers is involved in the potentiation of inflammatory pain in rats. Pain. 2002;99(1–2):133–43. https://doi.org/10.1016/s0304-3959(02)00070-2.
35. Wang D, Chen T, Gao Y, Quirion R, Hong Y. Inhibition of SNL-induced upregulation of CGRP and NPY in the spinal cord and dorsal root ganglia by the 5-HT(2A) receptor antagonist ketanserin in rats. Pharmacol Biochem Behav. 2012;101(3):379–86. https://doi.org/10.1016/j.pbb.2012.02.004.
36. van Hoogstraten WS, MaassenVanDenBrink A. The need for new acutely acting antimigraine drugs: moving safely outside acute medication overuse. J Headache Pain. 2019;20(1):54. https://doi.org/10.1186/s10194-019-1007-y.
37. Bruno AN, Pochmann D, Ricachenevsky FK, Fontella FU, Bonan CD, Dalmaz C, Barreto-Chaves ML, Sarkis JJ. Nociceptive response and adenine nucleotide hydrolysis in synaptosomes isolated from spinal cord of hypothyroid rats. Neurochem Res. 2005;30(9):1155–61. https://doi.org/10.1007/s11064-005-7867-3.
38. Tepper DE, Tepper SJ, Sheftell FD, Bigal ME. Headache attributed to hypothyroidism. Curr Pain Headache Rep. 2007;11(4):304–9. https://doi.org/10.1007/s11916-007-0208-2.
39. Giffin NJ, Kowacs F, Libri V, Williams P, Goadsby PJ, Kaube H. Effect of the adenosine A1 receptor agonist GR79236 on trigeminal nociception with blink reflex recordings in healthy human subjects. Cephalalgia. 2003;23(4):287–92. https://doi.org/10.1046/j.1468-2982.2003.00511.x.
40. Khawaja NM, Taher BM, Barham ME, Naser AA, Hadidy AM, Ahmad AT, Hamamy HA, Yaghi NA, Ajlouni KM. Pituitary enlargement in patients with primary hypothyroidism. Endocr Pract. 2006;12(1):29–34. https://doi.org/10.4158/EP.12.1.29.
41. Arafah BM, Prunty D, Ybarra J, Hlavin ML, Selman WR. The dominant role of increased intrasellar pressure in the pathogenesis of hypopituitarism, hyperprolactinemia, and headaches in patients with pituitary adenomas. J Clin Endocrinol Metab. 2000;85(5):1789–93. https://doi.org/10.1210/jcem.85.5.6611.
42. Levy MJ, Jäger HR, Powell M, Matharu MS, Meeran K, Goadsby PJ. Pituitary volume and headache: size is not everything. Arch Neurol. 2004;61(5):721–5. https://doi.org/10.1001/archneur.61.5.721.
43. Tasnim S, Wilson SG, Walsh JP, Nyholt DR. Cross-trait genetic analyses indicate pleiotropy and complex causal relationships between headache and thyroid function traits. Genes (Basel). 2022;14(1):16. Published 2022 Dec 21. https://doi.org/10.3390/genes14010016.
44. Tasnim S, Wilson SG, Walsh JP, Nyholt DR. Shared genetics and causal relationships between migraine and thyroid function traits. Cephalalgia. 2023;43(2) https://doi.org/10.1177/03331024221139253.
45. Tasnim S, Nyholt DR. Migraine and thyroid dysfunction: co-occurrence, shared genes and biological mechanisms. Eur J Neurol. 2003;30(6):1815–27.
46. Evans RW, Timm JS. New daily persistent headache caused by a multinodular goiter and headaches associated with thyroid disease. Headache. 2017;57(2):285–9.
47. Topliss DJ, White EL, Stockigt JR. Significance of thyrotropin excess in untreated primary adrenal insufficiency. J Clin Endocrinol Metab. 1980;50(1):52–6. https://doi.org/10.1210/jcem-50-1-52.
48. Wilson SA, Stem LA, Bruehlman RD. Hypothyroidism: diagnosis and treatment. Am Fam Physician. 2021;103(10):605–13.
49. Jonklaas J, Bianco AC, Bauer AJ, Burman KD, Cappola AR, Celi FS, Cooper DS, Kim BW, Peeters RP, Rosenthal MS, Sawka AM, American Thyroid Association Task Force on Thyroid Hormone Replacement. Guidelines for the treatment of hypothyroidism: prepared by the American Thyroid Association Task Force on Thyroid Hormone Replacement. Thyroid. 2014;24(12):1670–751. https://doi.org/10.1089/thy.2014.0028. PMID: 25266247; PMCID: PMC4267409.

Chapter 44
Cardiac Cephalalgia

Vinícius da Silva Lessa de Oliveira, Victor Alfonso Garcia Ortiz, and Vanise Grassi

44.1 Introduction

The term "cardiac headache" was initially introduced by Lipton et al. in 1997, following the report of two cases of exertional headache. Their study detailed two male patients, aged 57 and 67, who experienced headache developing 5–15 minutes after the onset of vigorous exercise, with improvement occurring minutes or hours after cessation of the activity [1]. A subsequent literature review identified similar case reports, demonstrating that symptoms either decreased or resolved completely with pharmacological and/or surgical interventions aimed at correcting myocardial ischemia [2].

Since it is a rare condition among headaches, the literature primarily consists of case reports, making it challenging to establish robust diagnostic criteria [3]. This is partly due to its atypical presentation, with an absence of specific neurological signs and variability in pain characteristics, which may mimic primary headaches [4]. Additionally, cardiac headache can be an isolated manifestation of myocardial

V. da Silva Lessa de Oliveira
Postgraduate Program in Medicine, Pediatrics, and Child Health, Pontifícia Universidade Católica do Rio Grande do Sul, Porto Alegre, Brazil

V. A. G. Ortiz
Pontifícia Universidade Católica do Rio Grande do Sul, Porto Alegre, Brazil

V. Grassi (✉)
Department of Neurology, Hospital São Lucas da Pontifícia Universidade Católica do Rio Grande do Sul, Porto Alegre, Brazil

D. Uludüz et al. (eds.), *Rare Causes of Headache Disorders*, Headache,
https://doi.org/10.1007/978-3-032-10242-3_44

ischemia, frequently underdiagnosed due to low awareness and its unconventional presentation. Unlike typical angina, which is characterized by oppressive chest pain radiating to the arm and jaw, cardiac headache can occur in isolation, triggered by physical exertion [5]. Therefore, a detailed clinical approach—based on medical history, cardiovascular risk factor assessment, and complementary exams such as stress tests and coronary angiography—is essential for differential diagnosis and appropriate treatment of these patients [2, 3, 6–10].

44.2 Pathophysiology

While the precise pathophysiology of cardiac cephalalgia remains incompletely understood, several key hypotheses are gaining increasing acceptance. First, referred pain is the most widely cited mechanism, supported by numerous articles and case reports. This theory posits that the association between headache and chest pain arises from the somatic nervous system via its visceral afferent and efferent fibers. Cardiac stimuli are detected by cardiac nociceptors and ascend through afferent pathways, including the spinothalamic and spinoreticular tracts, ultimately reaching the sensory cortex and manifesting as a headache [2, 5, 11]. The parasympathetic autonomic nervous system also plays a role, with vagal nerve (cranial nerve X) afferent fibers terminating in the nucleus of the solitary tract. These fibers connect with spinothalamic tract neurons, further contributing to cortical activation and headache generation [3]. Notably, some ascending neurons synapse at the C1–C2 levels, connecting with the trigeminal nerve (cranial nerve V) nucleus, which explains the potential for shoulder and jaw pain in these patients [5, 12].

Second, transient intracranial hypertension is proposed as another mechanism [13]. Following acute myocardial ischemia, reduced cardiac output diminishes the heart's pumping capacity, impacting systemic venous return, including cerebral venous drainage. This disruption alters cerebral blood flow, leading to increased cerebral perfusion pressure and, consequently, intracranial pressure [13].

The third and last hypothesis suggests that inflammatory mediators are implicated in cardiac cephalalgia. Acute myocardial injury triggers the release of pro-inflammatory substances from the cardiac muscle, such as bradykinin, serotonin, substance P, histamine, and adenosine. These mediators can induce cerebral edema, cerebral artery vasodilation, and cerebral cortical hypoperfusion, ultimately manifesting as a headache [2, 5].

44.3 Case Presentation

A 61-year-old male with a history of hypertension, managed with regular antihypertensive therapy, and obesity presented to the emergency department with acute precordial pain. The pain began approximately 30 minutes prior while the patient was at rest at home. He described the pain as oppressive, retrosternal, and radiating to the left shoulder and upper limb, accompanied by dyspnea, nausea, and a single episode of emesis. Concurrently, the patient experienced a severe, acute-onset headache localized to the vertex, characterized as oppressive and increasing in intensity with the worsening chest pain. Upon arrival, vital signs revealed a blood pressure of 145/80 mmHg; other vital signs were unremarkable. Neurological examination revealed no focal deficits or abnormalities. An electrocardiogram (ECG) demonstrated ST-segment elevation greater than 1.5 mm in leads II, III, and aVF. An ultrasensitive troponin level was elevated at 1500 ng/L. Laboratory investigations showed inflammatory markers within normal limits and no evidence of autoimmune or infectious etiologies. A computed tomography (CT) scan of the head revealed normal anatomical findings, without evidence of hemorrhage, mass lesions, or other abnormalities. The patient was transferred to the cardiac catheterization laboratory, where primary percutaneous coronary intervention (PCI) revealed a 90% occlusion of the right coronary artery. Following PCI, the patient reported significant improvement in both chest pain and headache.

44.4 Case Discussion

The rarity of cardiac cephalalgia makes its diagnosis complex, given its varied clinical presentation [3]. The literature suggests a patient profile typically over 50 years old male exhibiting established cardiovascular risk factors including systemic arterial hypertension, dyslipidemia, obesity, and a smoking history [14–19]. However, this is not absolute, as cases have been reported in younger individuals and in patients without cardiovascular risk factors [13, 20, 21].

Cardiac headache is frequently described as diffuse or localized to the vertex and can be either unilateral or bilateral. Its presentation is characterized by a rapid-onset, intense, and oppressive headache, sometimes described as a sensation that the head is about to explode [4, 10, 15, 18, 19, 22, 23]. Patients generally deny photophobia and phonophobia [11, 19, 24, 25]. Nausea and signs and symptoms of myocardial ischemia, such as retrosternal, epigastric, or left upper limb pain, may accompany the headache [4, 18, 24, 26]. Cardiac headache is usually triggered by physical exertion, including activities such as sexual activity or walking, and generally improves soon after stopping the activity [1, 8, 27].

Although age is a relevant factor in the anamnesis, other characteristics must be carefully assessed for proper patient identification. Gathering information about headache presentation, similarity to previous typical headache episodes, and response to commonly used headache medications is crucial [28]. Additionally, investigating the presence of comorbidities, as previously mentioned, should be part of the patient's evaluation.

The assessment of these patients involves stress testing, which usually reveals recurrent headaches associated with ST-segment depression, and coronary angiography [2, 3, 7–10]. A review, involving 30 patients, reinforced the importance of performing brain magnetic resonance imaging (MRI) to exclude other underlying pathological conditions [6]. Regarding treatment, the triptans, as selective 5-HT_{1B-1D} receptor agonists, promote vasoconstriction of extracerebral and intracranial arteries in migraine treatment, but they also exert a mild vasoconstrictive effect on coronary arteries [6]. This justifies why triptans are contraindicated for patients with cardiovascular disease, whereas improvement is seen with nitrate administration or surgical intervention (bypass, myocardial revascularization, percutaneous transluminal coronary angioplasty, stenting) [1, 6, 8, 22, 23]. Furthermore, the literature has emphasized that the immediate relief achieved with nitrate administration is a consistent characteristic linking headaches to myocardial ischemia [7]. The adverse reaction to triptan administration may aid in the identification of cardiac headache [13].

44.5 Headache Characteristics of Cardiac Cephalalgia

A summary of headache characteristics and associated symptoms from the literature is presented in Table 44.1.

Table 44.1 Case reports found in the literature review

Author (year)	Sex (Age)	Onset mode	Headache location	Character	Intensity	Triggering or aggravating factors	Relief factors	Associated signs and symptoms	ICHD-3 criteria	Intervention
Rambihar (2001) [29]	Female (56–60)	–	Occipital	–	–	Exertion	Rest; sublingual nitroglycerine	Pain radiating to the shoulders	C (1; 2a,b)	Multivessel bypass surgery
Blacky et al. (1987) [30]	Male (40)	–	Bilateral temporal	–	–	Exertion (running or cycling)	Rest	Associated symptoms denied	C (1; 2a,b)	Antianginal therapy
Ortiz et al. (2019) [11]	Female (74)	–	Vertex; bilateral frontal	Oppressive	Moderate	Mild exertion	Rest	Associated symptoms denied	C (1; 2a,b; 3c,d)	Two-stage revascularization with drug-eluting stents; individualized therapy with dual antiplatelet therapy combined with anticoagulant therapy
Martínez et al. (2002) [3]	Female (68)	Acute	Left hemicrania and facial headache	–	Severe (10 on the visual analogue scale)	Exertion	Rest	–	C (1; 2a,b; 3a,c,d)	Coronary angioplasty
Wang and Lin (2008) [25]	Female (81)	–	–	–	Severe	–	–	Dizziness, diaphoresis, nausea	C (1; 2a,b; 3a,b)	Stent

(continued)

Table 44.1 (continued)

Author (year)	Sex (Age)	Onset mode	Headache location	Character	Intensity	Triggering or aggravating factors	Relief factors	Associated signs and symptoms	ICHD-3 criteria	Intervention
Sathirapanya (2004) [19]	Male (58)	Acute	Occipital (left)	–	Severe	Exertion	–	Initially, he denied associated symptoms. In another episode, he reported the presence of chest tightness	C (1; 2a,b; 3a,c,d)	Myocardial revascularization
Cutrer and Huerter (2006) [14]	Male (55)	–	Bilateral parietal	Non-throbbing	–	–	–	–	C (1; 2a,b; 3c,d)	Stent
Lefkowitz and Biller (1982) [18]	Male (62)	–	Bregmatic	–	Severe	Stress and exertion	Sublingual nitroglycerin	Retrosternal pain and occasional numbness of both arms	C (1; 2a,b; 3a,d, 4)	Coronary artery bypass
Wang et al. (2017) [31]	Male (40)	–	Bilateral temporal	Pulsatile	Severe	Exertion, cold stimuli, and sexual activities	Nitrates	Occasionally radiating to upper limbs, chest discomfort, palpitations, cold sweating, and facial pallor	C (1; 2a,b; 3a,c, d)	Percutaneous transluminal coronary angiography, stenting of LAD, and bifurcation of the first diagonal and the RCA

Fleetcroft and Maddocks (1985) [12]	Female (78)	–	Frontal	–	–	Exertion, temperature variation	–	Radiated to the roof of the mouth and down both arms, tightness in the chest	C (1; 2a,b)	Nitrate and calcium channel blockers
Sun et al. (2021) [13]	Female (83)	–	–	–	–	–	–	–	C (1; 2a,b)	Percutaneous coronary angioplasty and thrombus aspiration
Lafitte et al. (1996) [26]	Male (40)	–	–	–	–	–	–	Severe, constrictive, retrosternal chest pain with malaise, pallor, reduced level of consciousness, and a mild sensorimotor deficit of the left upper and lower limb	C (1)	Sublingual nitroglycerin

(continued)

Table 44.1 (continued)

Author (year)	Sex (Age)	Onset mode	Headache location	Character	Intensity	Triggering or aggravating factors	Relief factors	Associated signs and symptoms	ICHD-3 criteria	Intervention
Gutiérrez-Morlote and Pascual (2002) [16]	Male (59)	–	Vertex; occipital	–	Moderate-to-severe	Rest	–	Chest discomfort and slight diaphoresis	C (2a)	Sublingual nitroglycerin
Lance and Lambros (1998) [17]	Male (62)	–	–	–	–	Exertion	–	–	C (1; 2a,b; 3d)	Coronary artery bypass
Wei and Wang (2008) [28]	Female, Male (36–85)	Acute	Vertex, bilateral occipital, eyeball	–	Severe	Exertion	Rest or sublingual nitroglycerin	Chest discomfort	B; C (1; 3a)	Stent
Famularo et al. (2002) [15]	Male (70)	Acute	–	Sharp or shooting	Severe (10 out of 10 in severity)	–	–	Symptoms such as shortness of breath and discomfort in the chest, arm, jaw, neck, or abdomen are denied	B; C (1; 3a, c, 4)	Nitroglycerin, aspirin, enoxaparin, captopril, and metoprolol
Lazari et al. (2019) [32]	Male (64)	Acute	–	Oppressive	Severe	–	–	Warm sensation in the chest	C (1; 2a,b; 3c)	Stent, aspirin, clopidogrel, atorvastatin, bisoprolol, ramipril and lansoprazole

Lipton et al. (1997) [1]	Male (57–67)	Acute	Vertex	Sharp	Severe (10 out of 10 in severity)	Exertion	Rest	Nausea	C (1; 2a,b; 3a,b,c,d)	Calcium channel blockers, aspirin, myocardial revascularization, rotational atherectomy, percutaneous transluminal coronary angioplasty
Shankar et al. (2016) [23]	Male (73)	–	–	Dull (oppressive)	Severe	Exertion or temperature	Rest	Chest discomfort	B; C (1; 2a,b; 3a,d)	Aspirin, enalapril, simvastatin, myocardial revascularization
Seow et al. (2007) [21]	Male (35)	Acute	–	Explosive	Severe	–	–	Cold sweat and vomiting	–	–
Mathew et al. (2015) [27]	Male (47)	Progressive	Vertex and bilateral occipital	Oppressive	Severe	Exertion	Rest	Chest discomfort denied	C (1; 3a,d)	Stent
Chen et al. (2004) [24]	Male (76)	–	Bilateral temporal	Nonpulsatile	Severe	Exertion	Rest or nitrates	Chest discomfort	B; C (1; 3a,b,d)	Nitrates
Grace et al. (1997) [9]	Male (59)	–	Vertex and occipital	–	Severe	Exertion	Rest	–	C (3a,d)	Saphenous vein grafts

(continued)

Table 44.1 (continued)

Author (year)	Sex (Age)	Onset mode	Headache location	Character	Intensity	Triggering or aggravating factors	Relief factors	Associated signs and symptoms	ICHD-3 criteria	Intervention
Costopoulos (2011) [8]	Male (55)	–	Vertex and occipital	–	–	Exertion	Rest	–	C (1,4)	Sublingual nitrate, aspirin, clopidogrel and heparin, myocardial revascularization
Cheng et al. (2010) [22]	Female (52–67)	Acute	Bilateral temporal, parietal	Throbbing	Severe	Local anesthesia, exertion	Rest	Chest pain	C (1; 3b; 4)	Nitroglycerin, aspirin and calcium channel blockers
Bowen and Oppenheim (1993) [7]	Male (59)		Bilateral temporal	Non-throbbing	Severe	–	Nitroglycerin	Left arm and chest pain	C (1,4)	Beta-blocker, calcium channel blocker, nitroglycerin and angioplasty
Takayanagi et al. (1990) [33]	Female, Male (64–67)	–	–	–	–	–	–	Headache and chest pain	–	Outcome: death
Wayne (1986) [34]	Female (>49)	–	–	–	–	Exertion	Nitroglycerin	Chest pain	B; C (1, 3d)	Beta-blocker, calcium channel blocker

Ishida et al. (1996) [10]	Male (64)	Acute	Occipital	Throbbing	Severe	Exertion	Rest	Chest pain denied	B; C (1, 3d)	Percutaneous transluminal coronary angioplasty
Auer et al. (2001) [20]	Male (47)	–	Occipital	–	–	–	–	–	–	Outcome: death
Broner et al. (2007) [35]	Female (72)	Acute	Bilateral occipital and frontal	Throbbing	Mild-to-moderate	Exertion or rest	Acetaminophen	Nausea, vomiting and facial pallor	C (1, 3d)	Aspirin, metoprolol, lisinopril, simvastatin, heparin

Age: years
ICHD-3 International Classification of Headache Disorders, 3rd edition

44.6 Diagnostic Approach

Accurate diagnosis of cardiac cephalalgia necessitates distinguishing its unique characteristics from other headache types, including migraine and secondary headaches [6]. Recognizing the epidemiological profile of this condition is crucial for clinical awareness in potentially affected patients. Cardiac cephalalgia primarily affects individuals over 50 years of age, and a male predominance is observed, attributed potentially to a higher prevalence of cardiovascular risk factors [4, 16]. Concurrent cardiovascular risk factors, such as hypertension, coronary artery disease, and diabetes mellitus, are common [14].

Distinguishing cardiac headache from other disorders can be challenging; however, the simultaneous onset of headache and cardiac symptoms is a key diagnostic clue. Cardiac headache typically presents with a sudden onset, reaching peak intensity rapidly and maintaining a stable severity. Autonomic symptoms, such as nausea, may be present, while photophobia and phonophobia are usually absent. Exacerbation can occur with both physical activity and rest [2, 3, 6]. These features should be meticulously documented in the patient's history. Clinical evaluation should focus on confirming the headache's characteristics, including onset, location, triggering, associated, and relieving factors, as previously described. Confirmatory diagnosis relies on demonstrating acute myocardial ischemia through ancillary testing. Resting or stress electrocardiography (ECG), stress testing, and myocardial perfusion imaging can reveal ischemic changes. Cardiac biomarkers, such as cretine kinase muscle brain (CK-MB) and troponins, further support the diagnosis [6, 11, 14, 19]. Definitive diagnosis is established by the resolution of headache following treatment of the underlying coronary artery disease. Therapeutic strategies include addressing the coronary pathology, which alleviates the headache [4, 16]. Triptans, commonly used for migraine, are contraindicated due to their vasoconstrictive effects, which can exacerbate coronary ischemia. Vasodilators, such as nitroglycerin, are preferred for their coronary vasodilatory properties and relief of referred pain. Revascularization procedures, including percutaneous coronary intervention (PCI) and coronary artery bypass grafting (CABG), restore coronary flow and promptly resolve the headache, confirming the diagnosis.

44.7 Management

Based on the synthesized pathophysiology, cardiac cephalalgia is characterized by headaches originating from underlying cardiac ischemia. Therefore, the primary therapeutic objective is to address acute cardiac ischemia, thereby alleviating the headache. Consequently, conventional treatments for primary headaches, such as non-steroidal anti-inflammatory drugs (NSAIDs), are not indicated. Triptans are formally contraindicated [2, 6]. Treatment modalities for cardiac cephalalgia range from intravenous medications, such as nitroglycerin, to invasive procedures, including percutaneous coronary intervention (PCI). Literature reviews consistently highlight nitrates, particularly nitroglycerin, as the first-line treatment for cardiac headache relief. Nitroglycerin can be administered via sublingual or intravenous routes [1, 6]. For sublingual administration, a 0.4 mg dose is recommended, with response observed within approximately 30 minutes. Intravenous administration should begin with 5–10 μg/minute, titrated based on patient response, utilizing an infusion pump. The maximum dose is typically 400 μg/minute. Continuous monitoring of blood pressure and heart rate is essential during administration. Nitroglycerin's efficacy stems from its vasodilatory properties, which reduce cardiac afterload and improve venous return. This enhances blood flow to ischemic myocardial cells, alleviating the referred headache [36]. The response to vasodilators, particularly nitrates such as nitroglycerin, is a pivotal aspect in supporting the diagnosis of cardiac headache and differentiating it from conditions like migraine [4, 16]. Cardiac headache, originating from myocardial ischemia, typically resolves with coronary vasodilation. This response contrasts sharply with migraine, where vasodilators are generally ineffective and usually trigger or exacerbate symptoms [4, 16]. Therefore, a positive response to vasodilators not only provides therapeutic benefit but also serves as a crucial diagnostic clue, helping to distinguish cardiac headache from other primary headache disorders. Additional treatments for acute myocardial ischemia, as described in the literature, include fibrinolytic agents and invasive procedures like PCI. These interventions aim to restore coronary blood flow, thereby resolving headaches through the previously described pathophysiological mechanisms [4].

44.8 Conclusion

Discussing cardiac cephalalgia is crucial for raising clinical awareness, particularly given that acute headache as the initial presentation of myocardial ischemia is exceedingly rare. This atypical presentation significantly increases the risk of missed diagnoses of acute cardiac ischemia, underscoring the importance of considering cardiac origins in patients presenting with sudden-onset headaches, even in the absence of typical chest pain. Furthermore, it is essential to recognize that cardiac cephalalgia is not necessarily an exertional headache, as it can occur at rest, further complicating its identification. A heightened index of suspicion, coupled with thorough clinical evaluation and appropriate ancillary testing, is paramount to ensuring timely and accurate diagnosis, thereby improving patient outcomes.

References

1. Lipton RB, Lowenkopf T, Bajwa ZH, Leckie RS, Ribeiro S, Newman LC, Greenberg MA. Cardiac cephalgia: a treatable form of exertional headache. Neurology. 1997;49:813–6. https://doi.org/10.1212/WNL.49.3.813.
2. Torres-Yaghi Y, Salerian J, Dougherty C. Cardiac cephalgia. Curr Pain Headache Rep. 2015;19:14. https://doi.org/10.1007/s11916-015-0481-4.
3. Martínez HR, Rangel-Guerra RA, Cantú-Martínez L, Garza-Gómez J, González HC. Cardiac headache: Hemicranial Cephalalgia as the sole manifestation of coronary ischemia. Headache. 2002;42:1029–32. https://doi.org/10.1046/j.1526-4610.2002.02233.x.
4. Providencia RA. Headache and cardiovascular disease: old symptoms, new proposals. Futur Cardiol. 2010;6:703–23. https://doi.org/10.2217/fca.10.76.
5. Navarro-Pérez MP, Bellosta-Diago E, Olesen J, Santos-Lasaosa S. Cardiac cephalalgia: a narrative review and ICHD-3 criteria evaluation. J Headache Pain. 2022;23:136. https://doi.org/10.1186/s10194-022-01508-7.
6. Bini A, Evangelista A, Castellini P, Lambru G, Ferrante T, Manzoni GC, Torelli P. Cardiac cephalgia. J Headache Pain. 2009;10:3–9. https://doi.org/10.1007/s10194-008-0087-x.
7. Bowen J, Oppenheim G. Headache as a presentation of angina: reproduction of symptoms during angioplasty. Headache. 1993;33:238–9. https://doi.org/10.1111/j.1526-4610.1993.hed3305238.x.
8. Costopoulos C. Acute coronary syndromes can be a headache. Emerg Med J. 2011;28:71–3. https://doi.org/10.1136/emj.2009.082271.
9. Grace A, Horgan J, Breathnach K, Staunton H. Anginal headaches and its basis. Cephalalgia. 1997;17:195–6. https://doi.org/10.1046/j.1468-2982.1997.1703195.x.
10. Ishida A, Sunagawa O, Touma T, Shinzato Y, Kawazoe N, Fukiyama K. Headache as a manifestation of myocardial infarction. Jpn Heart J. 1996;37:261–3. https://doi.org/10.1536/ihj.37.261.
11. Luiz Ortiz M, Bermejo Guerrero L, Martínez Porqueras R, González De La Aleja J. Cefalea cardíaca: cuando la isquemia miocárdica llega a la consulta del neurólogo. Neurologia. 2020;35:614–5. https://doi.org/10.1016/j.nrl.2019.09.003.
12. Fleetcroft R, Maddocks JL. Headache due to ischaemic heart disease. J R Soc Med. 1985;78(8):676. https://doi.org/10.1177/014107688507800817.
13. Sun L, Zhang Q, Li N, Bao S, Wang D, Li X. Case report: cardiac cephalalgia closely associated with acute myocardial infarction. Am J Emerg Med. 2021;47:350.e1–3. https://doi.org/10.1016/j.ajem.2021.03.019.
14. Cutrer FM, Huerter K. Exertional headache and coronary ischemia despite normal electrocardiographic stress testing. Headache. 2006;46:165–7. https://doi.org/10.1111/j.1526-4610.2006.00316_1.x.
15. Famularo G, Polchi S, Tarroni P. Headache as a presenting symptom of acute myocardial infarction. Headache. 2002;42:1025–8. https://doi.org/10.1046/j.1526-4610.2002.02232.x.
16. Gutiérrez-Morlote J, Pascual J. Cardiac cephalgia is not necessarily an exertional headache: case report. Cephalalgia. 2002;22:765–6. https://doi.org/10.1046/j.1468-2982.2002.00418.x.
17. Lance JW, Lambros J. Unilateral exertional headache as a symptom of cardiac Ischemia. Headache. 1998;38:315–6. https://doi.org/10.1046/j.1526-4610.1998.3804315.x.
18. Lefkowitz D, Biller J. Bregmatic headache as a manifestation of myocardial ischemia. Arch Neurol. 1982;39:130. https://doi.org/10.1001/archneur.1982.00510140064019.
19. Sathirapanya P. Anginal cephalgia: a serious form of exertional headache. Cephalalgia. 2004;24:231–4. https://doi.org/10.1111/j.1468-2982.2003.00632.x.
20. Auer J, Berent R, Lassnig E, Eber B. Headache as a manifestation of fatal myocardial infarction. Neurol Sci. 2001;22:395–7. https://doi.org/10.1007/s100720100071.
21. Seow V-K, Chong C-F, Wang T-L, Ong J-R. Severe explosive headache: a sole presentation of acute myocardial infarction in a young man. Am J Emerg Med. 2007;25:250–1. https://doi.org/10.1016/j.ajem.2006.11.014.

22. Cheng P-Y, Sy H-N, Chen W-L, Chen Y-Y. Cardiac cephalalgia presented with a thunderclap headache and an isolated exertional headache: report of 2 cases. Acta Neurol Taiwan. 2010;19:57–61.
23. Shankar A, Allan CLM, Smyth D, Jardine D. Cardiac cephalgia: a diagnostic headache. Intern Med J. 2016;46:1219–21. https://doi.org/10.1111/imj.13217.
24. Chen S-P, Fuh J-L, Yu W-C, Wang S-J. Cardiac cephalalgia case report and review of the literature with new ICHD-II criteria revisited. Eur Neurol. 2004;51:221–6. https://doi.org/10.1159/000078489.
25. Wang W, Lin C-S. Headache angina. Am J Emerg Med. 2008;26:387.e1–2. https://doi.org/10.1016/j.ajem.2007.07.029.
26. Lafitte C, Even C, Henry-Lebras F, De Toffol B, Autret A. Migraine and angina pectoris by coronary artery spasm. Headache. 1996;36:332–4. https://doi.org/10.1046/j.1526-4610.1996.3605332.x.
27. Mathew PG, Boes CJ, Garza I. A tale of two systems: cardiac cephalalgia vs migrainous thoracalgia. Headache. 2015;55:310–2. https://doi.org/10.1111/head.12373.
28. Wei J-H, Wang H-F. Cardiac cephalalgia: case reports and review. Cephalalgia. 2008;28:892–6. https://doi.org/10.1111/j.1468-2982.2008.01590.x.
29. Rambihar VS. Headache angina. Lancet. 2001;357(9249):72. https://doi.org/10.1016/S0140-6736(05)71575-0.
30. Blacky RA, Ritelmeyer JT, Wallace MR. Headache angina. Am J Cardiol. 1987;60:730–2. https://doi.org/10.1016/0002-9149(87)90394-8.
31. Wang M, Wang L, Liu C, Bian X, Dong Z, Yu S. Cardiac cephalalgia: one case with cortical hypoperfusion in headaches and literature review. J Headache Pain. 2017;18:24. https://doi.org/10.1186/s10194-017-0732-3.
32. Lazari J, Money-Kyrle A, Wakerley BR. Cardiac cephalalgia: severe, non-exertional headache presenting as unstable angina. Pract Neurol. 2019;19:173–5. https://doi.org/10.1136/practneurol-2018-002045.
33. Takayanagi K, Fujito T, Morooka S, Takabatake Y, Nakamura Y. Headache angina with fatal outcome. Jpn Heart J. 1990;31:503–7. https://doi.org/10.1536/ihj.31.503.
34. Wayne VS. A possible relationship between migraine and coronary artery spasm. Aust NZ J Med. 1986;16:708–10. https://doi.org/10.1111/j.1445-5994.1986.tb00020.x.
35. Broner S, Lay C, Newman L, Swerdlow M. Thunderclap headache as the presenting symptom of myocardial infarction. Headache. 2007;47:724–5. https://doi.org/10.1111/j.1526-4610.2007.00795.x.
36. Amsterdam EA, Wenger NK, Brindis RG, Casey DE, Ganiats TG, Holmes DR, Jaffe AS, Jneid H, Kelly RF, Kontos MC, Levine GN, Liebson PR, Mukherjee D, Peterson ED, Sabatine MS, Smalling RW, Zieman SJ. 2014 AHA/ACC guideline for the management of patients with non–ST-elevation acute coronary syndromes. J Am Coll Cardiol. 2014;64:e139–228. https://doi.org/10.1016/j.jacc.2014.09.017.

Part VIII
Headache or Facial Pain Attributed to Disorder of the Cranium, Neck, Eyes, Ears, Nose, Sinuses, Teeth, Mouth or Other Facial or Cervical Structure

Chapter 45
Cervicogenic Headache

Marcelo Valença and Juliana Ramos de Andrade

45.1 Introduction

Cervicogenic headache (CGH) is a secondary headache disorder characterized by pain referred from a source in the cervical spine or surrounding structures [1]. The condition has gained increasing recognition since it was first defined more clearly in the late twentieth century [1–3]. In the 1980s, Australian neurologist Dr. James Lance and British neurologist Dr. Martin Anthony played pivotal roles in establishing the foundational concept that cervical structures, especially the upper cervical nerves, could be sources of headache through convergent input onto the trigeminocervical complex. Their observations of head pain associated with cervical pathology laid the groundwork for subsequent clinical and anatomical studies.

The International Classification of Headache Disorders (ICHD) has progressively refined the diagnostic criteria for CGH, now listed in its third edition (ICHD-3) as a distinct clinical entity [4]. However, despite its formal recognition, CGH remains underdiagnosed and often misclassified, particularly due to its symptom overlap with primary headache disorders such as migraine and tension-type headache. The underlying mechanisms of CGH are believed to involve the convergence of afferent fibers from the upper cervical roots (C1–C3) and the trigeminal nerve within the trigeminocervical complex.

We present a case of a man who developed episodic occipital headaches during upper respiratory tract infections. The clinical features and presumed pathophysiological mechanisms of his pain are consistent with cervicogenic headache triggered by lymphadenopathy compressing the greater occipital nerve (GON). This case serves to explore a possible yet underrecognized etiology of CGH and to highlight the complex neuroanatomical interactions involved.

M. Valença (✉) · J. R. de Andrade
Federal University of Pernambuco, Recife, Pernambuco, Brazil

D. Uludüz et al. (eds.), *Rare Causes of Headache Disorders*, Headache,
https://doi.org/10.1007/978-3-032-10242-3_45

45.2 Pathophysiology

Cervicogenic headache (CGH) arises from nociceptive sources within the cervical spine, primarily involving structures innervated by the upper cervical nerves (C1–C3). The fundamental pathophysiological mechanism is the convergence of afferent fibers from the upper cervical spinal nerves and the trigeminal nerve within the trigeminocervical complex—a region in the upper cervical spinal cord where sensory input from both the cervical and trigeminal territories is integrated [5, 6]. This anatomical convergence enables nociceptive stimuli originating in the cervical spine to be perceived as pain in the head and face, explaining the referred nature of CGH.

Key anatomical sources of nociception implicated in CGH include:

- Zygapophyseal (facet) joints, especially the C2–C3 joint, which is the most commonly identified pain generator.
- Atlantoaxial (C1–C2) and atlanto-occipital joints, which can refer pain to the posterior fossa and occipital region.
- Cervical intervertebral discs, particularly at the C2–C3 level.
- Cervical muscles and ligaments, especially those innervated by C1–C3, such as the suboccipital muscles.
- Greater occipital nerve (GON), a significant branch of the C2 dorsal ramus, which is susceptible to irritation or compression, leading to occipital pain that may radiate anteriorly.
- Dura mater of the upper spinal cord and posterior cranial fossa, which can also contribute to pain referral.

Mechanisms of pain generation and referral [5, 6]:

- Peripheral sensitization: Local inflammation, trauma, degenerative changes, or mechanical irritation (e.g., by reactive lymphadenopathy, as in the presented case) can activate nociceptors in cervical structures.
- Central sensitization: Repeated or intense peripheral nociceptive input can sensitize second-order neurons in the trigeminocervical complex, amplifying pain perception and broadening the pain referral zone.
- Experimental evidence: Stimulation of the C2–C3 facet joint or the GON in humans can reproduce characteristic CGH pain patterns, including referral to frontal and orbital regions, supporting the clinical relevance of trigeminocervical convergence.

Triggering factors include:

- Degenerative changes (e.g., arthritis of the C2–C3 facet joint)
- Trauma (e.g., whiplash injury)
- Muscle dysfunction or trigger points in the upper cervical and suboccipital muscles
- Mechanical compression (e.g., by hypertrophied muscles, connective tissue, or reactive lymphadenopathy)

45.3 Case Presentation

The patient is a 58-year-old man with a prior diagnosis of migraine without aura. He reported experiencing occasional episodes of headache, typically once every year or two, associated with upper respiratory tract infections characterized by nasal congestion, pharyngitis with erythema, odynophagia, and palpable cervical and retroauricular lymphadenopathy.

During these episodes, he developed a unilateral occipital headache that radiated anteriorly toward the ipsilateral frontal region. The pain was described as fine, dull, and bothersome, with a continuous but fluctuating intensity rated between 3 and 6 out of 10. Palpation of the ipsilateral occipital or nuchal region exacerbated the pain. He noted that the pain was worsened by head and neck movement.

These episodes lasted between 1 and 3 days, coinciding with the peak of his infectious symptoms. Over time, he had experienced at least eight such episodes, more commonly on the right side. No diagnostic nerve block was performed. The headaches resolved spontaneously as his systemic symptoms improved.

Given the anatomical overlap between the pain distribution and the sensory territory of the GON, as well as the presence of enlarged lymph nodes during symptomatic periods, we hypothesize that reactive cervical lymphadenopathy caused intermittent compression of peripheral nerves such as C2, GON, or the lesser occipital nerve, contributing to his headache episodes.

45.4 Clinical Characteristics of Headache

Cervicogenic headache (CGH) presents with distinct clinical characteristics, although some features may overlap with other headache types. The hallmark symptom is a unilateral headache that typically does not shift sides. The pain often follows a characteristic "ram's horn" pattern, beginning in the occipital region and potentially radiating toward the frontal, temporal, or orbital areas [7, 8].

Patients almost always report ipsilateral neck pain or discomfort, which is frequently associated with tenderness over the upper cervical spine joints (C1–C3), restricted cervical range of motion (ROM), and worsening of headache with neck movement or prolonged awkward head positions. The quality of pain is usually described as dull, steady, and non-throbbing, with a tightening or pressing sensation, and pain intensity is often moderate [9].

Associated symptoms may include diffuse, vague shoulder, and arm pain on the same side, which can occasionally exhibit radicular features. There is often muscle tightness and myofascial trigger points in muscles such as the upper trapezius, levator scapulae, scalenes, and suboccipital muscles. Some patients may also present with weakness in the deep neck flexors and atrophy of suboccipital muscles. If the greater occipital nerve is involved, sensory changes in the occipital scalp may occur.

Neck movements, sustained postures, or external pressure over the upper cervical or occipital region typically exacerbate a headache. As a result, patients often adopt protective behaviors to minimize or avoid neck motion.

45.5 Diagnosis of Cervicogenic Headache

The diagnosis of cervicogenic headache (CGH) relies on a comprehensive approach that includes clinical evaluation, established diagnostic criteria, and, when necessary, confirmatory procedures. Because CGH often mimics primary headache disorders such as migraine or tension-type headache, careful clinical assessment is essential. The diagnostic process begins with a detailed history, focusing on the onset, duration, and characteristics of the headache, its relationship to neck movement or sustained postures, and the presence of neck pain, trauma, or known cervical pathology. Associated symptoms, such as ipsilateral shoulder or arm pain, are also essential to document [2, 9].

Physical examination should include palpation of the upper cervical spine and occipital region for tenderness, evaluation of cervical range of motion (often restricted), and observation of headache provocation by neck movements or pressure. A neurological exam helps rule out alternative causes. Manual diagnostic tests such as the cervical flexion–rotation test (CFRT), palpation for myofascial trigger points, and assessment of deep cervical muscle strength and function further support the clinical impression [2, 9, 10].

Diagnostic criteria from the International Classification of Headache Disorders (ICHD-3) [4] require (A) a headache fulfilling causation criteria, (B) clinical or imaging evidence of cervical pathology known to cause headache, (C) at least two indicators of a causal relationship—such as temporal correlation with cervical pathology, improvement with treatment, worsening with neck movement, or relief following a diagnostic nerve block—and (D) exclusion of other ICHD-3 diagnoses.

The Cervicogenic Headache International Study Group (CHISG) adds further specificity with criteria such as precipitation of headache by neck motion or pressure, restricted cervical motion, ipsilateral neck/shoulder/arm pain, consistent one-sided headache without shifting, and confirmation by anesthetic block.

Confirmatory diagnostic procedures include imaging techniques like magnetic resonance imaging (MRI) or computed tomography (CT) to identify cervical spine lesions or rule out other structural causes. Diagnostic nerve blocks targeting cervical joints or nerve roots are used to confirm the cervical origin if the headache is abolished. Lastly, differential diagnosis is essential to exclude primary headache disorders and other secondary causes such as vascular, neoplastic, infectious, or traumatic conditions.

45.6 Treatment

The diagnosis of cervicogenic headache is often complex due to its diverse etiologies and symptom overlap with primary headaches. In this case, the episodic nature of the pain, its occipital onset with frontal radiation, exacerbation by neck movement, and aggravation by occipital palpation support the diagnosis of CGH.

The convergence of cervical afferents (C1–C3) and trigeminal inputs within the trigeminocervical complex allows for the referral of cervical nociceptive input to cranial regions, particularly the orbit and forehead, as first proposed by Lance and Anthony [1, 11]. This neuroanatomical substrate provides a logical explanation for why cervical pathology can manifest as cranial pain.

Support for this mechanism comes from experimental studies such as that of Piovesan et al. [2], who investigated referred pain following stimulation of the GON. In their study, 2 mL of distilled water was injected near the right GON in three human subjects. Two of the three participants experienced referred pain extending beyond the anatomical territory of the GON, projecting into the ipsilateral ophthalmic division (V1) territory. This phenomenon is a direct clinical correlate to the patient described here, where presumed GON compression by lymphadenopathy elicited pain that radiated from the occipital to the frontal region.

Their study supports the concept that the convergence of cervical and trigeminal inputs within the spinal cord and brainstem facilitates the mislocalization of pain. This convergence theory has formed the basis for understanding not only cervicogenic headache but also its treatment modalities, which target cervical structures.

Interestingly, this case also highlights an underexplored cause of CGH—transient reactive lymphadenopathy that compresses the cervical nerves. Though not traditionally included in the differential diagnosis of CGH, reactive nodes may pose a potential entrapment point. The GON, for instance, exits the semispinalis capitis muscle and ascends through a dense network of connective tissue and musculature in the suboccipital region, which can be a site for entrapment or compression [8].

There is a growing trend among surgeons to perform decompression surgeries targeting cranial nerves, particularly the greater occipital nerve, in patients with refractory headache disorders [12]. Emerging evidence suggests that these nerves may be subjected to chronic compression from surrounding anatomical structures, such as hypertrophied muscles, fibrous bands, or aberrant vascular loops. These compressive phenomena are believed to contribute to the pathophysiology of certain chronic headaches, including cervicogenic headache and occipital neuralgia. Interestingly, a significant proportion of patients who undergo occipital nerve decompression procedures report substantial and lasting relief from pain, often after years of failed pharmacological treatments. This growing body of surgical outcomes is prompting a reevaluation of the role of peripheral nerve compression in chronic headache syndromes. It supports further investigation into targeted neurosurgical interventions as part of a comprehensive headache management strategy [13, 14].

The anatomical course of the GON and its susceptibility to mechanical irritation have led to surgical decompression being proposed as a treatment option for refractory occipital neuralgia and chronic migraine, particularly when physical findings correlate with tenderness over the nerve.

Although this patient did not undergo diagnostic nerve blockade, which is a requirement for CGH diagnosis per ICHD-3, the temporal relationship between infection, lymphadenopathy, and headache resolution supports a causal relationship.

45.7 Conclusion

This case illustrates a possible variant of cervicogenic headache triggered by mechanical irritation of the greater occipital nerve from reactive cervical lymphadenopathy. It highlights the need to consider uncommon yet plausible causes of cervicogenic pain, particularly in patients with episodic occipital-frontal headaches in the setting of infection.

Further studies are needed to validate whether lymph node-induced nerve compression should be formally considered among the etiologies of CGH. This case also underscores the importance of detailed anatomical and clinical assessment in the diagnosis and management of secondary headache disorders.

References

1. Lance JW, Anthony M. Neck-tongue syndrome on sudden turning of the head. J Neurol Neurosurg Psychiatry. 1980;43:97–101. https://doi.org/10.1136/jnnp.43.2.97.
2. Piovesan E, Kowacs P, Tatsui C, Lange M, Ribas L, Werneck L. Referred Pain After Painful Stimulation of the Greater Occipital Nerve in Humans: Evidence of Convergence of Cervical Afferences on Trigeminal Nuclei. Cephalalgia [Internet]. 2001;21(2):107–9. Available from: https://journals.sagepub.com/doi/10.1046/j.1468-2982.2001.00166.x
3. Bartsch T, Goadsby PJ. The trigeminocervical complex and migraine: current concepts and synthesis. Curr Pain Headache Rep. 2003;7:371–6. https://doi.org/10.1007/s11916-003-0036-y.
4. The International Classification of Headache Disorders, 3rd edition (beta version). Cephalalgia. 2013;33:629–808. https://doi.org/10.1177/0333102413485658.
5. Bogduk N, Govind J. Cervicogenic headache: an assessment of the evidence on clinical diagnosis, invasive tests, and treatment. Lancet Neurol. 2009;8:959–68. https://doi.org/10.1016/S1474-4422(09)70209-1.
6. Sjaastad O, Fredriksen TA, Pfaffenrath V. Cervicogenic headache: pathophysiology, diagnostic criteria and treatment. Agri. 2005;17(3):1–7.
7. Rubio-Ochoa J, Benítez-Martínez J, Lluch E, Santacruz-Zaragozá S, Gómez-Contreras P, Cook CE. Physical examination tests for screening and diagnosis of cervicogenic headache: a systematic review. Man Ther. 2016;21:35–40. https://doi.org/10.1016/j.math.2015.09.008.
8. Fredriksen TA, Hovdal H, Sjaastad O. "Cervicogenic headache": clinical manifestation. Cephalalgia. 1987;7:147–60. https://doi.org/10.1046/j.1468-2982.1987.0702147.x.

9. Leone M, D'Amico D, Grazzi L, Attanasio A, Bussone G. Cervicogenic headache: a critical review of the current diagnostic criteria. Pain. 1998;78(1):1–5. https://doi.org/10.1016/S0304-3959(98)00116-X.
10. Putilina MV. Cervicogenic headache: pathogenesis, clinical features, and diagnosis. Neurol Neuropsychiatr Pol. 2011;45(5):456–60.
11. Anthony M. Cervicogenic headache: prevalence and response to local steroid therapy. Clin Exp Rheumatol. 2000;18:S59–64.
12. Hammond S. Headache caused by neuralgias and structural disorders of the neck. In: Olesen J, Tfelt-Hansen P, Welch KMA, editors. The headaches. 2nd ed. Lippincott Williams & Wilkins; 2005.
13. Jansen J. Surgical treatment of non-responsive cervicogenic headache. Clin Exp Rheumatol. 2000;18:S67–70.
14. van Suijlekom JA, Weber WE, van Kleef M. Cervicogenic headache: techniques of diagnostic nerve blocks. Clin Exp Rheumatol. 2000;18:S39–44.

Chapter 46
Headache Attributed to Craniocervical Dystonia

Míriam Carvalho Soares and Pedro Augusto Sampaio Rocha-Filho

46.1 Introduction

Headache attributed to craniocervical dystonia (HACCD) is listed in the third edition of the International Classification of Headache Disorders (ICHD-3) among headaches attributed to disorders of the neck [1]. *This type of headache is closely related to dystonia*, which is a movement disorder characterized by sustained or intermittent muscle contractions that lead to abnormal, often repetitive movements and postures. These movements are typically patterned and twisting, and may include tremors. Diagnosis is primarily clinical, with distinctive features such as "sensory tricks"—specific maneuvers that temporarily alleviate dystonic symptoms—crucial in confirming the condition [2]. When muscle contractions extend to adjacent areas, such as the neck, oromandibular region, tongue, or larynx, the condition is termed craniocervical dystonia (CCD), a type of segmental dystonia [3]. CCD is a complex and often debilitating neurological disorder marked by sustained or intermittent abnormal postures and movements of the head and neck, typically accompanied by painful muscle contractions.

While the primary symptoms of CCD are motor disturbances, an often overlooked aspect of the condition is the significant presence of pain [4]. Headaches in individuals with dystonia are not well-documented in the literature, but they are commonly described as either starting or worsening in conjunction with dystonic episodes. HACCD can severely impact quality of life and present considerable challenges in terms of both diagnosis and treatment [1].

Several mechanisms may contribute to headaches in CCD patients. These include pain resulting from abnormal cervical muscle contractions, altered postural alignment, or potential involvement of the central nervous system and its sensitization [4,

M. Carvalho Soares · P. A. Sampaio Rocha-Filho (✉)
Federal University of Pernambuco (UFPE), Recife, Brazil
e-mail: pedro.rochafilho@ufpe.br

D. Uludüz et al. (eds.), *Rare Causes of Headache Disorders*, Headache,
https://doi.org/10.1007/978-3-032-10242-3_46

5]. In patients with cervical dystonia (CD), headache attributed to dystonia may present with a migraine-like or tension-type pattern. Additionally, headaches—such as migraine, tension-type, or cervicogenic headache—may coexist independently, without a temporal relationship to the dystonic movements, further complicating the diagnostic process [6]. Therefore, understanding the interplay between CCD and headache is essential for optimizing patient management and improving outcomes.

This chapter provides a comprehensive overview of HACCD, exploring its pathophysiology, diagnostic challenges, and treatment strategies. A clinical case will be presented to illustrate key aspects of HACCD. By examining this comorbidity, we aim to emphasize the importance of a multidisciplinary approach to managing both the motor and non-motor manifestations of this complex disorder.

46.2 Pathophysiology

The pathophysiology of pain in dystonia involves both "muscle-based" and "non-muscle-based" mechanisms. Preclinical studies suggest that sustained muscle contractions in dystonia can lead to muscle ischemia, triggering the release of inflammatory mediators, including substance P, bradykinin, and ATP. These mediators increase the excitability of A-delta and C fibers, potentially leading to abnormal nociceptive transmission and processing. Some hypotheses also propose that trigger points in dystonic muscles contribute to pain through excessive local release of these inflammatory mediators, which can further exacerbate muscle contractions [7].

Additionally, dysfunction in descending pain inhibitory pathways, as well as structural and functional changes in the basal ganglia, cortex, and other areas involved in sensorimotor integration, may contribute to the pain experience in CCD patients. Individuals with dystonia may experience abnormal cortical sensorimotor integration and processing, further complicating the pain experience. Pain in dystonia is likely multifactorial, influenced by factors such as the severity and chronicity of dystonic postures, as well as comorbid orthopedic complications (e.g., spinal degeneration, disc herniation, or radiculopathy), which may also contribute to the development of pain [8]. Nevertheless, pain does not always correlate with the severity of motor symptoms. Some individuals with severe dystonic movements report little or no pain, while others with similar levels of motor involvement experience significant discomfort [5].

Although the exact mechanisms linking dystonia and headache—particularly migraine—remain unclear, shared pathogenic pathways, such as cortical spreading depression and ion channel gene dysfunction (e.g., CACNA1A, ATP1A2, ATP1A3, PRRT2, PNKD), suggest a phenotypic overlap [9]. Additionally, pain may result from local muscle contraction, genetic susceptibility, and secondary sensitization.

46.3 Case Presentation

A 60-year-old male was diagnosed with cervical dystonia at the age of 32, initially presenting with involuntary movements in the cervical muscles. Over the past 20 years, he has been undergoing botulinum toxin type A therapy (BoNT-A). In addition to his dystonia, he has experienced cervical pain and headache for the past 10 years, coinciding with a worsening of the dystonic movements. Brain magnetic resonance imaging (MRI) did not show any structurally significant alteration. Cervical spine computed tomography (CT) was unremarkable as well. No alternative secondary etiologies for dystonia were found.

On physical examination, the patient exhibited right torticollis, left laterocollis, and anterocollis (Fig. 46.1). Latent trigger points were identified bilaterally in the superior trapezius and the left suboccipital region. The patient rated his pain as moderate, scoring 7 out of 10 on the Visual Analog Scale (VAS). The pain was primarily localized in the occipital and nuchal regions bilaterally coinciding with areas of greater muscle contraction. It was described as a pressing sensation, with additional descriptors of tiredness, annoyance, and tightness (McGill Pain Questionnaire). The Toronto Western Spasmodic Torticollis Rating Scale (TWSTRS) was administered, revealing scores of 19 in the severity subscale (indicating moderate severity); 11 in disability (moderate functional impact); and 5 in pain (minimal).

The patient reported experiencing headaches on an average of 20 days per month. He denied nausea or phonophobia but noted mild photophobia. He also indicated that his headaches were not exacerbated by physical exertion. Despite the frequency of his headache, he had not been using prophylactic treatment or overusing analgesics. His Headache Impact Test (HIT-6) score was 56, suggesting a significant impact on his quality of life due to headaches. The headache pattern was consistent with a tension-type headache.

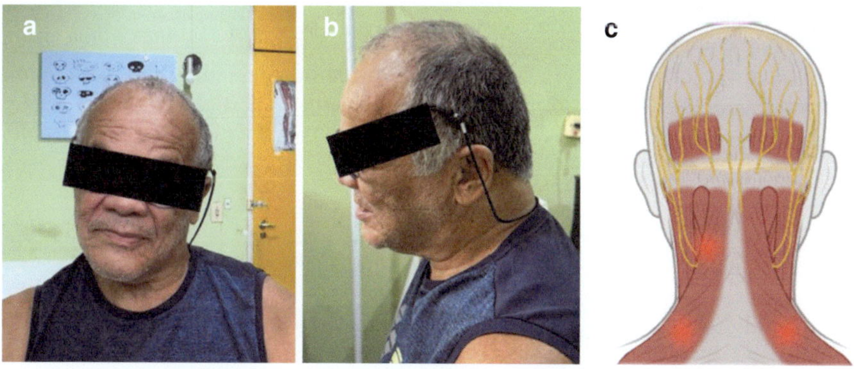

Fig. 46.1 Patient with cervical dystonia. (**a**) Right torticollis and left laterocollis (**b**) Noticeable anterocollis. (**c**) Latent trigger points in the bilateral superior trapezius and in the left suboccipital region. (Created in BioRender. Soares (2025) https://BioRender.com/2sllw1q)

Regarding his cervical dystonia, the patient reported a subjective improvement of approximately 70% in cervical movements with BoNT-A, with effects lasting around 4 months following previous injections. One month after his most recent BoNT-A injection, the patient reported no headaches, and his muscle contractions were notably improved, as reflected in his TWSTRS score—severity decreased to 7, disability to 6, and pain was reduced to 0. On physical examination, the trigger points in the trapezius muscles had resolved, though the trigger point in the left suboccipital region remained. The patient noted that as the effects of the BoNT-A began to wear off, his pain gradually returned. BoNT-A treatment was administered using abobotulinum toxin, with the specific injected muscles and dosages detailed in Table 46.1.

Cervical dystonia (CD) is more common in women than in men, with a prevalence ranging from 5 to 20 per 100,000 individuals. It is the most common form of focal dystonia and is often referred to as spasmodic torticollis when confined to the cervical region [10]. The heterogeneous nature of CD arises from the varied patterns of muscle involvement, which can significantly impact diagnosis and treatment [11]. Regarding etiology, primary CD may be idiopathic or, in approximately 12% of cases, hereditary. Secondary CD results from other underlying pathologies, which may be inherited or acquired. Secondary causes of CD include medication side effects, vascular injury, or neurodegenerative diseases such as Huntington's disease or Parkinson's disease [12].

CD can present as either painless or painful, with pain being a significant source of disability for many patients. Several instruments are used to assess the severity of dystonia, including the Toronto Western Spasmodic Torticollis Rating Scale (TWSTRS), a validated tool that evaluates the severity of cervical dystonic contractions, functional disability, and pain intensity [13]. The condition significantly impairs quality of life, causing both functional and psychosocial disabilities. Pain is often the primary reason patients seek treatment, with approximately two-thirds of CD patients requiring analgesics during the disease. Studies report that up to 66% of CD patients experience significant pain, and in some studies, pain prevalence is reported as high as 90% [4].

Given the high prevalence of pain among CD patients, recent studies have explored its specific manifestations and comorbidities, including the association with migraine. *Zolin et al.* examined 58 patients with comorbid CD and migraine. Most were female (88%), with migraine preceding CD in 72% of cases. Laterocollis

Table 46.1 Botulinum toxin dosage and muscles selected (abobotulinum toxin)

Muscles	Dosage (units)
Left splenius capitis	40
Left levator scapulae	60
Right sternocleidomastoid	20
Left sternocleidomastoid	60
Right trapezius (pars descendens)	20
Left trapezius (pars descendens)	60

was the most prevalent phenotype (98%), often coexisting with torticollis (60%) and no correlation was observed between migraine frequency and dystonia severity. Nonetheless, dystonic movements were common migraine triggers. Treatment with BoNT-A led to migraine improvement in 63% of patients at 12 months, suggesting a therapeutic role for botulinum toxin in this subgroup [14]. The study highlights how specific dystonic patterns may be linked to headache manifestations.

In this clinical case, the patient experienced a headache that began 18 years after the onset of cervical dystonia. The onset of this headache coincided with the worsening of the dystonia. The headache improved with the improvement in the dystonia, after each cycle of botulinum toxin. Therefore, we can classify it as HACCD. The treatment of this headache consisted of treating the dystonia with BoNT-A.

46.4 Clinical Characteristics

The ICHD-3 recognizes that CCD, in the context of HACCD, encompasses not only classical spasmodic torticollis (isolated cervical dystonia) but also other forms of segmental dystonia, such as pharyngeal, mandibular, and lingual dystonia, which may contribute to the headache [1]. The prevalence of HACCD varies between studies, ranging from 1.3 (using ICHD-2 criteria) [6] to 29% (using ICHD-3 criteria) [15]. This variability in prevalence may be partly attributed to evolving diagnostic criteria, as reflected in the current definition of HACCD in ICHD-3 [1] (Table 46.2).

46.5 Differential Diagnosis

HACCD is a secondary headache disorder that typically manifests in regions affected by dystonic muscle contractions—most commonly the occipital, suboccipital, or temporal areas. Diagnostic clues include the *temporal and topographical relationship* between the onset of headache and dystonic activity, as well as improvement in headache following effective dystonia treatment, most notably with BoNT-A

Table 46.2 HACCD diagnostic criteria by ICHD-3 [1]

A. Neck and posterior head pain fulfilling criterion C.
B. CCD is demonstrated by abnormal movements or defective posturing of the neck and/or head due to muscular hyperactivity.
C. Evidence of causation, as indicated by at least two of the following: 1. Pain has developed in close temporal relation to the onset of CCD. 2. Pain has significantly worsened in parallel with progression of the CCD. 3. Pain has significantly improved or resolved in parallel with improvement in or resolution of the CCD. 4. Pain location corresponds to the location of the dystonic muscle(s).
D. Not better accounted for by another ICHD-3 diagnosis.

[1]. The headache is often described as pressing or tightening in quality and may present features of *tension-type headache* or *migraine*. However, its association with dystonic muscle overactivity is a defining characteristic [19].

The differential diagnosis includes several primary and secondary headache types. *Cervicogenic headache* is a key condition to distinguish, as it is typically provoked by neck movement or sustained awkward postures, commonly unilateral and often relieved by anesthetic nerve blocks, features that are less characteristic of HACCD. An evidence of a cervical disorder or lesion capable of causing headache, based on clinical or imaging findings, is necessary for its diagnosis [1]. *Tension-type headache* is generally bilateral, dull, and non-pulsatile, and it does not exhibit a temporal relationship with dystonic movements. *Myofascial pain syndrome* may present with referred pain in the occipital or cervical region but is identified by the presence of palpable trigger points and absence of involuntary movements [8]. Also, it can coexist with HACCD and other headaches. Notably, HACCD may clinically resemble migraine or tension-type headache in characteristics, but the *temporal and anatomical correlation with dystonia* is the key feature that supports its diagnosis according to ICHD-3 [1]. Accurate recognition requires careful clinical correlation between headache features, its distribution, and timing of dystonic activity.

46.6 Treatment

Some studies have evaluated the effect on BoNT-A for treating CCD and associated headaches and have shown an improvement in pain [14–19]. A prospective cohort study compared patients with CCD with HACCD versus patients with CCD and other headaches. Only those with HACCD showed a decrease in the impact of headache after BoNT-A (measured by HIT-6 score) [15]. It is not clear whether the improvement in headache secondary to BoNT-A occurs due to the improvement in dystonia or due to the effect of botulinum toxin on pain itself.

Therapeutic responses to botulinum toxin in the context of CD-associated headaches remain variable. Hulzenga et al. noted limited efficacy of botulinum toxin for headache in CD, with only 3 of 19 patients receiving treatment, and only two reporting symptomatic relief [9]. Conversely, Barbanti et al. reported more favorable outcomes: among 45 patients with primary CCD, 12 (26.7%) experienced headache relief following botulinum toxin injection [6]. These findings highlight both the potential therapeutic role and the challenges in recognizing subtle forms of dystonia contributing to head pain.

Chemodenervation with BoNT-A remains the most effective and preferred treatment for CD, requiring a highly individualized approach to optimize outcomes. However, achieving the best outcomes depends on the precise and tailored application of injection techniques [7]. Nevertheless, no clinical trials evaluate the specific treatment of HACCD. While BoNT-A injections are generally well-tolerated, mild-to-moderate side effects such as dysphagia, local injection pain, and muscle weakness can occur, but these are typically manageable. The therapeutic effects of

BoNT-A may be mediated through multiple mechanisms. First, BoNT-A inhibits muscle contractions and subsequent peripheral release of neurotransmitters involved in pain regulation. Additionally, there is evidence suggesting that BoNT-A can be retrogradely transported into the central nervous system, where it may modulate pain-related pathways in the spinal cord, brainstem, and cerebral cortex [16]. These mechanisms likely help prevent or reverse peripheral and central sensitization, providing a possible explanation for the efficacy of BoNT-A in treating not only dystonia-related pain but also other painful conditions [8].

46.7 Conclusion

CCD is a complex and multifaceted neurological disorder that not only presents with debilitating motor symptoms but also with significant pain, often in the form of HACCD. Understanding the interplay between motor dysfunction and pain in CCD is crucial for developing effective, comprehensive treatment strategies. While BoNT-A remains the cornerstone of treatment for both the motor and pain symptoms associated with CCD, its efficacy in managing headache-related pain highlights the importance of addressing both peripheral and central mechanisms of pain in these patients. Although BoNT-A is highly effective for many patients, the individualized nature of its application requires careful consideration of injection techniques, muscle targeting, and patient response.

References

1. Olesen. Headache Classification Committee of the International Headache Society (IHS) The International Classification of Headache Disorders, 3rd edition. Cephalalgia. 2018;38(1):1–211.
2. Albanese A, Bhatia K, Bressman SB, DeLong MR, Fahn S, Fung VSC, Hallett M, Jankovic J, Jinnah HA, Klein C, Lang AE, Mink JW, Teller JK. Phenomenology and classification of dystonia: a consensus update. Mov Disord. 2013;28(7):863–73.
3. Balint B, Mencacci NE, Valente EM, Pisani A, Rothwell J, Jankovic J, Vidailhet M, Bhatia KP. Dystonia. Nat Rev Dis Primers. 2018;4(1)
4. Bezerra ME, Rocha-Filho PA. Headache attributed to Craniocervical dystonia—a little known headache. Headache J Head Face Pain. 2017;57(2):336–43.
5. Kutvonen O, Dastidar P, Nurmikko T. Pain in spasmodic torticollis. Pain. 1997;69(3):279–86.
6. Barbanti P, Fabbrini G, Pauletti C, Defazio G, Cruccu G, Berardelli A. Headache in cranial and cervical dystonia. Neurology. 2005;64(7):1308–9.
7. Lizarraga KJ, Al-Shorafat D, Fox S. Update on current and emerging therapies for dystonia. Neurodegener Dis Manag. 2019;9(3):135–47.
8. Rosales RL, Cuffe L, Regnault B, Trosch RM. Pain in cervical dystonia: mechanisms, assessment and treatment. Expert Rev Neurother. 2021;21(10):1125–34.
9. Hulzenga MA, Beumer D, Koehler PJ. Dystonic head tremor and the coexistence of headache. Tremor Other Hyperkinet Mov. 2017;7:485.
10. LaHue SC, Albers K, Goldman S, Lo RY, Gu Z, Leimpeter A, Fross R, Comyns K, Marras C, De Kleijn A, Smit R, Katz M, Ozelius LJ, Bressman S, Saunders-Pullman R, Comella C,

Klingman J, Nelson LM, Van Den Eeden SK, Tanner CM. Cervical dystonia incidence and diagnostic delay in a multiethnic population. Mov Disord. 2020;35(3):450–6.

11. Defazio G, Belvisi D, Comella C, Hallett M, Jinnah HA, Cimino P, Latorre A, Mascia MM, Rocchi L, Gigante AF, Ercoli T, Berardelli A. Validation of a guideline to reduce variability in diagnosing cervical dystonia. J Neurol. 2023;270(5):2606–12.
12. Comella C, Bhatia K. An international survey of patients with cervical dystonia. J Neurol. 2015;262(4):837–48.
13. Boyce MJ, Canning CG, Mahant N, Morris J, Latimer J, Fung VSC. The Toronto Western Spasmodic Torticollis rating scale: reliability in neurologists and physiotherapists. Parkinsonism Relat Disord. 2012;18(5):635–7.
14. Zolin A, Broner SW, Yoo A, Guan I, Lakhani S, Trabilsy M, Klebanoff L, Vo M, Sarva H. Dystonia phenomenology and treatment response in migraine. Headache J Head Face Pain. 2023;63(2):255–63.
15. Bezerra ME, Rocha-Filho PA. Headache attributed to craniocervical dystonia: a prospective cohort study. Eur J Pain. 2020;24(8):1484–94.
16. Ondo WG, Gollomp S, Galvez-Jimenez N. A pilot study of botulinum toxin a for headache in cervical dystonia. Headache J Head Face Pain. 2005;45(8):1073–7.
17. Dowson AJ, Kilminster SG, Salt R. Clinical profile of botulinum toxin a in patients with chronic headaches and cervical dystonia: a prospective, open-label, longitudinal study conducted in a naturalistic clinical practice setting. Drugs R D. 2008;9(3):147–58.
18. Winner PK, Sadowsky CH, Martinez WC, Zuniga JA, Poulette A. Concurrent OnabotulinumtoxinA treatment of cervical dystonia and concomitant migraine. Headache J Head Face Pain. 2012;52(8):1219–25.
19. Galvez-Jimenez N, Lampuri C, Patiño-Picirrillo R, Hargreave MJ, Hanson MR. Dystonia and headaches: clinical features and response to botulinum toxin therapy. Adv Neurol. 2004;94:321–8.

Chapter 47
Headache Attributed to Heterophoria Or Heterotropia

Caio Vinicius de Meira Grava Simioni

47.1 Introduction

Headache attributed to heterophoria or heterotropia represents a unique intersection between neurology and ophthalmology. From the start, heterophoria is a latent deviation of the eyes that surfaces when binocular fusion is disrupted. Heterotropia, in turn, is the overt misalignment observable during routine examination. In both pediatric and adult populations, ocular misalignment and related refractive issues play a significant role in headache pathogenesis.

Given that a considerable proportion of patients (especially children) with headaches are found to have ocular findings that might be causally related, clinicians must approach headache evaluation with an interdisciplinary mindset.

In this context, collaboration between neurologists and ophthalmologists is paramount. Timely identification and management of subtle ocular aberrations can be key to effective headache treatment.

47.2 Pathophysiology

Headaches in patients with heterophoria or heterotropia are associated with distinct neural and muscular processes related to binocular vision dysfunction [1]. Several studies report that altered neural control of vergence plays a role. For example, differences in the fast and slow fusional disparity systems, with associated activity changes in the secondary visual cortex, right cuneus, and oculomotor vermis, have

C. V. de Meira Grava Simioni (✉)
University of São Paulo, Faculdade de Medicina, Hospital das Clínicas, Departamento de Neurologia, São Paulo, SP, Brazil
e-mail: caiosimioni@gmail.com

D. Uludüz et al. (eds.), *Rare Causes of Headache Disorders*, Headache,
https://doi.org/10.1007/978-3-032-10242-3_47

been observed in patients with convergence insufficiency [2]. In migraine cases, activation of the trigeminovascular system and lateral inhibition in the visual cortex are noted during episodes of binocular dysfunction. At the same time, interruptions in sensory-motor feedback compromise the continuous calibration of vergence [3].

Muscular mechanisms are also implicated. Multiple reports describe how disruptions in the coordination between accommodation and convergence increase the effort required by extraocular muscles. In one study, associations between exophoria, convergence insufficiency, and inadequate positive fusional vergence at near fixation were identified in 150 headache patients [1]. Other observations reveal that in cases of vertical heterophoria, competition between a faulty vestibular reflex and a corrective fusional reflex leads to muscle overuse and fatigue [4]. These findings collectively suggest that both neural pathway alterations and compensatory muscular strain contribute to the pathogenesis of headaches in these patients.

Studies examined binocular anomalies and headaches in populations ranging from children to adults. In a sample with a mean age of 25 years, near-fixation assessments revealed 82% exophoria, 7.34% esophoria, and 10.7% orthophoria; this study also noted a statistically significant association between headache and female gender ($p < 0.0001$) [5]. In a young adult group (ages 20–30), exophoria correlated with headache, with frontal and hemicranial pain reported by 44 and 34% of patients, respectively [6]. A pediatric study (mean age 10 years) documented a 4.4% prevalence of strabismus, with no specific data on heterophoria [7]. Another study covering ages 5–36 years found that 26.2% of headache patients had convergence insufficiency, with 78.7% of these reporting frontal headaches [8]. In studies reporting gender, females constituted 60–79% of participants, with one study finding a ratio of 1.85:1 compared to males [5]. Heterotropia data were limited to the single pediatric study, and no study provided incidence rates [7]. While reports in adult and mixed-age populations consistently show high prevalences of heterophoria (notably exophoria) and associated headache symptoms, pediatric-specific data on heterophoria remain sparse, limiting definitive age-based comparisons [5].

47.3 Case Presentation

Sara, a 14-year-old female, presents to the neurologic clinic with complaints of frequent headaches, particularly when exposed to smartphone or computer screens. She reports that these headaches have been occurring for the past 6 months and have gradually increased in frequency and intensity.

She describes her headaches as dull, aching pain localized in her forehead and around her eyes. The headaches typically begin after about an hour of screen time and worsen with continued use. She denies any throbbing sensation, nausea, vomiting, photophobia, or phonophobia. She reports occasional blurred vision, especially when switching her gaze between the screen and distant objects. She also notes that her eyes feel tired and strained after prolonged use of screens. Sara has no significant past medical history and no known allergies. She does not have a personal or family history of migraine or other headache disorders. The patient occasionally takes over-the-counter ibuprofen for headache relief, which provides only temporary relief. Her mother has a history of refractive errors but no significant headache disorders. She is a healthy-appearing adolescent female. Her vital signs are within normal limits. Her neurological examination is normal, with no cranial nerve deficits, motor or sensory abnormalities, or reflex asymmetry. The patient's visual acuity was 20/25 in both eyes without correction. Subjective refraction revealed a mild hyperopic refractive error bilaterally. Extraocular movements were full and smooth, indicating normal ocular motility. The cover test demonstrated exophoria at near fixation, which became more pronounced with prolonged near work. Slit-lamp examination of the anterior segment was normal. Fundoscopic evaluation showed healthy optic nerves and retinal vessels, with no abnormalities noted.

Sara is prescribed a course of vision therapy to improve her fusional reserves and reduce the strain on her extraocular muscles. The therapy includes exercises to strengthen convergence and improve binocular coordination. She is advised to take frequent breaks during screen use, adjust her screen distance and lighting, and ensure proper posture.

Ultimately, Sara is prescribed glasses with a mild hyperopic correction and a small amount of prism to help align her eyes at nearby distances.

After 6 weeks of vision therapy, ergonomic adjustments, and wearing her prescribed glasses, Sara reports a significant reduction in the frequency and intensity of her headaches. She also notes improved visual comfort and less eye strain during screen use.

47.4 Case Discussion

Based on Sara's history and examination findings, she is diagnosed with a headache attributed to heterophoria, specifically exophoria, exacerbated by prolonged screen use. Sara's case illustrates the typical presentation of headaches associated with ocular misalignment. Her symptoms of frontal headache, blurred vision, and eye strain, which are exacerbated by screen time, are consistent with the strain on the extraocular muscles when compensating for exophoria. The absence of migraine features and a normal neurological examination further supports the diagnosis of headache attributed to heterophoria.

47.5 Clinical Presentations

Three pediatric studies ($n = 2904$) provided limited information on headache symptoms in patients with strabismus. No study reported headache frequency, intensity, or duration by specific strabismus subtype [7, 9, 10]. One study noted that 57.8% of a high-risk group experienced headaches, yet no quantitative measures of pain intensity were provided [10]. Headache duration was described only qualitatively, with one report linking shorter episodes and morning pain to ocular findings such as optic nerve elevation [7].

Siqueira et al. proposed a scale that can predict the likelihood of headache in pediatric patients with ophthalmic disorders, a tool called "HAMS Score". According to the HAMS score, strabismus is more likely to have headache (5.21), followed by hyperopia (3.10), myopia (2.67), and, finally, astigmatism (1.86) [10].

47.6 Diagnostic Algorithm

Step 1: Clinical Suspicion

- Identify Key Symptoms:
  - Headache related to visual effort
  - Aggravated by sustained visual tasks (i.e., prolonged exposure to screens).

Step 2: Initial Diagnostic Workup

- Refer the patient to an ophthalmologic examination
- Rule out other secondary headache disorders, based on "red flags" symptoms [11]; if necessary, order neuroimaging tests (i.e., magnetic resonance imaging [MRI] or computed tomography [CT] scan).

Step 3: Apply Third Edition of the International Classification of Headache Disorders (ICHD-3) Diagnostic Criteria [12]

A. Headache fulfilling criterion C
B. Heterophoria or heterotropia has been identified, with at least one of the following symptoms:
   1. Blurred vision
   2. Diplopia
   3. Difficulty switching from near to far focus and/or vice versa
C. Evidence of causation demonstrated by at least two of the following:
   1. Headache has developed in temporal relation to the onset of heterophoria and/or heterotropia, or led to its discovery
   2. Headache has significantly improved after correction of the heterophoria and/or heterotropia
   3. Headache is aggravated by sustained visual tasks
   4. Headache is alleviated by closing one eye and/or discontinuation of the visual task
D. Not better accounted for by another ICHD-3 diagnosis.

47.7 Differential Diagnosis

As mentioned earlier, the headache attributed to heterophoria and heterotropia should be distinguished from other secondary headaches, especially other ocular conditions that may cause headaches, such as glaucoma or uveitis.

It is worth noting that primary headaches, such as migraine and tension-type headache, have a high prevalence and can coexist with headaches attributed to heterophoria and heterotropia, which warrants a distinct approach and treatment.

Headache characteristics	Detailed description of headache frequency, duration, intensity, location, and associated symptoms.
Visual symptoms	Specific inquiries about blurred vision, double vision, eye strain, and difficulties with near or distance vision.
Ocular history	Prior diagnoses of refractive errors, strabismus, or other ocular conditions.
Triggers	Identification of factors that exacerbate headaches, such as prolonged reading, computer use, or specific visual tasks.
Impact on daily life	Assessment of how headaches and visual symptoms affect the patient's ability to perform daily activities, including work, school, and leisure.

47.8 Treatment

This case highlights the importance of considering ocular causes in the evaluation of pediatric headaches, particularly in the context of increased screen time. Sara's diagnosis of headache attributed to exophoria, a type of heterophoria, was made based on her history, symptoms, and ophthalmological examination findings. The successful management of her headaches with vision therapy, ergonomic adjustments, and corrective lenses underscores the effectiveness of addressing the underlying ocular misalignment. This vignette also emphasizes the importance of a multidisciplinary approach, involving collaboration between neurologists and ophthalmologists, to optimize patient outcomes.

In one study of 111 adults with vertical heterophoria, treatment with micro-prism lenses reduced headache disability. This study reported a decrease in the mean Headache Disability Inventory score from 37.55 to 22.13 (effect size $d = 0.54$) and similar reductions in dizziness and situational anxiety scores [13]. Two other studies—in adults with convergence insufficiency—evaluated office-based vision therapy (versus placebo or home-based pencil pushups) and a home-based computer orthoptic program. Although these studies demonstrated significant improvements in near point of convergence and positive fusional vergence, they did not report outcomes for headache frequency or intensity [14, 15].

Thus, among adults with heterophoria or heterotropia, only micro-prism lenses have documented benefits for reducing headache-related disability based on the available findings [13].

47.9 Conclusion

Headache attributed to heterophoria or heterotropia represents a complex clinical entity that requires a comprehensive and multidisciplinary approach. By integrating clinical history, physical examination findings, ophthalmological examination results, and diagnostic tools such as the HAMS Score, clinicians can effectively identify and manage these cases, leading to improved patient outcomes.

References

1. Saif Hassan Al-Rasheed. Clinical characteristics of patients presenting with headache at binocular vision clinic: a hospital based study. Pak J Ophthalmol. 2020:36(3):247–252. https://doi.org/10.36351/pjo.v36i3.1046.
2. Alvarez TL, Scheiman M, Morales C, Gohel S, Sangoi A, Santos EM, Yaramothu C, d'Antonio-Bertagnolli JV, Li X, Biswal BB. Underlying neurological mechanisms associated with symptomatic convergence insufficiency. Sci Rep. 2021;11(1):6545. https://doi.org/10.1038/s41598-021-86171-9. PMID: 33753864; PMCID: PMC7985149.
3. Sara L, Ruzda K, Shabeebz N, Meghana KH. Binocular vision function and migraine: a review. Int J Multidiscipl Res (IJFMR). 2022;4(6).
4. Rosner MS, Feinberg DL, Doble JE, Rosner AJ. Treatment of vertical heterophoria ameliorates persistent post-concussive symptoms: A retrospective analysis utilizing a multi-faceted assessment battery. Brain Inj. 2016;30(3):311–7. https://doi.org/10.3109/02699052.2015.1113564. Epub 2016 Feb 1. PMID: 26829465.
5. Alrasheed SH, Osman TM, Aljohani S, Alshammeri S. Clinical features of sudanese patients presenting with binocular vision anomalies: a hospital-based study. J Med Life. 2023;16(8):1251–57. https://doi.org/10.25122/jml-2023-0132. PMID: 38024832; PMCID: PMC10652681.
6. Kumar DG, Kumar DS. Evaluation of the relationship between binocular anomaly and headache: prospective cross-sectional study. Eur J Mol Clin Med (EJMCM). 2021;07(10).
7. Lin LY, Pan W, Ying GS, Binenbaum G. Ocular findings in children with headache. Ophthalmic epidemiology. 2022;30(4):392–99. https://doi.org/10.1080/09286586.2022.2125019.
8. Priya SV, Priya TV, Amudha P, Lalithambigai C. The relationship between headache and convergence insufficiency. Panacea J Med Sci. 2021;11(1):147–150.
9. Mo Y, Zhang W, Tang X, Zhang R, Wang Y, Zheng L. Evaluation of postoperative discomfort after strabismus surgery under general anesthesia in children: a prospective observational study. J Pain Res. 2024;17:2717–2726. https://doi.org/10.2147/JPR.S468977. PMID: 39188912; PMCID: PMC11346475.
10. Siqueira P de TVV, Andrade-Valença LPA de, Andrade JR, Valença MM. Pediatric patients at a high risk of headache of ocular origin: the HAMS Score (Hyperopia, Astigmatism, Myopia, and Strabismus). Headache Med [Internet]. 2021 Oct. 19 [cited 2025 Apr. 29];12(2):134-40. Available from: https://headachemedicine.com.br/index.php/hm/article/view/443.
11. Do TP, Remmers A, Schytz HW, Schankin C, Nelson SE, Obermann M, Hansen JM, Sinclair AJ, Gantenbein AR, Schoonman GG. Red and orange flags for secondary headaches in clinical practice: SNNOOP10 list. Neurology. 2019;92(3):134–144. https://doi.org/10.1212/WNL.0000000000006697. Epub 2018 Dec 26. PMID: 30587518; PMCID: PMC6340385.
12. Headache Classification Committee of the International Headache Society (IHS) the international classification of headache disorders, 3rd edition. Cephalalgia 2018;38(1):1–211 https://doi.org/10.1177/0333102417738202.

13. Rosner MS, Feinberg DL, Rosner AJ. Vertical Heterophoria Treatment Ameliorates Headache, Dizziness and Anxiety. Optometry & Visual Performance 2020;8(1):24–34.
14. Scheiman M, Mitchell GL, Cotter S, Kulp MT, Cooper J, Rouse M, Borsting E, London R, Wensveen J. A randomized clinical trial of vision therapy/orthoptics versus pencil pushups for the treatment of convergence insufficiency in young adults. Optom Vis Sci. 2005;82(7):583–95. https://doi.org/10.1097/01.opx.0000171331.36871.2f. PMID: 16044063.
15. Serna A, Rogers DL, McGregor ML, Golden RP, Bremer DL, Rogers GL. Treatment of symptomatic convergence insufficiency with a home-based computer orthoptic exercise program. J AAPOS. 2011;15(2):140–3. https://doi.org/10.1016/j.jaapos.2010.11.023. Epub 2011 Mar 31. PMID: 21458340.

Chapter 48
Meningotheliomatous Meningioma

Dilcan Kotan, Esen Çiçekli, and Derya Kara Genç

48.1 Introduction

Meningiomas are among the most common types of intracranial tumors, with an annual incidence of approximately 8 cases per 100,000. Although more than half of the cases have a benign course, meningiomas may become symptomatic due to mass effect on the adjacent parenchyma or peritumoral edema [1]. Olfactory groove meningiomas (OGM) account for 8–13% of all intracranial meningiomas. These space-occupying lesions located in the anterior cranial fossa often arise from arachnoid cells embedded in the ethmoid lamina cribrosa and midline dural covers of the frontosphenoidal suture. Rarely, it may also arise from meningeal precursor cells derived from mesoderm and neuronal crest [2]. It is more common in women than men and its frequency increases in the sixth decade [3].

Due to its benign and slow-progressing nature, OGMs, which do not cause symptoms until they reach large sizes, are diagnosed quite late. In OGMs, there are findings such as personality changes, anosmia, visual impairment, seizures, intracranial hypertension because of pressure on the frontal lobe, optic nerve, and optic chiasm, and the most common symptom is headache [2, 4]. The most important treatment approach in OGM is surgical resection, and radiotherapy (RT) can be performed in selected cases. RT is not as successful as surgery in relieving tumor-related neurological symptoms. For patients whose tumors cannot be

D. Kotan (✉)
Sakarya University, School of Medicine, Department of Neurology, Sakarya, Turkey

E. Çiçekli
Akyazı State Hospital, Neurology Department, Sakarya, Turkey

D. K. Genç
Sakarya University Education and Research Hospital, Neurology Department, Sakarya, Turkey

D. Uludüz et al. (eds.), *Rare Causes of Headache Disorders*, Headache,
https://doi.org/10.1007/978-3-032-10242-3_48

accessed surgically or are at risk for surgery, RT is frequently used to control local tumor growth [5].

In this section, a case of olfactory meningioma that presented with complaints of headache and visual impairment is described. It aims to increase the curiosity of clinicians and researchers in this subject by providing detailed clinical information about OGMs, which are not frequently considered among the causes of headache in clinical practice and whose diagnosis can be overlooked until they reach giant proportions.

48.2 Pathophysiology

Meningothelial meningiomas originate from arachnoidal cap (meningothelial) cells, which form part of the meninges and regulate cerebrospinal fluid absorption. The most frequent genetic facilitator involves loss-of-function mutations in the NF2 gene on chromosome 22q, leading to inactivation of its protein product, Merlin, a tumor suppressor that normally restrains multiple proliferative pathways. Neurofibromin 2 (NF2) inactivation results in disrupted cytoskeleton remodeling and cell–cell junction integrity, permitting unchecked cell growth and chromosomal instability [6]. Additional genomic alterations (e.g. TNF Receptor Associated Factor 7 (TRAF7), AKT Serine/Threonine Kinase 1 (AKT1), and Smoothened Frizzled Class Receptor (SMO)) may also play a role, though they are often mutually exclusive to NF2 mutations [7]. Histologically, meningothelial features include syncytial cell sheets with indistinct borders, whorled patterns, and occasional psammoma bodies—calcified concentric structures reflecting apoptotic debris. These tumors exhibit low mitotic activity and proliferation index (Ki-67), in line with their benign WHO Grade I classification and favorable prognosis [6].

48.3 Case Presentation

A 39-year-old female patient applied to the neurology clinic with a complaint of headache that started a few weeks ago, lasted 5–10 minutes, and recurred from time to time during the day. The headache was responsive to analgesics, was not accompanied by nausea and vomiting, had no photophobia or phonophobia, and was felt more intensely around the right eye. For the last week, blurry vision in both eyes was added to his headache. The patient, who was interned for further examination, had a history of allergic asthma and a family history of migraine in his mother. There was no regular medication use other than occasional inhaler asthma treatment.

In her neurological examination, her pupils were isochoric, and his light reflex was positive bilaterally. Bilateral eye movements were free in all directions. In fundus evaluation, optic disc borders were slightly blurred on the right and normal on the left. On vision examination, the right eye was 2/10 and the left eye was 6/10. On visual field examination, there was near-total vision loss in all quadrants in the right eye (Fig. 48.1a). There was a visual field defect in the left eye, more

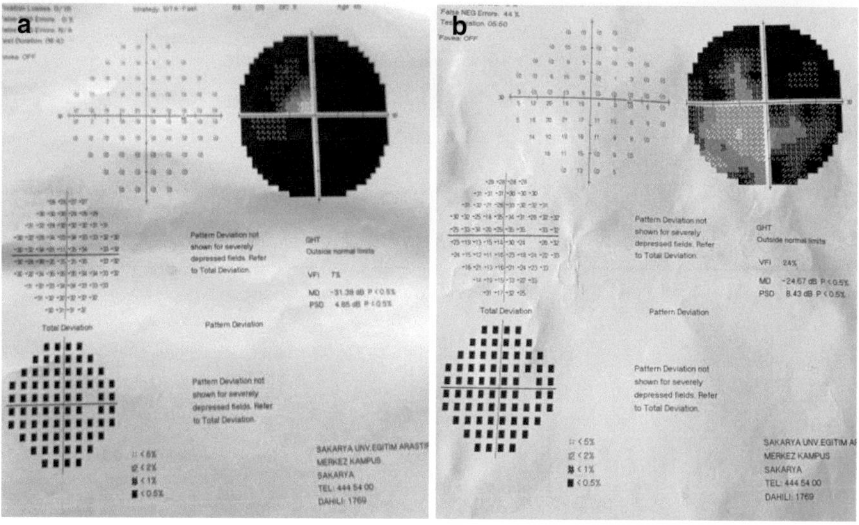

Fig. 48.1 (**a**) Right eye visual field test (**b**) Left eye visual field test

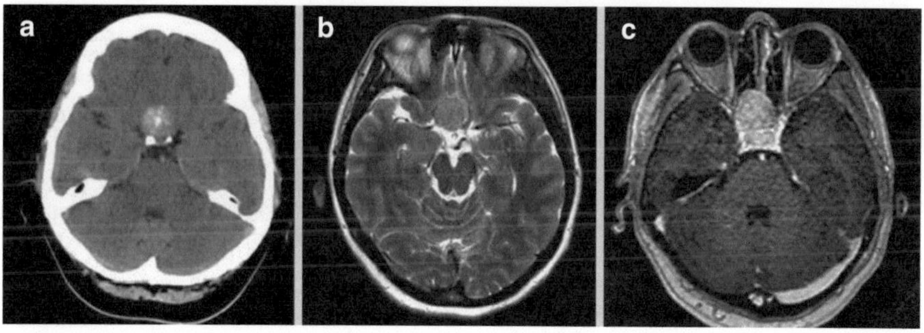

Fig. 48.2 From left to right (**a**) Cranial CT (**b**) T2-weighted MRI (**c**) Contrast-enhanced T1-weighted MRI images of the patient

prominent in the upper outer quadrants (Fig. 48.1b). There was no facial asymmetry. The patient's muscle strength examination was bilaterally normal, and his plantar skin reflex was bilateral flexor. Vital signs were stable, and laboratory parameters were normal.

Cranial computed tomography (CT) showed a hyperdense appearance with well-circumscribed 22 mm diameter and minimal calcification in the sellar-suprasellar region (Fig. 48.2a). Contrast-enhanced cranial magnetic resonance imaging (MRI) showed a well-circumscribed lesion in the sellar region, consistent with CT, isointense and sometimes minimally hyperintense in T2 sections, hypointense in T1 series, and with pathological contrast enhancement (Figs. 48.2b, c). When the neurological examination and current neuroimaging findings were evaluated together, it was evaluated as olfactory meningioma, which was thought to originate from the

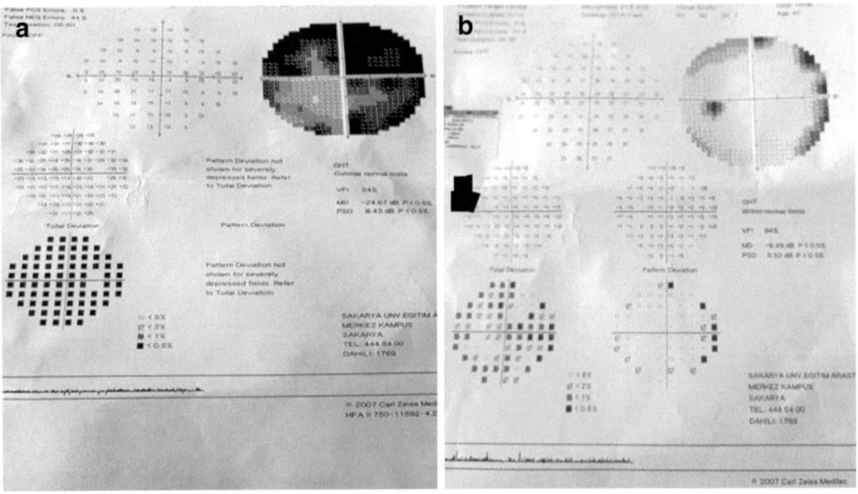

Fig. 48.3 From left to right (**a**) Postoperative right eye visual field test (**b**) Postoperative left eye visual field test

olfactory groove, and it was referred for neurosurgical intervention. The patient's tumor tissue was resected under elective conditions by the neurosurgery department. For this purpose, the mass was removed through a right frontal incision and sent for pathological examination. The pathology result was reported as meningotheliomatous meningioma, Grade 1.

At the first postoperative follow-up examination, visual acuity was recorded as 4/10 on the right and full on the left. In the visual field examination, although the defect continued in every quadrant of the visual field in the right eye, there was an improvement compared to the pre-operative period (Fig. 48.3a). Visual field examination was normal in the left eye (Fig. 48.3b). The patient's follow-up continues in the neurosurgery and ophthalmology outpatient clinics.

48.4 Case Discussion

OGMs most commonly present with symptoms of headache, anosmia, or personality changes. In our case, clinical findings first presented with headache, followed by visual impairment a few weeks later. The fact that the headache was located in the same region and unilateral. The accompanying symptom of visual impairment suggested an underlying organic cause, and the diagnosis was made after the requested cranial imaging. Imaging methods are used in the diagnosis of OGMs. Although diagnosis can be made with cranial CT or MRI, in cases where there is a choice, MRI provides better image quality and localization chance [8].

Due to its anatomical location, OGM may cause long-term psychiatric symptoms before the onset of significant neurological deficits. Because of these mild symptoms, olfactory groove meningiomas can grow insidiously and emerge as one of the largest intracranial tumors. Tumor size was categorized by neuroimaging assessment. As classification, they are small (0–2 cm in diameter), medium (2–4 cm in diameter), large (4–6 cm in diameter), and giant (>6 cm in diameter). Visual symptoms usually occur after an olfactory groove meningioma has reached a significant size but may also depend on the anatomical site of origin. Because olfactory groove meningiomas extend posteriorly, this extension may cause compression of one or both optic nerves or the chiasm. It may occur earlier in smaller tumors arising from the posterior half of the cribriform plate. Compression injury to the optic nerves can cause optic nerve head edema and eventually progress to optic atrophy [9]. The mechanism of damage in OGM is caused by the size of the tumor and creates a downward pressure on the nerve and chiasm from above, whereas in suprasellar meningioma, the chiasm rises, thus the cross fibers are stretched and optic atrophy and bitemporal hemianopsia occur. In our current case, which involved a medium-sized olfactory groove meningioma measuring 2.2 cm in axial diameter, there were complaints of headaches and visual findings that were attributed to chiasm involvement due to the suprasellar location.

OGMs must be distinguished from other midline meningiomas of the anterior cranial fossa, namely planum sphenoidale meningiomas, whose dural attachments lie behind the frontosphenoidal suture, and tuberculum sellae meningiomas, which arise from the dura anterior to the chiasmatic sulcus. This distinction is not only an anatomical application but also has clinical importance. Planum sphenoidale and tuberculum sellae meningiomas are generally diagnosed earlier in their clinical course due to visual impairment. It is smaller in size and easier to approach during surgery. Due to their large size, OGMs can sometimes be long and difficult to approach and require meticulous surgery to minimize tissue damage. Tumor size and location are also important in determining the surgical approach to be chosen on a patient-by-patient basis [10]. In addition to the transcranial approach, the endoscopic endonasal approach is also used in appropriate cases [11]. However, the chance of success after a good resection is quite high and complications can be easily controlled. In our case, resection was performed through a right frontal incision, which is the point where the tumor can be most easily reached. High patient age and large tumor size are considered poor prognostic factors [12]. Our patient's age was considered early according to the literature. The fact that the tumor size was detected when it was medium sized also suggests that our case will have a good prognosis.

Although most meningiomas are Grade 1 and benign tumors, up to 15% may be atypical and 2% may be anaplastic [13]. As in most cases, the pathology in our patient was Grade 1. This result suggests that the patient will have a good prognosis.

48.5 Clinical Characteristics

Headache is the most common presenting symptom in patients with meningothelial meningiomas. It is typically attributed to a combination of mass effect, irritation of pain-sensitive dural structures, and increased intracranial pressure (ICP). The headache usually develops insidiously over weeks or months and is often described as a dull, constant, pressure-like pain rather than a sharp or pulsating sensation. It frequently worsens in the early morning hours, likely due to overnight CO_2 retention and the supine position increasing cerebral blood flow and ICP. In some cases, the headache may be exacerbated by Valsalva maneuvers such as coughing or straining, further supporting the role of raised ICP. These headaches are often poorly responsive to standard analgesics and may be accompanied by additional signs such as nausea, vomiting, or transient visual disturbances like blurred vision or papilledema. Significantly, the location of the headache does not consistently correlate with the anatomical site of the tumor, reflecting the diffuse nature of pressure-related symptoms rather than localized cortical involvement [14, 15].

48.6 Diagnosis of Meningothelial Meningiomas

The diagnosis of meningothelial meningiomas involves a combination of clinical evaluation, neuroimaging, and histopathological confirmation. Clinically, patients may present with non-specific symptoms such as headache, seizures, or focal neurological deficits, depending on the tumor's location and mass effect. Radiologically, contrast-enhanced MRI is the modality of choice, typically revealing a well-circumscribed, extra-axial mass that shows homogeneous enhancement and is often associated with a dural tail sign. These tumors are usually isointense to gray matter on T1- and T2-weighted images. Definitive diagnosis is made via histopathological examination following surgical resection. Meningothelial meningiomas are characterized by lobules or whorls of polygonal cells with indistinct cell borders, eosinophilic cytoplasm, and round to oval nuclei. Psammoma bodies may also be present. Immunohistochemistry is supportive, with tumors typically positive for epithelial membrane antigen (EMA) and vimentin [8, 15, 16].

48.7 Treatment

The primary treatment of meningothelial meningiomas is surgical resection, aiming for complete removal of the tumor, including involved dura and any invaded bone. For WHO Grade I meningiomas, such as the meningothelial subtype, gross total resection is often curative, and adjuvant therapy is usually not required. However, in cases of subtotal resection, tumor recurrence, or when surgery is contraindicated due to location or patient factors, radiotherapy—particularly stereotactic radiosurgery or fractionated radiotherapy—may be employed as an adjunct or primary treatment. Observation (watchful waiting) is also an option in asymptomatic or incidental cases, especially when the tumor is small and not causing mass effect. Long-term follow-up with periodic imaging is essential, as even benign meningiomas may recur, particularly if resection is incomplete [13, 15, 17].

48.8 Conclusion

The importance of this case report is that when evaluating intracranial areas in patients presenting with headache, evaluation of the extracranial regions should not be overlooked. However, it is essential to draw attention to the diagnostic value of imaging, as well as a good anamnesis and examination, in the differential diagnosis of visual findings accompanying headache, which may occur in insidious tumors such as OGM. It is aimed to raise awareness about OGMs, as they can be successfully treated and prevented from becoming life-threatening by a surgical procedure performed before the tumor reaches giant sizes. The importance of prioritizing appropriate imaging in terms of early detection of pathologies in headache and accompanying vision problems in the young female population is emphasized.

References

1. Maggio I, Franceschi E, Tosoni A, Nunno VD, Gatto L, Lodi R, Brandes AA. Meningioma: not always a benign tumor. A review of advances in the treatment of meningiomas. CNS Oncol. 2021;10(2):CNS72. https://doi.org/10.2217/cns-2021-0003. Epub 2021 May 21. PMID: 34015955; PMCID: PMC8162186.
2. Ikhuoriah T, Oboh D, Abramowitz C, Musheyev Y, Cohen R. Olfactory groove meningioma: a case report with typical clinical and radiologic features in a 74-year-old Nigerian male. Radiol Case Rep. 2022;17(12):4492 7. https://doi.org/10.1016/j.radcr.2022.08.077. PMID: 36189154; PMCID: PMC9519506.
3. Ciurea AV, Iencean SM, Rizea RE, Brehar FM. Olfactory groove meningiomas: a retrospective study on 59 surgical cases. Neurosurg Rev. 2012;35(2):195–202. https://doi.org/10.1007/s10143-011-0353-2; discussion 202. Epub 2011 Sep 30.
4. Niklassen AS, Jørgensen RL, Fjaeldstad AW. Olfactory groove meningioma with a 10-year history of smell loss and olfactory recovery after surgery. BMJ Case Rep. 2021;14(8):e244145. https://doi.org/10.1136/bcr-2021-244145. PMID: 34433535; PMCID: PMC8388279.
5. Buerki RA, Horbinski CM, Kruser T, Horowitz PM, James CD, Lukas RV. An overview of meningiomas. Future Oncol. 2018;14(21):2161–77. https://doi.org/10.2217/fon-2018-0006. Epub 2018 Aug 7. PMID: 30084265; PMCID: PMC6123887.
6. Huntoon K, Toland AMS, Dahiya S. Meningioma: a review of clinicopathological and molecular aspects. Front Oncol. 2020;10:579599. https://doi.org/10.3389/fonc.2020.579599.
7. Dwianingsih EK, Krisnugraha YP, Bawono RG, Malueka RG. Molecular biomarkers in meningioma (review). Biomed Rep. 2025;22:56.

8. Timothy JH, Derek EK, Ivan M. The role of imaging in the follow up of meningiomas. J Neurol Neurosurg Psychiatry. 1995;59:545–7. https://doi.org/10.1136/jnnp.59.5.545.
9. Jung JJ, Warren FA, Kahanowicz R. Bilateral visual loss due to a giant olfactory meningioma. Clin Ophthalmol. 2012;6:339–42. https://doi.org/10.2147/OPTH.S30283.
10. Candy NG, Hinder D, Jukes AK, Wormald PJ, Psaltis AJ. Olfaction preservation in olfactory groove meningiomas: a systematic review. Neurosurg Rev. 2023;46(1):186. https://doi.org/10.1007/s10143-023-02096-z. PMID: 37500988; PMCID: PMC10374754.
11. Liu JK, Silva NA, Sevak IA, Eloy JA. Transbasal versus endoscopic endonasal versus combined approaches for olfactory groove meningiomas: importance of approach selection. Neurosurg Focus. 2018;44(4):E8. https://doi.org/10.3171/2018.1.FOCUS17722.
12. Pallini R, Fernandez E, Lauretti L, Doglietto F, D'Alessandris QG, Montano N, Capo G, Meglio M, Maira G. Olfactory groove meningioma: report of 99 cases surgically treated at the Catholic University School of Medicine, Rome. World Neurosurg. 2015;83(2):219–31.e1–3. https://doi.org/10.1016/j.wneu.2014.11.001. Epub 2014 Nov 8.
13. Apra C, Peyre M, Kalamarides M. Current treatment options for meningioma. Expert Rev Neurother. 2018;18(3):241–9. https://doi.org/10.1080/14737175.2018.1429920. Epub 2018 Jan 22.
14. Kilic T, Hanimoglu H, Borcek AO, Cengiz G, Soylemezoglu F, Pamir MN. Clinical presentation of intracranial meningiomas in the elderly. Acta Neurochir. 2008;150(6):589–95. https://doi.org/10.1007/s00701-007-1476-4.
15. Louis DN, Perry A, Wesseling P, Brat DJ, Cree IA, Figarella-Branger D, Hawkins C, Ng HK, Pfister SM, Reifenberger G. WHO classification of tumours of the central nervous system. 5th ed. Lyon: International Agency for Research on Cancer; 2021.
16. Wippold FJ II, Lubner M, Perrin RJ, Lämmle M, Perry A. Neuropathology for the neuroradiologist: meningioma. AJNR Am J Neuroradiol. 2006;27(3):553–64.
17. Goldbrunner R, Minniti G, Preusser M, Jenkinson MD, Sallabanda K, Houdart E, von Deimling A, Stavrinou P, Lefranc F, Lund-Johansen M, Weber DC, Reijneveld JC, Henriksson R, Soffietti R, Weller M. EANO guidelines for the diagnosis and treatment of meningiomas. Lancet Oncol. 2016;17(9):e383–91.

Chapter 49
Headache or Facial Pain Attributed to Inflammation of the Stylohyoid Ligament

Elder Sarmento

49.1 Introduction

Headache and facial pain are common complaints in neurological practice, with a wide range of etiologies. Among the less frequent causes, inflammation of the stylohyoid ligament emerges as a distinct clinical entity, although it is often underdiagnosed. Previously known as Eagle syndrome, this condition is now classified in the International Classification of Headache Disorders, third edition (ICHD-3) as 11.8 Headache or facial pain attributed to inflammation of the stylohyoid ligament [1]. This chapter aims to provide an in-depth analysis of this condition, exploring its anatomical bases, pathophysiological mechanisms, clinical manifestations, diagnostic approaches, and treatment options. In doing so, we aim to raise awareness of this rare cause of craniofacial pain and equip clinicians with the necessary tools for accurate recognition and management.

E. Sarmento (✉)
Sociedade Brasileira de Cefaleia, Barra Mansa, Brazil

UniFOA, Centro Universitário Fundação Oswaldo Aranha, Volta Redonda, Brasil

D. Uludüz et al. (eds.), *Rare Causes of Headache Disorders*, Headache, https://doi.org/10.1007/978-3-032-10242-3_49

49.2 Pathophysiology

The stylohyoid ligament is a fibrous structure that extends from the styloid process of the temporal bone to the lesser horn of the hyoid bone. Its primary function is to suspend and stabilize the hyoid bone, which plays a crucial role in swallowing, speech, and breathing. Inflammation of the stylohyoid ligament can result from a variety of factors, including trauma, infection, prior surgery (such as tonsillectomy), or systemic inflammatory conditions [2].

The pathophysiology of pain in inflammation of the stylohyoid ligament is multifaceted. Direct inflammation of the ligament can activate local nociceptors, leading to referred pain in the cervical, facial, or cranial region. Additionally, inflammation can cause compression or irritation of adjacent nerve structures, such as cranial nerves V, VII, IX, and X, resulting in neuropathic pain. Vascular compression may also play a role, especially in the context of Eagle syndrome, where an elongated styloid process or a calcified stylohyoid ligament can compress the internal or external carotid artery [3].

49.3 Case Presentation

A 34-year-old patient begins with incipient symptoms: difficulty in ingesting solid foods and odynophagia. Sudden intensification of symptoms includes dyspnea, homolateral cervicalgia, cervical edema with lymphadenomegaly, intense headache, leading to the first hospital admission. The evolution of the condition includes worsening of cervicalgia during neck rotation, otalgia, pain in the temporomandibular joint (TMJ), changes in dental occlusion, dizziness, and changes in facial and dental arch sensitivity on the homolateral side. Characteristic symptom includes lancinating pain in the topography of the submandibular gland and region posterior to the palatine tonsil. The patient relieved the pain by pressing the area with his finger. During an episode of intense pain, he applied excessive pressure, probably leading to a fracture of the styloid process, which significantly aggravated the clinical condition. Multiple hospitalizations occur due to the intensity of the symptoms, including difficulty swallowing, persistent cervical edema, and a foreign body sensation in the pharynx. Initial examinations (electroneuromyography, magnetic resonance imaging [MRI] of the skull and neck, cerebrospinal fluid [CSF]) do not reveal a specific cause. Cervical MRI shows degenerative changes, which were ruled out as the cause of the symptoms. Panoramic radiography suggests Eagle syndrome, revealing calcification of the right stylohyoid ligament (Fig. 49.1). Cone-beam computed tomography (CT) with three-dimensional (3D) reconstruction confirms calcification and elongation of the right stylohyoid ligament (50 mm) (Fig. 49.2). Cervical angiotomography shows contact of the styloid process with a branch of the external carotid artery. Surgery was performed to resect the right styloid process,

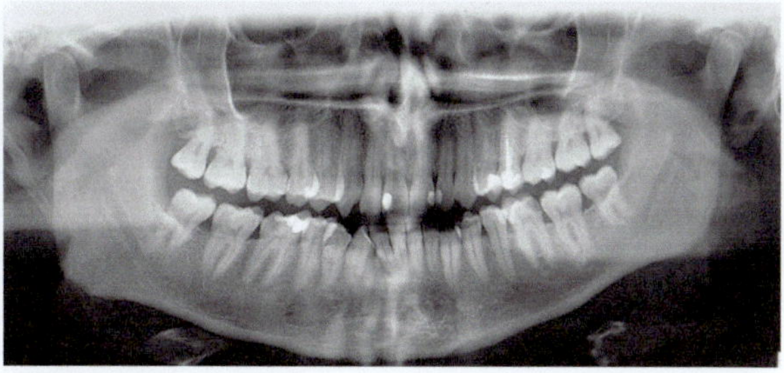

Fig. 49.1 Panoramic radiography suggests Eagle Syndrome, revealing calcification of the right stylohyoid ligament

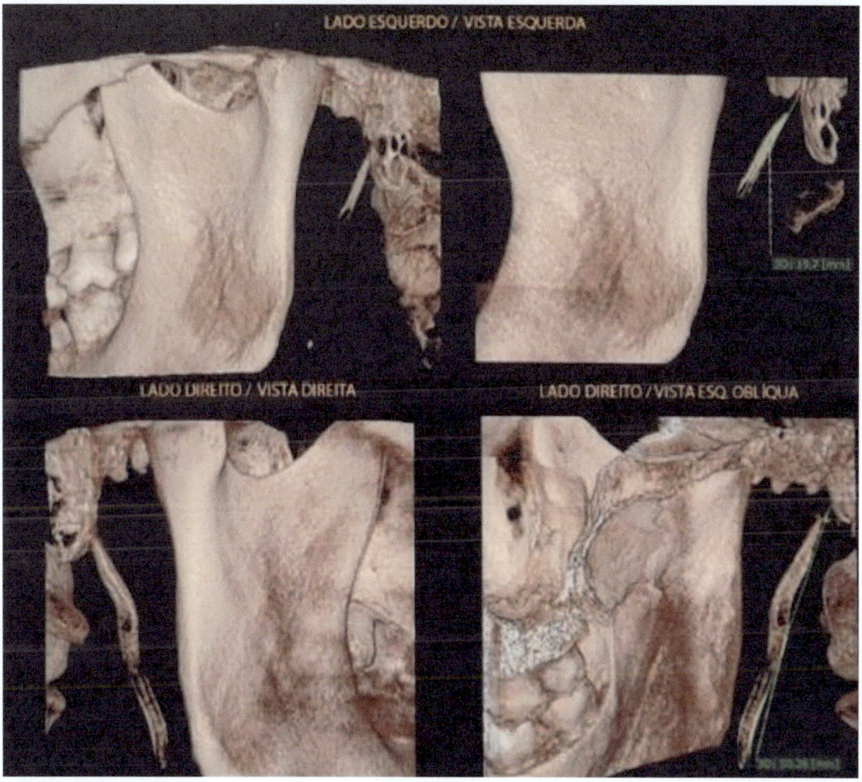

Fig. 49.2 Cone beam CT with 3D reconstruction confirms calcification and elongation of the right stylohyoid ligament (50 mm). The panels are labeled in Portuguese: Lado Esquerdo Vista Esquerda (Top Left), Lado Direito Vista Direita (Top Right), Lado Direito Vista Direita (Bottom Left), and Lado Direito Vista Esq. Obliqua (Bottom Right)

with intraoperative confirmation of the previously suspected fracture (Fig. 49.3). There was immediate resolution of the syndrome's symptoms after the procedure. The postoperative course includes peripheral facial paralysis on the right, showing significant improvement in 3 months.

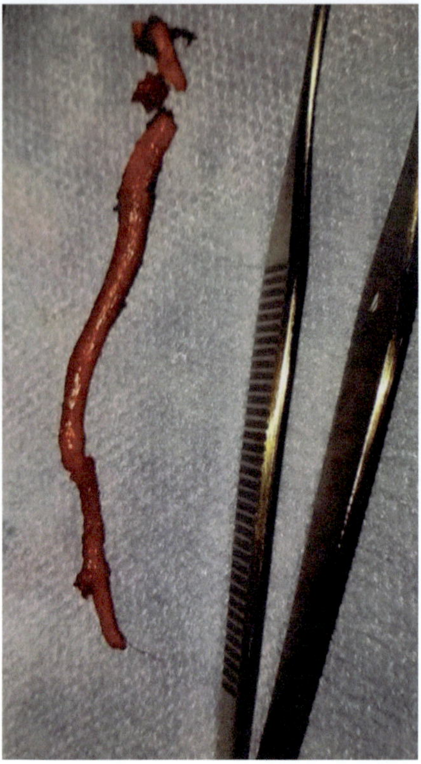

Fig. 49.3 The figure shows the styloid process after extraction and placed next to surgical forceps to aid visual comparison

49.4 Clinical Presentation

The clinical presentation of headache or facial pain attributed to inflammation of the stylohyoid ligament is variable, depending on the underlying cause, the extent of inflammation, and the adjacent structures involved. According to the ICHD-3 [1], this condition typically manifests as a unilateral headache, with pain in the neck, pharynx, and/or face.

Pain associated with inflammation of the stylohyoid ligament is typically localized to the lateral region of the neck, throat, face, ear, or skull. According to the ICHD-3 classification, while the pain is generally perceived in the oropharynx, neck, or face, some patients may report a more diffuse headache pattern. The quality of pain varies and is often described as sharp, lancinating, throbbing, burning, or dull. Movements of the head and neck, swallowing, speaking, or palpation over the stylohyoid ligament area may aggravate it. Patients commonly experience dysphagia, manifesting as difficulty in swallowing solids or liquids and a persistent sensation of a foreign body in the throat. Odynophagia, or pain during swallowing, is also frequently reported. Other associated symptoms may include tinnitus [3], vertigo, headache, facial pain, and restricted movement of the head and neck. Significantly, clinical presentations vary: while some patients may report only localized pain, others may experience a broader constellation of symptoms reflecting the extent of inflammation or mechanical irritation in the region.

49.5 Diagnosis

Diagnosing headache or facial pain attributed to inflammation of the stylohyoid ligament necessitates a high index of suspicion, particularly due to its rarity and frequent misclassification as temporomandibular joint disorders, dental pathologies, or idiopathic cervical pain. A systematic diagnostic strategy combining clinical assessment and imaging is essential for accurate identification.

A thorough clinical history should elicit the nature, location, and triggers of the pain, along with any history of trauma, infection, or head and neck surgeries. Patients typically report unilateral pain localized to the neck, submandibular region, or posterior tonsillar area, often exacerbated by head rotation or digital palpation. Associated symptoms may include dysphagia, odynophagia, otalgia, vertigo, and temporomandibular discomfort.

Physical examination should include targeted palpation along the styloid process and adjacent tissues to assess tenderness or replication of symptoms. A positive response here can be diagnostically suggestive.

The ICHD-3 diagnostic criteria for *11.8 Headache or facial pain attributed to inflammation of the stylohyoid ligament* (Headache Classification Committee of the International Headache Society, 2018) require:

A. Headache, neck, pharynx, and/or facial pain meeting criterion C.
B. Radiological evidence of a calcified or elongated stylohyoid ligament.
C. Evidence of causality by at least two of the following:

    1. Pain induced by digital palpation of the ligament.
    2. Pain exacerbated by head movement.
    3. Pain relief with local anesthetic injection or styloidectomy.
    4. Ipsilateral pain to the involved ligament.

D. Not better explained by another ICHD-3 diagnosis.

Imaging plays a critical role in confirming the diagnosis. While panoramic radiographs can reveal elongation or calcification of the styloid process, CT with 3D reconstruction offers superior anatomical detail, identifying the extent of calcification, elongation, or compression on adjacent neurovascular structures [4, 5]. MRI is valuable for assessing soft tissue inflammation and ruling out other pathologies. In select cases, cervical angiotomography may be warranted to evaluate vascular impingement. Additionally, a diagnostic anesthetic block into the stylohyoid ligament region can offer both therapeutic relief and confirm the source of pain [2, 5].

In the presented case, the patient met all ICHD-3 criteria. Imaging revealed a 50 mm elongated and calcified right stylohyoid ligament, with CT and angiotomography showing close contact with the external carotid artery. These findings, along with symptom provocation during palpation and movement, confirmed the diagnosis. Intraoperatively, a fracture of the styloid process was identified, likely caused by digital self-manipulation. Symptom resolution following styloidectomy provided strong evidence for the etiological role of the ligament pathology [3].

49.6 Treatment

The treatment of headache or facial pain attributed to inflammation of the stylohyoid ligament aims to relieve pain, reduce inflammation, and treat the underlying cause. Treatment options vary depending on the severity of symptoms and the cause of the inflammation.

The treatment of stylohyoid ligament-related pain can be approached conservatively or surgically, depending on the severity of symptoms and the patient's response to initial therapies. Conservative treatment typically begins with the use of analgesic medications, such as paracetamol, nonsteroidal anti-inflammatory drugs (NSAIDs), and, in more severe cases, opioids to manage pain. Muscle relaxants may also be prescribed to alleviate cervical muscle tension. Physical therapy plays a supportive role by incorporating stretching and strengthening exercises aimed at improving neck mobility and reducing discomfort. For temporary pain relief and diagnostic confirmation, anesthetic blocks involving the injection of local anesthetic into the stylohyoid ligament region may be utilized. If conservative measures fail to provide adequate relief or if there is significant compression of neural or vascular structures, surgical treatment in the form of a styloidectomy may be indicated. This procedure involves the removal of the elongated or calcified styloid process and can be performed using either an intraoral or extraoral surgical approach [6]. While surgery is often effective in alleviating symptoms, it carries potential risks, including bleeding, infection, nerve injury, and recurrence of pain.

49.7 Conclusion

Headache or facial pain attributed to inflammation of the stylohyoid ligament is a rare but important condition that can cause significant morbidity. Early recognition and proper management, following the diagnostic criteria of the ICHD-3 (Headache Classification Committee of the International Headache Society, 2018), are essential to improve patient outcomes. This chapter provided a case that gives a comprehensive overview of the condition and made a literature review of the topic including anatomy, pathophysiology, clinical manifestations, diagnostic approach, and treatment options. We hope that this information helps clinicians to better diagnose and treat this often-neglected cause of craniofacial pain.

References

1. Headache Classification Committee of the International Headache Society (IHS). The international classification of headache disorders, 3rd edition (ICHD-3). Cephalalgia. 2018;38(1):1–211.
2. Badhey A, Jategaonkar A, Anglin Kovacs AJ, Kadakia S, De Deyn PP, Ducic Y, Schantz S, Shin E. Eagle syndrome: a comprehensive review. Clin Neurol Neurosurg. 2017;159:34–8. https://doi.org/10.1016/j.clineuro.2017.04.021.
3. Pagano S, Ricciuti V, Mancini F, Barbieri FR, Chegai F, Marini A, Marruzzo D, Paracino R, Ricciuti RA. Eagle syndrome: an updated review. Surg Neurol Int. 2023;14:389. https://doi.org/10.25259/SNI_666_2023.
4. Murtagh RD, Caracciolo JT, Fernandez G. CT findings associated with Eagle syndrome. AJNR Am J Neuroradiol. 2001;22(7):1401–2.
5. Demirtaş N, Erdem T, Korkmaz H. Three-dimensional computed tomography in the diagnosis of Eagle's syndrome. Eur Arch Otorrinolaringol. 2008;265(10):1219–25.
6. Fusco DJ, Asteraki S, Spetzler RF. Eagle's syndrome: embryology, anatomy, and clinical management. Acta Neurochir. 2012;154(7):1119–26.

Part IX
Painful Lesions of the Cranial Nerves and Other Facial Pain

Chapter 50
Glossopharyngeal Neuralgia

Marcelo Valença

50.1 Introduction

Glossopharyngeal neuralgia (GPN) is a rare craniofacial pain syndrome characterized by paroxysmal, severe, unilateral pain in areas innervated by the glossopharyngeal nerve (cranial nerve [CN] IX) [1, 2]. The pain is typically described as lancinating, electric shock-like, and brief, often affecting the oropharynx, tonsillar fossa, posterior tongue, and sometimes radiating to the ear. It is frequently triggered by activities such as swallowing, chewing, coughing, talking, or yawning [3].

Although GPN is far less common than trigeminal neuralgia, it can cause significant disability. A particularly rare and dangerous subtype of GPN is the syncopal or vagal form, in which pain episodes are associated with autonomic symptoms, most notably bradycardia, hypotension, or even syncope. These events are thought to result from stimulation of the adjacent vagus nerve (cranial nerve X), which shares a close anatomical relationship with the glossopharyngeal nerve at the brainstem and jugular foramen. In such cases, early recognition and management are critical, as syncopal events may lead to life-threatening consequences.

The etiology of GPN includes idiopathic cases as well as secondary causes such as neurovascular compression, neoplastic lesions, demyelinating diseases, and post-surgical or post-infectious changes. Neurovascular compression at the root entry zone (REZ) of the glossopharyngeal or vagus nerves is often implicated, especially in refractory or atypical cases. It may be confirmed via high-resolution magnetic resonance imaging (MRI) with angiographic sequences.

M. Valença (✉)
Federal University of Pernambuco, Recife, Pernambuco, Brazil

Center of Excellence in the Treatment of Migraine and Other Headache Disorders, Hospital Esperança, Recife, Pernambuco, Brazil

D. Uludüz et al. (eds.), *Rare Causes of Headache Disorders*, Headache,
https://doi.org/10.1007/978-3-032-10242-3_50

This presents a case of glossopharyngeal neuralgia with associated bradycardia—representing the syncopal variant—occurring in an elderly patient, with partial response to pharmacological therapy and radiological evidence of bilateral neurovascular contact.

50.2 Pathophysiology

The glossopharyngeal and vagus nerves both emerge from the medulla and exit the skull via the jugular foramen, making them anatomically susceptible to simultaneous neurovascular compression. When compressed by arterial loops—typically posterior inferior cerebellar artery (PICA) or vertebral artery branches—these nerves may develop hyperexcitability or ephaptic transmission, resulting in pain paroxysms and, in the case of vagal stimulation, bradycardia or syncope.

The pathophysiology of glossopharyngeal neuralgia (GPN) involves paroxysmal activation of the glossopharyngeal nerve (cranial nerve IX), resulting in severe, episodic pain typically perceived in the posterior oropharynx, tonsillar region, base of the tongue, and sometimes radiating to the ear. These pain episodes are thought to arise from hyperexcitability or ephaptic transmission along the affected nerve fibers, often triggered by sensory stimuli such as swallowing, talking, coughing, or yawning [4].

A predominant underlying mechanism is neurovascular compression, particularly at the root entry zone (REZ) of the glossopharyngeal nerve, where it emerges from the medulla oblongata. The REZ is especially vulnerable to compression due to its transition from central (oligodendrocyte-myelinated) to peripheral (Schwann cell-myelinated) fibers. This histological interface is known to predispose to demyelination and aberrant synaptic activity. In many cases, the compressing vessel is a loop of the posterior inferior cerebellar artery (PICA) or another nearby artery, which exerts pulsatile mechanical pressure on the nerve, contributing to both structural irritation and functional sensitization.

In the vagal or syncopal variant of GPN, pathophysiological complexity increases due to involvement of the adjacent vagus nerve (cranial nerve X), which lies in close anatomical proximity to the glossopharyngeal nerve in the jugular foramen and medullary region. Noxious stimuli conducted through CN IX may cross-excite parasympathetic fibers of CN X, leading to cardioinhibitory reflexes such as bradycardia, hypotension, and in some cases, syncope. These autonomic manifestations are mediated via reflex arcs involving the nucleus tractus solitarius, dorsal motor nucleus of the vagus, and cardiac parasympathetic output pathways [5].

Secondary etiologies of GPN may include neoplastic compression, demyelinating disease (e.g., multiple sclerosis), inflammatory neuropathies, or iatrogenic injury following oropharyngeal or skull base procedures. However, in idiopathic or classic cases, neurovascular contact remains the most frequently identified structural abnormality—especially when detected via high-resolution MRI with angiographic sequences, which allow visualization of the nerve-vessel interface.

50.3 Case Presentation

A 78-year-old woman presented with a five-year history of paroxysmal right facial pain, described as acute, stabbing, electric shock-like, and unilateral. The pain lasted from a few seconds to up to 1 minute and occurred multiple times a day, both spontaneously and in response to specific triggers such as swallowing, speaking, or coughing. These episodes were localized to the right posterior oropharyngeal region, radiating occasionally to the ear.

Notably, during some of these episodes, the patient reported accompanying sensations of dizziness and lightheadedness. A 24-hour Holter monitor was performed and revealed episodes of significant bradycardia temporally associated with the pain paroxysms. These findings were consistent with the so-called vagal or syncopal variant of glossopharyngeal neuralgia. There were no episodes of syncope, but transient cardiovascular symptoms raised clinical concern.

Approximately 1 year after symptom onset, the patient experienced periods of spontaneous remission lasting between 6 and 12 months. During these intervals, she remained entirely asymptomatic without the need for pharmacological treatment. However, over the past 6 months, the pain recurred with the same intensity, quality, and frequency as previously reported. Treatment with carbamazepine (initiated at 200 mg/day and titrated up to 600 mg/day) provided only partial relief. The intensity and frequency of attacks decreased, but breakthrough pain continued to impact her activities. The drug was tolerated without significant side effects.

A brain MRI with angiographic sequences (angio-MRI) was performed, which demonstrated evidence of vascular contact with the lower cranial nerves bilaterally, more pronounced on the right side. The vessels involved appeared to be loops of the posterior inferior cerebellar artery (PICA), in close apposition to the glossopharyngeal-vagal complex at the root entry zone in the medulla oblongata. No mass lesions, demyelination, or inflammatory signs were detected. These findings supported the diagnosis of neurovascular compression as the underlying etiology.

50.4 Case Discussion

This case illustrates several key features of glossopharyngeal neuralgia, particularly the syncopal variant. While classic GPN is rare, the syncopal form is even more uncommon and may initially be misattributed to cardiac or psychiatric causes. In this patient, the presence of reproducible pain triggered by typical stimuli (swallowing, speaking) and the involvement of autonomic symptoms—demonstrated objectively by Holter monitoring—strongly indicated the vagal involvement associated with the glossopharyngeal nerve.

50.5 Clinical Characteristics

Glossopharyngeal neuralgia (GPN) is clinically characterized by paroxysmal, severe, and unilateral pain in regions innervated by the glossopharyngeal nerve (cranial nerve IX). The pain is classically described as sharp, lancinating, or electric shock-like, with each episode typically lasting a few seconds to 1 minute. Attacks can occur spontaneously or be triggered by innocuous stimuli, most commonly swallowing, chewing, talking, coughing, or yawning [6].

The pain localization includes the posterior oropharynx, tonsillar fossa, base of the tongue, and may radiate to the ipsilateral ear—a distribution that reflects the sensory territory of CN IX. Patients often report pain on one side only, and the episodes can occur several times per day, often without any warning [4].

A particularly important subset of patients presents with the syncopal (vagal) variant of GPN. In these individuals, paroxysmal pain is accompanied by autonomic symptoms, including:

- Bradycardia
- Hypotension
- Presyncope or syncope
- Dizziness or lightheadedness

These symptoms are attributed to concomitant activation or irritation of the adjacent vagus nerve (cranial nerve X), which shares close anatomical proximity with CN IX, especially at the jugular foramen and root entry zone in the medulla. This co-activation may lead to exaggerated cardioinhibitory reflexes, potentially resulting in life-threatening events if not recognized early.

GPN may also demonstrate periods of spontaneous remission, lasting weeks to months, followed by recurrent symptom flares. Between attacks, patients are typically asymptomatic and may not exhibit any neurological deficits. However, during active phases, the condition can be profoundly disabling and may significantly impair oral intake, speech, and quality of life.

In drug-responsive cases, medications such as carbamazepine or oxcarbazepine can reduce the frequency and severity of attacks, although partial or refractory responses are not uncommon. The presence of autonomic features often necessitates further cardiac evaluation and may influence treatment strategies, including the need for cardiac pacing in select cases or surgical decompression when neurovascular compression is confirmed.

50.6 Diagnosis

The diagnosis of glossopharyngeal neuralgia (GPN) is primarily clinical but requires a systematic approach to distinguish it from other craniofacial pain syndromes and to identify potentially treatable structural causes, especially in cases presenting with autonomic involvement.

1. Clinical History and Symptomatology

   A detailed patient history is paramount. Hallmark features include:

   - Unilateral, paroxysmal, electric shock-like pain
   - Distribution in the posterior oropharynx, tonsillar region, base of the tongue, and occasionally the ear
   - Pain episodes triggered by swallowing, talking, chewing, yawning, or coughing
   - Short duration (seconds to 1 minute), occurring multiple times daily

   In the syncopal or vagal variant, patients may also report:

   - Bradycardia, dizziness, presyncope, hypotension, or syncope during pain attacks. These autonomic symptoms suggest vagal nerve involvement, which carries a higher risk of misdiagnosis as a cardiac or psychiatric disorder.

2. Physical and Neurological Examination

   Physical examination is often normal between attacks, with no sensory deficits. Provocative maneuvers such as gentle palpation in the tonsillar fossa or posterior pharynx may occasionally reproduce symptoms. Neurological examination helps rule out other cranial nerve pathologies or mass lesions.

3. Cardiac Monitoring

   In suspected syncopal variants, electrocardiography (ECG) and 24-hour Holter monitoring are essential. Transient episodes of bradyarrhythmia temporally associated with pain paroxysms provide objective evidence of vagal involvement. In severe cases, additional autonomic testing or referral to cardiology may be required.

4. Neuroimaging

   To investigate possible secondary causes—particularly neurovascular compression high-resolution brain MRI with MR angiography is the imaging modality of choice. Key findings may include:

   - Vascular loops (commonly PICA) in contact with the root entry zone of CN IX or X
   - Absence of alternative etiologies such as neoplastic lesions, demyelination, or infectious/inflammatory changes

   Computed tomography (CT) angiography or three-dimensional (3D) constructive interference in steady state (CISS) sequences may be helpful in select cases for better visualization of nerve-vessel interfaces.

5. Differential Diagnosis

   Several other conditions may mimic GPN and should be excluded:

   - Trigeminal neuralgia (V2/V3 distribution, no oropharyngeal trigger)
   - Eagle syndrome (stylohyoid ligament elongation; may cause oropharyngeal pain)
   - Glossopharyngeal schwannoma or other cerebellopontine angle tumors
   - Multiple sclerosis, particularly in younger patients with dem

50.7 Treatment

The spontaneous remissions seen in this patient, followed by recurrence, is not unusual in cranial neuralgias [7]. Such patterns may delay diagnosis, especially when autonomic symptoms dominate the presentation. Furthermore, older adults may be more susceptible to cardiovascular consequences of vagal stimulation, increasing the potential severity of this syndrome.

In terms of management, carbamazepine remains the first-line treatment, as with trigeminal neuralgia. Other agents such as oxcarbazepine, gabapentin, pregabalin, or lamotrigine may also be tried, though evidence is limited. In this case, carbamazepine provided partial symptom relief, but persistent pain and bradycardia suggest the need to consider surgical intervention or microvascular decompression (MVD) [7–10], especially if quality of life is significantly impaired or syncopal episodes worsen.

MVD is the preferred surgical treatment for medically refractory GPN with demonstrable vascular compression. Success rates are high, and complications are relatively low in experienced hands. Alternatively, nerve sectioning, radiofrequency ablation, or stereotactic radiosurgery may be considered in selected cases, though with variable outcomes and higher risks of sensory or motor deficits [11, 12].

Given the bilateral neurovascular contacts observed in this patient's MRI, but the unilateral nature of symptoms, conservative management remains justified at this stage. However, progression or increased cardiovascular involvement would warrant neurosurgical evaluation.

50.8 Conclusion

Glossopharyngeal neuralgia is a rare but debilitating cranial neuropathy that may occasionally present with autonomic symptoms such as bradycardia or syncope—the so-called syncopal variant. In such cases, a comprehensive evaluation including cardiac monitoring and high-resolution neuroimaging is essential for accurate diagnosis.

This case underscores the importance of considering GPN in elderly patients with paroxysmal oropharyngeal pain and unexplained bradycardia. The finding of neurovascular contact on Angio-MRI supports a secondary etiology and strengthens the indication for surgical treatment in refractory cases.

Although carbamazepine remains the first-line therapy, partial response and recurrence over time may necessitate escalation of care. Clinicians should remain vigilant for potentially life-threatening autonomic manifestations in this underrecognized syndrome. Early diagnosis and appropriate treatment can significantly improve patient outcomes and quality of life.

References

1. Khan M, Nishi SE, Hassan SN, Islam MA, Gan SH. Trigeminal neuralgia, glossopharyngeal neuralgia, and myofascial pain dysfunction syndrome: an update. Pain Res Manag. 2017;2017:7438326. https://doi.org/10.1155/2017/7438326.
2. Allam AK, Larkin MB, Sharma H, Viswanathan A. Trigeminal and glossopharyngeal neuralgia. Neurol Clin. 2024;42(2):585–98. https://doi.org/10.1016/j.ncl.2023.12.011.
3. Shah RJ, Padalia D. Glossopharyngeal Neuralgia. In: StatPearls [Internet]. Treasure Island: StatPearls Publishing; 2023.
4. Han A, Montgomery C, Zamora A, Winder E, Kaye A, Carroll C, Aquino A, Kakazu J, Kaye AD. Glossopharyngeal neuralgia: epidemiology, risk factors, pathophysiology, differential diagnosis, and treatment options. Health Psychol Res. 2022;10(5):36042. https://doi.org/10.52965/001c.36042.
5. Singh PM, Chaturvedi A, Kaushik S. An uncommonly common: glossopharyngeal neuralgia. Ann Indian Acad Neurol. 2013;16(1):1–8.
6. Zakrzewska JM, Linskey ME. Glossopharyngeal neuralgia. In: Handbook of clinical neurology, vol. 139. Elsevier; 2016. p. 215–27.
7. Zhao H, Zhang X, Zhu J, Tang YD, Li ST. Microvascular decompression for glossopharyngeal neuralgia: long-term follow-up. World Neurosurg. 2017;102:151–6. https://doi.org/10.1016/j.wneu.2017.02.106.
8. Franzini A, Messina G, Franzini A, Marchetti M, Ferroli P, Fariselli L, Broggi G. Treatments of glossopharyngeal neuralgia: towards standard procedures. Neurol Sci. 2017;38(Suppl 1):51–5. https://doi.org/10.1007/s10072-017-2909-6.
9. Kuzucu P, Türkmen T, Ülkü G, Yaman ME, Aykol Ş. Glossopharyngeal neuralgia as initial symptom in combined hyperactive dysfunction syndrome: case report. Br J Neurosurg. 2023;37(3):309–12. https://doi.org/10.1080/02688697.2020.1817317.
10. Revuelta-Gutiérrez R, Piñon-Jiménez F, Contreras-Vázquez OR, Vales-Hidalgo LO, Martinez-Anda JJ. Glossopharyngeal and vagoglossopharyngeal neuralgia: long-term surgical outcomes in a single institution. Surg Neurol Int. 2023;14:267. https://doi.org/10.25259/SNI_518_2023.
11. Wu Z, Liu J, Fang Q, Yang Y, Fan Y. Safety and efficacy of radiofrequency treatment for glossopharyngeal neuralgia: a systematic review and single-arm meta-analysis. Neurosurg Rev. 2025;48(1):341. https://doi.org/10.1007/s10143-025-03490-5.
12. Zhang J, Li Z, Wang N, Zhang P, Li Y, Chen Y. Efficacy and safety of stereotactic radiosurgery for idiopathic glossopharyngeal neuralgia: a systematic review and meta-analysis. Clin Neurol Neurosurg. 2025;252:108878. https://doi.org/10.1016/j.clineuro.2025.108878.

Chapter 51
Nervus Intermedius Neuralgia

Raiza Borges

51.1 Introduction

Intermediate nerve neuralgia, also known as Ramsay Hunt syndrome, is named after Ramsay Hunt, who in 1908 identified the correlation between herpes zoster, the intermediate nerve, and geniculate neuralgia. Additionally, he described the "Ramsay Hunt zone," whose distribution corresponded to the innervation of the intermediate nerve, initially considered a branch of the facial nerve [1, 2]. This nerve has parasympathetic functions, contributing to the innervation of the lacrimal and salivary glands, in addition to transmitting sensory information from the tongue, nasal cavity, and auricular concha [3, 4].

Pain attributed to a lesion or disease of the nervus intermedius is a rare condition characterized by episodes of intense pain in the deep auricular region, which may radiate to the parieto-occipital area. In addition to the characteristic pain, associated symptoms may include dysgeusia, reduced lacrimation, and hyperacusis [5]. A literature review conducted by Robblee (2021) found that 2.6% of patients with intermediate nerve neuralgia reported hyperacusis, while 7.9% experienced reduced lacrimation [6].

Intermediate nerve neuralgia presents a diagnostic challenge due to its heterogeneous clinical presentation and the complex overlap of external ear innervation, which involves the trigeminal nerve (auriculotemporal branch), the facial nerve (intermediate nerve), the glossopharyngeal nerve, the vagus nerve, and upper cervical branches. In addition to being frequently mistaken for other cranial neuralgias, its differential diagnosis includes various otolaryngological conditions, such as otitis and temporomandibular joint dysfunction [7, 8].

R. Borges (✉)
Federal University of Pernambuco, Recife, Brazil

D. Uludüz et al. (eds.), *Rare Causes of Headache Disorders*, Headache,
https://doi.org/10.1007/978-3-032-10242-3_51

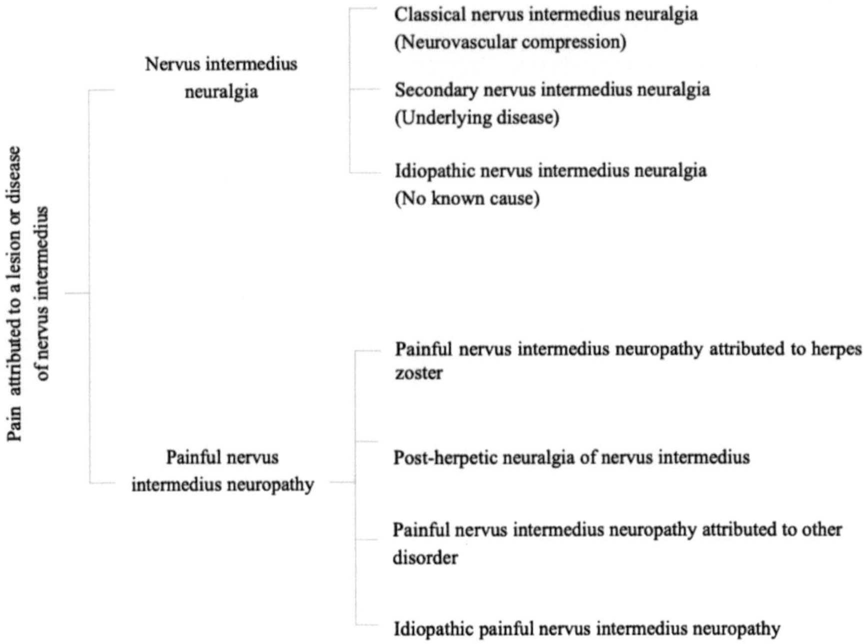

Fig. 51.1 Classification of painful syndromes of the nervus intermedius according to the *International Classification of Headache Disorders*, third edition (ICHD-3), with subdivisions into nervus intermedius neuralgia and painful nervus intermedius neuropathy

Previously, intermediate nerve neuralgia was considered a single entity. However, the International Classification of Headache Disorders, third edition (ICHD-3) revised this terminology, adopting the designation "Pain attributed to a lesion or disease of the nervus intermedius" [4]. This term has since been subdivided into distinct categories, allowing for a more precise characterization of the different etiologies and clinical presentations (Fig. 51.1).

According to the third edition of the International Classification of Headache Disorders, nervus intermedius neuralgia (NIN) is defined by brief paroxysms of pain felt deeply in the auditory canal, sometimes radiating to the parieto-occipital region (Panel 51.1).

Panel 51.1 Diagnostic criteria of nervus intermedius neuralgia according to the ICHD-3
ICHD-3

Description: A rare disorder characterized by brief paroxysms of pain felt deeply in the auditory canal, sometimes radiating to the parieto-occipital region. In the vast majority of cases, vascular compression is found at operation, occasionally with a thickened arachnoidea, but it may develop without apparent cause or as a complication of herpes zoster or, very rarely, multiple sclerosis or tumor. It is provoked by stimulation of a trigger area in the posterior wall of the auditory canal and/or periauricular region.

Criteria

A. *Paroxysmal attacks of unilateral pain in the distribution of nervus intermedius1 and fulfilling criterion B*
B. *Pain has all of the following characteristics:*
   1. *Lasting from a few seconds to minutes*
   2. *Severe in intensity*
   3. *Shooting, stabbing or sharp in quality*
   4. *Precipitated by stimulation of a trigger area in the posterior wall of the auditory canal and/or periauricular region*
C. *Not better accounted for by another ICHD-3 diagnosis.*

51.2 Case Presentation

A 58-year-old woman presented approximately 1 year ago with an episode of peripheral facial palsy on the left side. There was no report of blister formation or erythema in the ear. About 15 days after the event, she developed deep pain in the left ear, experiencing dozens of daily paroxysms, rated 9 to 10 on the pain scale. The pain could be triggered by stimulation of a periauricular trigger zone. In addition to the intense pain in the inner ear region, she also reported continuous pain in the left hemiface, consistent with the distribution of the trigeminal nerve.

Her medical, family, and social history was unremarkable. Magnetic resonance imaging (MRI) did not reveal any neurovascular conflict. After several weeks of treatment with pregabalin (75 mg, twice daily), followed by the addition of duloxetine (60 mg/day), there was a significant reduction in pain, leading to an improvement in quality of life.

51.3 Clinical Characteristics

The clinical evaluation begins with the characterization of pain, its location, and possible triggering factors. The physical examination should include inspection of the ear and auditory canal to rule out external otitis, foreign bodies, or visible lesions, as well as palpation of the mastoid and periauricular regions to assess for local inflammatory signs. The trigger test for intermediate nerve neuralgia should be performed by stimulating the posterior wall of the auditory canal and the periauricular region to check for pain reproduction. The evaluation of cranial nerves is essential, as deficits in the facial (VII), vestibulocochlear (VIII), or glossopharyngeal (IX) nerves may indicate associated pathologies such as pontocerebellar angle tumors or multiple neurovascular compressions. The Schirmer test can be used to assess lacrimal dysfunction, while taste evaluation may reveal alterations in taste perception and help localize the lesion.

51.4 Diagnosis

For an accurate assessment, a detailed anamnesis must be complemented by a thorough neurological examination, which is essential for detecting possible alterations in taste, lacrimation, and salivation, as well as for evaluating the involvement of other cranial nerves. This approach is crucial for differentiating between intermediate nerve neuralgia and other neurological conditions.

The diagnosis of intermediate nerve neuralgia is predominantly clinical, but neuroimaging is necessary for its subclassification. Brain magnetic resonance imaging (MRI) with angiographic sequences is the exam of choice for investigating associated structural causes. The FIESTA (Fast Imaging Employing Steady-State Acquisition) sequence is beneficial, as it provides a detailed visualization of the cranial nerves in the brainstem and facilitates the identification of possible neurovascular conflicts. The main finding in classic intermediate nerve neuralgia is neurovascular compression of the nerve, while MRI also plays a crucial role in detecting demyelinating lesions suggestive of multiple sclerosis and in identifying tumors such as schwannomas and meningiomas in cases of secondary neuralgia [9, 10].

51.5 Treatment

The initial management of intermediate nerve neuralgia generally involves the use of medications for neuropathic pain control, with a particular emphasis on anticonvulsants and antidepressants [11]. Among the anticonvulsants, the most commonly used include carbamazepine, oxcarbazepine, gabapentin, topiramate, phenytoin, and lamotrigine, due to their ability to modulate neuronal excitability. Carbamazepine and oxcarbazepine are widely cited in the literature for their efficacy in trigeminal neuralgia. Although studies on intermediate nerve neuralgia are limited, it is believed that they may offer similar benefits, making them the most frequently reported drugs for treating this condition [6, 12].

Tricyclic antidepressants, such as amitriptyline and nortriptyline, as well as dual-action antidepressants, are often prescribed due to their ability to inhibit serotonin and norepinephrine reuptake, thereby modulating pain transmission in the central nervous system. When pharmacological treatment does not provide adequate relief, minimally invasive interventions may be considered. Among these approaches, intermediate nerve block with local anesthetics and corticosteroids may offer pain relief, although evidence for sustained benefit remains limited [6, 13].

Another option described in the literature is the use of botulinum toxin type A, which has been extensively studied for the treatment of trigeminal neuralgia. However, to date, no clinical studies are proving its efficacy in intermediate nerve neuralgia, with only isolated case reports suggesting a possible benefit as an intermediate step before surgical intervention [13].

The surgical treatment of nervus intermedius neuralgia (NIN) is widely described in the literature and is indicated for cases refractory to pharmacological therapy and minimally invasive approaches. Microvascular decompression is the most commonly performed procedure, especially when there is evidence of neurovascular conflict involving the root of the nervus intermedius, with high success rates. This procedure aims to relieve vascular compression on the nerve, reducing irritation and, consequently, pain episodes [14–16].

In cases where microvascular decompression is not feasible or does not result in significant clinical improvement, more aggressive neurosurgical options may be considered, such as nerve sectioning, rhizotomy, and tractotomy. These procedures aim to interrupt the transmission of pain signals and are reserved only for highly refractory cases, due to the risk of permanent sensory deficits [14, 17].

51.6 Conclusion

Intermediate nerve neuralgia is a rare and challenging condition that is often underdiagnosed due to its symptomatic overlap with other cranial neuralgias. Early recognition of this syndrome is crucial for effective management, enabling the implementation of therapeutic strategies that alleviate pain and enhance patients' quality of life.

This chapter explored the pathophysiology, clinical presentation, diagnostic approach, and treatment options for intermediate nerve neuralgia, emphasizing the importance of detailed evaluation and advanced neuroimaging in identifying potential underlying causes.

Despite advancements in understanding intermediate nerve neuralgia, the available literature on this condition remains limited, highlighting the need for more robust studies to enhance knowledge of its mechanisms and validate therapeutic strategies.

References

1. Tubbs RS, Steck DT, Mortazavi MM, Cohen-Gadol AA. The nervus intermedius: a review of its anatomy, function, pathology, and role in neurosurgery. World Neurosurg. 2013;79:763–7.
2. Alfieri A, Strauss C, Prell J, Peschke E. History of the nervus intermedius of Wrisberg. Ann Anat-Anatomischer Anzeiger. 2010;192:139–44.
3. Rhoton AL Jr, Kobayashi S, Hollinshead WH. Nervus intermedius. J Neurosurg. 1968;29(6):609–18. https://doi.org/10.3171/jns.1968.29.6.0609.
4. Jordan DR. The nervus intermedius. Arch Ophthalmol. 1993;111(12):1691–2. https://doi.org/10.1001/archopht.1993.01090120115031.
5. Head Classification Committee of the International Headache Society (IHS). The International Classification of Headache Disorders, 3rd edition (beta version). Cephalalgia. 2013;33:629–808.
6. Robblee J. A pain in the ear: two case reports of nervus intermedius neuralgia and narrative review. Headache. 2021;61(3):414–21. https://doi.org/10.1111/head.14066. Epub 2021 Feb 15.
7. DeLange JM, Garza I, Robertson CE. Clinical reasoning: a 50-year-old woman with deep stabbing ear pain. Neurology. 2014;83:e152–7.
8. Harrison E, Cronin M. Otalgia. Aust Fam Physician. 2016;45:493–7.
9. Oh JH, Chung JH, Min HJ, Cho SH, Park CW, Lee SH. Clinical application of 3D-FIESTA image in patients with unilateral inner ear symptom. Korean J Audiol. 2013;17(3):111–7. https://doi.org/10.7874/kja.2013.17.3.111.
10. Martínez ER, Gredilla Molinero J, Arevalo N, Carretero M, Azpeitia Armán FJ. Study of lower cranial nerves by MRI Fiesta sequence. Madrid: European Congress of Radiology; 2012. https://doi.org/10.1594/ecr2012/C-0566.
11. McQuay HJ, Carroll D, Jadad AR, Wiffen P, Moore A. Anticonvulsant drugs for management of pain: a systemic review. BMJ. 1995;311:1047–52.
12. Bendtsen L, Zakrzewska JM, Heinskou TB, Hodaie M, Leal PRL, Nurmikko T, Obermann M, Cruccu G, Maarbjerg S. Advances in diagnosis, classification, pathophysiology, and management of trigeminal neuralgia. Lancet Neurol. 2020;19(9):784–96. https://doi.org/10.1016/S1474-4422(20)30233-7.
13. Erdocia-Goñi A, Hernando de la Bárcena I. The use of botulinum toxin type a in nervus intermedius neuralgia. Neurología (English Edition). 2020;35(8):618–9.
14. Peris-Celda M, Oushy S, Perry A, Graffeo CS, Carlstrom LP, Zimmerman RS, Meyer FB, Pollock BE, Link MJ. Nervus intermedius and the surgical management of geniculate neuralgia. J Neurosurg. 2019;131(2):343–51. https://doi.org/10.3171/2018.3.JNS172920.
15. Saers SJF, Han KS, de Ru JA. Microvascular decompression may be an effective treatment for nervus intermedius neuralgia. J Laryngol Otol. 2011;125:520–2.
16. Lovely TJ, Jannetta PJ. Surgical management of geniculate neural gia. Am J Otol. 1997;18:512–7.
17. Holste KG, Hardaway FA, Raslan AM, Burchiel KJ. Pain-free and pain-controlled survival after sectioning the nervus intermedius in nervus intermedius neuralgia: a single-institution review. J Neurosurg. 2018;131:352–9.

Chapter 52
Occipital Neuralgia

Ida Fortini

52.1 Introduction

Occipital neuralgia (ON) was first described in 1821 by Benito Lentijo and Martinez Ramos. It is a condition marked by neuropathic pain affecting the distribution of the occipital nerves, including the greater occipital nerve (GON), lesser occipital nerve (LON), and third occipital nerve (TON), either singly or in combination. Although relatively rare, ON predominantly affects women and is considered an uncommon cause of head and neck pain [1].

ON is a relatively rare condition, with an estimated prevalence of approximately 3 per 100.000 people [2]. In a Dutch population, ON comprised 8.3% of facial pain cases. The total incidence was 3.2 per 100,000 people, with a mean age of diagnosis of 54.1 years [3]. In a headache outpatient clinic, ON was diagnosed in 1.2% of patients [4].

This condition predominantly affects women, as evidenced by studies showing a higher female prevalence among patients diagnosed with ON [4, 5].

Several risk factors can influence the development of ON, with a higher prevalence observed in women, as indicated by research. This condition is prevalent in individuals with multiple sclerosis, where demyelinating lesions in the upper cervical spinal cord, especially at the C2–3 vertebral level, can lead to ON [5]. The patients tend to present with unilateral and episodic symptoms, with associated sensory loss. The response to treatment may vary depending on the clinical phenotype of multiple sclerosis [5]. While rare in children, ON can occur with trauma [6].

I. Fortini (✉)
University of São Paulo, São Paulo, Brazil

D. Uludüz et al. (eds.), *Rare Causes of Headache Disorders*, Headache,
https://doi.org/10.1007/978-3-032-10242-3_52

52.2 Pathophysiology

Figure 52.1 illustrates the occipital nerves and highlights their complex relationship with the occipital muscles. The greater occipital nerve (GON) originates from the dorsal ramus of the C2 spinal nerve. It then passes medially to the lower border of the obliquus capitis inferior muscle and crosses the suboccipital triangle. From there, it travels along the rectus capitis posterior major muscle, innervating it, before piercing the semispinalis capitis muscle and the tendon of the trapezius. The GON continues to ascend, passing the superior nuchal line of the occipital bone and proceeding toward the apex of the scalp, near the occipital artery [7, 8].

The lesser occipital nerve (LON) originates from the ventral ramus of C2 and loops inferiorly to the spinal accessory nerve. It ascends along the posterior border of the sternocleidomastoid muscle, piercing the deep cervical fascia. The nerve then passes across the posterior edge of the sternocleidomastoid insertion and enters the superficial fascia of the scalp. It divides into three branches: the auricular, mastoid, and occipital branches [7, 8].

The third occipital nerve (TON) originates from the dorsal ramus of C3, which divides into lateral and medial branches. The medial branch gives rise to both superficial and deep branches, with the superficial branch becoming the TON. The TON

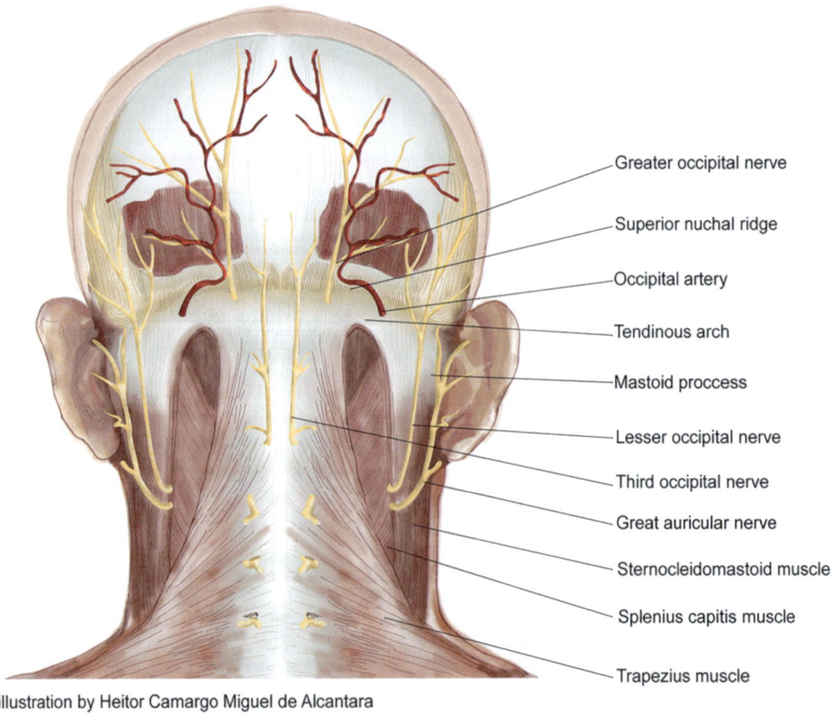

Fig. 52.1 Occipital nerves

curves around the dorsolateral surfaces of C2 and C3, travelling along the semispinalis capitis muscle. It then turns dorsally at the C2 spinous process, piercing the semispinalis capitis, splenius capitis, and trapezius muscles. After exiting these muscles, the TON innervates a small cutaneous area just below the nuchal line. Additionally, the TON sends branches to the greater occipital nerve (GON) and lesser occipital nerve (LON) [7, 8].

Both structural and non-structural causes can lead to ON. Still, almost always it results from the compression or irritation of one of the nerves at one of several anatomic points, the great occipital nerve (GON) being responsible for the great majority of the cases. Anatomical variations, such as the course of the greater occipital nerve through the obliquus inferior capitis muscle, may lead to nerve compression. Other causes of compression of the occipital nerves include hypertrophic ligaments, fibrosis, and bone spurs [9].

Multiple possible compression points of the GON exist that may result in ON [10].

These points include the C2 nerve root, the obliquus capitis inferior muscle, the semispinalis capitis muscle, points where the GON penetrates the trapezius muscle, and points of intersection between the GON and the occipital artery [8, 10].

Muscle hypertrophy or spasms can also contribute to nerve compression. Men, due to increased exposure to physical activities or occupations that heighten the risk of neck injuries, may be more prone to developing ON. Additionally, postural issues, particularly those related to prolonged use of computers or mobile devices, can cause tension in the neck muscles and contribute to nerve compression [11]. Trauma to the occipital region, such as whiplash injuries, may lead to ON either through direct nerve damage or secondary changes like fibrosis that result in nerve compression [12].

A less common cause of ON is vascular compression of the nerves by arteries, such as the posterior inferior cerebellar artery or the occipital artery [8, 13].

Degenerative diseases of the cervical spine, such as cervical spondylosis, may be more prevalent in middle-aged and older men, increasing the risk of occipital neuralgia. Arthritic changes, such as C1–C2 arthrosis syndrome and atlantoaxial lateral mass osteoarthritis, can cause nerve compression [12].

Other pathologies can also be associated with ON, such as cervical cord tumors, Chiari malformation, arteriovenous malformation, and neurosyphilis, which may cause secondary nerve compression or irritation [10, 14]. Systemic diseases such as diabetes can affect nerve health, increasing susceptibility to neuropathic conditions, including ON [11].

Familial cases of ON are extremely rare but have been reported, with an autosomal dominant or X-linked inheritance pattern. These cases often involve neuralgia of multiple cranial nerves, suggesting potential peripheral sensory anastomoses or central convergence of afferent pathways [15, 16].

52.3 Case Presentation

A 65-year-old female with a medical history of well-controlled arterial hypertension and hypothyroidism presented to the headache clinic with complaints of severe, acute, stabbing pain in the right occipital region. The pain, which started approximately 10 months ago, initially occurred four times a week. However, over the last five months, the frequency of the episodes increased to daily occurrences, often with multiple attacks per day, occasionally extending into the nighttime. The patient denied any positional influence on the pain and reported no associated symptoms, though tenderness over the affected region was present most of the time. The patient had been treated with a combination of non-steroidal anti-inflammatory drugs (NSAIDs), venlafaxine, pregabalin, and carbamazepine, but none provided significant relief. Occipital nerve blocks with lidocaine offered temporary pain relief.

Neurological examination was unremarkable, and systemic diseases other than hypertension and hypothyroidism were ruled out. Magnetic resonance imaging (MRI) revealed no abnormalities. The patient also underwent acupuncture and transcutaneous electrical nerve stimulation (TENS) sessions, but there was no improvement. Subsequently, she underwent rhizotomy of the right greater occipital nerve. No tissue abnormalities were observed during the procedure, and immediate pain relief was achieved, which persisted during follow-up visits.

52.4 Case Discussion

This case is characteristic of ON with a prolonged duration of symptoms. The positive response to the anesthetic block further supports the diagnosis. In some cases, a Tinel's sign may be present at the site of the greater occipital nerve emergence, but it was not noted in this case.

It is crucial to rule out systemic, cranial, and cervical causes of ON during diagnosis. While non-invasive treatments such as acupuncture, TENS, and nerve blocks are commonly attempted, they do not always provide sufficient relief. In such cases, more invasive treatments, such as occipital nerve stimulation (ONS) or radio frequency ablation, may be necessary to achieve sustained pain relief.

52.5 Clinical Characteristics

The pain associated with this condition is typically paroxysmal, sharp, and intense, often originating from the posterior region of the head. It lasts from seconds to minutes and may radiate toward the front of the head and face [10, 17]. Tenderness over the affected nerve area is commonly present, along with a Tinel's sign at the point where the nerve emerges. The pain may be exacerbated by movement or pressure applied to the posterior region of the head.

52.6 Diagnosis

The diagnosis of occipital neuralgia (ON) is primarily clinical, based on the presence of intermittent, typically unilateral, painful episodes of stabs in the occipital region. However, bilateral involvement can occur in some cases. The individual pain episodes can last seconds to minutes, and physical examination often reveals tenderness over the affected occipital nerves [10, 17].

The diagnostic criteria for occipital neuralgia (ON) according to the International Classification of Headache Disorders, 3rd edition (ICHD-3), are as follows [18]:

A. Unilateral or bilateral pain in the distribution(s) of the greater, lesser and/or third occipital nerves and fulfilling criteria B–D
B. Pain has at least two of the following three characteristics:
   1. Recurring in paroxysmal attacks lasting from a few seconds to minutes
   2. Severe in intensity
   3. Shooting, stabbing or sharp in quality
C. Pain is associated with both of the following:
   1. Dysesthesia and/or allodynia apparent during innocuous stimulation of the scalp and/or hair
   2. Either or both of the following:
      (a) Tenderness over the affected nerve branches
      (b) Trigger points at the emergence of the greater occipital nerve or in the distribution of C2
D. Pain is eased temporarily by local anesthetic block of the affected nerve(s)
E. Not better accounted for by another ICHD-3 diagnosis.

Pain usually begins unilaterally and may extend into a bilateral distribution over time. Bilateral symptoms are present in one-third of cases. A positive Tinel's sign may be present over the nerve's distribution, especially where the GON emerges at the base of the skull over the greater occipital notch [7, 8].

According to ICHD-3 standards, diagnosis of occipital neuralgia requires confirmation through a local anesthetic blockade of the suspected nerve. Pain relief following the nerve block should last for at least the duration of the local anesthetic. Since single diagnostic blocks can yield false-positive rates of up to 40%, performing a second block may help improve diagnostic accuracy [7, 8].

Occipital neuralgia (ON) can be easily confused with several other neurological conditions due to overlapping symptoms, particularly pain in the occipital region. While these conditions share similar symptoms, they have distinct etiologies and treatment approaches. Therefore, a thorough clinical evaluation, along with the use of imaging tests when necessary, is essential for accurate diagnosis. Conditions that may be mistaken for occipital neuralgia include:

52.6.1 Cervicogenic Headache

In cervicogenic headache, the pain is referred to the occipital region and is caused by dysfunction in the cervical spine. While it shares similarities with occipital neuralgia (ON), cervicogenic headache is a secondary headache disorder typically linked to mechanical issues in the cervical spine. Unlike the sharp, excruciating pain of ON, cervicogenic headache pain tends to be more constant and less paroxysmal, lacking the intense, sudden episodes characteristic of occipital neuralgia [19].

52.6.2 Migraine

Migraine has distinct features such as photophobia, phonophobia, and nausea, but occasionally occipital pain may be a symptom, leading to confusion with ON. Additionally, migraine pain is usually throbbing, unlike the stabbing pain of ON [2].

52.6.3 Neck Pain

Pain in the neck, especially when associated with muscle spasms and stiffness, can radiate to the occipital region, mimicking ON. Neck pain generally does not present the paroxysmal, stabbing pain typical of ON [20].

52.6.4 Demyelinating Lesions

Multiple sclerosis and the neuromyelitis optica spectrum of disorders may present with neuralgiform pain in the occipital region due to lesions in the cervical spinal cord, which may be confused with ON. Still, it is often associated with other neurological symptoms, such as sensory loss or weakness, which help differentiate it from isolated ON [5].

52.6.5 Cervical Myelitis

Inflammation of the cervical spinal cord may present as occipital neuralgia, especially when there are lesions at high levels of the cervical spine, such as C2, but is often associated with additional neurological deficits, such as sensory or motor changes, that are not typical of ON [5, 21].

A thorough differential diagnosis is essential and can be supported by anesthetic occipital nerve blocks, which help confirm occipital neuralgia (ON) if pain relief is achieved [2, 22]. In addition, there are less common symptoms of ON that may be present and can be useful in distinguishing this condition from others:

52.6.6 Occipital Allodynia

Increased sensitivity to light touch in the occipital region, which may be indicative of occipital neuralgia.

52.6.7 Cervical Muscle Spasms

Although pain is the predominant symptom, some patients may experience spasms in the cervical muscles, which can contribute to pain and stiffness in the region.

52.6.8 Radiation of Pain to Frontal Areas

Pain from occipital neuralgia can radiate to areas innervated by the trigeminal nerve, leading to migraine-like symptoms such as photophobia and nausea, especially when the pain extends to the frontal region. These less common symptoms can complicate the diagnosis, necessitating careful clinical evaluation to differentiate occipital neuralgia from other neurological conditions [5, 23].

52.7 Treatment

Treatment of occipital neuralgia is multimodal and may include both conservative interventions and more invasive procedures, depending on the severity and the patient's response to initial therapies. Non-steroidal anti-inflammatory drugs, tricyclic antidepressants, serotonin-norepinephrine reuptake inhibitors, and anticonvulsants may help to alleviate symptoms.

52.7.1 Conservative and Complementary Treatments

Conservative treatments are often recommended as first-line treatment and include pain education, self-care, physical therapy to reduce muscle tension and improve posture, and the use of transcutaneous electrical nerve stimulation (TENS) [24, 25].

Complementary therapies that have demonstrated effectiveness in treating occipital neuralgia include acupuncture and transcutaneous electrical nerve stimulation (TENS). These alternative therapies can be integrated into a multimodal treatment plan, especially in patients who do not respond well to conventional interventions. However, it is important to consider that more research is needed to validate the long-term effectiveness and safety of these approaches.

52.7.2 Acupuncture

Studies indicate that acupuncture can be effective in treating occipital neuralgia, showing a significantly higher effectiveness rate compared to drug treatment alone. Acupuncture has also been associated with a significant reduction in adverse events compared to medications. Side effects are generally mild and may include pain or bruising at the needle insertion site, dizziness, or fatigue [26, 27].

Acupuncture has been assessed in systematic reviews and meta-analyses, demonstrating significantly higher efficacy compared to drug treatment alone. It is associated with a notable reduction in pain on the visual analogue scale and fewer adverse events [26].

52.7.3 Transcutaneous Electrical Nerve Stimulations (TENS)

Although evidence is limited, TENS is a conservative option that can be used to relieve muscle tension and improve posture, contributing to the management of pain associated with ON [24, 25].

Immobilization of the neck by the cervical collar, physiotherapy, and cryotherapy have not been shown to perform better than placebo [28].

52.8 Minimally Invasive Treatment

52.8.1 Nerve Blocks

Injections of local anesthetics, such as lidocaine or bupivacaine, with or without corticosteroids, are often used for short-term pain relief and may have diagnostic value [11, 12, 17].

Ultrasound guidance was introduced to increase the effectiveness of the procedure. Greher et al. (2010) described the original ultrasound-guided technique for injection of the GON. It targets the nerve as it courses superficial to the obliquus capitis inferior muscle at the C1–C2 level [29].

52.8.2 Botulinum Toxin A

Botulinum toxin A injection has emerged as a treatment with a relatively lower side effect profile compared to many other approaches. Recent trials have shown that it can result in a 50% or greater improvement in symptoms [10, 28].

52.8.3 Radio Frequency

Pulsed radio frequency (PRF) ablation of the occipital nerves is effective in providing long-term pain relief in refractory patients. Studies indicate that PRF may provide greater pain relief compared to steroid injections [24, 30].

52.8.4 Occipital Nerve Stimulation

Occipital nerve stimulation (ONS) is a valuable option for treating refractory cases of occipital neuralgia and can provide significant pain relief in some patients. This minimally invasive procedure has shown promising results, though further studies are needed to confirm its long-term effectiveness [24, 31].

Salmasi et al. (2020) followed three patients for an average of eight months, with an average pain reduction of approximately 50% [31].

Occipital nerve stimulation (ONS) is both safe and effective, with response rates ranging from 63 to 100% in patients with occipital neuralgia. Furthermore, a high percentage of patients continue to respond positively to ONS over the long term [32].

52.9 Surgical Treatments

In very refractory cases, surgical procedures such as occipital nerve decompression or neurectomy may be considered, but there are associated risks [11, 33, 34].

Occipital neuralgia can be difficult to manage, and treatment options should be carefully considered based on the patient's unique clinical presentation and their response to previous interventions. Treatment decisions must be personalized, weighing factors such as efficacy, potential risks, and the patient's preferences. A systematic review investigated 12 articles on the surgical management of occipital neuralgia and did not find sufficient evidence to recommend neurolysis versus neurotomy [35].

52.10 Conclusions

Occipital neuralgia is an uncommon but significant cause of intense, paroxysmal, sharp headaches that typically last from seconds to minutes. These headaches are localized in the areas innervated by the greater occipital nerve (GON), lesser occipital nerve (LON), or third occipital nerve (TON). The primary etiologies include anatomical, traumatic, iatrogenic, and vascular causes. Diagnosis is based on a thorough patient history, clinical examination, and a positive response to an anesthetic block of the occipital nerves. Other conditions may mimic occipital neuralgia and can also respond to nerve blocks, so these must be ruled out through careful clinical assessment and, if necessary, imaging studies. Conservative treatments, such as pharmacological therapy combined with physical therapy, are often effective. Minimally invasive interventions, such as occipital nerve blocks, can be both diagnostic and therapeutic. In cases that are refractory to these treatments, additional options like radio frequency (RF) ablation or neuromodulation may be required for long-term relief. Surgical decompression, neurotomy, and neurolysis are considered last-resort options for particularly challenging cases.

References

1. Belvís R, Guerrero ÁL. Benito's neuralgia: the first description of the occipital neuralgia was made by Spanish doctors at the beginning of the nineteenth century. Neurol Sci. 2019;40(11):2425–9. https://doi.org/10.1007/s10072-019-03734-5. Epub 2019 Feb 15. PMID: 30771022.
2. Dougherty C. Occipital neuralgia. Curr Pain Headache Rep. 2014;18(5):411. https://doi.org/10.1007/s11916-014-0411-x. PMID: 24737457.
3. Koopman JS, Dieleman JP, Huygen FJ, de Mos M, Martin CG, Sturkenboom MC. Incidence of facial pain in the general population. Pain. 2009;147(1–3):122–7. https://doi.org/10.1016/j.pain.2009.08.023. Epub 2009 Sep 26. PMID: 19783099.
4. Martínez-Pías E, Trigo-López J, García-Azorín D, McGreal A, Peral ÁLG. Clinical characteristics and therapeutic results in a series of 68 patients with occipital neuralgia. Pain Med. 2021;22(2):396–401. https://doi.org/10.1093/pm/pnz199. PMID: 31498395.
5. Kissoon NR, Watson JC, Boes CJ, Kantarci OH. Occipital neuralgia associates with high cervical spinal cord lesions in idiopathic inflammatory demyelinating disease. Cephalalgia. 2019;39(1):21–8. https://doi.org/10.1177/0333102418769953. Epub 2018 Apr 8. PMID: 29629601.
6. Villeneuve LM, Coulibaly NJ, Raza SM, Poinson B, Chrusciel D, Desai VR. Surgical management of pediatric occipital neuralgia: a single-center experience of an uncommon pathology. J Neurosurg Pediatr. 2023;32(4):514–21. https://doi.org/10.3171/2023.5.PEDS22554. PMID: 37548543.
7. Djavaherian DM, Guthmiller KB. Occipital Neuralgia. 2023. In: StatPearls [Internet]. Treasure Island: StatPearls Publishing; 2024. PMID: 30855865.
8. Cesmebasi A, Muhleman MA, Hulsberg P, Gielecki J, Matusz P, Tubbs RS, Loukas M. Occipital neuralgia: anatomic considerations. Clin Anat. 2015;28(1):101–8. https://doi.org/10.1002/ca.22468. Epub 2014 Sep 22. PMID:2524419.
9. Janjua MB, Reddy S, El Ahmadieh TY, Ban VS, Ozturk AK, Hwang SW, Samdani AF, Passias PG, Welch WC, Arlet V. Occipital neuralgia: A neurosurgical perspective. J Clin Neurosci.

2020;71:263–70. https://doi.org/10.1016/j.jocn.2019.08.102. Epub 2019 Oct 9. PMID: 31606286.
10. Choi I, Jeon SR. Neuralgias of the head: occipital neuralgia. J Korean Med Sci. 2016;31(4):479–88. https://doi.org/10.3346/jkms.2016.31.4.479. Epub 2016 Mar 9. PMID: 27051229; PMCID: PMC4810328.
11. Pan W, Peng J, Elmofty D. Occipital Neuralgia. Curr Pain Headache Rep. 2021;25(9):61. https://doi.org/10.1007/s11916-021-00972-1. PMID: 34287719.
12. Narouze S. Occipital neuralgia diagnosis and treatment: the role of ultrasound. Headache 2016;56(4):801–7. https://doi.org/10.1111/head.12790. Epub 2016 Mar 21. PMID:26997206.
13. White JB, Atkinson PP, Cloft HJ, Atkinson JL. Vascular compression as a potential cause of occipital neuralgia: a case report. Cephalalgia. 2008;28(1):78–82. https://doi.org/10.1111/j.1468-2982.2007.01427.x. Epub 2007 Nov 16. PMID: 18021267.
14. Ducic I, Felder JM 3rd, Janis JE. Occipital artery vasculitis not identified as a mechanism of occipital neuralgia-related chronic migraine headaches. Plast Reconstr Surg. 2011;128(4):908–912. https://doi.org/10.1097/PRS.0b013e3182174229. PMID: 21921766.
15. Riederer F, Sándor PS, Linnebank M, Ettlin DA. Familial occipital and nervus intermedius neuralgia in a Swiss family. J Headache Pain. 2010;11(4):335–8. https://doi.org/10.1007/s10194-010-0207-2. Epub 2010 Mar 28. PMID: 20349261; PMCID: PMC3476342.
16. Wang Y, Yu CY, Huang L, Riederer F, Ettlin D. Familial neuralgia of occipital and intermedius nerves in a Chinese family. J Headache Pain. 2011;12(4):497–500. https://doi.org/10.1007/s10194-011-0350-4. Epub 2011 May 24. PMID: 21607730; PMCID: PMC3139053.
17. Swanson D, Guedry R, Boudreaux M, Muhlenhaupt E, Kaye AD, Viswanath O, Urits I. An update on the diagnosis, treatment, and management of occipital neuralgia. J Craniofac Surg. 2022;33(3):779–83. https://doi.org/10.1097/SCS.0000000000008360. Epub 2021 Nov 9. PMID:34753868.
18. Headache Classification Committee of the International Headache Society (IHS) The International Classification of Headache Disorders, 3rd edition. Cephalalgia. 2018;38(1):1–211. https://doi.org/10.1177/0333102417738202. PMID: 29368949.
19. Barmherzig R, Kingston W. Occipital neuralgia and Cervicogenic headache: diagnosis and management. Curr Neurol Neurosci Rep. 2019;19(5):20. https://doi.org/10.1007/s11910-019-0937-8. PMID: 30888540.
20. Noh SM, Kang HG. Cervical myelitis presenting as occipital neuralgia. Int J Neurosci. 2018;128(7):682–3. https://doi.org/10.1080/00207454.2017.1403917. Epub 2017 Nov 23. PMID: 29124999.
21. Nikakis P, Koutsis G, Potagas C, Mandellos D, Sfagos C. Occipital neuralgia as an isolated symptom of C2 myelitis. Headache. 2006;46(8):1304–6. https://doi.org/10.1111/j.1526-4610.2006.00543_2.x. PMID: 16942479.
22. Vanelderen P, Lataster A, Levy R, Mekhail N, van Kleef M, Van Zundert J. 8. Occipital neuralgia. Pain Pract. 2010;10(2):137–44. https://doi.org/10.1111/j.1533-2500.2009.00355.x. PMID: 20415731.
23. Blake P, Burstein R. Emerging evidence of occipital nerve compression in unremitting head and neck pain. J Headache Pain. 2019;20(1):76. https://doi.org/10.1186/s10194-019-1023-y. PMID: 31266456; PMCID: PMC6734343.
24. Lefel N, van Suijlekom H, Cohen SPC, Kallewaard JW, Van Zundert J. 11. Cervicogenic headache and occipital neuralgia. Pain Pract. 2025;25(1):e13405. https://doi.org/10.1111/papr.13405. Epub 2024 Sep 1. PMID: 39219023; PMCID: PMC11680101.
25. Deuel D, Sandgren A, Nelson EO, Cropes M, Deacon A, Houdek T, Abd-Elsayed A. Conservative management of occipital neuralgia supported by physical therapy: a review of available research and mechanistic rationale to guide treatment. Curr Pain Headache Rep 2024;28(12):1321–31. https://doi.org/10.1007/s11916-024-01288-6. Epub 2024 Jul 3. PMID: 38958920.

26. Zheng H, Li C, Hu J, Zeng L. Effects of acupuncture in the treatment of occipital neuralgia: a systematic review and meta-analysis. Medicine (Baltimore). 2022;101(48):e31891. https://doi.org/10.1097/MD.0000000000031891. PMID: 36482655; PMCID: PMC9726333.
27. Yun JM, Lee SH, Cho JH, Kim KW, Ha IH. The effects of acupuncture on occipital neuralgia: a systematic review and meta-analysis. BMC Complement Med Ther. 2020;20(1):171. https://doi.org/10.1186/s12906-020-02955-y. PMID: 32493452; PMCID: PMC7268636.
28. Finiels PJ, Batifol D. The treatment of occipital neuralgia: review of 111 cases. Neurochirurgie. 2016;62(5):233–40. https://doi.org/10.1016/j.neuchi.2016.04.004. Epub 2016 Aug 18. PMID: 27546882.
29. Greher M, Moriggl B, Curatolo M, Kirchmair L, Eichenberger U. Sonographic visualization and ultrasound-guided blockade of the greater occipital nerve: a comparison of two selective techniques confirmed by anatomical dissection. Br J Anaesth. 2010;104(5):637–42. https://doi.org/10.1093/bja/aeq052. Epub 2010 Mar 18. PMID: 20299347.
30. Cohen SP, Peterlin BL, Fulton L, Neely ET, Kurihara C, Gupta A, Mali J, Fu DC, Jacobs MB, Plunkett AR, Verdun AJ, Stojanovic MP, Hanling S, Constantinescu O, White RL, McLean BC, Pasquina PF, Zhao Z. Randomized, double-blind, comparative-effectiveness study comparing pulsed radiofrequency to steroid injections for occipital neuralgia or migraine with occipital nerve tenderness. Pain. 2015;156(12):2585–94. https://doi.org/10.1097/j.pain.0000000000000373. PMID: 26447705; PMCID: PMC4697830.
31. Salmasi V, Olatoye OO, Terkawi AS, Hah JM, Ottestad E, Pingree M. Peripheral nerve stimulation for occipital neuralgia. Pain Med. 2020;21(Suppl 1):S13–7. https://doi.org/10.1093/pm/pnaa083. PMID: 32804226.
32. Sweet JA, Mitchell LS, Narouze S, Sharan AD, Falowski SM, Schwalb JM, Machado A, Rosenow JM, Petersen EA, Hayek SM, Arle JE, Pilitsis JG. Occipital nerve stimulation for the treatment of patients with medically refractory occipital neuralgia: congress of neurological surgeons systematic review and evidence-based guideline. Neurosurgery. 2015;77(3):332–41. https://doi.org/10.1227/NEU.0000000000000872. PMID: 26125672.
33. Robinson IS, Salibian AA, Alfonso AR, Lin LJ, Janis JE, Chiu ES. Surgical management of occipital neuralgia: a systematic review of the literature. Ann Plast Surg. 2021;86(3S Suppl 2):S322–31. https://doi.org/10.1097/SAP.0000000000002766. PMID: 33651020.
34. Keifer OP Jr, Diaz A, Campbell M, Bezchlibnyk YB, Boulis NM. Occipital nerve stimulation for the treatment of refractory occipital neuralgia: a case series. World Neurosurg. 2017;105:599–604. https://doi.org/10.1016/j.wneu.2017.06.064. Epub 2017 Jun 17. PMID: 28634063.
35. McNutt S, Hallan DR, Rizk E. Evaluating the evidence: is neurolysis or neurectomy a better treatment for occipital neuralgia? Cureus. 2020;12(11):e11461. https://doi.org/10.7759/cureus.11461. PMID: 33329959; PMCID: PMC7733770.

Chapter 53
Painful Optic Neuritis

João José Freitas de Carvalho, Raimundo Neudson Maia Alcantara, and Renata De Oliveira Carvalho

53.1 Introduction

Painful optic neuritis (PON) is an acute inflammatory disorder of the optic nerve frequently associated with demyelinating diseases of the central nervous system, especially multiple sclerosis (MS) and, to a lesser frequency, diseases such as neuromyelitis optica spectrum disorder (NMOSD) and myelin oligodendrocyte glycoprotein (MOG) antibody-associated disease (MOGAD) [1–3]. PON is classically characterized by unilateral retro-orbital pain, exacerbated by eye movement, which precedes or accompanies subacute visual loss.

The International Classification of Headache Disorders, third edition (ICHD-3), defines PON as a secondary headache, characterized by pain in the retro-orbital, orbital, frontal, and/or temporal regions, and meeting specific diagnostic criteria (code 13.6) [4]. The onset of pain must be temporally related to the episode of optic neuritis (ON), and its intensity increases with eye movement, reflecting inflammation in the optic nerve sheaths and adjacent tissues.

Population and clinical studies indicate that pain is present in about 90% of cases of optic neuritis and may precede vision loss by days [3, 5]. In the United States and Europe, idiopathic or multiple sclerosis-associated optic neuritis is the most prevalent form, while infectious or autoimmune etiologies are more common in developing countries [2, 6].

Early diagnosis of PON is essential, not only for the immediate management of visual and pain symptoms but also because it can be the first clinical sign of a chronic demyelinating disease. Contrast-enhanced magnetic resonance imaging is a

J. J. F. de Carvalho (✉) · R. De Oliveira Carvalho
Unichristus School of Medicine, Fortaleza, Brazil

R. N. M. Alcantara
Department of Neurology, Hospital Geral de Fortaleza, Fortaleza, Brazil

D. Uludüz et al. (eds.), *Rare Causes of Headache Disorders*, Headache,
https://doi.org/10.1007/978-3-032-10242-3_53

crucial diagnostic tool, with optic nerve enhancement observed in more than 90% of cases [1, 7].

This chapter explores the pathophysiological basis, clinical features, differential diagnosis, and therapeutic management of PON, integrating recent literature with a representative clinical case.

53.2 Pathophysiology

PON represents an acute inflammatory process that affects the optic nerve, usually of autoimmune origin, with segmental destruction of the myelin sheath and, to a lesser extent, the axons. This demyelination interferes with the conduction of visual impulses, leading to decreased visual acuity, scotomas, and loss of color discrimination [2, 3].

The immunological basis of optic neuritis varies according to etiology. In multiple sclerosis (MS), lymphocyte activation triggers an immune-mediated attack against myelin components, primarily myelin basic protein, leading to the infiltration of T-cells, macrophages, and the production of inflammatory cytokines [5]. In cases of NMOSD, the main target is aquaporin-4 (AQP4), a protein expressed in astrocytes, which leads to primary astrocytopathy. In contrast, in MOGAD, the target is myelin oligodendrocyte glycoprotein, causing a distinct clinical and evolutionary phenotype [8].

The pain linked to optic neuritis arises from the inflammation of the optic nerve sheath and its surrounding structures, especially the dura mater, which is innervated by nociceptive fibers of the trigeminal nerve [5, 9]. Eye movements typically worsen this pain due to the stretching of the inflamed nerve within the orbit, a characteristic feature [2].

Histopathological and imaging studies demonstrate perivascular infiltration and disruption of the blood-brain barrier in the acute phase of the disease. Contrast-enhanced magnetic resonance imaging usually shows enhancement of the optic nerve in intraorbital or intracanalicular segments, reflecting active inflammation [10]. Optical coherence tomography (OCT) studies demonstrate progressive reduction of the retinal nerve fiber layer (RNFL), particularly in patients with MS, reflecting chronic axonal loss [6, 11].

Understanding the different immunopathological mechanisms is essential not only for the differential diagnosis between the variants of optic neuritis but also for defining the prognosis and the best therapeutic approach.

53.3 Characteristics of Pain

Pain is one of the most prominent and early features of optic neuritis (ON), particularly in its demyelinating form. It is present in approximately 90% of cases and often precedes visual symptoms by several hours to days [2, 3, 5]. The typical pain is described as deep, dull, and retro-orbital, sometimes radiating to the frontal or temporal regions. It is characteristically worsened by eye movement, a hallmark that helps distinguish ON from other causes of visual loss [2, 9].

This pain, as already mentioned, results from inflammatory involvement of the optic nerve sheath and surrounding dura mater, which is innervated by nociceptive fibers of the ophthalmic branch of the trigeminal nerve. The intraorbital portion of the optic nerve is particularly vulnerable, as it is mobile and subjected to mechanical traction during ocular motility [2]. This explains why pain associated with eye movement is a highly specific indicator for optic neuritis and serves as an essential diagnostic clue.

Unlike other optic neuropathies, such as non-arteritic anterior ischemic optic neuropathy (NAION) or Leber hereditary optic neuropathy (LHON), which are typically painless, the presence of periocular or retro-orbital pain is a critical feature suggestive of an inflammatory demyelinating process [5, 12].

For some patients, pain might be the sole symptom at the initial presentation, particularly in the early stages, which can result in diagnostic delays. This underscores the importance of maintaining a high index of suspicion when evaluating patients with unilateral orbital pain of unclear etiology—even in the absence of immediate visual complaints [1, 3].

Although pain usually resolves spontaneously within a few days, it can significantly impair quality of life. Fortunately, it is generally responsive to corticosteroid therapy, which reduces inflammation and hastens symptom resolution [2, 13].

53.4 Case Presentation

A 25-year-old woman presented to the Neurology Outpatient Clinic at Hospital Geral de Fortaleza, Brazil. She reports experiencing a sudden onset of decreased visual acuity in the left eye on August 27, 2024, initially presenting with ocular pain upon horizontal eye movement and a left-sided frontotemporal headache, dyschromatopsia, associated with a progressive reduction in visual acuity over one week.

Neurological examination was normal except for a left afferent pupillary defect and decreased visual acuity on the left eye limited to hand motion. Ocular motility was intact but painful in the left eye.

Magnetic resonance imaging (MRI) of the brain and orbits demonstrate increased T2-weighted signal intensity in the posterior intraorbital segment of the left optic nerve, which, even in the absence of enhancement on post-gadolinium images, was interpreted as consistent with acute inflammatory left optic neuritis. There is no evidence of significant optic nerve atrophy, orbital inflammation, or involvement of extraocular muscles. No additional intracranial lesions or demyelinating plaques were identified on the available sequences (Fig. 53.1).

Cerebrospinal fluid (CSF) analysis was unremarkable, with normal protein and cell count, negative infectious screening, and no intrathecal IgG synthesis. AQP4 and MOG antibodies tested after treatment initiation were negative. The ophthalmologic evaluation revealed left eye visual acuity of 20/100 with questionable slight optic disk edema. Laboratory results were largely normal.

The patient received intravenous (IV) methylprednisolone 1 g/day for five days. Due to the persistence of the severity of vision loss on the fifth day, plasmapheresis was initiated but limited to one session due to logistical constraints. At discharge two weeks later, her left eye's visual acuity had improved partially, and the pain had subsided.

She was diagnosed with unilateral PON as a clinically isolated syndrome (CIS), with no evidence of MS, NMOSD, or MOGAD. A follow-up plan included outpatient neuroimmunology review, prednisone tapering, and repeat AQP4 and MOG testing.

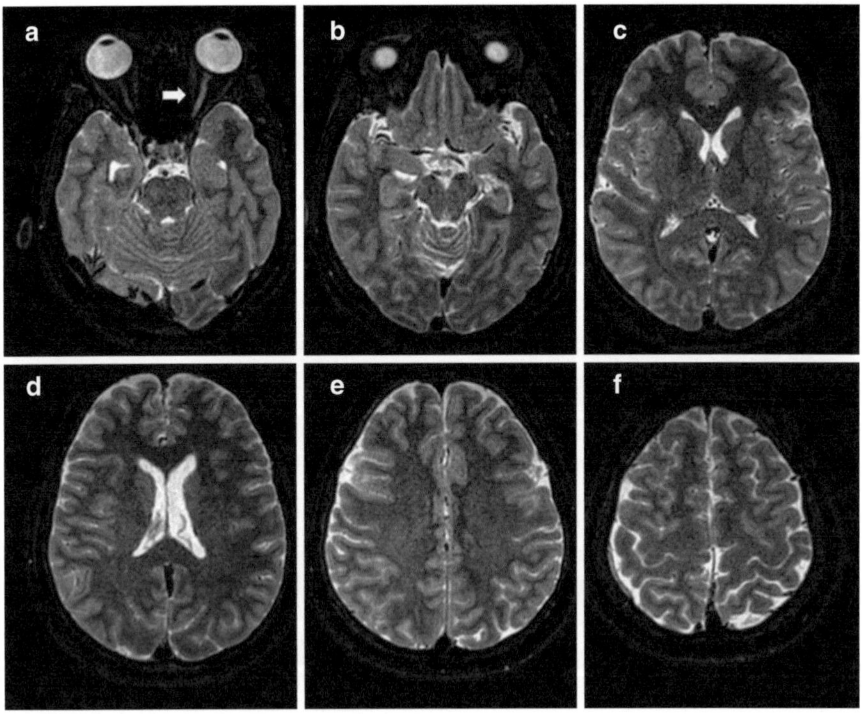

Fig. 53.1 MRI findings demonstrate increased T2-weighted signal intensity in the posterior intraorbital segment of the left optic nerve (white arrow), consistent with acute left optic neuritis (**a**). No additional intracranial abnormalities or demyelinating lesions are identified on this axial enhanced T2-weighted 3D sequence (**b**–**f**)

53.5 Case Discussion

This case fulfils the ICHD-3 criteria for PON [4]. The temporal relationship between retro-orbital pain and subsequent visual decline, with pain exacerbated by eye movement, is typical of demyelinating optic neuritis. MRI findings of increased T2-weighted signal intensity in the posterior intraorbital segment of the left optic nerve is consistent with acute inflammatory left optic neuritis. The absence of gadolinium enhancement does not rule out optic neuritis [7]. Although the patient's AQP4 and MOG antibody tests were negative, the timing of testing—after corticosteroid initiation—may have reduced their diagnostic sensitivity [8]. The absence of oligoclonal bands in the CSF and a normal brain MRI suggest a diagnosis of clinically isolated syndrome (CIS), with no current criteria for MS, NMOSD, or MOGAD [2, 11].

53.6 Clinical Characteristics

This case highlights several key aspects of painful optic neuropathies. First, the differential diagnosis of painful visual loss must consider optic neuritis, especially in young adults, but also include compressive lesions, infectious optic neuritis (e.g., syphilitic or viral), sarcoidosis, and perioptic neuritis secondary to systemic autoimmune diseases. Pain in optic neuropathies typically results from inflammation of the optic nerve sheath and its meningeal covering, both of which are innervated by the ophthalmic branch of the trigeminal nerve [2, 14]. The presence of pain with eye movement is particularly useful in distinguishing inflammatory causes from ischemic or compressive etiologies, which are usually painless.

In compressive optic neuropathies, caused by orbital masses, aneurysms, or optic canal lesions, pain may occur if adjacent tissues are involved; however, the progression is typically subacute or chronic, with less sudden visual decline. Ischemic optic neuropathy (e.g., NAION) is usually painless and occurs in older individuals with vascular risk factors. Hereditary optic neuropathies, such as Leber hereditary optic neuropathy (LHON), also tend to present with painless bilateral vision loss [12].

The partial visual recovery after corticosteroid therapy in this patient is consistent with demyelinating optic neuritis. While one session of plasmapheresis was administered, its clinical necessity is uncertain in cases that begin to improve promptly. Nonetheless, it is noteworthy that early consideration of escalated therapy in severe visual loss may preserve vision when steroid response is inadequate [13, 14].

Close outpatient follow-up is essential for monitoring recurrence and determining the need for long-term immunomodulatory therapy, especially if new symptoms or lesions emerge on follow-up imaging. Repeat AQP4 and MOG antibody testing is appropriate, ideally in a steroid-free window, to rule out antibody-mediated demyelinating syndromes. This case highlights the importance of a structured diagnostic approach to managing painful optic neuropathies, integrating clinical, radiological, and serological data to inform both immediate management and long-term surveillance.

53.7 Diagnostics and Differential Diagnosis

The diagnosis of PON is primarily clinical, guided by a thorough history and neurological examination. However, neuroimaging and electrophysiological studies are essential for confirmation and to exclude alternative etiologies.

Key clinical findings include:

- Subacute onset of monocular vision loss.
- Pain exacerbated by eye movement.
- Central scotoma or visual field defects.
- Dyschromatopsia (especially red desaturation).
- Relative afferent pupillary defect (RAPD), unless bilateral.

Fundoscopy is often normal in retrobulbar neuritis—the most common form—but may show optic disk swelling (papillitis) in up to one-third of cases [9, 15].

MRI of the orbits with gadolinium contrast is the imaging modality of choice. Enhancement of the optic nerve, especially in the intraorbital segment, confirms active inflammation and supports the diagnosis [1]. Optic nerve enhancement is present in approximately 90% of typical ON cases and may persist for several weeks after symptom onset [14]. Brain MRI is also performed to assess for demyelinating lesions suggestive of multiple sclerosis (MS) or other central nervous system inflammatory diseases [1].

Typical radiological findings include:

- T2 hyperintensity and contrast enhancement of the optic nerve.
- Absence of mass effect or compressive lesions.
- Periventricular or juxtacortical lesions in MS.

Visual Evoked Potentials (VEP) testing can reveal delayed P100 latency in the affected eye, reflecting demyelination along the visual pathway. While less specific than MRI, it remains useful when imaging is inconclusive or unavailable [15].

Optical Coherence Tomography (OCT) provides structural information on the peripapillary retinal nerve fiber layer (RNFL) and the ganglion cell layer. RNFL thinning becomes evident weeks after the acute phase and correlates with axonal loss and long-term visual prognosis [1, 6].

CSF examination is recommended in atypical cases or when an inflammatory or infectious etiology is suspected. The presence of oligoclonal bands is an established biomarker for MS and predicts increased risk of disease conversion in clinically isolated syndromes (CIS) [16].

Several conditions may mimic the clinical picture of optic neuritis and must be excluded [17]:

- *Non-arteritic anterior ischemic optic neuropathy (NAION)*: Typically occurs in older patients with vascular risk factors, and presents with painless vision loss and altitudinal field defects. The optic disk is swollen and pale.
- *Compressive optic neuropathies*: Caused by tumors or aneurysms. These evolve slowly and rarely present with pain or acute visual decline.
- *Leber hereditary optic neuropathy (LHON)*: Painless, bilateral visual loss in young males, often with a family history. Mitochondrial inheritance.
- *Infectious optic neuritis*: Associated with syphilis, Lyme disease, tuberculosis, or viral infections (e.g., herpes zoster, Cytomegalovirus (CMV)), particularly in immunocompromised individuals.
- *Autoimmune optic neuropathies*: Sarcoidosis, systemic lupus erythematosus, and Behçet's disease can cause optic nerve inflammation, often accompanied by systemic signs.
- *Neuromyelitis optica spectrum disorder (NMOSD)*: Frequently bilateral, severe, and relapsing. Serum AQP4-IgG positivity helps confirm the diagnosis.
- *MOG antibody disease (MOGAD)*: Often indistinguishable from typical ON at onset, but more likely to involve bilateral or recurrent optic neuritis and better visual recovery [8].

A comprehensive diagnostic workup incorporating clinical features, imaging, and laboratory testing is essential to distinguish PON from these conditions and guide appropriate management.

53.8 Treatment

The PON management is designed to reduce inflammation, accelcrate visual recovery, alleviate pain, and, in select cases, initiate long-term immunomodulatory therapy. Treatment decisions are based on clinical presentation, imaging findings, serological markers, and the likelihood of progression to chronic demyelinating disease [18].

High-dose intravenous corticosteroids are the mainstay of treatment for acute demyelinating optic neuritis. The standard regimen consists of methylprednisolone 1 g/day intravenously for 3–5 consecutive days, optionally followed by an oral taper with prednisone (typically 1 mg/kg/day for 11–14 days) [3, 5].

The pivotal Optic Neuritis Treatment Trial (ONTT) demonstrated that intravenous corticosteroids significantly hasten visual recovery but do not improve long-term visual acuity compared to placebo [13]. Additionally, oral corticosteroids alone (without initial IV treatment) were associated with a higher rate of recurrence and are therefore not recommended as monotherapy in typical ON [7, 13].

Corticosteroids usually lead to rapid pain resolution by suppressing inflammation. In cases where pain is severe or persists despite treatment, adjunctive use of non-steroidal anti-inflammatory drugs (NSAIDs) may be beneficial. However, more potent analgesics are rarely indicated, as pain generally resolves within a few days [3, 5].

In severe or steroid-refractory cases, particularly those with profound visual loss or bilateral involvement, plasma exchange (PLEX) may be considered. Evidence supports its use in NMOSD-related optic neuritis and in a subset of severe MS-related optic neuritis unresponsive to steroids [19].

Intravenous immunoglobulin (IVIG) has limited evidence for efficacy in optic neuritis and is generally reserved for select cases, including those associated with MOG-antibody disease or when PLEX is contraindicated [20].

Patients with CIS and high-risk features—such as abnormal brain MRI or positive oligoclonal bands in CSF—should be evaluated for early initiation of DMTs to reduce the risk of conversion to multiple sclerosis [15]. Options include interferon-beta, glatiramer acetate, or newer oral and monoclonal antibody agents, depending on patient-specific factors and risk stratification [18].

In cases of NMOSD, long-term immunosuppression with agents such as rituximab, eculizumab, or inebilizumab is critical to prevent relapses and severe disability (19). Similarly, MOGAD may require long-term immunotherapy in recurrent cases, often using corticosteroid-sparing agents like azathioprine or mycophenolate mofetil [20].

Follow-up includes serial assessment of visual function, OCT to monitor axonal loss, and MRI if there is suspicion of new demyelinating lesions. Visual rehabilitation, including contrast sensitivity training and low-vision aids, may be beneficial for patients with residual deficits [1, 3].

53.9 Conclusion

PON remains one of the most common and clinically significant causes of acute monocular vision loss in young adults. Recognizing the typical presentation—retro-orbital pain exacerbated by eye movement followed by subacute visual impairment—is crucial for timely diagnosis and management. The diagnostic process should integrate careful clinical assessment with magnetic resonance imaging, visual evoked potentials, and, when indicated, cerebrospinal fluid analysis and antibody testing.

While corticosteroids remain the cornerstone of acute management, they primarily accelerate recovery rather than improve long-term visual outcomes. Identifying patients at higher risk for progression to MS, NMOSD, or MOGAD is essential to guide early initiation of disease-modifying therapy and prevent future relapses.

Differentiating PON from other causes of optic neuropathy—such as ischemic, compressive, hereditary, or infectious etiologies—requires a structured, multidisciplinary approach. Advances in imaging and biomarker detection have significantly enhanced the clinician's ability to establish an early and accurate diagnosis.

Ultimately, the effective management of PON depends not only on controlling the acute inflammatory episode but also on a long-term strategy that includes risk stratification, neuroimmunological evaluation, patient education, and, when necessary, visual rehabilitation.

References

1. Alshahrani Y, Korkoman A, Alghamdi A, Alshehri M, Alremthi F, Alshahrani M. Optic neuritis: a review of diagnostic imaging modalities and effective management approaches. Int J Med Dev Countries. 2024;8(4):1776–80.
2. Ayuso Blanco T, Aliseda D, Ajuria I, Zandio B, Mayor S, Navarro MC. Inflammatory optic neuritis. An Sist Sanit Navar. 2009;32(2):249–63.
3. Spillers NJ, Luther PM, Talbot NC, Kidder EJ, Doyle CA, Lutfallah SC, Derouen AG, Tirumala S, Ahmadzadeh S, Shekoohi S, Kaye AD, Varrassi G. A comparative review of typical and atypical optic neuritis: advancements in treatments, diagnostics, and prognosis. Cureus. 2024;16(3):e56094. https://doi.org/10.7759/cureus.56094.
4. Headache Classification Committee of the International Headache Society (IHS). The International Classification of Headache Disorders, 3rd edition. Cephalalgia. 2018;38(1):1–211.
5. Bennett JL. Optic neuritis. Continuum (Minneap Minn). 2019;25(5):1236–64.
6. de Seze J, Blanc F, Jeanjean L, Zéphir H, Labauge P, Bouyon M, Ballonzoli L, Castelnovo G, Fleury M, Defoort S, Vermersch P, Speeg C. Optical coherence tomography in neuromyelitis optica. Arch Neurol. 2008;65(7):920–3. https://doi.org/10.1001/archneur.65.7.920.
7. Hickman SJ, Dalton CM, Miller DH, Plant GT. Management of acute optic neuritis. Lancet. 2002;360(9349):1953–62.
8. Cacciaguerra L, Flanagan EP. Updates in NMOSD and MOGAD diagnosis and treatment: a tale of two central nervous system autoimmune inflammatory disorders. Neurol Clin. 2024;42(1):77–114.
9. Toosy AT, Mason DF, Miller DH. Optic neuritis. Lancet Neurol. 2014;13(1):83–99.
10. Pleşa A, Antochi FA, Macovei ML, Vîrlan AG, Georgescu R, Beuran DI, Bucurica SN, Sîrbu CA, Axelerad A, Pleşa FC. Eyes as windows: unveiling neuroinflammation in multiple sclerosis via optic neuritis and Uhthoff's phenomenon. Diagnostics (Basel). 2024;14(19):2198. https://doi.org/10.3390/diagnostics14192198.
11. Tong B, Zhang X, Hu H, Yang H, Wang X, Zhong M, Yang F, Hua F. From diagnosis to treatment: exploring the mechanisms underlying optic neuritis in multiple sclerosis. J Transl Med. 2025;23(1):87. https://doi.org/10.1186/s12967-025-06105-1.
12. Petzold A, Fraser CL, Abegg M, Alroughani R, Alshowaeir D, Alvarenga R, Andris C, Asgari N, Barnett Y, Battistella R, Behbehani R, Berger T, Bikbov MM, Biotti D, Biousse V, Boschi A, Brazdil M, Brezhnev A, Calabresi PA, Cordonnier M, Costello F, Cruz FM, Cunha LP, Daoudi S, Deschamps R, de Seze J, Diem R, Etemadifar M, Flores-Rivera J, Fonseca P, Frederiksen J, Frohman E, Frohman T, Tilikete CF, Fujihara K, Gálvez A, Gouider R, Gracia F, Grigoriadis N, Guajardo JM, Habek M, Hawlina M, Martínez-Lapiscina EH, Hooker J, Hor JY, Howlett W, Huang-Link Y, Idrissova Z, Illes Z, Jancic J, Jindahra P, Karussis D, Kerty E, Kim HJ, Lagrèze W, Leocani L, Levin N, Liskova P, Liu Y, Maiga Y, Marignier R, McGuigan C, Meira D, Merle H, Monteiro MLR, Moodley A, Moura F, Muñoz S, Mustafa S, Nakashima I, Noval S, Oehninger C, Ogun O, Omoti A, Pandit L, Paul F, Rebolleda G, Reddel S, Rejdak K, Rejdak R, Rodriguez-Morales AJ, Rougier MB, Sa MJ, Sanchez-Dalmau B, Saylor D, Shatriah I, Siva A, Stiebel-Kalish H, Szatmary G, Ta L, Tenembaum S, Tran H, Trufanov Y, van Pesch V, Wang AG, Wattjes MP, Willoughby E, Zakaria M, Zvornicanin J, Balcer L, Plant GT. Diagnosis and classification of optic neuritis. Lancet Neurol. 2022;21(12):1120–34. https://doi.org/10.1016/S1474-4422(22)00200-9.
13. Beck RW, Cleary PA, Anderson MM Jr, Keltner JL, Shults WT, Kaufman DI, Buckley EG, Corbett JJ, Kupersmith MJ, Miller NR, et al. A randomized, controlled trial of corticosteroids

in the treatment of acute optic neuritis. The Optic Neuritis Study Group. N Engl J Med. 1992;326(9):581–8. https://doi.org/10.1056/NEJM199202273260901.
14. Hickman SJ, Petzold A. Update on optic neuritis: an international view. Neuro-Ophthalmology. 2022;46(1):1–18.
15. Jamali Dogahe S, Pakravan P, Pakravan M. Acute optic neuritis: an update on approach and management. J Ophthalmic Vis Res. 2023;18(4):433–40.
16. Tintore M, Rovira À, Río J, Otero-Romero S, Arrambide G, Tur C, Comabella M, Nos C, Arévalo MJ, Negrotto L, Galán I, Vidal-Jordana A, Castilló J, Palavra F, Simon E, Mitjana R, Auger C, Sastre-Garriga J, Montalban X. Defining high, medium and low impact prognostic factors for developing multiple sclerosis. Brain. 2015;138(Pt 7):1863–74. https://doi.org/10.1093/brain/awv105.
17. Benard-Seguin E, Costello F. A practical approach to the diagnosis and management of optic neuritis. Ann Indian Acad Neurol. 2022;25(Suppl 2):S48–53.
18. Montalban X, Gold R, Thompson AJ, Otero-Romero S, Amato MP, Chandraratna D, Clanet M, Comi G, Derfuss T, Fazekas F, Hartung HP, Havrdova E, Hemmer B, Kappos L, Liblau R, Lubetzki C, Marcus E, Miller DH, Olsson T, Pilling S, Selmaj K, Siva A, Sorensen PS, Sormani MP, Thalheim C, Wiendl H, Zipp F. ECTRIMS/EAN guideline on the pharmacological treatment of people with multiple sclerosis. Eur J Neurol. 2018;25(2):215–37. https://doi.org/10.1111/ene.13536. Epub 2018 Jan 19. Erratum in: Eur J Neurol. 2018 Mar;25(3):605. doi: 10.1111/ene.13590.
19. Wingerchuk DM, Banwell B, Bennett JL, Cabre P, Carroll W, Chitnis T, de Seze J, Fujihara K, Greenberg B, Jacob A, Jarius S, Lana-Peixoto M, Levy M, Simon JH, Tenembaum S, Traboulsee AL, Waters P, Wellik KE, Weinshenker BG. International Panel for NMO Diagnosis. International consensus diagnostic criteria for neuromyelitis optica spectrum disorders. Neurology. 2015;85(2):177–89. https://doi.org/10.1212/WNL.0000000000001729.
20. Jurynczyk M, Messina S, Woodhall MR, Raza N, Everett R, Roca-Fernandez A, Tackley G, Hamid S, Sheard A, Reynolds G, Chandratre S, Hemingway C, Jacob A, Vincent A, Leite MI, Waters P, Palace J. Clinical presentation and prognosis in MOG-antibody disease: a UK study. Brain. 2017;140(12):3128–38. https://doi.org/10.1093/brain/awx276.

Chapter 54
Paratrigeminal Oculosympathetic (Raeder's) Syndrome

Renan Domingues

54.1 Introduction

Raeder's syndrome is defined by the triad of unilateral headache (typically periorbital or temporal) and partial Horner's syndrome (ptosis and miosis without facial anhidrosis). It is caused by lesions affecting the postganglionic oculosympathetic fibers adjacent to the internal carotid artery (ICA), particularly in the region of the cavernous sinus or middle cranial fossa. First described in 1924 by Johan Georg Raeder, the syndrome remains a relevant differential diagnosis in patients with painful Horner's syndrome [1].

The most common structural etiologies include tumors, inflammation, and vascular abnormalities such as dissection or aneurysm of the internal carotid artery [2–5]. The clinical presentation often mimics trigeminal autonomic cephalalgias (TACs), such as cluster headaches, but with distinctive neuro-ophthalmologic findings [6].

54.2 Pathophysiology

Raeder's syndrome results from injury or compression of postganglionic oculosympathetic fibers that travel along the internal carotid artery (ICA), particularly within its petrous and cavernous segments. These fibers originate from preganglionic neurons located in the intermediolateral gray matter of the spinal cord (levels T1–T3). After synapsing in the superior cervical ganglion, postganglionic fibers form a

R. Domingues (✉)
Headache Clinic, Neurology Section, Santa Casa de Misericórdia, São Paulo, Brazil
e-mail: contato@renandomingues.med.br

D. Uludüz et al. (eds.), *Rare Causes of Headache Disorders*, Headache,
https://doi.org/10.1007/978-3-032-10242-3_54

pericarotid plexus and ascend within the carotid canal, closely adherent to the arterial wall [2].

In the petrous portion, these fibers are especially vulnerable due to their intimate contact with the ICA and the surrounding bony canal. After ascending through the cavernous sinus, they reach ocular structures to innervate the pupillary dilator, and along this pathway, they maintain close anatomical proximity to the ophthalmic artery and cranial nerves III, IV, and VI. Lesions in this pathway result in ptosis and miosis, but not anhidrosis, since sudomotor fibers travel with branches of the external carotid artery. Contemporary evidence, particularly from anatomical and immunohistochemical studies, supports the existence of a lateral sellar plexus formed by sympathetic, parasympathetic, and trigeminal fibers around the ICA wall [3, 5, 6].

Raeder's syndrome is classically subdivided into two types: Type I, in which the oculosympathetic paresis is accompanied by cranial nerve involvement (typically III, IV, or VI), indicating a more extensive lesion in the parasellar region; and Type II, characterized by isolated hemicranial pain and partial Horner's syndrome without other cranial neuropathies, often reflecting more selective involvement of postganglionic sympathetic fibers adjacent to the ICA [3, 5]. Mechanical compression or ischemic injury to this region, regardless of the etiology, can activate nociceptive trigeminovascular pathways. This leads to pain referred to the orbital, nasal, or deep facial areas without sensory loss. Neurogenic inflammation may contribute to pain generation through the release of antidromic peptides (e.g., substance P, Calcitonin gene-related peptide (CGRP)), thereby enhancing pain perception and autonomic dysfunction [2].

54.3 Case Presentation

A 41-year-old woman presented to the emergency department with the acute onset of severe left-sided periorbital and temporal headache, associated with drooping of the left eyelid and photophobia. She denied visual loss, trauma, or systemic symptoms. On neurological examination, she had left-sided ptosis and miosis without anhidrosis or ophthalmoplegia. Extraocular movements and visual acuity were normal. The rest of the neurological exam was unremarkable.

Computed tomography angiography (CTA) and magnetic resonance imaging/magnetic resonance angiography (MRI/MRA) of the brain and cervical vessels revealed a dissection with pseudoaneurysm of the left internal carotid artery in its paraclinoid segment (Figs. 54.1 and 54.2). No signs of infarction or subarachnoid hemorrhage were present. The imaging findings, together with the clinical features of unilateral headache and partial Horner's syndrome without cranial nerve involvement, were consistent with Raeder's syndrome type II due to an ICA lesion compressing postganglionic oculosympathetic fibers traveling along this artery.

The patient was treated conservatively with analgesics and antiplatelet therapy. Follow-up imaging confirmed stabilization of the vascular lesion. Over the

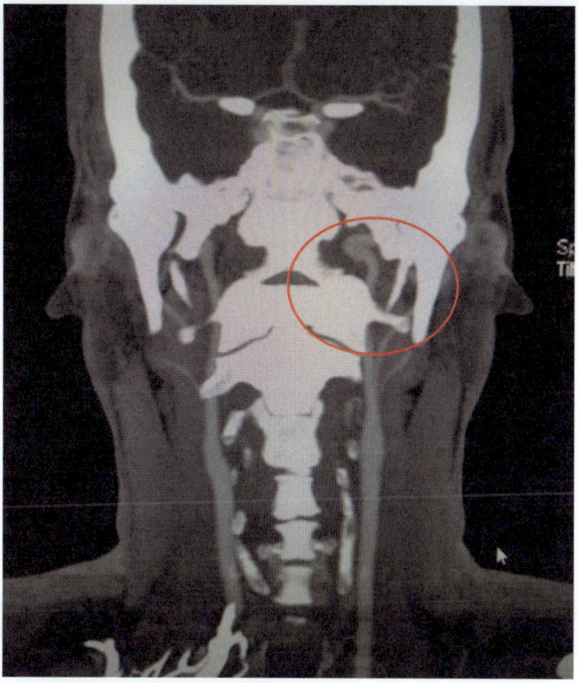

Fig. 54.1 Cranial and cervical arterial angiotomography coronal view. The red circle shows a left artery carotid artery pseudoaneurysm

following weeks, the ptosis gradually improved, and headache episodes became less frequent and less intense.

54.4 Case Discussion

Raeder's syndrome is a painful oculosympathetic paresis due to involvement of sympathetic fibers distal to the bifurcation of the common carotid artery. The first case reports were associated with parasellar masses or inflammatory lesions [1]. Some of the first cases did not have an obvious structural etiology when investigated using the methods available at the time. They were therefore classified as idiopathic or benign Raeder's syndrome, but these cases were most likely associated with some involvement of the ICA [7]. One of the most critical and potentially life-threatening causes of this syndrome is ICA dissection occurring in the paraclinoid or cavernous segment [2, 4].

The anatomical proximity of the postganglionic sympathetic fibers to this artery in the cavernous sinus explains how vascular wall disruption can result in partial Horner's syndrome and ipsilateral trigeminal pain. The sympathetic fibers are affected by direct compression, perivascular inflammation, or ischemia [2, 6].

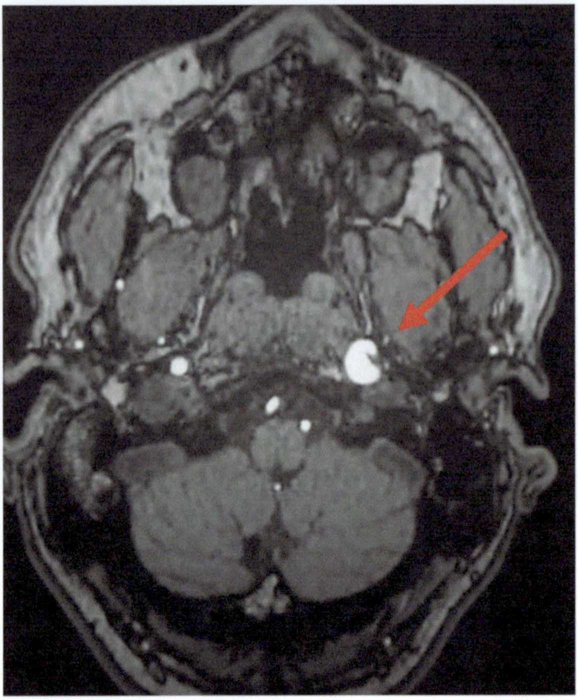

Fig. 54.2 Magnetic resonance angiography. The red arrow shows a left artery carotid artery pseudoaneurysm

54.5 Clinical Characteristics

Dissection of the internal carotid artery is an underrecognized cause of painful Horner's syndrome and is often missed unless actively investigated with high-resolution MRI/MRA or CTA [7]. Importantly, the clinical presentation may resemble cluster headache, leading to initial misdiagnosis. However, unlike primary headaches, Raeder's syndrome secondary to vascular lesions often has an acute or subacute onset, is persistent rather than paroxysmal, and may be associated with warning signs such as ptosis or focal neurological symptoms [6, 7]. In the present case, timely imaging investigations enabled the identification of the underlying etiology. The pseudoaneurysm represented a consequence of the spontaneous ICA dissection [8]. This evolution of the dissection further increases the risk of secondary complications such as embolic stroke or subarachnoid hemorrhage. Therefore, the recognition of Raeder's syndrome as a neuro-ophthalmological emergency in the context of carotid pathology is critical.

54.6 Diagnostic Algorithm

Step 1: Clinical evaluation

- Unilateral periorbital or temporal headache
- Ptosis and miosis without anhidrosis
- Cranial nerve palsies investigation

  Step 2: Neuroimaging

- MRI/MRA or CTA of intracranial and cervical arteries to evaluate for dissection or pseudoaneurysm

  Step 3: Classification

- Type I: Raeder's syndrome with cranial nerve involvement
- Type II: Isolated oculosympathetic paresis with hemicranial pain

54.7 Management

Treatment is directed by etiology:

- Vascular (e.g., dissection, aneurysm):
  - Antiplatelet or anticoagulant therapy
  - Neurological monitoring
  - In selected cases, endovascular intervention
- Idiopathic/Benign forms:
  - Non-steroidal anti-inflammatory drugs (NSAIDs), indomethacin, verapamil
- Neoplastic or inflammatory causes:
  - Immunosuppression or surgery as indicated

Spontaneous resolution is the most common outcome of spontaneous internal carotid artery dissection, as observed in this patient, who improved clinically over time without the need for invasive intervention [9].

54.8 Conclusion

Raeder's syndrome lies at the intersection between trigeminal autonomic cephalalgias and painful cranial neuropathies. While first associated with parasellar masses or inflammatory lesions in the first reports, one of the most critical and potentially life-threatening causes is the ICA dissection, especially when it occurs in the paraclinoid or cavernous segment [1–5].

Raeder's syndrome is not currently included in the International Classification of Headache Disorders, third edition (ICHD-3) [10], and this reflects the fact that it is not a headache disorder per se, but rather a topographical and syndromic description of a lesion affecting the postganglionic oculosympathetic pathway adjacent to the trigeminal nerve. The term “Raeder’s syndrome” designates a specific anatomical pattern rather than a single pathophysiological mechanism. As such, it encompasses different etiologies, including vascular, neoplastic, or infectious, that share the same neuroanatomical distribution of symptoms. Despite its absence from formal classifications, recognizing this pattern remains highly valuable in clinical neurology and neuro-ophthalmology.

Raeder’s syndrome exemplifies the clinical anatomical methodology of early twentieth-century neurology, in which disease patterns were mapped to anatomical topographies rather than etiological categories. Raeder’s detailed description of oculopupillary sympathetic dysfunction due to the middle cranial fossa lesions provided an early framework for understanding painful Horner’s syndromes, long before the advent of modern neuroimaging. Whether viewed as a historical term or anatomically grounded description, Raeder’s clinical insight represents a significant contribution to the understanding of the pathways connecting cranial pain and autonomic dysfunction.

References

1. Shoja MM, Tubbs RS, Ghabili K, Loukas M, Oakes WJ, Cohen-Gadol AA. Johan Georg Raeder (1889-1959) and paratrigeminal sympathetic paresis. Childs Nerv Syst. 2010;26(3):373–6. https://doi.org/10.1007/s00381-009-0965-9.
2. Tatsui CE, Prevedello DM, Koerbel A, Cordeiro JG, Ditzel LF, Araujo JC. Raeder’s syndrome after embolization of a giant intracavernous carotid artery aneurysm: pathophysiological considerations. Arq Neuropsiquiatr. 2005;63(3A):676–80. https://doi.org/10.1590/s0004-282x2005000400024.
3. Solomon S. Raeder syndrome. Arch Neurol. 2001;58(4):661–2. https://doi.org/10.1001/archneur.58.4.661.
4. Higa Lee AA, Montouro Stoarri AC, Domingues R. Internal carotid artery dissection associated with acute dengue virus infection: a case report. Headache Med. 2024;15(1):38–40. https://doi.org/10.48208/HeadacheMed.2024.10.
5. Salvesen R. Raeder’s syndrome. Cephalalgia. 1999;19(Suppl 25):42–5. https://doi.org/10.1177/0333102499019s2511.
6. Goadsby PJ. Raeder’s syndrome: paratrigeminal paralysis of the oculopupillary sympathetic system. J Neurol Neurosurg Psychiatry. 2002;72(3):297–9. https://doi.org/10.1136/jnnp.72.3.297.
7. Solomon S, Lustig JP. Benign Raeder’s syndrome is probably a manifestation of carotid artery disease. Cephalalgia. 2001;21(1):1–11. https://doi.org/10.1046/j.1468-2982.2001.00139.x.
8. Chaves C, Estol C, Esnaola MM, Gorson K, O’Donoghue M, De Witt LD, Caplan LR. Spontaneous intracranial internal carotid artery dissection: report of 10 patients. Arch Neurol. 2002;59(6):977–81. https://doi.org/10.1001/archneur.59.6.977.
9. Rao AS, Makaroun MS, Marone LK, Cho JS, Rhee R, Chaer RA. Long-term outcomes of internal carotid artery dissection. J Vasc Surg. 2011;54(2):370–5. https://doi.org/10.1016/j.jvs.2011.02.059.
10. Headache Classification Committee of the International Headache Society (IHS) The International Classification of Headache Disorders, 3rd edition. Cephalalgia. 2018;38(1):1–211. https://doi.org/10.1177/0333102417738202

Chapter 55
Burning Mouth Syndrome

Daniela Aparecida de Godoi Gonçalves, Juliana Stuginski Barbosa, and Marlon Ferreira Dias

55.1 Introduction

Burning mouth syndrome (BMS) is a condition characterized by persistent intraoral burning or dysesthetic sensation without a medical or dental cause, recurring for more than two hours per day for more than three months [23]. It is classified as a neuropathic pain disorder [1], more frequently occurring among women than men, with studies reporting female-to-male ratio ~7:1 [2]. The prevalence rates range from 0.7% up to 15%, being higher among postmenopausal women and increasing with age in both sexes [2, 3].

The symptoms involve the anterior two-thirds of the tongue, lips, and palate [4], and it is commonly accompanied by xerostomia and taste disturbances. The condition significantly impacts the patients' daily activity as speaking and eating [5], reducing the quality of life and leading to emotional distress and sleep disturbances [6–8].

The diagnosis is primarily clinical, requiring the exclusion of other conditions that may cause similar discomfort [9]. It is a diagnostic challenge because its symptoms overlap with various systemic and local conditions, including oral candidiasis, vitamin deficiencies, diabetes mellitus, and autoimmune disorders like Sjögren's syndrome. Therefore, it is crucial to observe the characteristics of pain (onset, duration, location, exacerbating/ameliorating factors) and psychological and sleep profile [10].

D. A. de Godoi Gonçalves (✉) · M. F. Dias
São Paulo State University, School of Dentistry, Araraquara, Brazil
e-mail: daniela.g.goncalves@unesp.br

J. S. Barbosa
Bauru Orofacial Pain Group, University of São Paulo, School of Dentistry, Bauru, Brazil

D. Uludüz et al. (eds.), *Rare Causes of Headache Disorders*, Headache,
https://doi.org/10.1007/978-3-032-10242-3_55

55.2 Pathophysiology

The etiology of BMS is multifactorial and may include neuropsychological factors (nervous system dysfunction and psychological disturbances), local factors (inappropriate dentures, salivary gland diseases), and systemic factors (malnutrition, anemia, thyroid disease, menopause syndrome, diabetes mellitus, and immune system deficiency) [1, 11]. The pathophysiology, in turn, is complex, encompassing neuropathic, endocrinological, and psychoneuroimmunological mechanisms.

A growing body of evidence indicates BMS is, at least in part, a neuropathic pain condition. Quantitative sensory testing (QST) reveals that many BMS patients have altered somatosensory function in the oral mucosa as decreased sensitivity to warmth and cold [12]. Besides, there is evidence of atrophy of the tongue's epithelium resulting in a reduced number of fibers innervating the taste buds and variations in the trigeminal innervation of the fungiform papillae that may contribute to a decrease in afferent nerve impulses [13–15]. It has also been demonstrated an increased expression of pain-associated neuroreceptors (TRPV1, P2X3) and sodium channels (Nav1.7) in mucosal nerves [15, 16]. Such changes indicate damage or dysfunction in small trigeminal nerve fibers and are suggestive of small-fiber neuropathy [12]. Additionally, brain function in the processing of nociceptive input is altered and has patterns like those of patients who had other neuropathic pain conditions [17, 18].

Regarding endocrinological factors, the striking female predominance and typical onset around menopause suggest that hormonal factors contribute to BMS. Estrogen withdrawal has been hypothesized to play a role in the thickening and keratinization of the tongue, increased expression of proteins that intensify pain, as well as dysfunction of salivary glands, resulting in dry mouth and burning pain [14]. Another hormonal factor that can contribute is related to a dysfunction of the hypothalamic–pituitary–adrenal axis (HPA axis), also known as the stress axis. Cortisol (a glucocorticoid hormone) levels are often elevated in BMS patients under basal conditions, which might reflect chronic stress or altered diurnal rhythm. Notably, recent findings point to possible circadian rhythm disruptions in BMS pathology [2, 14].

Psychological factors, such as chronic stress, anxiety disorder, and depression, have been widely reported by patients with BMS. They also report poorer overall health and complain of more illnesses, gastrointestinal (GI) problems, chronic fatigue, disturbed sleep patterns, headaches, and pain in other locations [19, 20]. The psychological distress closely relates to the activation of the HPA axis, which consists of the hypothalamic, the anterior pituitary, and the adrenal cortex. In situations of chronic stress, the hypothalamus releases corticotropin-releasing hormone (CRH), which stimulates the pituitary gland to secrete adrenocorticotropic hormone (ACTH). This, in turn, prompts the adrenal cortex to release cortisol into the bloodstream. Cortisol is a hormone that regulates growth, development, metabolism, and immunity [21]. When elevated due to chronic stress, cortisol disrupts the balance of immune cells, resulting in decreased cellular immunity, increased humoral immunity, and, consequently, immune dysfunction [22]. Together, these findings show that BMS is a condition where chronic pain, emotional stress, and immune dysregulation interact. Pain leads to stress and triggers immune responses, while pre-existing anxiety or immune changes may reduce the pain threshold. This intricate psychoneuroimmunological interaction likely explains the absence of a single trigger for BMS and why patients often need a multifaceted treatment approach.

55.3 Case Presentation

A 65-year-old female patient presented with a chief complaint of a persistent oral burning sensation, predominantly affecting the tongue. The symptoms had begun six months before consultation and were reminiscent of a similar episode experienced in 2018, which was then attributed to a period of intense emotional stress.

The burning sensation was described as constant in frequency but with intermittent fluctuations in intensity, with an average pain score of 8/10 on the Visual Analog Scale (VAS). The discomfort was aggravated by prolonged speaking, consumption of hot foods, chewing, and smoking. Relief was noted with cold stimuli, particularly ice cream, cold water, and sweet foods.

The patient's medical history was notable for irritable bowel syndrome and dyslipidemia, which were well-managed with pitavastatin 2 mg/day. She also reported significant anxiety, with a Generalized Anxiety Disorder 7-item scale (GAD-7) score of 14/21, exacerbated by ongoing financial difficulties and the recent cessation of psychological therapy.

Dental history was unremarkable, with regular dental follow-ups and no relevant oral alterations noted. The patient reported satisfactory sleep quality, with sporadic use of benzodiazepines, and intense awake and sleep bruxism, which she managed effectively with the regular use of an occlusal splint. Additionally, she engaged in regular physical activity, which she felt had a positive impact on her well-being.

Clinical examination revealed no visible lesions in the oral mucosa, buccal mucosa, or on the tongue. However, hyperalgesia was identified on the left lateral border of the tongue during qualitative sensory testing (QualST). There was no pain upon muscular or articular palpation, and sialometry results were normal.

Laboratory investigations, including a complete blood count, fasting glucose, vitamin panel, lipid profile, thyroid function tests, ferritin, zinc, iron levels, creatinine, C-reactive protein (CRP), antinuclear antibodies (ANA), and erythrocyte sedimentation rate (ESR), were all within normal limits.

A diagnostic anesthetic block of the left lingual nerve resulted in partial symptomatic relief, supporting the diagnosis of burning mouth syndrome (BMS).

Treatment was initiated with a multimodal approach. To manage awake bruxism, we used Ecological Momentary Intervention (EMI) with random smartphone prompts to classify real-time jaw states, and aggregated data then guided habit-reversal strategies, cue-based reminders, and brief breathing resets to reinforce a relaxed jaw posture and reduce daytime parafunctional activity. The intervention also included breathing exercises, mindfulness techniques, yoga, and guided meditation. The patient was referred for cognitive-behavioral therapy (CBT). Additionally, oral rinses with diluted sucralose solution were prescribed three times daily, and duloxetine 30 mg/day was initiated for neuropathic pain modulation and anxiety control.

After 30 days, the patient reported significant clinical improvement, with a decrease in burning intensity to VAS 3/10. Duloxetine was well tolerated after adjusting the timing of administration to minimize initial sleep disturbances. Over a six-month period, the patient achieved sustained clinical stabilization, closely associated with emotional improvement and reduced anxiety. After one year, duloxetine was gradually discontinued, with the patient maintaining satisfactory symptom control without pharmacologic support.

55.4 Case Discussion

This case report exemplifies the typical presentation of burning mouth syndrome (BMS). The patient's symptoms align with the classic features of BMS, including persistent oral burning without visible lesions on the oral mucosa, which is exacerbated by certain foods and stress and relieved by cooling agents. The lack of identifiable systemic or local pathology supports the BMS diagnosis, which was confirmed by diagnostic nerve anesthesia. The multidisciplinary approach applied—including pharmacological (duloxetine), psychological (cognitive-behavioral therapy), and behavioral (mindfulness, yoga, ecological momentary intervetion for bruxism management) methods—shows effectiveness in line with current literature and emphasizes the necessity of concurrently addressing neuropathic, psychological, and behavioral factors. This approach addresses the complex pathophysiology of BMS involving neuropathic pain, neuropsychological distress, and hypothalamic–pituitary–adrenal axis dysfunction. The substantial improvement and sustained symptomatic control observed after treatment highlight the importance of individualized and integrative care strategies in the effective treatment of BMS.

55.5 Clinical Characteristics

Burning mouth syndrome (BMS) presents with a distinct clinical profile characterized by chronic intraoral burning sensations in the absence of visible mucosal lesions or identifiable local or systemic pathology. The hallmark symptom is a burning, stinging, or scalding pain, most commonly localized to the anterior two-thirds of the tongue, but also involving the lips, palate, and buccal mucosa. The discomfort is typically bilateral and symmetrical, though it may sometimes present unilaterally in early or atypical cases.

Pain is described as persistent or intermittent, often waxing and waning throughout the day. In many cases, symptoms are mild or absent upon waking, gradually intensify as the day progresses, and reach peak intensity in the late afternoon or evening. A subset of patients, however, report no circadian variation and experience constant discomfort.

Typical pain descriptors include:

- Burning
- Tingling
- Tenderness
- Rawness
- Sensations of dryness or numbness

These symptoms may be exacerbated by talking, eating, consuming spicy or acidic foods, or emotional stress, while relief is often reported with cold stimuli, eating, or distraction.

In addition to pain, BMS is commonly accompanied by other sensory disturbances, including:

- Xerostomia (dry mouth), despite normal salivary flow rates on testing
- Taste alterations, such as dysgeusia (metallic, bitter, or altered taste perception) or hypogeusia
- Paresthesia or altered oral tactile sensitivity

Approximately 30–50% of BMS patients report sleep disturbances, difficulty concentrating, and mood alterations, including anxiety and depression. The relationship between emotional distress and symptom severity is well documented, often forming a vicious cycle where chronic pain exacerbates psychological symptoms, which in turn amplify pain perception.

On clinical examination, the oral mucosa appears normal, without signs of inflammation, trauma, or infection. This absence of objective findings often adds to patient frustration and contributes to diagnostic delays. However, qualitative sensory testing (QST) may reveal hyperalgesia or altered thermal thresholds, supporting the diagnosis of a small-fiber neuropathy in a significant subset of patients.

The temporal profile of BMS is chronic, with symptoms typically persisting for more than three months. Many patients report a gradual onset of symptoms, often coinciding with life stressors, hormonal changes (e.g., menopause), or after dental interventions, though no specific trigger is identified in most cases.

55.6 Diagnostic Criteria

BMS remains a diagnosis of exclusion, which implies that all local and systemic causes have been excluded [23]. Therefore, diagnostic process should be comprehensive including a detailed clinical history, a thorough oral examination, laboratory tests, and psychosocial assessments. According to the International Classification of Orofacial Pain (ICOP), the diagnostic criteria are as follows:

A. Oral pain fulfilling criteria B and C
B. Recurring daily for >2 hours per day for >3 months
C. Pain has both of the following characteristics:
   1. Burning quality
   2. Felt superficially in the oral mucosa
D. Oral mucosa is of normal appearance, and local or systemic causes have been excluded
E. Not better accounted for by another ICOP or ICHD-3 diagnosis

Yet, the "6.1 Burning Mouth Syndrome diagnosis" indicates that quantitative sensory testing (QST) has not been conducted. QSTs are specialized test that evaluates somatosensory abnormalities, such as altered thermal and pain thresholds. Therefore, they allow to identify one of the following subtypes: "6.1.1 Burning Mouth Syndrome without somatosensory changes" or "6.1.2 Burning Mouth Syndrome with somatosensory changes" [23]. Thus, QST is not feasible for use in clinical settings. However, QualST can be applied chairside and shows agreement with QST for detecting changes in orofacial somatosensory sensitivity.

As mentioned before, for a consistent clinical diagnosis a detailed symptom assessment should be conducted, including the onset, duration, and progression of symptoms, as well as possible exacerbating or relieving factors identified (Table 55.1). Clinicians must assess the tongue, gingiva, palate, and buccal mucosa to rule out conditions such as oral candidiasis, erosive lichen planus, or mucosal trauma. Additionally, laboratory tests and blood tests are often conducted to exclude vitamin deficiencies (e.g., B12, folate), iron deficiency anemia, diabetes, and thyroid dysfunction. The psychological assessment may include screening for mood disorders, chronic stress, and somatization, which is crucial, as these factors can influence symptom perception and treatment response [2, 6].

55.7 Treatment

Therapeutic approaches to BMS primarily focus on symptomatic relief and involve a multidisciplinary strategy. Recent clinical trials have identified the most promising therapies. Generally, treatments fall into two categories: pharmacologic (including systemic or topical medications and supplements) and non-pharmacologic (covering behavioral therapies, physical therapies, and devices). A combination of these therapies is often recommended to achieve the maximum benefit.

55.7.1 Alpha-Lipoic Acid (ALA)

ALA is an antioxidant with potential neuroprotective effects in BMS. Clinical studies report symptom improvement rates ranging from 64 to 87%, particularly in short-term use (≤3 months) [23, 24]. However, systematic reviews suggest only

Table 55.1 Clinical features of BMS

BMS: Clinical signs and symptoms
Pain characteristics
Burning, painful, tender, tingling, hot, scalding, or numb sensations Usually bilateral and symmetrical
Common locations
Anterior two-thirds of the tongue (71–78%) Dorsum and lateral borders of the tongue (72%) Anterior aspect of the hard palate (25%) Labial mucosa of the lips (24%)
Associated sensory symptoms
Positive symptoms:
Altered taste (dysgeusia) Dysesthesia
Negative symptoms:
Taste loss Paresthesia
Pain pattern
Constant with fluctuations in intensity Approximately one-third experience symptoms both day and night Minimal upon awakening, gradually intensifying throughout the day, peaking in the evening
Aggravating factors
Stress Fatigue Hot, spicy, or acidic foods
Alleviating factors
Eating Drinking Distraction techniques
Additional reported symptoms
Dry mouth Increased thirst Taste disturbances
Clinical examination
Typically, no observable changes in oral mucosa or dental conditions compared to healthy individuals

moderate and inconsistent benefits, especially when compared to placebo [25]. Combining ALA with gabapentin or B-complex vitamins (e.g., B1, B6, B12, folic acid) appears more effective, with up to 70% improvement in some cases. Despite short-term relief, long-term efficacy remains uncertain. ALA is generally well tolerated; side effects are mild (nausea, GI discomfort, dizziness). Further high-quality studies are needed to clarify its sustained benefits and optimal combinations.

55.7.2 Anticonvulsants

- *Clonazepam*: Clonazepam has been administered in doses ranging from 0.5 to 2 mg per day for periods of 4 to 6 months. It can be used either orally or topically, with the latter often producing better results. Significant reductions in pain, burning, taste alterations, and dry mouth have been observed. While some patients report mild drowsiness, this does not necessitate discontinuing therapy. Current evidence suggests that clonazepam (especially when used topically) is the only drug to consistently show superior results compared to a placebo in alleviating pain associated with burning mouth syndrome [14, 26, 27].
- *Gabapentin*: Gabapentin, at a dose of 300 mg per day for 2 months, showed improvement in pain symptoms in approximately 50% of patients with burning mouth syndrome (BMS), indicating a probability of improvement three times greater than placebo and four times greater than alpha-lipoic acid (ALA). It exerts analgesic effects by interacting with descending signaling related to serotonin (5-HT), norepinephrine (NA), gamma-aminobutyric acid (GABA), and enkephalins [28, 29].
- *Pregabalin*: Studies on pregabalin indicate that administering 150 mg/day for 4 months significantly reduces pain as measured by the visual analog scale. However, side effects like increased appetite, dizziness, mild nausea, and diarrhea were reported A network meta-analysis found that pregabalin may help alleviate BMS pain, and achieve the minimum important difference, but the low certainty of evidence hinders its definitive recommendation [26, 29].

55.7.3 Antidepressants

- *Trazodone*: The administration of 100 mg/day of trazodone for the first 4 days, followed by 200 mg for 8 weeks, significantly reduced pain intensity in patients compared to the control group [30]. However, a review also indicated moderate efficacy alongside a high placebo effect. Additionally, reported side effects such as dizziness and drowsiness may limit its use [29].

55.7.4 Non-Pharmacological Interventions

- *Low-Level Laser Therapy (LLLT)*: Applying LLLT to oral mucosa promotes tissue healing and modulates nerve function. Previous studies have shown that this therapy in patients with BMS reduces pain scores often for months without any systemic adverse effects [31, 32]. This non-pharmacological intervention typically requires multiple sessions (e.g., two to three times per week for several weeks), being an option for patients who prefer to avoid medications or in whom medications have failed [31].

- *Cognitive-Behavioral Therapy (CBT) and Counseling*: BMS has frequently been associated with psychological disorders such as depression, anxiety, hypochondriasis, and cancerphobia [33]. Despite this context, CBT improves patients' quality of life by allowing them to perform their daily activities without limitations and redirecting their focus on the pain and psychological demands, facilitating the development of adaptive coping behaviors and cognitive restructuring [34, 35]. A previous study indicated that after 1 hour of weekly behavioral therapy sessions for 12–15 weeks, patients with resistant BMS reported a significant improvement in their pain score [36]. Other studies also support CBT as an effective therapy for BMS patients [37].
- *Transcranial Magnetic Stimulation (TMS)*: In cases where BMS is refractory to pharmacologic treatments, TMS could represent an innovative treatment approach, aiming to recalibrate central pain networks non-invasively. Data suggest that BMS-related pain was significantly improved after two weeks of high-frequency repetitive TMS treatment [38]. However, due to the limited number of studies in this area, the effectiveness of this therapy for BMS remains unclear. Further research is needed to determine the optimal TMS protocol for BMS.
- *Acupuncture*: Studies have shown that after long-term follow-up (18–24 months after the initial acupuncture treatment), a decreased level of burning sensation and improved quality of life were maintained in patients who underwent acupuncture [39, 40]. A recent study also showed similar pain relief when comparing acupuncture over 4 weeks (three times per week) to pharmacological treatment with clonazepam [41]. It suggests that acupuncture may increase BMS patients' lip microcirculation, which in turn reduces the localized collection of inflammatory mediators, thereby providing relief from the burning pain.

55.8 Conclusion

BMS remains a complex and challenging condition, requiring a precise diagnostic framework and targeted therapeutic strategies to mitigate patient suffering. Advancements in understanding its neuropathic mechanisms, alongside integrative approaches that address hormonal and psychological factors, are essential for developing more effective interventions. A multidisciplinary treatment model not only enhances symptom management but also fosters an improvement in the quality of life for individuals affected by BMS, offering a pathway toward more personalized and evidence-based care.

References

1. Mao F, Cai L, Pan D, Huang M, Wang Q, Chen Q, Ai R, Zhou Y. Burning mouth syndrome may essentially be related to psychoneuroimmunology: mechanism hypothesis. J Oral Rehabil. 2025;52(2):199–207. https://doi.org/10.1111/joor.13893.
2. Klasser GD, Grushka M, Su N. Burning mouth syndrome. Oral Maxillofac Surg Clin North Am. 2016;28(3):381–96. https://doi.org/10.1016/j.coms.2016.03.005.
3. Forssell H, Jääskeläinen S, List T, Svensson P, Baad-Hansen L. An update on pathophysiological mechanisms related to idiopathic oro-facial pain conditions with implications for management. J Oral Rehabil. 2015;42(4):300–22. https://doi.org/10.1111/joor.12256.
4. Grushka M. Clinical features of burning mouth syndrome. Oral Surg Oral Med Oral Pathol. 1987;63(1):30–6. https://doi.org/10.1016/0030-4220(87)90336-7.
5. Klasser GD, Fischer DJ, Epstein JB. Burning mouth syndrome: recognition, understanding, and management. Oral Maxillofac Surg Clin North Am. 2008;20(2):255–71, vii. https://doi.org/10.1016/j.coms.2007.12.012.
6. Adamo D, Pecoraro G, Fortuna G, Amato M, Marenzi G, Aria M, Mignogna MD. Assessment of oral health-related quality of life, measured by OHIP-14 and GOHAI, and psychological profiling in burning mouth syndrome: a case-control clinical study. J Oral Rehabil. 2020;47(1):42–52. https://doi.org/10.1111/joor.12864.
7. Browning S, Hislop S, Scully C, Shirlaw P. The association between burning mouth syndrome and psychosocial disorders. Oral Surg Oral Med Oral Pathol. 1987;64(2):171–4. https://doi.org/10.1016/0030-4220(87)90085-5.
8. Ducasse D, Courtet P, Olie E. Burning mouth syndrome: current clinical, physiopathologic, and therapeutic data. Reg Anesth Pain Med. 2013;38(5):380–90. https://doi.org/10.1097/AAP.0b013e3182a1f0db.
9. Pereira SR, Tello Velasquez J, Duggan S, Ivanisevic B, McKenna JP, McCreary C, Downer EJ. Recent advances in the understanding of the aetiology and therapeutic strategies in burning mouth syndrome: focus on the actions of cannabinoids. Eur J Neurosci. 2022;55(4):1032–50. https://doi.org/10.1111/ejn.14712.
10. Canfora F, Calabria E, Pecoraro G, D Aniello L, Aria M, Marenzi G, Sammartino P, Mignogna MD, Adamo D. The use of self-report questionnaires in an analysis of the multidimensional aspects of pain and a correlation with the psychological profile and quality of life in patients with burning mouth syndrome: a case-control study. J Oral Rehabil. 2022;49(9):890–914. https://doi.org/10.1111/joor.13343.
11. Khawaja SN, Alaswaiti OF, Scrivani SJ. Burning mouth syndrome. Dent Clin North Am. 2023;67(1):49–60. https://doi.org/10.1016/j.cden.2022.07.004.
12. Madariaga VI, Tanaka H, Ernberg M. Psychophysical characterisation of burning mouth syndrome-a systematic review and meta-analysis. J Oral Rehabil. 2020;47(12):1590–605. https://doi.org/10.1111/joor.13028.
13. Eliav E, Kamran B, Schaham R, Czerninski R, Gracely RH, Benoliel R. Evidence of chorda tympani dysfunction in patients with burning mouth syndrome. J Am Dent Assoc. 2007;138(5):628–33. https://doi.org/10.14219/jada.archive.2007.0234.
14. Imamura Y, Shinozaki T, Okada-Ogawa A, Noma N, Shinoda M, Iwata K, Wada A, Abe O, Wang K, Svensson P. An updated review on pathophysiology and management of burning mouth syndrome with endocrinological, psychological and neuropathic perspectives. J Oral Rehabil. 2019;46(6):574–87. https://doi.org/10.1111/joor.12795.
15. Yilmaz Z, Renton T, Yiangou Y, Zakrzewska J, Chessell IP, Bountra C, Anand P. Burning mouth syndrome as a trigeminal small fibre neuropathy: increased heat and capsaicin receptor TRPV1 in nerve fibres correlates with pain score. J Clin Neurosci. 2007;14(9):864–71. https://doi.org/10.1016/j.jocn.2006.09.002.
16. Kouri M, Adamo D, Vardas E, Georgaki M, Canfora F, Mignogna MD, Nikitakis N. Small fiber neuropathy in burning mouth syndrome: a systematic review. Int J Mol Sci. 2024;25(21):11442. https://doi.org/10.3390/ijms252111442.

17. Albuquerque RJC, de Leeuw R, Carlson CR, Okeson JP, Miller CS, Andersen AH. Cerebral activation during thermal stimulation of patients who have burning mouth disorder: an fMRI study. Pain. 2006;122(3):223–34. https://doi.org/10.1016/j.pain.2006.01.020.
18. Hagelberg N, Forssell H, Rinne JO, Scheinin H, Taiminen T, Aalto S, Luutonen S, Någren K, Jääskeläinen S. Striatal dopamine D1 and D2 receptors in burning mouth syndrome. Pain. 2003;101(1–2):149–54. https://doi.org/10.1016/s0304-3959(02)00323-8.
19. Al Quran FA. Psychological profile in burning mouth syndrome. Oral Surg Oral Med Oral Pathol Oral Radiol Endod. 2004;97(3):339–44. https://doi.org/10.1016/j.tripleo.2003.09.017.
20. Lamey PJ, Freeman R, Eddie SA, Pankhurst C, Rees T. Vulnerability and presenting symptoms in burning mouth syndrome. Oral Surg Oral Med Oral Pathol Oral Radiol Endod. 2005;99(1):48–54. https://doi.org/10.1016/j.tripleo.2004.01.021.
21. Timmermans S, Souffriau J, Libert C. A general introduction to glucocorticoid biology. Front Immunol. 2019;10:1545. https://doi.org/10.3389/fimmu.2019.01545. PMID: 31333672; PMCID: PMC6621919.
22. Elenkov IJ, Chrousos GP. Stress system--organization, physiology and immunoregulation. Neuroimmunomodulation. 2006;13(5–6):257–67. https://doi.org/10.1159/000104853.
23. International Classification of Orofacial Pain, 1st edition (ICOP). Cephalalgia. 2020;40(2):129–221. https://doi.org/10.1177/0333102419893823.
24. Femiano F, Scully C. Burning mouth syndrome (BMS): double blind controlled study of alpha-lipoic acid (thioctic acid) therapy. J Oral Pathol Med. 2002;31(5):267–9. https://doi.org/10.1034/j.1600-0714.2002.310503.x.
25. Alvarenga-Brant R, Costa FO, Mattos-Pereira G, Esteves-Lima RP, Belém FV, Lai H, Ge L, Gomez RS, Martins CC. Treatments for burning mouth syndrome: a network meta-analysis. J Dent Res. 2023;102(2):135–45. https://doi.org/10.1177/00220345221130025.
26. Çınar SL, Kartal D, Pergel T, Borlu M. Effectiveness and safety of clonazepam, pregabalin, and alpha lipoic acid for the treatment of burning mouth syndrome. Erciyes Med J. 2018;40(1):35–8.
27. Heckmann SM, Kirchner E, Grushka M, Wichmann MG, Hummel T. A double-blind study on clonazepam in patients with burning mouth syndrome. Laryngoscope. 2012;122(4):813–6. https://doi.org/10.1002/lary.22490.
28. López-D'alessandro E, Escovich L. Combination of alpha lipoic acid and gabapentin, its efficacy in the treatment of Burning Mouth Syndrome: a randomized, double-blind, placebo controlled trial. Med Oral Patol Oral Cir Bucal. 2011;16(5):e635–40. https://doi.org/10.4317/medoral.16942.
29. Tan HL, Smith JG, Hoffmann J, Renton T. A systematic review of treatment for patients with burning mouth syndrome. Cephalalgia. 2022;42(2):128–61. https://doi.org/10.1177/03331024211036152.
30. Tammiala Salonen T, Forssell H. Trazodone in burning mouth pain: a placebo-controlled, double-blind study. J Orofac Pain. 1999;13(2):83–8.
31. de Pedro M, López-Pintor RM, Casañas E, Hernández G. Effects of photobiomodulation with low-level laser therapy in burning mouth syndrome: a randomized clinical trial. Oral Dis. 2020;26(8):1764–76. https://doi.org/10.1111/odi.13443.
32. Spanemberg JC, López López J, de Figueiredo MA, Cherubini K, Salum FG. Efficacy of low-level laser therapy for the treatment of burning mouth syndrome: a randomized, controlled trial. J Biomed Opt. 2015;20(9):098001. https://doi.org/10.1117/1.JBO.20.9.098001.
33. Scala A, Checchi L, Montevecchi M, Marini I, Giamberardino MA. Update on burning mouth syndrome: overview and patient management. Crit Rev Oral Biol Med. 2003;14(4):275–91. https://doi.org/10.1177/154411130301400405.
34. Hofmann SG, Asnaani A, Vonk IJ, Sawyer AT, Fang A. The efficacy of cognitive behavioral therapy: a review of meta-analyses. Cognit Ther Res. 2012;36(5):427–40. https://doi.org/10.1007/s10608-012-9476-1.

35. Lim JA, Choi SH, Lee WJ, Jang JH, Moon JY, Kim YC, Kang DH. Cognitive-behavioral therapy for patients with chronic pain: implications of gender differences in empathy. Medicine (Baltimore). 2018;97(23):e10867. https://doi.org/10.1097/MD.0000000000010867.
36. Bergdahl J, Anneroth G, Perris H. Cognitive therapy in the treatment of patients with resistant burning mouth syndrome: a controlled study. J Oral Pathol Med. 1995;24(5):213–5. https://doi.org/10.1111/j.1600-0714.1995.tb01169.x.
37. Miziara ID, Filho BC, Oliveira R, Rodrigues dos Santos RM. Group psychotherapy: an additional approach to burning mouth syndrome. J Psychosom Res. 2009;67(5):443–8. https://doi.org/10.1016/j.jpsychores.2009.01.013.
38. Umezaki Y, Badran BW, DeVries WH, Moss J, Gonzales T, George MS. The efficacy of daily prefrontal repetitive transcranial magnetic stimulation (rTMS) for burning mouth syndrome (BMS): a randomized controlled single-blind study. Brain Stimul. 2016;9(2):234–42. https://doi.org/10.1016/j.brs.2015.10.005.
39. Franco FR, Castro LA, Borsatto MC, Silveira EA, Ribeiro-Rotta RF. Combined acupuncture and Auriculotherapy in burning mouth syndrome treatment: a preliminary single-arm clinical trial. J Altern Complement Med. 2017;23(2):126–34. https://doi.org/10.1089/acm.2016.0179.
40. Scardina GA, Ruggieri A, Provenzano F, Messina P. Burning mouth syndrome: is acupuncture a therapeutic possibility? Br Dent J. 2010;209(1):E2. https://doi.org/10.1038/sj.bdj.2010.582.
41. Jurisic Kvesic A, Zavoreo I, Basic Kes V, Vucicevic Boras V, Ciliga D, Gabric D, Vrdoljak DV. The effectiveness of acupuncture versus clonazepam in patients with burning mouth syndrome. Acupunct Med. 2015;33(4):289–92. https://doi.org/10.1136/acupmed-2015-010759.

MIX
Papier aus verantwortungsvollen Quellen
Paper from responsible sources
FSC® C105338

If you have any concerns about our products,
you can contact us on
ProductSafety@springernature.com

In case Publisher is established outside the EU,
the EU authorized representative is:
Springer Nature Customer Service Center GmbH
Europaplatz 3, 69115 Heidelberg, Germany

Printed by Libri Plureos GmbH
in Hamburg, Germany